Research for Development

Series Editors

Emilio Bartezzaghi, Milan, Italy

Giampio Bracchi, Milan, Italy

Adalberto Del Bo, Politecnico di Milano, Milan, Italy

Ferran Sagarra Trias, Department of Urbanism and Regional Planning, Universitat Politècnica de Catalunya, Barcelona, Barcelona, Spain

Francesco Stellacci, Supramolecular NanoMaterials and Interfaces Laboratory (SuNMiL), Institute of Materials, Ecole Polytechnique Fédérale de Lausanne (EPFL), Lausanne, Vaud, Switzerland

Enrico Zio, Politecnico di Milano, Milan, Italy, Ecole Centrale Paris, Paris, France

The series Research for Development serves as a vehicle for the presentation and dissemination of complex research and multidisciplinary projects. The published work is dedicated to fostering a high degree of innovation and to the sophisticated demonstration of new techniques or methods.

The aim of the Research for Development series is to promote well-balanced sustainable growth. This might take the form of measurable social and economic outcomes, in addition to environmental benefits, or improved efficiency in the use of resources; it might also involve an original mix of intervention schemes.

Research for Development focuses on the following topics and disciplines:

Urban regeneration and infrastructure, Info-mobility, transport, and logistics, Environment and the land, Cultural heritage and landscape, Energy, Innovation in processes and technologies, Applications of chemistry, materials, and nanotechnologies, Material science and biotechnology solutions, Physics results and related applications and aerospace, Ongoing training and continuing education.

Fondazione Politecnico di Milano collaborates as a special co-partner in this series by suggesting themes and evaluating proposals for new volumes. Research for Development addresses researchers, advanced graduate students, and policy and decision-makers around the world in government, industry, and civil society.

THE SERIES IS INDEXED IN SCOPUS

Antonella Valeria Penati
Editor

In-Home Medication

Integrating Multidisciplinary Perspectives in Design-Driven Pharma Practices

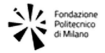

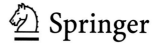

Editor
Antonella Valeria Penati
Department of Design
Politecnico di Milano
Milan, Italy

ISSN 2198-7300　　　　　　ISSN 2198-7319　(electronic)
Research for Development
ISBN 978-3-031-53293-1　　　ISBN 978-3-031-53294-8　(eBook)
https://doi.org/10.1007/978-3-031-53294-8

Politecnico di Milano

© The Editor(s) (if applicable) and The Author(s) 2025. This book is an open access publication.

Open Access This book is licensed under the terms of the Creative Commons Attribution 4.0 International License (http://creativecommons.org/licenses/by/4.0/), which permits use, sharing, adaptation, distribution and reproduction in any medium or format, as long as you give appropriate credit to the original author(s) and the source, provide a link to the Creative Commons license and indicate if changes were made.
The images or other third party material in this book are included in the book's Creative Commons license, unless indicated otherwise in a credit line to the material. If material is not included in the book's Creative Commons license and your intended use is not permitted by statutory regulation or exceeds the permitted use, you will need to obtain permission directly from the copyright holder.
The use of general descriptive names, registered names, trademarks, service marks, etc. in this publication does not imply, even in the absence of a specific statement, that such names are exempt from the relevant protective laws and regulations and therefore free for general use.
The publisher, the authors and the editors are safe to assume that the advice and information in this book are believed to be true and accurate at the date of publication. Neither the publisher nor the authors or the editors give a warranty, expressed or implied, with respect to the material contained herein or for any errors or omissions that may have been made. The publisher remains neutral with regard to jurisdictional claims in published maps and institutional affiliations.

This Springer imprint is published by the registered company Springer Nature Switzerland AG
The registered company address is: Gewerbestrasse 11, 6330 Cham, Switzerland

If disposing of this product, please recycle the paper.

Contents

1   **Towards In-Home Medication: Medicinal Products as Daily Objects**   1
Antonella Valeria Penati

Part I   Objects of Science: The Pharmaceutical Industry as a Place of Preciseness

2   **Medicine Packaging Legislation and Its Evolution According to Technological Innovation for Better Healthcare Support**..........   37
Simona Cazzaniga

3   **Primary Medicine Packaging and Quality Control**...............   57
Elena Piovosi

4   **Pharmaceutical Forms and Primary Packaging: A Glossary**.......   75
Elena Piovosi

5   **Secondary Packaging of Medicines: Design Processes for the Pharmaceutical Industry**.....................................   101
Marcello Mariani

6   **Secondary Packaging and Leaflets: A Glossary**..................   117
Marcello Mariani

Part II   Prescribing and Dispensing: Accompanying the Patient to the Correct Use of Medicines

7   **Moving the Care Process in the in-Home Context: The Therapeutic Prescription**   131
Carlo Emilio Standoli, Milena Giovanna Guarinoni, and Enrico Morello

8   **Dispensing Medicines: A Necessary Link Between Doctor and Patient**   143
Antonella Valeria Penati

9 **The Future Digital Pharmacological Prescriptions Between Therapy Adherence and Integrated Healthcare Personal Plans** 177
Giuseppe Andreoni

10 **Navigating the Complexities of the OTC Medicine Ecosystem** 189
Elena Caratti

11 **Dealing with Medicines Through Online Platforms and Communities** 205
Carlo Emilio Standoli and Umberto Tolino

Part III The Daily Life as a Place of Inaccuracy: The Domesticity of Therapy

12 **Medicines as Designed Objects** 223
Silvia Pizzocaro and Antonella Valeria Penati

13 **The In-Home Place of Medications: Perspectives of Domestication** 247
Silvia Pizzocaro

14 **In-Home. Medicinal Treatment as a Learning Process** 269
Antonella Valeria Penati

15 **Use Phenomenologies. Observing the User While Taking Pharmaceutical Therapies** 295
Antonella Valeria Penati

16 **Use Phenomenologies: Oral Solid Forms in Blister Packs** 313
Antonella Valeria Penati

17 **Use Phenomenologies: What Does the User Do with the Secondary Medicine Packaging and Package Leaflet?** 337
Antonella Valeria Penati

Part IV The Pharmaceutical Product System: Premises for the Definition of a Repertory of Good Practices

18 **How Political and Cultural Situations Are Impacting Pharma Industries** 363
Annabella Amatulli

19 **Medicinal Products: When Innovation Meets the Patient** 379
Lamberto Dionigi

20 **Pharmaceutical Packaging According to the "Packaging Ethics Charter"** 395
Valeria Bucchetti

21	**Sensory Qualities of the Medicines: From Problems to Proposals** .... Dina Riccò	411
22	**Compendium: Step Toward Design-Oriented Practices in the Pharma Industry in a Multidisciplinary Perspective** .... Antonella Valeria Penati	429

Addendum 1 Regulatory References 519

Addendum 2 Medication Errors Data................................ 523

Addendum 3 The Name of Medicines: LASA Medicines 531

Addendum 4 Methods of User Involvement........................... 543

Addendum 5 Undesirable Effects or Product Defects Reporting Procedures... 547

References.. 551

Chapter 1
Towards In-Home Medication: Medicinal Products as Daily Objects

Antonella Valeria Penati

1.1 Introduction

Alberto has difficulties with swallowing, which means he needs to break large and rough pills when taking medications. Additionally, he must smooth the jagged edges that result from splitting the pills. Unfortunately, this process leads to a loss of the active ingredient, which is dispersed into the environment. Due to his self-learned habits in the treatment process, Alberto happened to inadvertently split 'slow-release' tablets of a potent painkiller. The active ingredient entered his bloodstream abruptly and triggered a severe cholinergic crisis.

Maria consumes numerous medications daily, and, in the morning, her son organizes them in separate containers for the different times she needs them. However, once these pills are removed from their original blister pack and mixed in the containers, Maria struggles to identify the drugs correctly, leading to insecurity and occasional decisions to skip doses to avoid errors.

Jenny, a young mother, faces challenges when administering an antibiotic to her six-month-old son, Ryan when having a temperature. Although she attentively listens to the paediatrician's instructions, Jenny encounters difficulty when faced with the antibiotic bottle. She struggles to understand the instructions in the accompanying leaflet on measuring grams of antibiotic powder and decilitres of sterile solution for mixing. Furthermore, determining the appropriate dosage based on Ryan's weight poses another hurdle, ultimately leading Jenny to opt for a visit to the emergency room to ensure no mistakes are made.

Benny's situation involves the use of an anticoagulant with varying daily doses, which can be ¼, ½, or ¾ of a tablet as per the medical prescription. His challenge lies in accurately dividing the medication and storing the remaining fragments effectively.

Cristina uses artificial tears to alleviate dry eye symptoms but faces difficulty in exerting the necessary pressure to release the eye drops from the bottle. Consequently, she routinely requires assistance from a family member to properly care for her eyes.

A. V. Penati (✉)
Department of Design, Politecnico di Milano, Milan, Italy
e-mail: antonella.penati@polimi.it

© The Author(s) 2025
A. V. Penati (ed.), *In-Home Medication*, Research for Development,
https://doi.org/10.1007/978-3-031-53294-8_1

> Marco, who has diabetes, encounters challenges managing his blood glucose levels and medication when he's away from home due to work commitments. Administering the necessary procedures while outdoors proves to be a significant hurdle for him.
>
> Dina is leaving for the weekend. Dina's primary concern revolves around transporting a temperature-sensitive drug that must be kept below 15 degrees. She usually carries a small piece of ice with her, but airport staff often prohibit her from bringing it. This creates a dilemma for her in ensuring the drug's proper preservation during travel.
>
> Carlo uses cortisone and diligently reads the medication leaflet to understand its potential side effects. However, he struggles to grasp some of the medical terminology used, hindering his full comprehension of the treatment's potential adverse effects.
>
> Elisabeth buys a much-publicized over-the-counter analgesic for her 13-year-old son, Peter, who is suffering from a severe headache. She believes that over-the-counter medications pose no specific contraindications. However, upon returning home and reading the package, she finds not instructions about what to do. She opens the package and reads the leaflet inside. She discovers that the medicine is unsuitable for people under 16 years of age. Unfortunately, the packaging has now been opened, rendering it non-returnable. Elisabeth decides to buy a different medicine, and this time to seek guidance from the pharmacist for an alternative solution.
>
> Marcel's experience involves an omission in the discharging letter from the emergency room, which fails to specify the antibiotic treatment recommended by the doctor during their conversation. After Marcel returns to inquire about the oversight, the doctor explains that he had forgotten to insert the prescribed treatment. Since Marcel's 'emergency room folder' is now closed and archived, he provides Marcel with a prescription for the required antibiotic. However, Marcel realizes that he hasn't received instructions about the daily dosage and the duration of the therapy.

For the reflections presented in this text, we have chosen to begin by considering the lives of people dealing with medications through the vivid recounting of microstories, which serve as glimpses into common experiences related to medical treatment. While not exhaustive, they offer insights into the theoretical significance of the implications that can be drawn from these brief narratives. Through these stories, we have highlighted their theoretical relevance, recognizing the epistemological value of the implications that can be deduced from these short stories.

The primary focus of this book revolves around the practices associated with the daily in-home use and consumption of pharmaceuticals. The examination of patients navigating through pharmaceutical therapies within the confines of their homes incorporates perspectives from both medical and pharmaceutical research traditions. This approach is complemented by an examination of the relationship between users and products, a characteristic feature of design studies and user studies. It reveals the errors, discomforts, difficulties, doubts, and misunderstandings that punctuate the different moments of therapy, from when the medicine is prescribed, dispensed, taken, or administered, to when—at the end of its life cycle—it is disposed of. The communicative elements, formal and informal, of the medicine and the accompanying artifacts—prescriptions, recipes, therapeutic plans, calendars, package leaflets, packaging, containers, intake, and dosage devices to which the patient refers to manage the treatment practices—are examined here in their 'object' nature and in their propensity to express, more or less effectively, the function they must perform: to be understood and easily accessible to the user who must use them.

1 Towards In-Home Medication: Medicinal Products as Daily Objects

The cultural assumptions underpinning this book's exploration of the dynamics between patients and medications encompass several key aspects, which express the disciplinary interests from which the book takes its cue:

- A focus on the tangible and artifact-driven aspects of medications;
- An emphasis on the 'form' of medications and their role in treatment activities;
- Acknowledgment of the complex nature of the interaction of the medication throughout the therapy process;
- Recognition of the skills required of patients or their caregivers in the context of care activities;
- An understanding of the challenges associated with individual medications versus the therapy as a whole;
- The importance of considering therapy as a procedural journey;
- Awareness of the impact of everyday contexts on patient behavior during treatment;
- Acknowledgment of the potential pitfalls when medications are treated as 'everyday' objects.

These premises serve as the foundation for an exploration that considers the behavior and relationships users establish with products, free from idealistic or stereotypical notions. They also provide a springboard for generating ideas and incentives to foster user-centred innovation in the pharmaceutical industry.

Several clarifications are pertinent in this context. First, research into the relationship between patients and medications must revolve around what can be considered the 'fundamental principle' for pharmaceutical companies. This principle underpins all considerations for the effective management and use of medications by patients: the components of each medication package, as they are placed on the market, should remain inextricably linked throughout their life cycle. The pharmaceutical industry derives its criteria for the design of formal and communicative aspects of medications from this principle.

Any assumptions are based on the premise that the primary pack, secondary pack, package leaflet, and medicine form an inseparable and cohesive unit from the moment of purchase to the end of the product's lifecycle. From this principle, the pharmaceutical company derives all subsequent criteria for the design of the formal and communicative aspects of the medicine. These are conceived taking for granted that primary pack, secondary pack, package leaflet, and medicine remain united and integral from purchase to the end of life.

However, real-world experiences often challenge this principle, prompting an investigation into the instances and reasons for deviations, as well as the potential risks associated with adhering to this principle when user behavior contradicts it.

Despite this theoretical foundation, everyday experiences frequently demonstrate a widespread disregard for this principle. Current research endeavours to shed light on the specific times and causes for such deviations, exploring the potential dangers associated with steadfastly adhering to this principle, acknowledging that in everyday use, user behavior frequently contradicts the assumed unity of the primary pack, secondary pack, package leaflet, and medicine.

This recognition of the disparity between theoretical principles and actual user behavior underscores the importance of understanding the factors influencing deviations and the associated risks. Such insights contribute to a more nuanced comprehension of user interactions with medical products and can inform strategies to enhance user adherence and safety.

Second, the medicamentous function of medications—namely, their role in treating specific medical conditions or the active ingredient—is not within the scope of analysis in this book. The authors consider this a subject of study specific to the medical and pharmaceutical domains. Instead, this text focuses on a complementary objective: that medications, to be effective, must be stored and taken correctly. Taking medication is not a simple, one-time action but a multifaceted process that engages the user cognitively, sensory, physically, and emotionally. The observations in this book centre on these points, concluding when medications begin to show their therapeutic effects.

Please note that this book also adopts an editorial method that avoids direct reference to specific medications (to prevent discrediting or improper advertising). Instead, the 'active ingredient' is used as the reference element in textual parts, and fictional packaging is used in illustrated sections to represent the information, graphics, and formal elements under scrutiny. Any reference to the problems encountered has here the sense of wanting to contribute to the reflection on possible improvements to medicine, one of the most complex and, at the same time, consolidated products in terms of design and production quality. It is important to clarify that, due to the authors' expertise and research goals, each medication used as an example has never been examined from a medical-pharmaceutical perspective regarding its active ingredient's benefits and effects. The focus remains on the "medicine system," encompassing the medication and the set of physical and informational artifacts that make it usable, with a focus on "usability" as a set of formal, textual, and visual qualities and characteristics that simplify access to treatment information and cure-related products.

Third, this book does not delve into what the literature terms "radical" or "fundamental" forms of innovation (Schumpeter 1977 [Op. Ed. 1939]). In an industry constrained by production and regulatory challenges, where innovation for improving the patient's user experience is limited, attention is directed toward "minor" product improvements (Rosenberg 1991, p. 202 [Op. Ed. 1982]). While radical innovations are already transforming traditional medication forms to enhance the efficiency of active ingredients and usability, this book primarily concentrates on minor enhancements. The pharmaceutical industry is actively developing medicines to incorporate electronic technologies, such as information dissemination, recognition, tracking, and more, to make them more contemporary and user-friendly.

In short, the book primarily considers the interactions between patients and medications, shedding light on the challenges and opportunities for improving the usability of medications in everyday life.

This is not a remissive position. From a cultural standpoint, the authors prefer to focus on forms of micro-innovation characterized by 'tidying up', 'reordering', and 'retouching' to update a product without fundamentally altering or replacing it. This perspective aligns with an established body of literature, beginning with the seminal work of Arrow (1962), which emphasizes the economic impact of incremental improvements achieved through micro modifications, additions, and adjustments made to a product after it is on the market. These forms of innovation can stem from user experiences (not limited to end-users but encompassing all individuals involved with the product throughout its life cycle) and can significantly enhance a product's performance and usability. They may also result from enhancements in production, logistics, or distribution processes aimed at increasing efficiency. Additionally, they can arise from improvements in product materials or components that are more technologically advanced (Rosenberg 1991 [Op. Ed. 1982]).

These performance enhancements are distinct from the innovations stemming from Basic Research and Research and Development activities. Instead, they are a result of the growing expertise of those involved in production, distribution, and usage, cultivated through "learning by doing" and "learning by using" practices that drive improvements at all stages of the product's life cycle (Georghiou 1986). In this book, the focus will be on issues observed in the product's use by the end-user, which can trigger modifications or optimizations of the product and its functionalities.

By integrating a diverse range of expertise, this book aims to emphasize the interconnected issues that span from regulatory matters to production, encompassing activities such as prescription and dispensation, ultimately placing the drug and the essential information for its use in the hands of the patient. It serves as a round table where experts from various fields converge, including the pharmaceutical sector, product design, communication, user studies, regulatory compliance, production engineering, chemistry, biotechnology, bioengineering, and medical professionals.

Through this multidisciplinary approach, the book tentatively demonstrates the potential for a dialogue between a culture of design and a culture of healthcare. The collection of 'good practices' drawn from exemplary instances, innovative micro-experiments, pilot projects, and user experiences presented in the final section of the book is not intended to serve as a definitive conclusion of the study but as a potential starting point for future collaborative efforts and endeavours in this domain.

1.2 Medicines in a Design-Oriented Framework

In our everyday lives, we are all aware of the crucial role that medicines play. They often serve as the first line of defence for treating many of the health conditions that affect our bodies. Despite their ubiquity in our domestic landscape, there remains a relative absence of design thinking regarding medications as objects of use and consumption.

Within the realm of a 'culture of care', a growing focus is emerging on patients' behavior in the daily use of medications. This focus underscores the importance of adherence to therapy and addresses the errors that can occur during treatment.

Taking a perspective from both design studies and user studies, we begin by considering that a significant portion of the errors and difficulties associated with the assumption of pharmacological therapies, particularly within the context of self-care behaviours and in-home medication, may be linked to a research tradition that has not extensively embraced the idea of framing medications and pharmaceutical therapies within a design-oriented framework.

In our shared experiences, the importance of drugs in our lives is undeniable. However, despite being integral to our domestic landscape and often serving as the initial remedy for various pathologies, there remains a relative deficiency in design thinking concerning medications as objects of use and consumption.

The underlying hypothesis of the research that forms the basis of this text posits that a range of errors, discomforts, and challenges in adhering to pharmacological therapies can be elucidated by examining the content and presentation of information on the medicine's packaging and package leaflet. Additionally, it considers the insufficient presence of identifying signs on the medicine and the lack of design attention to the formal characteristics crucial in the processes of understanding, use, and memory of the experience associated with the medicine and its packaging. Well-designed features in these aspects have the potential to guide the user's experience and facilitate access to medicine.

Built upon these assumptions, the present research explores the feasibility of transferring, integrating, and adapting methodologies and theoretical reflections central to the design discourse to a product typology—medicine—that exhibits a stringent relationship between form and function. Medicines are characterized by a complex interplay between content and container, a strong complementarity between material artifact and communicative artifact, and a unique user—the patient—whose psycho-physical conditions, abilities, skills of use, motivations for purchase and use, create a distinctive backdrop for innovative research. This endeavour serves as not only an experimental test bed but also a theoretical exploration.

Approaching the world of medicines from a design-oriented perspective seeks to investigate the potential connections between the 'form of the medicine' and the errors or discomforts experienced by the user. This involves assessing the effectiveness and efficiency that the packaging and the medicine itself contribute in terms of identity, comprehension, and usability.

What is more, this perspective encourages us to contextualize medications and the treatment process within the broader cultural and social systems. These systems carry significance, meaning, and values that transcend the medication as a purely functional object. Therefore, it is essential to consider the cultural and social context in which medications are used, recognizing that their roles and connotations extend beyond their basic utility.

Such a perspective also induces one to place the medicine and the treatment process within its concrete context of use: in this text, the authors' attention is focused on the therapy in the home context, which has specific logic and gives rise to behaviours, different, for example, from those that take place in the hospital context. Again, from a design-oriented perspective, it seems relevant to place medicine within cultural and social systems.

The following paragraphs represent an initial step toward constructing a theoretical framework that underpins the reflections of this book's contributors, starting with the role played by the formal aspects of medication in facilitating therapy management and medication adherence. Subsequent chapters explore more deeply the issues raised here, providing a more comprehensive exploration of this topic.

Such a perspective prompts an exploration of placing the medicine and the treatment process within its tangible context of use. In this book, the authors specifically direct their attention to therapy in the home context, which adheres to a distinct logic and gives rise to behaviours different from those observed in a hospital setting. From a design-oriented viewpoint, it becomes pertinent to situate medicine within cultural and social systems that carry significance, meaning, and values, transcending the object's purely functional dimension—even in the case of medicine.

1.3 Design and Medicinal Products Shape

Design culture has generated various theoretical perspectives to delineate the design activity of 'giving shape,' emphasizing its character as an "interpreter" (Arnheim 1985), "translator" (Baule and Caratti 2016), and "configurator" (Maldonado 1976). These terms incorporate the cultural component, underscoring the reliance of formal outcomes on the subjectivity and discretion of those involved in the processes of formal construction, as well as the contextual factors such as socio-historical, technical-productive, economic, and geographical contexts.

While the intent of this book is not to revisit these positions, they are referenced here to underscore the significance of formal aspects in pharmaceutical products. Formal elements contribute to the construction of their identity and recognizability as objects, and the formal element plays a crucial role in either facilitating or hindering the processes of access, use, and interaction with the user. For more information about these, see Chap. 12.

The question of how abstract scientific principles take on the semblance of a tangible "technical individual" (Simondon 1958) has long characterized speculative thought surrounding the processes that give objects their distinct identities. From a philosophical point of view, the path that leads science to translate into technology and this, in turn, to take on an artefactual physiognomy of its own represents only a partially explored field. Various theoretical positions view the concept of form differently, whether as a result of an objective process inscribed in scientific principles; or as an 'internal' necessity influenced by the material composition, or as a blend of technological objectivity and subjective creativity, or as the result of a compositive equilibrium, or as the expression of a specific function, even considering the user's experience. Form can finally be seen as the result of social forces that shape science and its processes of objectification (Penati 2016).

It is important to clarify that the concept of 'form' in the world of objects and within the discipline of design, while broader, only partially overlaps with the concept of 'pharmaceutical form' as used in the medical-pharmacist culture.

We will limit ourselves here to pointing out that, in the realm of medicine and pharmacopoeia, it is notable that the 'reasons' for the form are predominantly attributed to technical reasons. It is assumed, in essence, that 'pharmaceutical forms' primarily stem from scientific principles, from the 'internal' necessity dictated by the unique characteristics and transformative constraints of the 'active ingredient,' and from the specific function that the medicine is intended to fulfil.

The term 'function' in the medical and pharmaceutical perspective is declined prioritizing the curative purpose of the medication, focusing on its ability to intervene, modifying certain physiological functions; controlling the times and ways in which this can occur, making the treatment's efficiency maximum and side effects minimum. The body and the patient, in this view, are also subordinated to technical reasons. The body is translated in terms of 'route of intake', 'organ to be treated' etc. (Borgna 2005).

The same notion of 'therapeutic adherence' is often assessed based on 'measuring', 'weighting' the patient's ability to correspond to the doctor's instruction, overlooking individual reasons like personal tastes, fears, anxieties, discomforts, pain, and emotional factors, but also incapacities, forgetfulness. Elements that translate bodies into persons.

And furthermore, it is the very concept of usability (and the resulting product validation tests and protocols) that embodies this scientific approach, which cleanses the validation processes of the 'interferences' of the context of use and the idiosyncrasies of the subjects.

From a design perspective, these different aspects are seen as complementary rather than in opposition to the interpretation conducted in medical disciplines.

In the context of design, which is central to this book, the ultimate functionality of medicine, peculiar to the medical field, is recognised, which includes its curative properties and mechanisms of action, is acknowledged, but the focus is accentuated on all the steps constituting the care process—understanding, recognition, remembering, organizing, handling, taking, and proper and conscious disposal. We pay close attention to aspects that ensure the correct usage of the medicine by the user, considering the influence of the context of use and consumption. Additionally, the book welcomes the symbolic and cultural values that transcend its strict functionality. These dimensions imbue medicine with meaning and value that extend beyond individual experiences of use, connecting it to broader interpretations of the body, illness, care, life, and death. These meanings are socially constructed from experiences of a universal nature.

Moreover, in design cultures, the focus is on how tangible elements give identity to objects and facilitate their use.

And so, if we look at medicines from a medical point of view, we can safely say that we are faced with a wide range of 'pharmaceutical forms' (solid, semi-solid, liquid, or gaseous). These depend on the chemical-physical composition (which may result in tablets, powders, granules, gels, creams, syrups, or liquids); on the 'route of intake' (oral, rectal, vaginal, dermal, etc.); on the intensity of the dosage required; on the context of domestic or hospital use, etc. (Caprino 2011).

But from a design perspective, medications often lack the attributes necessary to ensure correct methods of use; for recognizability and ease of use typical of designed objects. Despite their simplicity, medications may present complexities in use. Medicines are the evidence of a world made up mostly of primary forms, weak forms, which are nevertheless loaded with complexity of use.

Largely lacking in modal and identity qualities, the form of a medicine still does not meet the minimum requirements of recognisability and ease of understanding and use, typical of the world of objects.

Their 'way of being' (Simondon 1958) still belongs to the world of scientific discoveries and the formal images they evoke. Medicine—as an object—still appears to be too anchored in the realm of raw materials and does not adequately meet users' needs for usability (van der Geest et al. 1996). On these aspects, see Chap. 12.

The pharmaceutical product then seems extraneous to use morphological variants to adapt to the progressive refinement of user needs but, above all, as a guarantee of recognisability and identity.

In design cultures, moreover, the patient is not exclusively referable to the 'body of care', to the 'clinical body' which, insofar as it is the object of rigorous, precise, rational, logical, irrefutable experimentation—necessary to attribute to the medicine the license of scientificity –, becomes a scientificised body itself.

In observing the body in its relationship with therapy, one cannot ignore the fact that, in addition to the body of medicine, biology, anatomy, and genetics, the body lends itself to a kaleidoscopic reading depending on the points of view from which it is observed (Borgna 2005): the sociological body, the political body, the technological body, the ethical body, the aesthetic body, the cultural body, etc. The body is also physicality, sensitivity, and sensoriality, with related feelings, which play a significant role in the activities of care and its acceptance or rejection, just as there is the body in the state of suffering and pain, the body and the various sensitivities for hygiene, shame, feelings of embarrassment, inadequacy, the need for autonomy, the sense of disgust or aversion. But also, the body concerning the possession of abilities, aptitudes, skills, and techniques that allow or do not allow accessibility to the medicine and its correct use.

The concept of therapeutic adherence, which is central to medical discussion, is further explored by design culture investigating the motivations, causes, and contingencies that may lead a patient to comply with or deviate from medical prescriptions. Causes that can be linked to the reasons associated with the patient's body and its influence on their willingness to adhere to treatment. Moreover, these can be connected to the user's interactions with the medication as a tangible object with physical characteristics and signs that can either facilitate or hinder its use. And finally, the concept of usability also appears to be complementary. Compared to the same concept used in the pharmaceutical product world to validate the 'functioning' of a product, here the context and the concrete conditions of use in which the patient finds himself assume relevance; the effectiveness and not only the efficiency of the devices and accessory and auxiliary objects that convey the medicine, as well as the physical, cognitive, and cultural characteristics of the patient (Pizzocaro 2015).

1.4 The Relationship Between Users and Medicines as a Design Topic

The significance of medicines in our lives is undeniable, but the care provided for them does not currently reflect mature design thinking. This extends to both the objects themselves and the interactions and experiences of users, especially those who may lack the necessary training in effectively managing their medications.

We argue that adopting a design-oriented perspective toward medicine and therapy can provide unique stimuli for innovation, addressing users' difficulties in recognizing connections between shape and function, comprehending products, and ensuring ease of use (affordance) (Norman 2015). These stimuli can also contribute to interpreting the product interface for improved user-product interaction (i.e., interface design, interaction design), enhancing the role of past and present experiences in memory and cognitive mechanisms governing the user-product relationship (i.e., experience design).

A design-oriented approach can further investigate 'shape features' guiding the user's cognitive processes, focus on the product system and life cycle with specific considerations for different phases and the diverse users involved, draw on theoretical reflections and design experiences in packaging design and the role of info-communication in facilitating access to the product (i.e., access design), and promote research on multi-channel, multi-modal, multi-cultural processes that transform information based on the user's cultural traits (Baule and Caratti 2016).

This comprehensive approach aims to address various dimensions of the user-product interaction and contribute to the advancement of design thinking in the realm of medicines and therapy.

In a landscape centred around objects, where technological possibilities endow them with functions ranging from sophisticated to hypertrophic to useless, and where subject-object interactions have evolved (e.g., unlocking with a gaze, paying with the voice, remote surgery), and developed objects to which we assign human characteristics (intelligent, sentient, sensitive, sound objects endowed with sex appeal) (Perniola 2004), medicine appears to be in a process of formal renewal. However, medicine possesses a unique characteristic that sets it apart from most everyday objects: it is accompanied by a substantial 'body of prescriptions', predominantly expressed through verbal texts. In the world of objects, the prescription of correct behavior occurs, in part, through the form of the object itself.

Significant signs inscribed in the body of the object guide the user's actions, provide information, and ensure the safety of their gestures. This distinction highlights a particular challenge in the design of medicine, where the guidance and communication of correct usage are primarily conveyed through textual information, requiring a thoughtful approach to ensure effective user understanding and interaction.

How prescriptions are communicated, whether through linguistic forms in package leaflets or secondary packaging, can also be brought closer to the user's world. The field of communication design offers insights into text readability, enriching vocabulary with images, and replacing words with visual aids. Despite the widespread availability of medicines, they are not always easily usable, and this need for greater accessibility is further emphasized as healthcare shifts from hospitals to domestic settings, placing more responsibility on end users. The elderly, in particular, face challenges due to their personalities, physical and cognitive abilities, and language barriers.

The consideration of elderly users emphasizes the potential for increased safety through comprehensible information and interaction with accessible objects designed for both care and management processes. Redesigning medicines and related artifacts to guide and influence users' behavior in the care pathway is a task to which designers can significantly contribute. This collaboration with specialists in the medicine sector aims to ensure maximum patient safety, especially in the context of contemporary care, which has shifted from hospitals to domestic settings, placing more responsibility on end users. Prescriptions, in their linguistic forms and rhetoric in package leaflets or secondary packaging, can also be brought closer to the reality of the user. The field of communication design, with its theories and experiences, can contribute reflections on the readability of text, on how to enrich the vocabulary plane with that of the image, or how to replace a word with an image. Despite the widespread dissemination of medicines, their easy usability does not always correspond to their pervasiveness. In the context of contemporary care, the need to intervene in the formal connotations of medicine for greater accessibility becomes more crucial, especially with the increasing responsibility placed on end users. The elderly constitute the most fragile element in this transformation. Users often interpret objects, sometimes generating alternative uses beyond their intended purpose. In the case of medicines, the absence of precise and comprehensible usage protocols can lead to incorrect behaviours borrowed from interactions with products in other categories, posing significant health risks. Delegating responsibility for care management to users presupposes appropriate education on both the languages of care and interaction with supporting products and tools (Pizzocaro 2015). The absence of precise and comprehensible protocols of use for medicines, including indications on postures, handling techniques, storage methods, and disposal, can lead to behaviours not always correct and often borrowed from interactions with products in other categories. Learning to use medicines similarly to other objects poses an objective health risk for the user.

1.5 The Object Nature of Medicinal Products

The pharmaceutical product presents a unique challenge when viewed from a design perspective, deviating from the conventional idea of an '*object per se*'. Nevertheless, the undertaking here is to consider the medicine, including its packaging and the associated communication and information apparatus, as an object that can be observed, analysed, and studied (Akrich 1996). This approach aligns with the study perspectives typical of design investigations into products, as detailed in Chap. 12.

Understanding the 'meaningfulness' that objects assume in our lives, grasping their density of significance, and attributing theoretical importance to the cores of relationships and actions around the object are not always straightforward tasks. For those not directly engaged with "the world of objects" and even for those practicing theoretical reflection in design disciplines, the object often faces challenges due to its 'materiality' and 'ordinary' and 'commonplace' nature, which have historically led to its exclusion from critical reflection (Semprini 1999).

Fields such as sociology, anthropology, and semiotics, leveraging the concept of 'material culture,' have integrated the object into universes of meaning—functional, technical, instrumental, as well as symbolic, metaphorical, identitarian, and relational—contributing to the construction of their complex 'biography' (Fiorani 2001). The acknowledgment that an object can have an identity biography implies the intricate relationships between the object and the subject: in contact with each other, the object becomes humanized, and the subject becomes artificialized. This hybridization, not always consciously recognized, between body and machine, person, and instrument (Pizzocaro 2004), holds relevance for objects nearby, such as those in our domestic surroundings or those we wear.

When it comes to treatment objects, especially those in direct contact with our bodies and pervade our daily lives, there is a common tendency to emphasize, or even singularize, their utilitarian and instrumental nature. This applies not only to the medicine itself but also, particularly, to the system of therapy support devices. Often overlooked is the considerable emotional investment that each patient places in the hope of recovery, to the extent that the medicine is sometimes attributed to the characteristics and potentialities of a magical (Dorfles 1988), salvific, miraculous object.

A design-oriented analysis does not underestimate the impact of embedding medicine and the treatment process within cultural and social systems (Fainzang 2003). It explores the symbolic and meaning attributions related to these objects and their usage behavior. Medical practices intersect with various cultural, political, ideological, and bodily aspects. In this sense, medicine is not just an object with a function; it also becomes a 'social object'.

As already argued elsewhere, "*Drugs are the meeting point of production interests and a health-related ethic that has been pervaded by economic values. They carry ideologies about recovery and care, and so also about what constitutes an admissible and acceptable therapeutic object. They embody scientific principles, social values, forms of exclusion from or the right to treatment, and conceptions about health policies. As a socio-technical apparatus, they contain forms of hidden power. As a socio-semiotic apparatus* (Landowski and Marrone 2002), *they pave the way for signification processes that follow trajectories back and forth between the society level and individual level, between the level of scientific precision and the level of approximation of daily life, between technical-specialist level and the level of daily incompetence*" (Penati et al. 2021).

In other words, the concrete form and instrumental requirements of objects become enveloped in a halo of meaning that surpasses their immediate use, as discussed by Barthes (1957) and Baudrillard (1968). Viewing the medicine object as a product of social thought and its transformations suggests an enrichment of the instrumental perspective alone. Society and its manifestations play a crucial role in propelling medicine towards continual updates, aligning it with new behaviours and lifestyles. When necessary, this involves integration with the potential offered by new technological supports, bringing medicine closer to the evolving needs and requirements of patients. Interpreting the medicine object as a product of social thought and its evolution implies an enrichment even from a purely instrumental perspective. Society and its influences play a crucial role in propelling medicine towards updates, aligning it with emerging behaviours and lifestyles. This integration, when necessary, involves leveraging the potential offered by new technological supports, bringing medicine closer to the needs and requirements of patients.

Examining medicine from a design perspective, solely in the dimension of its use, reveals a lack of comprehensive reflection on the potential correlation between formal characteristics, functional or informational deficiencies, and their connection to errors in therapy. This gap is intended to be filled by the myriad of physical and communicative artifacts surrounding medicinal types, including recipes, prescriptions, instructions, outer packaging, inner packaging, containers, dispensers, and application accessories, among others. However, regrettably, this integration is not always achieved. Addressing the open topic of 'medicine-as-object' design necessitates outlining research trajectories and providing fundamental clarifications that remain unexplored. This underscores the current under-exploration of this research field.

1.6 Medicine in the Folds of Everyday Life

Another perspective through which the relationship between patients and medicines is investigated concerns the observation scale of the 'everyday', a distinct category of inquiry that demands a specific cognitive style. The everyday represents a unique instance with its statutory code. Michel Maffesoli (2012 [1990]), in his Preface to the Italian edition of Michel De Certeau's *L'invention du quotidien*. 1 *Arts de faire* [The invention of the everyday. Arts of doing], peremptory expressed the necessity of being on the level of the everyday (p. XII) to effectively investigate it. In essence, the perception of the nuances of ordinary things, let we appreciate them in their exceptional qualities.

This implies adapting one's perspective to the realm of the usual and customary, allowing one to observe these aspects in their exceptionality, in the literal sense of being an exception, even within the recurring and routine events of everyday life.

Interest in the everyday challenges the tradition of focusing on differences and extraordinary events, emphasizing the importance of ordinary, day-to-day activities that are often overlooked.

These are often anonymous and informal practices that are performed hastily.

And yet, the everyday is also a realm where unconventional and non-standard and non-canonical approaches of doing things can solidify and can become stable practices. These practices are absorbed into operational schemes, in the system of norms and repertoires of procedures that offer ready-made solutions to everyday challenges.

In this sense, everyday life involves the construction of its own rules, which, once ritualized, become the standard (De Certeau 2012 [1990]).

The act of taking medicine, when assimilated into the spectrum of household chores, can become part of the 'inaccuracy' and be handled carelessly and inattentively. Like other recurring actions typical of domestic life, once the most suitable method for managing this practical activity—whether deemed right or wrong—has been established, even in a personal or impromptu manner, it can integrate into repetitive behavioural patterns.

Everyday life is a realm of a do-it-yourself ethos and embraces a certain craftsmanship. It embodies the concept of "bricolage," involving practical and concrete intelligence, highlighting "a thousand different ways of doing the same thing" (De Certeau 2012 [1990], p. 63), as the everyday constitutes a space for experimentation, self-management, and self-determination.

Moreover, everyday life is a realm of small tactics and cleverness, where occasions and circumstances dominate (Giard 2012 [1990], p. XLIII). Many everyday practices, such as cooking, tidying up, and shopping, possess tactical dimensions. De Certeau suggests that the forms of pragmatic intelligence, the wit of 'here and now' solutions, and the 'buzz of ways of proceeding' inherent in these activities give rise to behavior that is not entirely programmed and predictable (De Certeau 2012 [1990], p. 21). The 'minute tactics' of everyday life seem to exhibit their forms of rationality, where technical knowledge, internalized rules, and creative decisive acts shape 'common knowledge.'

Care activities, within the spaces of everyday life, also rely on these forms of knowledge that only partly draw on formalised and institutionalised knowledge. In caring practices, within the home, in everyday life, we also find ways of doing and contributions derived from self-learned knowledge; solutions 'discovered' in practice; inventions derived from experiments; transcriptions of codes of use transferred from everyday life activities, to caring practices.

Medicines, introduced into everyday life within the logic of 'more or less' governing the authenticity of domestic practices, assimilate into the diverse world of goods and products that inhabit our homes, adopting the habitual patterns of use and consumption typical of everyday objects.

Moreover, everyday life constructs its etiquette, distinct from formal rules. Giard, in describing the informality governing everyday practices, refers to 'interstitial freedom' (2012 [1990], p. XXXV).

This freedom, complementing the tricks and stratagems of the art of making do (De Certeau 2012 [1990], p. 16), encompasses spontaneity and discretion in adhering to or contravening the sense of hygiene, modesty, and good manners that govern relationships with the body and corporeality—socially constructed principles that permeate care practices.

Daily life is indeed the realm of the sensitive body, the material world, and the experience through and on the body. It encompasses the prosaic and, in certain aspects, even the trivial dimensions of life. These elements are intrinsic and crucial in every act of care, which necessarily involves operating and establishing a relationship with concrete bodies. Care interventions may employ techniques that are invasive and intrusive, using tangible objects that require manipulation and direct interaction.

Everyday life is the domain of proximity, of the familiar, seemingly requiring no additional knowledge. It is the realm of the unspoken, where knowledge is embedded in shared practices, linguistic and behavioural slang prevails, and learning occurs by observing others and gaining familiarity with the world in this manner. Consequently, it becomes a space for improper, unvalidated knowledge, often not extending beyond the confines of the familiar world. This aspect has direct implications for the validity of care, encompassing its gestures, forms, and the beliefs that underpin it.

In constructing a practical and relational culture, often divergent from socially learned codes, the everyday discards common stereotypes to develop its own. This includes practices like 'showcasing', 'hiding', or 'staging' for guests (De Certeau 2012 [1990], p. 52). It involves attributing meaning to objects based on personal or, at most, familiar experiences, and memories, following logic that defies socially constructed attributions of meaning and value. These 'local' value stereotypes are also mirrored in care practices and objects, influencing the organization of the domestic pharmacy and the display or concealment of medicine and illness.

We can perceive the everyday as a place with a distinct level of civilization, where efforts are made to assimilate the foreign and external, rendering it familiar through processes of 'domestication.' Domestication, as an outcome, can yield more spontaneous, less formalized, and consequently, more raw, and unrefined knowledge.

For a product such as medicine, which is the result of scientific, technical, and hyper-normalized thinking, the entry into everyday life has outcomes that are anything but harmless. What is lacking, to date, is a perspective of studies that can precisely grasp this context of use in its peculiarities, in its ability to override the norms and codes of use of objects—in our case, medicines—taken for granted.

Everyday spaces ultimately prove to be places able to unveil "what consumers do with products" (De Certeau 2012 [1990], p. 7); what real use and consumption practices—often out of the ordinary—they put into practice; how much it is, in the end, the user's prerogatives to re-interpret (and often re-invent) products precisely under being inside the home: a perimeter in which the user feels free to activate forms of appropriation and re-appropriation of objects to the point of transforming their form and functions (De Certeau 2012 [1990]).

Everyday is also the place of "disseminated technologies" (De Certeau 2012 [1990], p. 85), pervasive, embedded in objects that are an integral part of our daily lives and that we take for granted. Technologies that enter our homes through objects, in an obvious form, thus become invisible. Everyday life is therefore also a place where technology is banalized (Nacci 1998); a place where, in the object, the scientific and technical world is made more friendly, domesticated, and simple (Lie and Sørensen 1996). In the case of medicine, one must ask what expedients can be used to bring the world of science into the universe of everyday life, reconciling the friendliness proper to objects of use with its scientific aura: medicine, if perceived in the same way as an object of everyday use, may lead the user to superficial and irresponsible attitudes, exposing him to the risk of error.

1.7 Medicine Remedies and Poison

The term 'medicine' encompasses the dual nature of being a remedy, a medicine, and a potentially dangerous substance or poison. This inherent dichotomy is rooted in the etymology of the term, reflecting its healing power linked to therapeutic properties and, conversely, its potentially lethal effects due to misuse.

A substantial body of literature and an increasing number of research studies focus on the purchasing and consumption behavior of pharmaceuticals, particularly the use (and abuse) of medicinal substances. Predominantly situated in the medical-pharmaceutical realm, major studies consider the side effects induced by the active ingredient and its interactions with other drugs or substances, such as food or drink, which may alter therapeutic properties. The exploration of these 'side-effects' and interactions is rigorously pharmacological, using methods from clinical pharmacology and pharmaco-epidemiology to enhance existing active ingredients and explore new ones.

Pharmacovigilance activities play a pivotal role, managed, for example, by the Italian Medicines Agency (https://www.aifa.gov.it/), encompassing the gathering of patient reports on side effects, preventing damage caused by adverse reactions, providing information to patients and healthcare professionals, and promoting research programs for increased knowledge about medicines, their usage, and patient characteristics. In addressing intake errors, the activities of Pharmacovigilance Centres play a crucial role as true 'observatories of the drug' and its effects. These observatories primarily engage in the collection of reports and the issuance of rules, conduct guidelines, prohibitions, and suggestions. These take the form of "Ministerial Recommendations," "Quality Control Standards" (especially in the hospital sector), and guidelines that primarily influence the behavior expected from various stakeholders in the system, including doctors, pharmacists, nursing staff, the drug industry, and sometimes patients. It is noteworthy that these measures rarely propose design interventions aimed at incorporating prescriptive aspects into the drug's form, packaging, and information system extending from the prescription to the package leaflet. For further details on regulatory aspects, please refer to Chap. 2 and Addendum 1 of this book.

International studies indicate that the causes of medication errors are multifactorial, involving both healthcare and non-healthcare professionals who interact at various stages of the drug management process (Hepler and Segal 2003). Despite an increasingly literate population, medication and medication management errors are on the rise and contribute to high mortality rates in some diseases (Davis et al. 2006). The causes of errors in medication administration are intricate and extend beyond individual behavior. An inclusive examination of potential error origins calls for the study of demographic and social changes, coupled with evolving lifestyles, which augment the risk of errors. A notable illustration is the transformative impact of shifts in work and study dynamics on time spent outside the home. This alteration affects medication management throughout the day, influencing our relationship with meals that have traditionally structured daily rituals, including those related to care.

The shift from home introduces pertinent themes in the realm of care, such as transportability, wearability, and the execution of traditionally home-based actions in informal settings. Beyond these considerations, the need for correct therapy administration outdoors encourages the separation of primary packaging from secondary packaging, along with the package leaflet, risking the loss of vital information. Global economic and cultural factors further accentuate the challenges. The associated linguistic amalgamation significantly hinders the comprehension of medicine usage information, creating difficulties in recognizing or adapting medicine names across different geographical contexts. This issue has intensified with the rise in international travel for study, work, and leisure purposes.

Due to changes in lifestyles, the subject of medication errors has emerged as a public health emergency, impacting healthcare expenditures substantially. This book strategically positions itself at a critical juncture, aiming to complement the existing regulatory framework. It interstitially integrates into the established guidelines, proposing additions and showcasing exemplary practices in pharmaceutical product valorisation. The stated objective is to contribute to enhancing treatment process safety by recommending micro-design interventions on drugs and packaging that ensure clarity, easy access to information, comprehension, and ease of use.

1.8 Innovation in the Pharma Industry

Addressing the challenge of reducing errors through the redesign of the form, morphology, and communication content of pharmaceuticals poses a significant hurdle for an industry primarily focused on research into discoveries and their development (Horrobin 2000). The economic returns of this expensive research are strongly influenced by the unique dynamics of supply and demand in the pharmaceutical market.

Pharmaceutical products, considered "meritorious goods" (Musgrave 1959) by economists, are essential assets for the community, often financed to some extent by the State, which plays a dual role as both controller and validator of product quality for public health assurance. Except for so-called over-the-counter drugs, drug purchases are largely influenced by specific acquisition modalities, typically intermediated by the doctor who plays a pivotal role in guiding most treatment choices. In essence, the doctor becomes a significant actor in determining demand, distinct from the traditional consumer. Consequently, the design of drug packaging, including its shape, information notes, and other elements, is only partially oriented towards the patient. Instead, it is conceived partly for the doctor-prescriber, the individual shaping the demand for the product, and partly for the pharmacist-dispenser. This situation deviates from the design logic of consumer goods, impacting the company's focus on the end user's needs and the microdynamics of the patient-product interaction.

The company's attention to addressing issues such as recognizability, comprehension, ease of use, satisfaction, and loyalty is consequently affected. These concerns typically guide contemporary design in meeting individual needs. The process of forming purchase demand also results in drug packaging losing many of the attributes associated with its persuasive function (Bucchetti 1999), particularly for prescription drugs. Instead, greater emphasis is placed on strictly functional values related to storage, disability, and dispensing. However, there is a relatively modest reflection on the processes of physical and cognitive interaction, the variety of contexts in which product use occurs, and the actual modes of assumption within the treatment ritual, where patients often ingeniously seek customized solutions.

The complexity of markets, characterized by global active ingredient dynamics but local fragmentation in pharmaceutical form, distribution, and sales methods, adds to the difficulty of rethinking the drug's form and packaging. Regulations acting on a national scale, even with supranational harmonization efforts, reduce market sizes, hindering economies of scale in packaging production.

It is essential to consider that the industry responsible for the primary packaging of pharmaceuticals is part of the allied sectors associated with the pharmaceutical industry. In many instances, it forms a distinct sector leveraging economies of diversification (Chandler 1994; Temin 1979) derived from the use of knowledge, resources, and equipment not only for pharmaceutical production but also for the manufacture of packaging products across various industrial domains. For instance, a manufacturer of glass test tubes may also produce containers for cosmetics or food, and a producer of ointment tubes may extend their production to the cosmetics industry. This organizational characteristic significantly influences strategies for packaging redesign and the development of new formats, making the industry less inclined to innovate without input from pharmaceutical companies or external regulatory influences (Carli Lorenzini et al. 2018).

Similarly, within the supply chain providing goods and services to the pharmaceutical industry (Singh et al. 2016), there is a diminished presence of highly specialized entities exclusively serving the pharmaceutical sector, particularly in areas like graphic design. Instead, the prevailing entities offer services across multiple industries, sometimes lacking the necessary focus on the specific challenges of the pharmaceutical sector. This industry, along with its industrial supply chain, stands out as one of Italy's and the world's best in terms of research investment, turnover, number of employees, and innovation capacity (Atella et al. 2008).

Finally, it is important to recognize that this is a private industry operating within a complex system of stakeholders (Malerba and Orsenigo 2015): the National Health System, Drug Agencies, the hospital system, general practitioners, industrial research centres, independent pharmacological research institutes, pharmacies, the broader distribution system, and citizens/patients. This system embodies both private interests, such as the capacity to innovate for competition and business sustenance, and public interests, such as responsiveness to health demands, safety of care, prevention, and optimal utilization of social security resources. Negotiating the diverse private and public needs within this system influences the construction of relationships among stakeholders, making it challenging to easily reconcile their interests for the promotion of design-oriented research and design experiences.

The book explores these challenges, presenting a thorough exploration of the issues highlighted in the introductory paragraphs. It aims to offer in-depth studies and analyses that contribute to the ongoing discourse on the redesign of pharmaceuticals, with a focus on enhancing safety and efficacy.

1.9 Overview of Book Contents

This book introduces the topic of medicines and pharmaceutical therapies, highlighting the gap between the supposed precision of the processes that characterize the production phase, and the difficulties that punctuate all of the subsequent stages that, from prescriptive to dispensing, bring the medicine inside the patient's daily home.

It identifies packaging as the point of contact between medicine, doctor, pharmacist, and patient, and identifies its main functions: preserving, protecting, dispensing, portioning, communicating, and informing. It describes the priorities of the pharmaceutical industry from drug quality assurance to patient safety and process optimisation. It notes how a new set of social demands (an aging population, an increase in chronic diseases, a new concept of quality of life, body culture, health, and illness), and new cultural values (multi-ethnic societies, networked societies, life outside the home, new environmental sensitivities) are intervening, enriching and directing the innovation processes within this industry.

> *A drug or medicine is any substance capable of inducing a biological effect, which can be used for prophylactic, curative or diagnostic purposes. A medicine consists of one or more active ingredients, to which are added auxiliary substances, called excipients, which enable the medicine to be used and which determine, in some cases, the speed and site of absorption of the active ingredient. The medicine may be used after the active ingredient has been given a form that allows it to be administered by the chosen route and dosage. […] The preparation of the active ingredient, which is rightfully among the process steps of pharmaceutical production, is generally carried out by specialised companies that do not produce finished drugs […]*
>
> *At a general level, the production cycle of the pharmaceutical industry can be summarised in the following phases:*
>
> - *Arrival of raw materials and storage;*
> - *Washing and sterilisation of working environments before production;*
> - *Weighing of raw materials;*
> - *Preparation of granulate;*
> - *Production of the different pharmaceutical forms (solid, semi-solid and liquid);*
> - *Packaging;*
> - *Storage and shipping* (Brusco et al. 2011, p. 890).

A pharmaceutical product is the outcome of a complex process that involves the collaboration of various industries to bring it to the market and make it accessible to patients. In alignment with the objectives outlined in this volume, our focus is directed towards a specific phase within the production process of the pharmaceutical industry. This phase involves the decision-making process in which the company selects the packaging for its products.

Like other products in the market, a drug, to enter the distribution system, needs packaging that can contain, protect, preserve its integrity, ensure safety throughout its life cycle, and facilitate its use and dosage. From production to patient use, packaging assumes crucial and varied roles. Every medicine exits the pharmaceutical industry shielded by three layers of packaging: primary packaging (the container directly in contact with the drug), secondary packaging (the external packaging encountered by the user at the time of purchase), and tertiary packaging designed for transport and storage. Given the focus on the patient's interaction with the medicine, this book exclusively addresses primary and secondary packaging, along with the package leaflet and auxiliary products intended to enhance the use of medicines.

The selection of primary packaging and its constituent materials depends on the drug's chemical characteristics, storage requirements, and method of administration (Figs. 1.1, 1.2, and 1.3). Commonly used materials include glass, plastic, and aluminium, with primary packaging taking various forms, such as bottles, vials, blisters, ampoules, pre-filled syringes, aluminum, or plastic tubes, etc. Formats must adhere to regulations and be tailored to each drug's characteristics and potential risks associated with incorrect dosage, especially overdose.

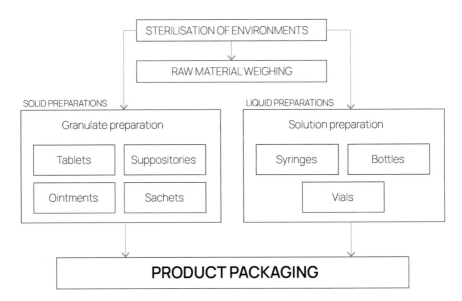

Fig. 1.1 Diagram of the production cycle of the pharmaceutical industry as a whole (Brusco et al. 2011, p. 910)

Fig. 1.2 Packaging components. Overview of packaging of oral solid forms (Brusco et al. 2011, p. 911)

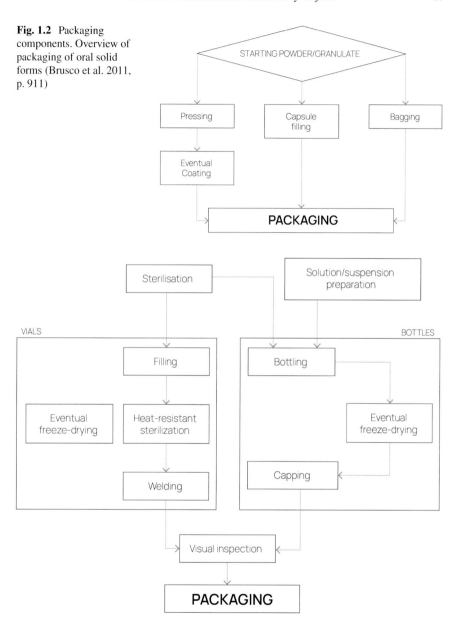

Fig. 1.3 Packaging components. Summary diagram of the preparation of liquid pharmaceutical forms (Brusco et al. 2011, p. 912)

Secondary packaging chiefly comprises cases designed in close relation to the chosen primary packaging. Paper and cardboard are preferred materials, and the design aims to ensure transport protection, efficient use of space in pharmacies, easy identification of the medicine, and effective communication elements.

In both primary and secondary packaging, the choice of materials and the design are critical for proper functionality, including protection, collection, recycling, disposal, user experience enhancement, and streamlining storage, transport, and sales phases. The formal characteristics of the primary and secondary packaging can significantly impact patient adherence to therapy, influencing treatment effectiveness. Therefore, meticulous design attention is devoted to these aspects. Compliance with regulatory and legal standards for safety and quality is imperative, necessitating information inclusion on prescriptions, usage instructions, precautions, warnings, expiration dates, and production batch numbers. The communicative function of pharmaceutical packaging is a strategic consideration in its design.

Effective communication is vital within production facilities to prevent confusion, in distribution and sales to avoid dispensing errors, and during the usage phase to provide patients with all necessary information for correct drug administration.

The primary and secondary packaging must be imprinted with the expiration date and the production 'batch' number. Additionally, the outer packaging must feature a self-adhesive label with progressive, machine-readable numbering, essential for tracing each unit of the drug from its placement on the market through the entire distribution chain to the point of sale. This traceability is a crucial tool in preventing the counterfeiting of medicines.

Equally important and strategically integral to the design of pharmaceutical packaging is its communicative function. Communication plays a vital role within production facilities to prevent the confusion of different drugs. In the distribution and sales phase, effective communication is essential to avoid dispensing errors. Furthermore, during the use phase, the packaging serves to provide patients with all the necessary information for the correct administration of the drug.

In addition to primary and secondary packaging, various devices that, although not part of the sales packaging, encounter the drug during the administration phase to facilitate its use must also be considered as objects of design.

The pharmaceutical packaging sector, encompassing both primary and secondary aspects, typically outsources its operations to entities external to the pharmaceutical industry. These external entities, while strongly interacting with the pharmaceutical sector, are answerable to various stakeholders across the production, distribution, regulatory, and other processes. The definition of drug packaging characteristics is contingent upon multiple factors. These include constraints within the production system, such as productivity, costs, and quality; characteristics of the drug itself, including pharmaceutical form, route of administration, and chemical attributes; requirements imposed by the distribution chain; and regulatory standards outlined by regulatory authorities. Additionally, societal macro-trends, such as safety and anti-counterfeiting concerns, environmental considerations, product redesign for the elderly population, and gender medicine, also influence packaging system adaptation. Technological advancements contribute to innovation within the sector.

While contemporary dynamics affecting the pharmaceutical industry are vast and diverse, this book maintains its focus on the role of physical and communicative artifacts—specifically packaging and package leaflets—in facilitating drug accessibility and supporting users in the correct usage process. Notably, users within the pharmaceutical industry often struggle to find formal and effective spaces to express their needs, with their voices frequently remaining in the background or being considered post-decision-making processes.

The first section of the book, "*Objects of Science: The Pharmaceutical Industry as a Place of Preciseness*," underscores the distinctive nature of pharmaceutical products characterized by accuracy, precision, and scientific rigor. This precision governs every step of the process, but its efficacy lies in emphasizing efficacy in non-expert user applications. Part I delves into issues of safety, quality, production standards, and compliance with regulations that guide the entire process from design to market, connecting directly with the end user—the patient.

Given the unique impact of pharmaceutical products on consumer health, the pharmaceutical sector operates within a highly regulated environment. The misuse of medicines, a well-known issue, leads to numerous deaths annually, often due to misunderstanding or underestimation of prescriptions. The regulation of packaging, both functionally and communicatively, involves multiple regulatory levels at the national, EU, and international scales. This book presents relevant legislation in Simona Cazzaniga's chapter "Medicine packaging legislation and its evolution according to technological innovation for better healthcare support," emphasizing its evolution according to technological innovation and its role in driving innovation within the pharmaceutical industry.

Regulation, for instance, plays a pivotal role in propelling the development of smart packaging. Such packaging allows for tracking and monitoring medicines, counteracting counterfeiting, ensuring tamper resistance, preventing contamination, providing understandable patient instructions, and enhancing user-friendliness.

The chapter "*Primary Medicine Packaging and Quality Control*" elaborates on the crucial role of primary packaging in preserving the quality of medicines throughout their lifetime. The choice of packaging material depends on various factors, including the type of use and market demands. Therefore, the choice of the type of container and its material is of paramount importance for both the pharmaceutical company that has to manufacture it and the patient who uses it.

In this chapter, Elena Piovosi relies on authoritative European and American manuals that meticulously regulate every facet of the production process through stringent standards. The chapter illuminates the intricate constraints and criteria governing the selection of primary packaging and the materials used, considering the pharmaceutical form and the chemical-physical characteristics of the active ingredient. Furthermore, the author addresses another chapter "*Pharmaceutical forms and primary packaging: a glossary*". While not exhaustive in providing a complete 'collection' of the primary types of pharmaceutical forms and their corresponding primary packaging available in the market, it does elucidate how progressive specialization has fostered the proliferation of morphological variants for each type of primary packaging. This phenomenon has given rise to a substantial array of objects dedicated to the preservation and administration of drugs.

Marcello Mariani contributes two chapters in this first section. "*Secondary Medicine Packaging: Design Processes for the Pharmaceutical Industry*" outlines the decision-making process leading from design to testing of secondary packaging and package leaflets. The chapter highlights critical steps in meeting the needs of various actors, such as the pharmaceutical industry, distribution system, and patients. An example of innovation—substituting primary packaging materials to reduce environmental impact—is presented as evidence of possible transformations in a heavily regulated industry. The subsequent chapter, *"Secondary Packaging and Leaflets: A Glossary"*, explains the main types of secondary packaging and commonly used leaflets in the pharmaceutical industry.

The second part of the book, *"Prescribing and Dispensing: Accompanying the Patient to the Correct Use of Medicines"*, delves into the prescription and dispensing processes, emphasizing the roles of healthcare professionals—doctors and pharmacists—in delivering medications from the places of production to the patient. This section reveals the lack of a seamless connection between prescription, dispensing, and use, highlighting communication gaps that often lead to improper drug use. Incomplete and sometimes incomprehensible information further compounds the issue, with package leaflets unable to fully address these gaps. The significance of artifacts, specifically prescription and secondary packaging, is underscored in facilitating these critical phases for the patient.

Chapter 7, *"Moving the care in the in-home context: the therapeutic prescription"*, edited by Enrico Morello, Milena Guarinoni and Carlo Emilio Standoli explores strategies for ensuring better adherence and continuity of therapy as patients transition to everyday life post-medical consultation or hospitalization. The focus is on multidimensional treatments and the challenges patients face in precisely following doctors' instructions. Communication strategies, therapeutic tools, and the dialogue between physicians and patients are examined to ensure appropriate prescriptions that consider the patient's clinical and lifestyle needs.

Antonella Penati's chapter, *"Dispensing Medicines: A Necessary Link Between Doctor and Patient"*, scrutinizes the critical moment of drug dispensing in pharmacies. This activity is recognized as a critical link between the prescriptive activity of the doctor and the essential need for instruction in use, health education, and information required by patients. The chapter underscores various challenges related to the organization of activities, the layout of the workspace, and a role that may not be perfectly defined, potentially resulting in misunderstandings and dispensing errors. These observations are grounded in a comprehensive review of international literature.

Particular emphasis is placed on secondary packaging and its role as an informational artifact. It is highlighted that the similarity of drug names (Look-Alike and Sound-Alike drugs being examples) and the resemblance of packaging graphics significantly impact the dispensing process. This similarity can lead to easy confusion, potentially resulting in serious errors during dispensing. The chapter sheds light on these issues, providing insights into the complexities and potential risks associated with the dispensing of medicines.

The chapter also considers the challenges of the current prescriptive recipe. Giuseppe Andreoni explores this theme in *"The Future Digital Pharmacological Prescription Between Therapy Adherence and Integrated Healthcare Personal*

Plans". In the context of prevalent strategies in the medical field that aim to minimize the impact of non-adherence to drug therapy through processes of patient empowerment and active participation in the treatment process, the author introduces critical elements essential for a correct prescription.

These elements include ensuring the prescription is dispensed at the right time, for the right patient, with the correct drug, and the proper dosage (customized to the standard one in the packet). Additionally, factors such as the correct dosage (quantity per day/week), the accurate intake over time (type of intake and distribution per day/week), and the correct duration (drug intake and washout) are crucial considerations.

The chapter underscores the importance of patient empowerment, emphasizing a comprehensive understanding of the pathology, therapy, and the correct treatment plan. To achieve this, the author advocates for more effective communication tools among the involved stakeholders, such as patients, specialists or hospital doctors, family doctors, pharmacists, nurses, therapists, and family caregivers, among others. The evolution of medical prescription is detailed in this context, and the potential for its redesign is explored.

In her chapter, "*Navigating the Complexities of the OTC Medicine Ecosystem*", Elena Caratti raises a crucial question: What information does a patient have when purchasing a non-prescription medicine? The chapter explores the challenges associated with over-the-counter (OTC) medicines and the information available to consumers during the purchase process.

Caratti notes that during an OTC medicine purchase, the patient's ability to inform themselves about the curative properties and contraindications of the drug relies solely on the secondary packaging. Given the absence of prior medical advice during the purchase of non-prescription medications, it becomes imperative for patients to access richer information through the drug's packaging compared to what is traditionally provided for prescribed medicines. However, the chapter observes that, currently, secondary packaging does not exhibit significant informative differences.

Moreover, the package insert, which can only be accessed after the purchase, does not offer additional or more specific information than typically found in the package leaflets of prescription drugs. The chapter explores this issue, offering an in-depth analysis of the challenges encountered when translating descriptive and prescriptive content through both verbal and visual language. Caratti's exploration sheds light on the complexities surrounding OTC medicine information and the need for enhanced communication strategies to better inform consumers.

In the realm of drug information, beyond the formal sources represented by healthcare professionals and pharmaceutical companies communicating through package leaflets, there exists a proliferation of non-institutional discourses. These are generated by the users themselves, engaging in the exchange of opinions and advice on treatments. The advent of online information has significantly amplified these informal exchanges. The chapter "*Dealing with medicines through online platforms and communities*" by Carlo Emilio Standoli and Umberto Tolino examines this side of drug communication.

The chapter investigates the current landscape of medicines on online platforms, including websites, forums, and social networks. Through an analysis of the content published on these platforms, it illuminates the dialogues, interactions, and communication modes among different users. The examination highlights the presence of diverse user types, such as content creators (pharmaceutical companies, med-influencers, expert users, etc.) and content consumers (patients, healthcare professionals, etc.) on the web. The authors emphasize that the content on these platforms is sometimes managed by pharmaceutical institutions or companies, and formally presented under government and international standards. Conversely, at other times, this content is generated by users with varying levels of knowledge and awareness regarding medicines, their use, and their effects.

Part III *"The Daily Life as a Place of Inaccuracy: The Domesticity of Therapy"* signifies a departure from the realm of norms, protocols, and adherence rules that govern the production, prescription, and dispensing of medications. Once the drug enters the domestic setting, it sheds its scientific aura and becomes reintegrated into everyday practices when handled by users. This section emphasizes the importance of observing people's behaviours to enhance the design of commonly used medications for daily use. It presents reflections, from both a product design and communication design perspective, that revolve around the broader theme of people-centeredness in the daily in-home use of medications.

The proposed reflection delves into medications as tangible, technical, and social objects—critical devices that materialize the meaning of medication within the prosaic dimension of domesticity. The theoretical framework embedded in the discipline of design guides the discussion, addressing issues related to product shape, affordance, and user-centeredness to enhance product accessibility and usability.

Throughout this section, a theoretical approach is used to examine real behaviours associated with medications in everyday life, particularly within the home environment. The goal is to bring forth gestures, corporeality, habits, routines, and even rituals. The reflection underscores the need for increased attention to user-centred design properties of drugs themselves.

The opening chapter, *"Medicines as Designed Objects"*, takes on the task of delineating the nature of the drug object by employing categories of analysis inherent to design in the interpretation of its characteristics. The authors Silvia Pizzocaro and Antonella Penati observe that despite the scientific sophistication of the pharmacological principle, the drug remains somewhat traditional in its nature as an object. This is due to its limited exploration as a product characterized by practical uses and user behavior (Akrich 1998). According to the authors, the drug seems to be more aligned with the world of chemical formulas than with the world of concrete forms designed to fulfil specific use requirements.

The absence of a theoretical perspective reflecting on the drug in its object dimension inevitably leads to a similar lack of theoretical interest in the interactions between the patient-user, the drug, and the myriad of formal and informal objects used by the patient to complete the act of treatment. This act involves the patient cognitively in activities of comprehension and memory, physically in the skills required for acts of care, and emotionally because the drug and care are imbued with symbolic and ideological meanings.

By relegating the analysis of the drug to the medical-pharmaceutical realm, there has been a neglect of the daily lives of patients, their vulnerabilities, and the highly personal ways in which they interact with the objects of treatment. These interactions are not scientific but imprecise and approximate, mirroring the imprecise and approximate logic and manners that govern our daily lives. The chapter calls for a broader perspective that encompasses the patient's experiences and behaviours with medications, recognizing their complexity and intertwining them with various aspects of daily life.

In her chapter, "*The In-Home Place of Medications: Perspectives of Domestication*", Silvia Pizzocaro engages in a reflection on the disposition of medicines in the domestic sphere, particularly in the context of the home pharmacy. Employing a theoretical approach that draws from the anthropology of medicine, the author revisits and integrates well-established literature. The chapter explores several key themes, including the logic influencing the definition of the home pharmacy, self-determination in private space, the exclusivity and promiscuity of spaces allocated to drugs, the domestication of drugs, and viewing drugs as things.

However, Pizzocaro goes beyond the physical arrangement of medications and explores the emotional aspects surrounding in-home medication use. Elements such as inattention, embarrassment, privacy, attraction, resistance, fear, and rejection are addressed. The chapter also shifts the focus from the typical medical perspective of examining the effects of therapeutic adherence on the patient to exploring the causes that can generate it. The author challenges the underestimation of the peculiarities of domestic drug use in determining discomfort and errors in use, which can ultimately lead to non-adherence. Additionally, attention is given to the process aspect of care, revealing various orders of difficulty in the domestic context of medication use.

The chapter "*In-home: Medicinals Treatment as a Learning Process*" by Antonella Penati focuses on observing the management of drug therapy throughout the process, shedding light on the tactics and strategies employed by patients as they navigate the complexities of drug treatment at home. In this domestic setting, where patients operate as non-experts, they are tasked with learning the practices of care. The chapter emphasizes the learning dimension of organizational techniques (Carlsson-Wall et al. 2011), body techniques (Mauss 2017), memory techniques, discipline and self-discipline techniques, and various devices.

In the course of this learning process, a type of training emerges that involves instructing the body in the ways of doing, saying, recurring gestures (Denham 2003), and cognitive expedients necessary to acquaint the patient with the practical actions at the heart of the care experience. The chapter examines the complexities of this educational journey, shedding light on how patients adapt and learn the diverse techniques and strategies needed to effectively manage their medication regimens within the home environment.

The subsequent chapters, specifically "*Use Phenomenologies: Observing the User While Taking Pharmaceutical Therapies*", "*Use Phenomenologies: Oral Solid*

Forms in Blister Packs" and "*Use Phenomenologies: What Does the User Do with the Secondary Medicine Packaging and Package Leaflet?*" draw from concrete investigative experiences related to elderly people's therapies in everyday life. These chapters provide insights into the gap between codified care models developed by pharmaceutical industries and the actual lifestyles of users (Carli Lorenzini and Olsson 2021; Carli Lorenzini et al. 2021, 2022). The investigations focus on the qualitative aspects of care phenomenology, supporting theoretical considerations and international literature studies.

Using evidence and examples documented through photographic shoots and interviews, these chapters illustrate how users interpret, translate, and integrate care information. Users may modify the shape of packaging or medication, add handwritten notes, or personalize their home care spaces with objects and signs to aid in actions like remembering, preparing, and taking medications.

Their contributions underscore how a design culture grounded in observing real user behavior, rather than reducing users to a specific type, can reveal design possibilities not immediately apparent in the pharmaceutical sector.

The section employs a rich array of images to depict the challenges in medication use, derived from observing patients' experiences in managing therapy at home. The chapters also analyze the formal and communicative characteristics of care objects, with a particular focus on the secondary and primary packaging of oral solid forms.

The fourth and final part of the book, "*The Pharmaceutical Product System: Premises for the Definition of a Repertory of Good Practices*," delves into various insights on innovation in the pharmaceutical industry, specifically focusing on improvements that can enhance the patient's life in therapy management.

The observations in the first two chapters are at the macro level, addressing phenomena affecting society due to technological development. These transformations necessitate continuous adjustments from pharmaceutical industries, and while they may initially manifest as micro-innovations, they possess the potential to become disruptive and profoundly alter the conception of drugs and treatment in the long term. It is well-known that the driving force of innovation tends to be restrained in the initial phase. New ideas require recognition and understanding to be accepted, and so, very often, innovation moves incrementally and interstitially. This pattern is particularly valid in industries like pharmaceuticals, constrained by regulations and standards. Additionally, the pharmaceutical industry primarily targets its products at the elderly population, known for being less inclined to change. Coupled with the fact that the industry is strongly influenced by silent and long-gestation social transformations, this makes the acceptance of innovation a gradual process.

The chapter "*How Political and Cultural Challenges Impact Pharma Industries*" by Annabella Amatulli focuses precisely on these aspects. Amatulli delves into an exploration of how pharmaceutical companies can effectively respond to societal demands for change while navigating established norms. The author defines the complex dynamics of interaction between the drug industry and health authorities, emphasizing the need to give substance to the voice of the real world in this complex interplay. More than ever, pharmaceutical industries are challenged to respond to the evolving landscape shaped by changes in cultural and social behavior. This is evidenced by emerging themes and initiatives encompassing gender medicine, personalized and individualized medicines/treatments, rare diseases, and the development of 'orphan drugs.' Additionally, there are activities aimed at supporting patients and families in need, such as drug donation and patient support programs. Initiatives also target prescribing the appropriate amount of medicines to address the urgent need to protect the environment and avoid the wastage of valuable drugs. These endeavours represent a renewal of strategies within pharmaceutical companies, despite facing challenges in innovation due to the numerous regulations and requirements set by health authorities worldwide. The chapter particularly explores these challenges by focusing on 'gender medicine' and the potential ramifications in the research and testing phases leading to marketing approval of new active ingredients.

In the chapter "*Medicinal Products: When Innovation Meets the Patient*", Lamberto Dionigi examines technological innovations in the contemporary context aimed at ensuring the proper use of drugs and optimizing the benefit/risk ratio for patients. The author specifically highlights innovations focused on drug administration and enhancing patient compliance with therapy, underscoring the growing importance of these advancements. Not only do they provide a competitive advantage for companies, but they may also attract incentives from drug agencies. The presented solutions extend beyond packaging, proposing a model of 'passive compliance' to treatment, especially in chronic cases or when incorrect dosage poses a risk to the patient's life. These solutions range from extended-release tablets for less frequent intake to reminder apps detailing how and for how long therapy should be taken, and even edible chips printed on the tablet surface to track intake. Dionigi emphasizes that such incremental innovations have the potential to create value for patients with established molecules comparable to the identification of a new drug.

The chapter "*Pharmaceutical Packaging According to the "Packaging Ethics Charter*", edited by Valeria Bucchetti, is grounded in the Packaging Ethics Charter (Baule et al. 2015). This charter serves as a 'tool for a system culture,' intending to relate obligations and rights linking the moment of production with that of use and consumption. The examination of medicine, as a product, and its packaging is conducted through the lens of the ten key points of the document. These principles act as interpretative filters, allowing a critical re-evaluation of medicine as an artifact with mature forms of packaging stemming from a consolidated design attitude. This design approach not only orchestrates complexity but also assesses implications and refines reference models.

In this context, the principles of the Charter of Ethics offer a conceptual tool and reference coordinates for self-reflexivity. They guide an analysis of medicine packaging that, beyond its technical-functional result, transfers models of interaction, offers degrees of freedom, imposes constraints, and establishes a relationship with the end user. This necessitates a re-examination of responsibilities and a renewal of the vision of the world promoted by the pharmaceutical product.

Dina Riccò's chapter, "*Sensory Qualities of Medicines: From Problems to Proposals*", shifts focus to the perceptual aspects of medicine, particularly oral solid forms. Through a systematic review of studies on the sensory qualities of medicines, Ricco examines medicines as design objects, assessing their tertiary qualities—the experienced object (Bozzi 1990). This examination includes visual qualities (colour, and shape), taste (being bitter, sweet, pleasant etc.), surface characteristics (smooth, rough etc.), alongside their impact on adherence to treatment.

The concluding chapter functions as a compendium of the text, resulting from a collective operation involving critical elements extracted from authors' contributions. It addresses the formal concreteness of the drug, the accompanying objects facilitating its use, and the challenges encountered in therapy management by patients. The 'collection' includes examples and cases, showcasing good solutions, improvements, and innovative details present in some products already on the market. Some of these solutions are devised by patients themselves, presented here as 'exemplars'—literal examples for drawing inspiration. Although formally derived from the author's drafting by the editor, the concluding chapter, *"Compendium: Step Towards Design-oriented Practices in the Pharma Industry in a Multidisciplinary Perspective"*, can be considered a multi-voice contribution. Some authors, as specified in the notes to the chapter, have supplemented specialized paragraphs. However, any liability for inaccuracies or omissions rests with the author. The chapter aims to define an initial repertoire of good practices—experiences, procedures, actions, and design indications—deduced during the research.

Discomfort, inattention, embarrassment, incomprehension, and incapacity contribute to errors in daily medicine intake and may reduce patient adherence to prescribed therapy. This book highlights that these errors occur throughout the entire therapeutic process, involving not only the interaction between the patient and the medicine but also the entire system of actors operating in the field of pharmaceutical therapy in various contexts and procedural phases.

Building on the critical issues identified in the analysis by various authors, we have tried to lay the groundwork for a future systematic collection of design recommendations, and organizational or procedural solutions aimed at enhancing and ensuring the safety of the medicine usage experience.

Currently, the pharmaceutical industry operates within a substantial framework of norms, codes of conduct, prohibitions, and guidelines that manifest as laws, ministerial recommendations, quality control standards, and guidelines. These regulations are active in production processes, prescription and dispensing activities, and the use of medicines. They reflect an increasing attention to considering the user/patient as a fundamental stakeholder of the pharmaceutical product (European Parliament 2001; Ministero della salute 2008, 2010). Quality Function Deployment (QFD) processes themselves define more structured ways of transforming customer requirements into design, production, and production process characteristics. This compendium aligns with these different regulatory plans to translate them into initial design indications and/or suggestions for correct behavior, providing a systemic view and supplementing them with recommendations that extend to the entire life cycle of therapy (Rodgers et al. 2019).

The writer hopes that the observations on drug-user interactions and the identified problems may foster a new sensitivity among those working in the field of care. This applies to both the design and production of pharmaceutical products and the roles of doctors and pharmacists who act as intermediaries between drugs and patients. Additionally, the book addresses regulatory institutions responsible for overseeing and governing the market placement of drugs, urging renewed attention to the tangible characteristics of the product that users have to deal with, including the features of the devices facilitating its intake (dispensers, containers, integrated measuring devices for regulation, conservation, portioning, supply, and information) and contributing to safer pharmaceutical usage for all.

Acknowledgements The reflections contained in this book stems from the activities of the *Pharma Design Studies* research group, based at the Department of Design—Politecnico di Milano, within the research project named—Curati con cura!—*Care for Care! Shaping Medication to Avoid Treatment Inaccuracy. Design Culture between Identity, Communication and Use Handling.* Are members of the research group: Giuseppe Andreoni, Valeria Bucchetti, Elena Caratti, Valeria Iannilli, Antonella Penati, Silvia Pizzocaro, Agnese Rebaglio, Dina Riccò, Carlo Emilio Standoli, and Umberto Tolino.

The work presented here is the result not only of the research group just named, but also of professionals and consultants working in the pharmaceutical industry or in the world of hospital care as well as figures who, in their legal professions, have paid special attention to the world of pharmaceuticals. Finally, the book, especially in the part investigating and observing the behaviour of elderly patients in home care, has benefited from the contribution of students and thesis writers who, for several years, have turned their design attention to the world of patients and their difficulties in using drugs.

The graphic editing of diagrams, illustrations, and photographic images was carried out by Alice Belardinelli and Mattia Tafel with the coordination of Carlo Emilio Standoli and Elena Caratti.

Carlo Emilio Standoli also did the overall editing of the volume.

We would like to thank the *Laboratorio Immagine—Image Lab.* of the School of Design at Politecnico di Milano.

References

Akrich M (1996) Le médicament comme objet technique [Medicines as a technical object]. Revue Int de Psychopathol 21:135–158. Available from: https://halshs.archives-ouvertes.fr/halshs-00081737 [Accessed November 2022]

Akrich M (1998) Les utilizateurs, acteurs de l'innovation. Educ Perm 134:79–90. Retrieved from: https://halshs.archives-ouvertes.fr/halshs-00082051. Accessed 27 July 2019

Arnheim R (1985) La dinamica della forma architettonica. Feltrinelli, Milano. [Original Ed. (1967) The dynamics of architectural form. University of California Press, Berkeley]

Arrow KJ (1962) The economic implications of learning by doing. Rev Econ Stud 29:155–173

Atella V, Bhattacharya J Carbonari L (2008) Drug quality and regulation: evidence from US and Italy. National bureau of economic research, working paper series pharmaceutical industry, n. 145657, http://www.nber.org/papers/w14567

Barthes R (1957) Mythologies. editions du Seuil, Paris. (trad. It. Miti d'oggi. (1974). Torino: Einaudi)

Baudrillard J (1968) Le système des objects. editions gallimard, Paris. (trad. It. Il sistema degli oggetti. (2007). Bompiani, Milano)

Baule G, Bucchetti V, Guidotti L, Lavorini S (2015) Carta etica del packaging [Ethical packaging charter]. Edizioni Dativo, Milano

Baule G, Caratti E (2016) Design è traduzione. Il paradigma traduttivo per la cultura del progetto, [Design is translation. The translation paradigm for design culture]. FrancoAngeli, Milano

Borgna P (2005) Sociologia del corpo. [Sociology of the body]. Laterza, Bari

Bozzi P (1990) Fisica ingenua. Studi di psicologia della percezione [Naive physics. Studies in the psychology of perception]. Garzanti, Milano

Brusco A, Menicocci FR, Mignacca F, Venanzetti F (2011) Il ciclo lavorativo e i rischi nell'industria farmaceutica italiana, rivista degli infortuni e delle malattie professionali. Fascicolo 3:899–933

Bucchetti V (1999) La messa in scena del prodotto. Packaging identità e consumo [The staging of the product. Packaging identity and consumption]. FrancoAngeli, Milano

Caprino L (2011) Il farmaco. settemila anni di storia. dal rimedio empirico alle biotecnologie. [The drug. Seven thousand years of history. From the empirical remedy to biotechnology]. Armando, Roma

Carli Lorenzini G, Bell A, Olsson A (2022) You need to be healthy to be sick': exploring older people's experiences with medication packaging at home. Age Ageing 51:1–10

Carli Lorenzini G, Mostaghel R, Hellström D (2018) Drivers of pharmaceutical packaging innovation: a customer-supplier relationship case study. J Bus Res 88:363–370

Carli Lorenzini G, Olsson A (2021) Exploring how and why to develop patient-centered packaging: a multiple-case study with pharmaceutical companies. Ther Innov Regul Sci 56:117–129

Carli Lorenzini G, Olsson A, Larsson A (2021) Listening to current practice: patient involvement in the pharmaceutical packaging design process. J Appl Packag Res 13(1):4

Carlsson-Wall M, Kraus K, Lind J (2011) The interdependencies of intra- and inter-organisational controls and work practices-The case of domestic care of the elderly. Manag Account Res 22:313–329

Chandler AD Jr (1994) Dimensione e diversificazione. Le dinamiche del capitalismo industriale. Il Mulino, Bologna. [Original Edition (1990) Scale and scope: the dynamics of industrial capitalism. The Belknap Press of Harvard University Press, Harvard]

Davis TC II et al (2006) Literacy and misunderstanding prescription drug labels. Ann Intern Med 145(12):887–894

De Certeau M (2012) L'invenzione del quotidiano [The invention of everyday life. Arts of doing]. Edizioni Lavoro, Roma. [Original edition (1990): L'invention du quotidien. L'ars de faire. Éditions Gallimard, Paris]

Denham SA (2003) Relationships between family rituals, family routines, and health. J Fam Nurs 9(3):305–330

Dorfles G (1988) Il feticcio quotidiano [The daily fetish]. Feltrinelli, Milano

European Parliament and of the Council (The) (2001) Directive 2001/83/EC of 6 November 2001 on the community code relating to medicinal products for human use. OJEC: Official Journal of the European Communities. 28.11.2001. Retrieved from: https://eur-lex.europa.eu/legal-content/EN/TXT/PDF/?uri=CELEX:32001L0083

Fainzang S (2003) Les médicaments dans l'espace privé. Gestion individuelle ou collective [Medicines in the private area. Individual or collective management]. Anthropologie et Sociétés 27(2):139–154. https://doi.org/10.7202/007450ar

Fiorani E (2001) Il mondo degli oggetti [The object world]. Lupetti, Milano

van der Geest S, Reynolds Whyte S, Hardon A (1996) The anthropology of pharmaceuticals: a biographical approach. Annu Rev Anthropol 25:153–178. https://doi.org/10.1146/annurev.anthro.25.1.153

Georghiou L et al (1986) Post-innovation performance: Technological development and competition. Macmillan, London

Giard L (2012) Storia di una ricerca [Story of a research]. In: De Certeau M (ed) L'invenzione del quotidiano [The invention of everyday life. Arts of doing]. Edizioni Lavoro, Roma, pp XXIII–XLIX. [Original edition: L'invention du quotidien. L'ars de faire. Éditions Gallimard, Paris

Hepler CD, Segal R (2003) Preventing medication errors and improving drug therapy outcomes. In: A management systems approach. CRC Press, London

Horrobin DF (2000) Innovation in the pharmaceutical industry. J R Soc Med 93(7):341–345

Landowski E, Marrone G (2002) La società degli oggetti. problemi di interogettività [The society of objects. problems of interogectivity]. Meltemi, Roma

Lie M, Sørensen K (1996) Making technology our own, domesticating technology into everyday life. Scandinavian University Press, Oslo

Maffesoli M (2012) Prefazione [Preface]. In: De Certeau M (ed) L'invenzione del quotidiano [The invention of everyday life. Arts of doing]. Edizioni Lavoro, Roma, pp IX–XIV. [Original edition: L'invention du quotidien. L'ars de faire. Éditions Gallimard, Paris

Maldonado T (1976) Disegno industriale: un riesame [Industrial design: a review]. Feltrinelli, Milano

Malerba F, Orsenigo L (2015) The evolution of the pharmaceutical industry. Bus Hist 157(5):664–687

Mauss M (2017) Le tecniche del corpo. Edizioni ETS, Pisa. (Les Techniques du Corps). (1936). Journal de psychologie, XXXII(3-4)

Ministero della salute—Dipartimento della qualità—Direzione generale della programmazione sanitaria, dei livelli di assistenza e dei principi etici di sistema—Ufficio III (march 2008) Raccomandazione n. 7—Raccomandazione per la prevenzione della morte, coma o grave danno derivati da errori in terapia farmacologica [Recommendation 7— Recommendation for the prevention of death, coma or serious harm resulting from medication errors]. Retrieved from https://www.salute.gov.it/imgs/c_17_pubblicazioni_675_allegato.pdf

Ministero della salute—Dipartimento della qualità—Direzione generale della programmazione sanitaria, dei livelli di assistenza e dei principi etici di sistema—Ufficio III (August 2010) Raccomandazione n. 12—Raccomandazione per la prevenzione degli errori in terapia con farmaci "lookalike/sound-alike" [Recommendation 12—Recommendation for the prevention of errors in look-alike/sound-alike medicine therapy]. Retrieved from https://www.salute.gov.it/imgs/C_17_pubblicazioni_1307_allegato.pdf

Musgrave RA (1959) The theory of public finance. McGraw Hill, New York

Nacci M (1998) Oggetti d'uso quotidiano. Rivoluzioni tecnologiche nella vita d'oggi [Objects of everyday use. Technological revolutions in today's life]. Marsilio, Venezia

Norman D (2015) La caffettiera del masochista. Il design degli oggetti quotidiani. Giunti, Firenze. [Original edition, (2013). The design of everyday things: Revised and expanded edition. Basic books, New York]

Penati A (2016) Forma degli oggetti [Object shape]. In: Pizzocaro S (ed) Artefatti concreti. Temi di fondamento per il design di prodotto [Concrete artefacts. Foundation themes for product design]. Edizioni Unicopli, Milano

Penati A, Pizzocaro S, Standoli CE, Iannilli VM (2021) The shape of drugs: a matter of human-centred design. In: Design Culture(s) Conference, Cumulus Conference Proceedings Rome, pp 1364–1375

Perniola M (2004) Il sex appeal dell'inorganico [The sex appeal of inorganic]. Einaudi, Torino

Pizzocaro S (2004) Pensare insieme "corpi e macchine", "tecnica e cultura", "natura e artificio" [Thinking together 'bodies and machines', 'technique and culture', 'nature and artifice']. In: Bertoldini M (ed) La cultura politecnica [The polytechnic culture]. Milano, Mondadori, pp 103–121

Pizzocaro S (2015) Introduzione agli studi sull'utente. Conoscere gli utenti tra ricerca e design dei prodotti. [Introduction to user studies. Knowing users between research and product design]. Unicopli, Milano

Rodgers P et al (2019) The Lancaster Care Charter. Design Issues 35(1):73–77. https://doi.org/10.1162/desi_a_00522

Rosenberg N (1991) Dentro la scatola nera: tecnologia ed economia. Il Mulino, Bologna. [Inside the black-box: technology and economy (1982). Cambridge University Press, Cambridge]

Schumpeter JA (1977) Il processo capitalistico. Cicli economici. ed. ridotta. Bollati-Boringhieri, Torino. [Business cycles: a theoretical, historical, and statistical analysis of the capitalist process. (1939). Martino Publishing, Mansfield, Connecticut]

Semprini A (ed) (1999) Il senso delle cose [The sense of things]. Franco Angeli, Milano

Simondon G (1958) Du mode d'existence des objets techniques [On the mode of existence of technical objects]. Aubier, Paris

Singh RK, Kumar R, Kumar P (2016) Strategic issues in pharmaceutical supply chains: a review. Int J Pharm Healthcare Mark 10(3):234–257

Temin P (1979) Technology, regulation, and market structure in the modern pharmaceutical industry. Bell J Econ 10(2):429–446

Open Access This chapter is licensed under the terms of the Creative Commons Attribution 4.0 International License (http://creativecommons.org/licenses/by/4.0/), which permits use, sharing, adaptation, distribution and reproduction in any medium or format, as long as you give appropriate credit to the original author(s) and the source, provide a link to the Creative Commons license and indicate if changes were made.

The images or other third party material in this chapter are included in the chapter's Creative Commons license, unless indicated otherwise in a credit line to the material. If material is not included in the chapter's Creative Commons license and your intended use is not permitted by statutory regulation or exceeds the permitted use, you will need to obtain permission directly from the copyright holder.

Part I
Objects of Science: The Pharmaceutical Industry as a Place of Preciseness

Chapter 2
Medicine Packaging Legislation and Its Evolution According to Technological Innovation for Better Healthcare Support

Simona Cazzaniga

Abstract If directives, laws, and regulations play a fundamental role in constraining the pharmaceutical sector's production, distribution and communication policies and practices, regulatory devices have also had and are also playing a role in incentivising innovation and orienting it towards socially and environmentally sustainable practices. The chapter builds a review of the principal regulations that, starting from the EU level, are raising awareness in the various countries of the community (here, the Italian case is analysed) towards the issues of the environment (e.g., reduction of the source of packaging materials and redesigning the pack by favouring the use of recyclable materials), traceability for anti-counterfeiting purposes; safety; and the ethics of medicine communication both in advertising and online. The regulatory review constitutes a starting point, deepened in other chapters, through the review of guidelines, recommendations, and soft law tools, to which those involved in design and innovation activities in the sector must refer.

2.1 Pharmaceutical Packaging: Traceability as the Summa Ratio of the System

From a legal point of view, the pharma industry—given the peculiarity of the products in question and their impact on consumer health—has always been hyper-regulated. This results in a strong stratification of regulations and standars (UNI EN ISO 15378: 2017), that often lead to the coexistence of several national, EU and international regulations overlapping with each other, even concerning a specific issue.

Regarding medicine packaging, the reference legislation at the European level is first and foremost Delegated Regulation 2016/161, which supplements Directive 2001/83/EC, as amended by Directive 2004/27/EC (The European Parliament and of the Council 2001), on the Community code relating to medicinal products for human use. The Regulation entered into force on 9 February 2019 for all Member

---

S. Cazzaniga (✉)
Studio Legale Sutti, Milan, Italy
e-mail: simona.cazzaniga@sutti.com

States except Belgium, Greece, and Italy, for which application is postponed until 9 February 2025. This is because at the time of the entry into force of the Directive, Italy and the other two Member States mentioned, already had a system for verifying the authenticity of medicines and the identification of individual packs, in place since 2006 thanks to the provisions of Legislative Decree No. 219 (Presidente della Repubblica 2006a). The Decree defines the procedure necessary to obtain authorisation for the production, marketing, and importation of medicinal products; it regulates the labelling and advertising procedures, both of which are subject to supervision and sanctions.

In Italy, the essential information for the identification of a medicine and the identification of each of its packages is contained in the pharmaceutical sticker, a multi-layered adhesive paper support produced by the *Istituto Poligrafico e Zecca dello Stato*, which functions as an instrument to guarantee the authenticity of medicines on the market (Fig. 2.1).

In Article 73, the same Decree defines all the information that must necessarily be given on the carton or—in the absence of the latter—on the primary packaging of each medicinal product. In this case, the information considered essential by the legislation appears to be:

- the name of the medicinal product, followed by the strength and the pharmaceutical form, adding, if appropriate, the terms "early childhood", "children" or "adults" [...];
- the qualitative and quantitative composition in terms of active substances per posological unit or, concerning the pharmaceutical form, per volume or weight, using common names;
- the pharmaceutical form and package contents expressed by weight, volume or posological units;
- a list of excipients with known action or effect, included in the guidelines published according to Article 65 of Directive 2001/83/EC; however, in the case of an injectable product or a preparation for topical or ocular use, all excipients shall be listed;
- the method of administration and, if necessary, the route of administration [...];
- the warning: "Keep out of the reach and sight of children";
- any special warnings which may be necessary in respect of the medicinal product concerned, with particular reference to the side-effects of the interaction of the medicinal product with alcoholic and non-alcoholic drinks and any dangerous effects on driving resulting from the medicinal product;
- the month and year of expiry, indicated by words or numbers;

Fig. 2.1 Example of a pharmaceutical vignette, including both barcode and QR code

- special storage precautions, if needed;
- special precautions for the disposal of unused medicinal products or waste materials derived from them, if any, and a reference to any appropriate collection system in place;
- the name and address of the *Autorizzazione Immissione in Commercio—* Marketing Authorization (AIC) holder preceded by the words *Titolare AIC;*
- the AIC number;
- the production batch number;
- for non-prescription medicinal products, the therapeutic indications, and principal instructions for the use of the medicinal product;
- the supply arrangements […];
- the retail price of the medicinal product […];
- an indication of the conditions for reimbursement by the National Health Service.[1]

A partial derogation is provided in cases where the primary packaging of the medicinal product is so oversized that it does not allow all the above information to be stated; in these cases, Italian legislation provides for a reduced number of indications specified in Article 74.[2]

It should be noted that there is a Period After Opening (PAO) (Fig. 2.2) requirement in the cosmetics sector,[3] but not for pharmaceutical products (Table 2.1).

Back to the European legislation, the aim of Regulation 2016/161 (The European Parliament and of the Council 2016) is to introduce perfect traceability of every medicine package, to curb the risk of falsified medicines entering the distribution chain, as well as to facilitate any urgent action for the withdrawal of a specific batch of a pharmaceutical product from the market.

---

[1] Art. 73 Legislative Decree No 219/2006 (Presidente della Repubblica 2006a).

[2] Art. 74 Legislative Decree No 219/2006 (Presidente della Repubblica 2006a): (1). Primary packaging other than that provided for in paragraphs 2 and 3 shall bear the particulars listed in Article 73. (2). Provided that they are contained in an outer packaging that complies with the requirements of Articles 73 and 79, primary packaging in blister form may bear only the following particulars: (a) the name of the medicinal product in accordance with point (a) of Article 73; (b) the name of the marketing authorisation holder; (c) the month and year of expiry indicated by words or numbers; (d) the production batch number. (3). Smaller primary packaging, on which it is impossible to mention the particulars provided for in Articles 73 and 79, shall bear at least the following particulars: (a) the name of the medicinal product, in accordance with Article 73 (a), and, if necessary, the route of administration; (b) the method of administration; (c) the month and year of expiry indicated by words or numbers; (d) the production batch number; (e) the contents by weight, by volume or by posology units.

[3] In the European Union, the PAO symbol was introduced by Directive 2003/15/EC and has been mandatory since 2005 (The European Parliament and of the Council 2003) for all cosmetic products with a shelf life of more than 30 months. Products in single-dose packs are exempt. It is represented on the container and packaging by the symbol shown in Annex VII of Regulation (EC) 1223/2009 (The European Parliament and of the Council 2009), which depicts an open jar with the number of months followed by the letter "M".

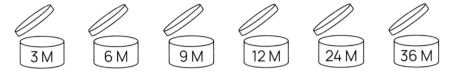

Fig. 2.2 Period after opening (PAO) graphic symbol, placed on cosmetics packaging to indicate the time during which the product, once opened, can be used without harmful effects on the consumer

Table 2.1 Indicative expiry date of different pharmaceutical forms after opening (source: https://www.federfarma.it/Home.aspx)

Pharmaceutical form	Validity (unless otherwise indicated)
Eye drops (vial)	15–20 days
Eye drops (single-dose)	Pack expiration date
Blister tablets	Pack expiration date
Bottle tablets	4–6 months
Intravenous vials	Few minutes
Intramuscular vials	Few minutes
Drops	1–2 months
Nose drops	15–20 days
Granulates can	1–2 months
Granulates sachet	5 days
Melting powders	5 days
Tube ointments	2–3 months
Ophthalmic ointments	15 days
Ointments vaso	5–7 days
Syrups	1–2 months
Syringes	Few minutes
Nose spray	15–20 days

It establishes a system in which—through the affixing of what is termed a unique identifier—the identification and authentication of medicinal products are ensured by an upstream and downstream verification of all healthcare products with safety features, supplemented by the guarantee by wholesalers of certain medicinal products with a higher risk of falsification. This makes it possible to verify the authenticity and integrity of the safety features placed on the packaging of a medicinal product from the beginning of the supply chain until the moment it is offered to the public.

Always to strengthen and make the traceability of medicines more efficient, Directive 2011/62/EU (The European Parliament and of the Council 2011) had already intervened by requiring the introduction of:

- elements identifying the medicine on the outer packaging of the product;[4]
- elements that guarantee against tampering with the medicine's packaging (e.g., safety seals);

---

[4] See Italian "Linee guida per la Tracciabilità del Farmaco e la predisposizione e la trasmissione dei file alla banca dati centrale"—Ministero della Salute, Ufficio Generale digitalizzazione sistema sanitario—March 2023 (Ministero della salute 2023).

- a common European logo identifying online pharmacies legally authorised to operate[5] (Fig. 2.3);
- stricter rules for controls and inspections of manufacturers of active ingredients of medicines;
- strengthening historical controls on registers and documents on the distribution channels used.

In line with the provisions of the European Medicines Agency (EMA) indications, acknowledged by Agenzia Italiana del Farmaco (AIFA), which recommend the use of electronic and digital technologies to support the improvement of medicine information, in recent years, companies have begun to reinterpret the *traditional* medicine pack by implementing it and inserting elements—such as special QR codes—aimed at simplifying the communication to patients of the correct use and dosage of the medicine itself.[6]

The most advanced technological solutions have not been slow in arriving, such as blisters equipped with a microchip that monitors the patients' use of the medicine, reminding them when to take the next dose, when the expiry date is approaching, when the packaging has been tampered with, or even when storage conditions are unsafe.[7]

Among the innovations to guarantee the quality and integrity of pharmaceutical products, European legislation 2011/62/EU (The European Parliament and of the Council 2011) requires that, from 2019, all pharmaceutical products sold in Europe must be equipped with anti-tampering devices. In this sense, therefore, the medicine pack must be equipped with special security systems that make it possible to verify the integrity of the packaging—and consequently of the product inside it—by implementing mechanisms such that, once opened, the pack can no longer be resealed as it was initially and thus reveal its tampering. In this context, creativity,

---

[5] On 24/06/2014, the EU Commission adopted this logo to "certify" the websites of pharmacies and other establishments authorised by member states to sell medicines online.

[6] For instance, a project launched in 2019 by an Italian pharmaceutical company included a QR code in the pack that —when specifically scanned with a smartphone—linked directly to the medicine's package leaflet and interactive videos describing how to take it (http://www.farmacista33.it/packaging-farmaci-intelligente-qr-code-per-video-su-uso-farmaco-progetto-chiesi-italia/pianeta-farmaco/news%2D%2D50434.html).

In some cases, technology has been used as a solution to specific needs: already in early 2016, a well-known Italian pharmaceutical company chose to introduce on all its medicines based on ibuprofen and naproxen a QR code allowing access to the relevant package leaflet, which can be printed in 10 of the most widely spoken languages in the world and in Italy. This is the first multilingual service available and quickly accessible on the package of a self-medication medicine. A useful service not only for residents, but also for foreigners passing through our country for tourism or work, some 50 million each year.

[7] In 2012, a wireless chip for automated intake of medicines was developed by MIT.

Embedded under the skin, it can be loaded with several medicines at the same time and can release them automatically at a predefined time or on command via a radio trigger. See https://www.aifa.gov.it/-/fda-approva-primo-sensore-digitale-commestibile- and https://www.quotidianosanita.it/scienza-e-farmaci/articolo.php?articolo_id=7503

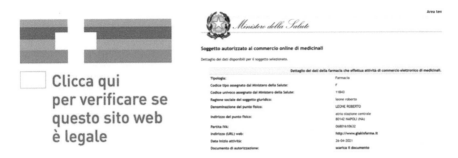

Fig. 2.3 On the left, the logo adopted by the European Commission as access to the webpage (on the right) that allows the user to check pharmacies and shops authorised to sell medicines online

design, and technology must cooperate and integrate to create tamper-proof packaging.[8]

2.2 The Disposal of Pharmaceutical Products

The disposal of pharmaceuticals and their packaging, whether primary or secondary, is another specific issue.

In this regard, Directive 2018/851/EU (The European Parliament and of the Council 2018a) amending Directive 2008/98/EC (The European Parliament and of the Council 2008) on waste, and Directive 2018/852/EU (The European Parliament and of the Council 2018b) amending Directive 1994/62/EC (The European Parliament and of the Council 1994) on packaging and waste materials have recently intervened at European level.

On the other hand, in Italy, the management of medical waste is regulated by Presidential Decree No. 254 of 15 July 2003 (Presidente della Repubblica 2003), while the management of waste more generally—and therefore also of pharmaceutical packaging—is regulated by Legislative Decree No. 152/2006 (Presidente della Repubblica 2006b), now amended by Legislative Decree No. 116/2020 (Presidente

---

[8] For many years, many companies have adopted various anti-tampering systems, using solutions such as:

- secondary pack with unique adhesive gripping labels that have to be removed in order to open the pack in order to be able to extract the contents, or with hot or cold glue dots or both hot and cold glue dots at the same time; all these methods must leave visible traces of the opening;
- secondary pack protected by an additional cellophane wrapping that makes it impossible to open the secondary pack without removing the transparent film wrapping it;
- secondary pack with cardboard devices designed with peculiar chromatic elements and/or removable flaps that, upon the first opening of the case, make evident or reveal any alteration or first opening.

della Repubblica 2020) implementing the aforementioned Directives No. 851 and 852 of 2018.

For waste disposal, the national system provides for each waste to be assigned an identification code according to the European Waste List (EWC), whereby waste produced by the healthcare sector is identified with the number 18, followed by further numbering that varies according to the specific type of healthcare waste and its components.

Entering the question of how to dispose of medicinal products for domestic use, then, it is necessary to distinguish between two significant cases: on the one hand, the case of disposing of products that still contain medicinal products inside them and, on the other hand, the case in which the sanitary products are now empty.

Concerning the former, defined as hazardous urban waste, the legislation provides that the outer packaging or, failing that, the primary packaging of medicines must display—among other necessary indications and information—*special precautions to be taken for the disposal of unused medicines or waste derived from them, as well as a reference to the appropriate existing collection systems*.[9]

Unused or expired medicines must be disposed of in special collection containers, which generally can be found near pharmacies or healthcare facilities.[10]

On the other hand, concerning the disposal of the individual elements that make up the packaging of medicines, precisely to reduce the amount of healthcare waste that must be disposed of, Article 5 of Presidential Decree 254/2003 (Presidente della Repubblica 2003) had already intervened, calling for the recovery of specific categories of materials (e.g., glass, plastic, cardboard, metal) through differentiated collection, encouraging the stipulation of special agreements by the Regions or individual municipalities directly with healthcare facilities.

Currently, to encourage the proper disposal of the different materials composing packaging, which also includes the packaging of pharmaceutical products, Article 219 of Legislative Decree no. 152/2006 (Presidente della Repubblica 2006b)—whose effective date has been extended several times until 1 January 2023—stipulates the obligation for packaging intended for the end consumer to indicate:

- the material coding, as laid down in Decision 97/129/EC (Commission Decision 28 January 1997);
- indications for disposal by separate collection.

In the case of multi-component packaging, then, it is not obligatory, but highly recommended by the Guidelines on the Labelling of Packaging of the Ministry for the Ecological Transition of 27 July 2022, the identification of the individual

---

[9] Article 73, letter l), Legislative Decree No 219/2006 (Presidente della Republica 2006a).

[10] Regarding the location of sanitary waste collection containers on the territory, several initiatives have emerged from companies that deal with waste collection, transport and disposal on a provincial scale, aimed at facilitating their identification. One example is the G-app created by Gelsia ambiente, a company of the A2A group, which with the help of a map, makes it possible to find the nearest collection point (https://www.gelsiambiente.it/farmaci-scaduti-ecco-come-vanno-raccolti/)

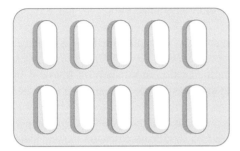

RECOMMENDED INFORMATION
Packaging type (e.g., blister)

REQUIRED INFORMATION
Material (e.g., C/ALU 90)
Directions for disposal (e.g., aluminum and metal collection. Check your local's regulations)

RECOMMENDED INFORMATION
Process of disposal (e.g., empty the packaging of its contents before disposing)

Fig. 2.4 Example of environmental labelling of a plastic/aluminium blister. Revised source CONAI

components, using a written description or graphic representation that facilitates the consumer in their separation and disposal[11] (Fig. 2.4).

All these information, whether mandatory or highly recommended, can be made available by physically affixing it to the packaging clearly and legibly or through digital channels, replacing or supplementing the information directly on the packaging. If digital channels are chosen, the obliged party is obliged to display on the packaging or at the point of sale to which the consumer has access the instructions for accessing the platform (e.g., App, QR code, website, etc.) specifically dedicated to conveying the environmental labelling content relating to the specific packaging, always guaranteeing easy, direct, timely and not difficult to interpret information.[12]

2.3 Healthcare Advertising

As is the case regarding packaging and disposal, pharmaceutical products are also subject to specific regulations regarding advertising. Health advertising has always been strongly regulated to protect the consumer, who—even more in promoting health-related products—must receive the information in a simple and easily understandable form. Also, in this case, the reference regulation at the European level is Directive 2001/83/EC (The European Parliament and of the Council 2001), implemented by Legislative Decree No. 219/2006 (Presidente della Repubblica 2006a). In this regard, it is necessary to clarify that direct advertising to consumers is only permitted for medicines without a prescription (so-called SOP—*Senza Obbligo di Prescrizione*) and Over The Counter (OTC) medicines.[13]

---

[11] Measure effective from 1 January 2023 (Ministero della transizione ecologica 2022). See: https://www.mase.gov.it/sites/default/files/archivio/normativa/rifiuti/Linee_guida_etichettatura_ambientale_27.09.2022.pdf.

[12] The Guidelines on Packaging Labelling (Ministero della transizione ecologica 2022).

[13] Art. 115 Legislative Decree No 219/2006 (Presidente della Repubblica 2006a).

The limits identified by the legislator concerning the advertising of these products to the public are manifold; in particular, the purpose of the advertising is defined both positively, by identifying the minimum content,[14] and negatively, by explaining in detail the content that is not permitted.[15]

In any case, the advertising is always subject to the authorisation of the *Ministero della Salute*, which is issued by the latter within forty-five days from the application submission by the manufacturer or person responsible for placing the medicinal product on the market, accompanied by the appropriate documentation.

If they are granted, the authorisations—which may also imply a modification of the advertising material applied for—are valid for 24 months *without prejudice to the possibility of the Ministero della Salute to establish a shorter period of validity, with justified reasons, about the characteristics of the message disseminated*, which run from the date indicated by the applicant for the start of the advertising campaign or—in the absence thereof—from the date of authorisation.[16]

---

[14] Art. 116 Legislative Decree No 219/2006 (Presidente della Repubblica 2006a): "Characteristics and minimum advertising content to the general public 1. Without prejudice to the provisions of Article 115, the advertising of a medicinal product to the general public: (a) shall be carried out in such a way that the advertising nature of the message is clear and the product is clearly identified as a medicinal product; (b) shall include at least: (Agenzia Italiana del Farmaco (AIFA) 2012) the name of the medicinal product and the common name of the active substance; mention of the latter shall not be compulsory if the medicinal product consists of several active substances; (Berardi 2012) information essential for the proper use of the medicinal product; (Commission Decision 129 of 28 1997) an express and clear invitation to read carefully the warnings on the package leaflet or the outer packaging, as the case may be; in written advertising, the invitation must be easily legible from a normal point of observation; in advertising in the daily and periodical press, it must, in any case, be written in characters no smaller than body size nine."

[15] Art. 117 Legislative Decree No. 219/2006 (Presidente della Republica 2006a): "Prohibited advertising content 1. Advertising to the general public of a medicinal product may not contain any element that: (a) makes it appear unnecessary to consult a doctor or undergo surgery, in particular by offering a diagnosis or proposing treatment by correspondence; (b) leads to the belief that the efficacy of the medicinal product is free of undesirable effects or is superior or equal to another treatment or medicinal product (c) induces the belief that the medicinal product is likely to improve the subject's normal state of good health; (d) induces the belief that the non-use of the medicinal product is likely to have a detrimental effect on the subject's normal state of good health; this prohibition shall not apply to the vaccination campaigns referred to in Article 115 (Berardi 2012); (e) is directed exclusively or predominantly at children (f) it includes a recommendation by scientists, health professionals or persons widely known to the public; (g) it likens the medicinal product to a foodstuff, cosmetic or other consumer product; (h) it leads to the belief that the safety or efficacy of the medicinal product is due to the fact that it is a 'natural' substance; (i) is likely to induce erroneous self-diagnosis; (l) improperly, impressively or misleadingly refers to claims of healing; (m) improperly, impressively or misleadingly uses visual representations of changes in the human body due to disease or injury, or of the action of a medicinal product on the human body or part of it. 2. Similarly, consistent with Article 116 (Agenzia Italiana del Farmaco (AIFA), 2012) (a), disseminating messages and texts whose advertising intent is concealed by the redundancy of other information shall not be permitted. 3. By decree of the Ministero della Salute, it may be established that advertising messages authorised according to Article 118 shall contain the marketing authorisation number of the medicinal product".

[16] Art. 118, (The European Parliament and of the Council, 2001), Legislative Decree No 219/2006 (Presidente della Republica 2006a).

The Legislature also intervened on the subject at the sanction level, providing that if health advertising were to be carried out in violation of the provisions of the law, the Ministero della Salute would intervene by ordering the immediate cessation of the advertising and the dissemination, at the expense of the offender, of rectification and clarification.

Lastly, concerning specifically online advertising via social networks, the position taken by the legislator through the Guidelines of 25 July 2017 (Ministero della Salute 2017) is one of total prohibition. The rationale for this exclusion lies in the authorisation of the Ministero della Salute is issued in respect of an advertising message that must nevertheless remain static and thus not be changed in any way as a result. This requirement of static nature, however, contrasts with the characteristics that characterise communications on social networks, which are changeable as they are subject to user observations, comments, and discussions, which could in this sense, blur or alter the content of the original communication. It is always based on this reasoning that the use of Facebook for advertising purposes is instead considered lawful, to the extent that the advertising message appears as a static or dynamic ones,[17] and of YouTube, always provided that the interactivity features are deactivated (e.g., like, share, comment, etc.).

Advertising of drugs that can only be purchased with a medical prescription or that can only be used with the help of a health professional, on the other hand, is only possible with health professionals and is defined as scientific information. The latter does not require any prior authorisation, but the legislation represents a minimum content requirement and generally stipulates that it must:

- present the product in an objective manner;
- contain accurate and proven information;
- specify that the advertising material is intended exclusively for specialised healthcare personnel and cannot be conveyed to the end consumer in any way.

As a conclusion to the presented reflections, we refer to the Code of Self-Discipline for Commercial Communication, in force since 1 June 2023, the first edition of which dates to 12 May 1966. We quote in full some of its articles relevant to pharmaceuticals.

- Article 23a—Food supplements and dietetic products.
- Marketing communication relating to food supplements and dietetic products must not claim properties inconsistent with the characteristics of the products, or properties not actually possessed by the products themselves. Furthermore, such marketing communication must be carried out so that it does not mislead consumers about nutrition and must avoid references to medical recommendations or claims. These rules also apply to infant dietary foods, those that replace all or part of breastfeeding, and those used for weaning or supplementing children's diets. Marketing communication relating to food supplements offered for weight

---

[17] See:https://www.pharmaretail.it/archivio/pubblicita-via-internet-dei-farmaci-di-automedicazione-linee-guida-ministeriali-aggiornate.

control or weight reduction and other specific types of accessories, the rules contained in the appropriate Regulations, which form an integral part of this Code, shall apply. […]
- Art. 25—Medicinal products and curative treatments.
- Marketing communication relating to medicinal products and curative treatments must consider the subject matter's particular importance and be carried out with the utmost sense of responsibility as well as following the technical data sheet summarising the product characteristics.
- Such marketing communication must draw the consumer's attention to the need for appropriate precautions in using the products by clearly and explicitly inviting the consumer to read the packaging warnings and not inducing product misuse. In particular, the commercial communication to the consumer relating to OTC medicinal products must include the name of the medicinal product and the common name of the active ingredient; the latter is not mandatory if the medicinal product consists of several active ingredients, or if the communication is intended only as a generic reminder of the name of the product.

Furthermore, marketing communication relating to over-the-counter medicinal products or curative treatments must not:

- suggest that the efficacy of the medicinal product is without side effects or that its safety or efficacy is since it is a natural substance;
- attribute to the medicine or treatment an efficacy equal to or superior to that of others;
- make it appear unnecessary to consult a doctor or undergo surgery or induce an erroneous self-diagnosis;
- target exclusively or predominantly children or induce minors to use the product without adequate supervision;
- making use of recommendations of scientists, health professionals or persons widely known to the public, or of the fact that the medicinal product has been authorised for marketing, or referring to certificates of cures improperly or misleadingly;
- likening the medicinal product to a food, cosmetic or other consumer product;
- mislead into believing that the medicine or curative treatment can improve the normal state of good health, as well as the lack thereof can have—detrimental effects; unless it is a vaccination campaign;
- make improper, misleading, or striking use of representations of changes in the human body due to disease or injury or of the action of the medicine.

In particular, the advertising of veterinary medicinal products, and the rules contained in the relevant Regulation, which forms an integral part of this Code, shall apply.

2.4 Counterfeiting and Forgery in the Pharmaceutical Field

In the pharmaceutical field, counterfeiting has a broad significance. In this regard, Article 1 of Directive 62/2011/EU (The European Parliament and of the Council 2011), which modifies the previous Directive 2001/83/EC (The European Parliament and of the Council 2001), defines a falsified medicinal product as:

> *any medicinal product which contains a misrepresentation of:*
>
> (a) *its identity, including its packaging and labelling, name or composition […];*
> (b) *its origin, including its manufacturer, country of manufacture, country of origin and marketing authorisation holder; or*
> (c) *its history, including records and documents relating to the distribution channels used.*[18]

Thus, based on this definition, a *falsified medicinal product* includes those whose contents or packaging have been deliberately and/or consciously altered, but likewise, any medicinal product that bears a false representation of even one of the aforementioned elements and even if it is accidental. One might refer to counterfeiting or falsification in the strict and broad sense: the former is where the medicinal product has been knowingly falsified, and the latter is falsified due to an accidental and/or fortuitous mistake.

This phenomenon generally involves all medicines, irrespective of brand name, generic status, and qualification. Depending on the concrete case, it is possible to distinguish different types of counterfeiting in the strict sense. The latter, for example, may be linked to the active ingredients or excipients present in the medicine, which may be potentially absent or underdosed, of poor quality or simply different from those declared. Each specific case brings different and severe consequences from a health point of view. In the case of absence or under-dosing, therapeutic efficacy will be lacking or reduced, and this will contribute to the spread of microbial strains resistant to antibiotics; the case of poor quality may imply the presence of synthetic impurities or potentially toxic degradation products, and if the active ingredients or excipients differ from those declared at the time of purchase. This may cause reactions due to individual intolerances or interactions with concomitant therapies.

Similarly, counterfeiting linked to the timing and method of storage of the pharmaceutical product could lower the titre, meaning a decrease in the content of the active ingredient with consequent therapeutic ineffectiveness or its degradation with the potential formation of toxic by-products.

Counterfeiting may also relate to the packaging, an essential element in ensuring medicines' quality, efficacy, and safety. In this case, using an unsuitable material could cause physical or chemical interaction between the packaging and its contents, altering its quality. The counterfeiting of medicines brings considerable consequences in the global market, involving different subjects and interests. First, there is damage to people's health: every year, between 72,000 and 169,000

---

[18] Art. 1, part 1—letter C, Directive 62/2011/EU (European Parliament and Council 2011).

Table 2.2 Counterfeit drugs in the world: unofficial estimates from OMS and CENSIS

Geographical area	Percentage of counterfeit drugs on the market
World	6–7%
Developing countries	20–30% (with peaks over 50% in times of crisis)
Europe	1%
Italy	0,1% (from illegal channels only)

children may die of pneumonia after taking counterfeit medicines; counterfeit antimalarial medicines may cause 116,000 deaths.[19] At the same time, counterfeiting causes severe damage in terms of lost sales and reputation to legitimate manufacturers, depriving pharmaceutical companies of revenues that could be invested in research and, in this sense, undermining innovation. This translates into enormous costs for governments and economies. The cost to EU governments for lost revenue from counterfeit medicines is around EUR 1.7 billion, to which must be added the costs for the treatment of patients who have suffered adverse health consequences from the consumption of counterfeit medicines.

Finally, counterfeiting affects environmental pollution and generates significant job losses when it originates from incorrect practices by unregulated criminal activities using potentially toxic chemical substances.

In recent years, data on counterfeiting have reached increasingly alarming numbers, with the *USA Food & Drug Administration* (FDA) reporting that the percentage of counterfeit medicines worldwide is around 10%, with an average of more than 25% in developing countries[20] (Table 2.2).

A report published on the official website of the *Agenzia Italiana del Farmaco* (AIFA) presents the most effective tools used to combat the counterfeiting phenomenon; among these, in the first place, we find international operations that involve several competent authorities collaborating.[21]

Among the many conducted in recent years, surprising results were achieved thanks to the 15th edition of *Pangea*, an international operation coordinated by Interpol to combat the online trade in illegal or falsified medicines. Ninety-four countries worldwide participated in the initiative from 23 to 30 June 2022.[22]

The balance recorded three million units of seized drugs and medical devices, more than four thousand websites closed, and arrested a considerable number of individuals involved in the trafficking of potentially harmful medicines. In Italy, the increased surveillance led to the identification and seizure of almost 43,000 units of illegal and falsified medicines, with an estimated value of over EUR 150,000. In this regard, the *Agenzia Dogane e Monopoli* (ADM) specified that the surveillance made

---

[19] See: https://www.ansa.it/europa/notizie/proprieta_intellettuale/2020/03/24/farmaci-giro-daffari-contraffatti-in-ue-da-44-miliardi_91953c78-bf3b-40df-b679-99191c35788d.html.

[20] See: https://www.aifa.gov.it/documents/20142/516919/i_capitolo.pdf

[21] See: https://www.aifa.gov.it/documents/20142/0/Farmaci_Contraffatti_2010.pdf

[22] See: https://www.salute.gov.it/portale/news/p3_2_1_2_1.jsp?lingua=italiano&menu=notizie&p=nas&id=2404

it possible to intercept illegal shipments of medicines because unauthorised persons made them and posed severe health risks because they were not stored at the prescribed temperature.

2.5 The Protection under Criminal Law

The legal assets protected concerning pharmaceutical counterfeiting are physical integrity and life.

The nature of these legally protected goods requires the intervention of criminal protection regardless of the occurrence of the damaging event; consequently, the offences provided for by the legislator to combat this phenomenon are configured as danger offences.

Counterfeiting can integrate many different types of offences depending on the individual case.

First and foremost is the case of *trade in or administration of defective medicinal products*, which punishes anyone who holds for trade, places on the market or administers defective or imperfect medicinal products with imprisonment from six months to three years and a fine of not less than EUR 103 (Art. 443 of the Criminal Code). For this purpose, a medicinal product is considered defective if it is corrupted or deteriorated due to natural causes, without human intervention, as in the case of poor preservation. In contrast, a medicinal product is considered imperfect if it lacks the necessary elements or the correct dosage or is otherwise affected by any other defect, whether original or supervening, making it unsuitable for its purpose.

Because of these definitions, the offence described in Article 443 of the Italian Codice Penale differs from the one set out in Article 440, concerning *adulteration and counterfeiting of foods*.

By *adulteration*, the article intends *the modification of the genuine nature of a medicinal substance through a process by which its essential therapeutic constituents are removed, added or replaced, without such modification having an outward appearance*. By *counterfeiting*, the article intends *the ex-novo formation of a substance that is dangerous to public health*; this means that the medicinal product is composed of wholly or partly different substances, in quality or quantity, from those that generally constitute it.

The adulteration or counterfeiting of foods typically carries a term of three to ten years' imprisonment, increased if the activities in question involve medicinal substances.

To confirm the seriousness of the offence just described, moreover, Article 446 of the Italian Criminal Code provides that, in the event of conviction under Article 440, if the death or serious or very serious injury of a person results from the offence, the confiscation of the offence is mandatory.

Article 445 of the Italian Criminal Code regulates the hypothesis of *administering medicines in a manner dangerous to public health*. In this case, *anyone who, even illegally, trades in medicinal substances, administers them in a species, quality and/or quantity that does not correspond to the medical orders [...] shall be punished by imprisonment from six months to two years and a fine ranging from one hundred and three euros to one thousand and thirty-two euros.*

The application of this offence hypothesis requires, on closer inspection, that we are dealing with medicinal substances, understood as those which—if introduced into the body—have a diagnostic, prophylactic, therapeutic or anaesthetising effect (thus also including herbal and/or cosmetic products, provided they have curative or therapeutic properties), and that the administration deviates from the medical prescription, whether written or oral.

In addition, Legislative Decree 17/2014 (Presidente della Repubblica 2014) intervened by dwelling in more detail on the online trade and sale of pharmaceutical products.

This Decree transposes the Directive 2011/62/EU (The European Parliament and of the Council 2011). On the one hand, it allows the online sale and purchase of medicines for those not requiring a doctor's prescription, aligning the Italian market with other European countries; on the other hand, it introduces new criminal offences relating to the online sale of medicines subject to such prescription. It provides that *unless the act constitutes a more severe offence, the owners of pharmacies and commercial establishments [...] who offer for sale to the public at a distance, using information society services, medicinal products subject to medical prescription shall be punished by imprisonment of up to one year and a fine of between two thousand and ten thousand euro.* This liability is then also extended to anyone who manufactures, distributes, imports, exports, trades, and sells falsified medicinal products remotely to the public using information society services, as well as who brokers falsified medicines, shall be punished by imprisonment of one to three years and a fine of between 2.600 and 15.600 euros.

2.6 Opportunities and Risks in the Intellectual Property World

As far as the IP world is concerned, the protection of the medicine, as packaging and brand, can be traced back to three distinct legal cases: pure counterfeiting, the danger of confusion, and parasitic competition.

Pure counterfeiting occurs when the packaging of the medicine is counterfeited identically to the original due to the counterfeiting of the pharmaceutical product itself; the medicine is counterfeited because it does not entirely or adequately contain the ordinary active ingredient. This is the most dangerous type of counterfeiting for the health of the end consumer and, consequently, for the image of the company producing the original medicine. This type of counterfeiting usually occurs in cases where it is possible to reproduce—often abroad—an 'identical' medicine economically while selling it at a lower price.

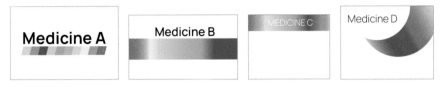

Fig. 2.5 Example of graphic signs used in different drugs with minimal variance

On the other hand, the danger of confusion and errors in administration is linked to the existence of so-called LASA medicines (an acronym for Look Alike/Sound Alike), used to indicate those medicines that can be mistaken for others due to their graphics and/or phonetic similarity of name.[23] Medicines with names spelled and pronounced similarly, and similar packaging in size and colour can be misleading at all stages of medicine management, whether in the hospital (procurement, storage and preservation, prescription, transcription and interpretation of the prescription, preparation/fitting, distribution, administration) or at home, for instance in General Practitioners' (GPs) and Family Paediatricians' (FOPs) surgeries, community pharmacies, nursing homes or at the patient's home.

Still different is the case that occurs when a person decides to adopt the shapes, colours, and dimensions of the pack of a well-known drug—almost always on the shelf—in bad faith, namely to mislead the consumer and sell their product in place of the competitor's well-known product, having the 'shrewdness' of slavishly copying the pack (often not registered as a design and model), but not the trade mark.

Concerning the latter, case law has been stringent in assessing the second type of offence, the requirement of confusability between products. On this point, the Italian Suprema Corte di Cassazione has long since intervened, emphasising that *not every slavish imitation of another's packaging is liable to be punished, but only that imitation which concretely poses a danger of diversion, to the imitator's advantage, of the imitated entrepreneur's customers.*[24]

Multivitamin supplements often have multicoloured bands (Fig. 2.5).

---

[23] The Lazio Regional Administrative Court (TAR) also intervened on this point (no. 9050 of 29/08/2018), arguing that: "AIFA may decide to change the name of a parallel imported medicine to avoid confusion with other already authorised medicinal specialities, applying the Guideline on the acceptability of names for human products (European Medicines Agency 2014)".

The EMEA Guideline of 11 December 2007 already recommended avoiding the use of names whose similarity could lead to safety problems in the use of products (https://www.ema.europa.eu/en/documents/annual-report/summary-european-medicines-agencys-annual-report-2007_it.pdf). EMA (2018); see also the Guideline on quality, non-clinical and clinical requirements for investigational advanced therapy medicinal products in clinical trials. Lastly, see Italian Ministero della Salute—Recommendation No. 12 of August 2010 (Ministero della Salute 2010). In other words, it must be a matter of potential risk of confusion by consumers with other medicinal products, or possible errors in therapy with Look-Alike/Sound-Alike medicines.

[24] Corte di Cassazione, no. 15761/2003 and, *ex multis*, subsequently Tribunale. Milano 18/06/2016 (RG 50940/12) and 11/04/2016 (RG 53702/12) and Tribunal of Turin 10/08/2021 (RG13800/19).

In such a complex context, where protection is elusive, and the possibility of confusion and imitation is very high, companies must develop proprietary packaging systems for all their products to distinguish themselves in the market strongly.[25]

References

Agenzia Italiana del Farmaco (AIFA) (2012) FDA approva primo sensore digitale commestibile. Retrieved from https://www.aifa.gov.it/-/fda-approva-primo-sensore-digitale-commestibile

Berardi L (2012) Messo a punto dal Mit un chip wireless per l'assunzione automatizzata di farmaci [MIT develops a wireless chip for automated medicine intake]. Quotidianosanità.it, published in 19 Feb 2012, retrieved from https://www.quotidianosanita.it/scienza-e-farmaci/articolo.php?articolo_id=7503

Commission Decision 129 (1997) Establishing the identification system for packaging materials pursuant to European Parliament and council directive 94/62/EC on packaging and packaging waste. Off J Eur Communities. 20.2.97, Retrieved from https://eur-lex.europa.eu/legal-content/EN/TXT/PDF/?uri=CELEX:31997D0129

EMA (2018) Guideline on quality, non-clinical and clinical requirements for investigational advanced therapy medicinal products in clinical trials—EMA/CAT/852602/2018

EMEA (2007) (11 dicembre 2007), Sintesi della XIII relazione annuale dell'EMEA, retrieved from https://www.ema.europa.eu/en/documents/annual-report/summary-european-medicines-agencys-annual-report-2007_it.pdf

European Medicines Agency (EMA) (2014) Guideline on the acceptability of names for human medicinal products processed through the centralised procedure – Scientific guideline 22 May 2014 EMA/CHMP/287710/2014—Rev. 6 Committee for Medicinal Products for Human Use (CHMP), Retrieved from https://www.ema.europa.eu/en/documents/regulatory-procedural-guideline/guideline-acceptability-names-human-medicinal-products-processed-through-centralised-procedure_en.pdf

The European Parliament and of the Council (1994) 94/62/EC of 20 December 1994 on packaging and packaging waste. Off J Eur Communities. 31.12.94, retrieved from https://eur-lex.europa.eu/legal-content/EN/TXT/PDF/?uri=CELEX:31994L0062

The European Parliament and of the Council (2001) Directive 2001/83/EC of 6 November 2001 on the Community code relating to medicinal products for human use. Off J Eur Communities. 28.11.2001, retrieved from https://eur-lex.europa.eu/legal-content/EN/TXT/PDF/?uri=CELEX:32001L0083

The European Parliament and of the Council (2003) Directive 2003/15/EC of 27 February 2003 amending Council Directive 76/768/EEC on the approximation of the laws of the Member States relating to cosmetic products. Off J Eur Union. 11.3.2003, retrieved from https://eur-lex.europa.eu/legal-content/EN/TXT/PDF/?uri=CELEX:32003L0015

The European Parliament and of the Council (2008) Directive 2008/98/EC of 19 November 2008 on waste and repealing certain Directives. Off J Eur Union. 22.11.2008. Retrieved from https://eur-lex.europa.eu/legal-content/EN/TXT/PDF/?uri=CELEX:32008L0098

The European Parliament and of the Council (2009) Regulation (EC) No 1223/2009 of 30 November 2009 on cosmetic products. Off J Eur Union. 22.12.2009. Retrieved from https://eur-lex.europa.eu/legal-content/EN/TXT/PDF/?uri=CELEX:32009R1223

The European Parliament and of the Council (2011) Directive 2011/62/EU of 8 June 2011 amending Directive 2001/83/EC on the Community code relating to medicinal products for human

---

[25] The author would like to thank Dr. Chiara Biffi of Studio Legale Sutti for her cooperation in the drafting and proofreading this contribution.

use, as regards the prevention of the entry into the legal supply chain of falsified medicinal products Text with EEA relevance. Off J Eur Union. 1.7.2011, Retrieved from https://eur-lex.europa.eu/legal-content/EN/TXT/PDF/?uri=CELEX:32011L0062

The European Parliament and of the Council (2016) Commission delegated regulation (EU) 2016/161 of 2 October 2015 supplementing Directive 2001/83/EC of the European Parliament and of the Council by laying down detailed rules for the safety features appearing on the packaging of medicinal products for human use. Off J Eur Union. 9.2.2016, Retrieved from https://eur-lex.europa.eu/legal-content/EN/TXT/PDF/?uri=CELEX:32016R0161

The European Parliament and of the Council (2018a) Directive (EU) 2018/851 OF 30 May 2018 amending Directive 2008/98/EC on waste – 14.6.2018. Off J Eur Union. 14.6.2018, retrieved from https://eur-lex.europa.eu/legal-content/EN/TXT/PDF/?uri=CELEX:32018L0851

The European Parliament and of the Council (2018b) Directive (EU) 2018/852 of 30 May 2018 amending Directive 94/62/EC on packaging and packaging waste. Off J Eur Union. 14.6.2018, retrieved from https://eur-lex.europa.eu/legal-content/EN/TXT/PDF/?uri=CELEX:32018L0852

Ministero della salute (2010) Raccomandazione Ministeriale. n. 12, retrieved 18 Oct, 2022 from https://www.salute.gov.it/imgs/C_17_pubblicazioni_1307_allegato.pdf

Ministero della Salute – Direzione Generale dei Dispositivi Medici e del Servizio Farmaceutico – Ufficio II (2017) Aggiornamento delle Linee guida per la pubblicità a mezzo Social network degli OTC, retrieved from: https://www.salute.gov.it/imgs/C_17_pubblicazioni_3344_allegato.pdf

Ministero della Salute, Ufficio Generale digitalizzazione sistema sanitario (2023) Linee guida per la Tracciabilità del Farmaco e la predisposizione e la trasmissione dei file alla banca dati centrale, retrieved from https://www.salute.gov.it/imgs/C_17_pubblicazioni_1066_allegato.pdf

Ministero della transizione ecologica (2022) Linee Guida sull'etichettatura degli imballaggi ai sensi dell'art. 219 comma 5 del D.Lgs. 152/2006 e ss.mm, del 27/7/2022, retrieved from https://www.mase.gov.it/sites/default/files/archivio/normativa/rifiuti/Linee_guida_etichettatura_ambientale_27.09.2022.pdf

Presidente della Repubblica (2003) Decreto del 15 luglio 2003, n. 254 – Regolamento recante disciplina della gestione dei rifiuti sanitari a norma dell'articolo 24 della legge 31 luglio 2002, n. 179. Gazzetta Ufficiale – Serie Generale n. 211 del 11.09.2003. Retrieved from https://www.gazzettaufficiale.it/eli/id/2003/09/11/003G0282/sg

Presidente della Repubblica (2006a) Decreto Legislativo 24 aprile 2006, n. 219 – Attuazione della direttiva 2001/83/CE (e successive direttive di modifica) relativa ad un codice comunitario concernente i medicinali per uso umano, entrata in vigore il 6-7-2006, Gazzetta Ufficiale n.142 del 21-06-2006 – Suppl. Ordinario n. 153, retrieved from https://www.gazzettaufficiale.it/eli/id/2006/06/21/006G0237/sg

Presidente della Repubblica (2006b) Decreto Legislativo 3 aprile 2006, n. 152 – Norme in materia ambientale. Gazzetta Ufficiale Serie Generale n.88 del 14-04-2006 – Suppl. Ordinario n. 96, retrieved from https://www.gazzettaufficiale.it/dettaglio/codici/materiaAmbientale

Presidente della Repubblica (2014) Decreto legislativo 19 febbraio 2014, n. 17 – Attuazione della direttiva 2011/62/UE, che modifica la direttiva 2001/83/CE, recante un codice comunitario relativo ai medicinali per uso umano, al fine di impedire l'ingresso di medicinali falsificati nella catena di fornitura legale. Gazzetta Ufficiale n. 55 del 07.03.2014, retrieved from https://www.normattiva.it/uri-res/N2Ls?urn:nir:stato:decreto.legislativo:2014;017

Presidente, della Repubblica (2020) Decreto legislativo 3 settembre 2020, n. 116 – Attuazione della direttiva (UE) 2018/851 che modifica la direttiva 2008/98/CE relativa ai rifiuti e attuazione della direttiva (UE) 2018/852 che modifica la direttiva 1994/62/CE sugli imballaggi e i rifiuti di imballaggio. Gazzetta Ufficiale Serie Generale n. 226 del 11-09-2020, retrieved from https://www.gazzettaufficiale.it/eli/id/2020/09/11/20G00135/sg

Open Access This chapter is licensed under the terms of the Creative Commons Attribution 4.0 International License (http://creativecommons.org/licenses/by/4.0/), which permits use, sharing, adaptation, distribution and reproduction in any medium or format, as long as you give appropriate credit to the original author(s) and the source, provide a link to the Creative Commons license and indicate if changes were made.

The images or other third party material in this chapter are included in the chapter's Creative Commons license, unless indicated otherwise in a credit line to the material. If material is not included in the chapter's Creative Commons license and your intended use is not permitted by statutory regulation or exceeds the permitted use, you will need to obtain permission directly from the copyright holder.

Chapter 3
Primary Medicine Packaging and Quality Control

Elena Piovosi

Abstract In the case of pharmaceuticals, packaging has moved from being the last step in the production chain to influencing the whole product design process, bounding a series of strict production standards. Why is the primary packaging of a medicine important? The primary packaging encounters the product, and its function is not only to be able to contain, protect or transport the medicine. Above all, packaging preserves the product, guaranteeing its quality throughout the self-life period. Furthermore, the choice also depends on the type of use and market demands. The typology of packaging and its material is of fundamental importance both for the pharmaceutical company that use it and for the patient. The chapter presents an abacus with the principal pharmaceutical form and packaging types.

3.1 Dosage Form

"A dosage form is a pharmaceutical preparation consisting of medicine substance(s) and/or excipient(s) to facilitate dosing, administration, and delivery of the content of the medicine product or placebo to the patient. The design, materials, manufacturing, and testing of all dosage forms target medicine product quality" (United States Pharmacopeia (2021b).

According to the principles of biopharmaceutics, the pharmaceutical form must ensure (Lai 2023, pp. 7–12):

- chemical and physical stability;
- adequate protection against contamination;
- uniformity of dosage;
- acceptability for the patient;
- appropriate packaging and labelling.

It ensures the physical appearance of a medicinal product so that the chosen route can administer it.

E. Piovosi (✉)
Scandolara S.p.A, Ascoli Piceno, Italy

© The Author(s) 2025
A. V. Penati (ed.), *In-Home Medication*, Research for Development,
https://doi.org/10.1007/978-3-031-53294-8_3

The pharmaceutical form can be classified according to the following:

- physical state: solid, semi-solid, liquid;
- route of administration;
- dosage modality: single dose or multidose;
- medicine release mode: instantaneous or modified.

3.2 Classification by Route of Administration

Among the several classifications in literature, delving into indispensable aspects for the correct knowledge and management of pharmaceutical forms, here we choose to deepen the one referring to the route of administration. We believe this is the description closest to the end user's experience. Since the topic is the result of consolidated manuals to which all pharmaceutical companies refer, we will include extensive excerpts from scientific references describing the various pharmaceutical forms. All the following pharmaceutical forms and their description follow the guidance provided by the Council of Europe (Council of Europe 2019b).

3.2.1 Oral Pharmaceutical Forms

Capsules: […] Capsules are solid preparations with hard or soft shells of various shapes and capacities, containing a single dose of active substance(s). […] The capsule shells are made of gelatin or other substances, the consistency of which may be adjusted by the addition of substances such as glycerol or sorbitol. […] (p. 906);

Tablets: Tablets are solid preparations each containing a single dose of one or more active substances. They are obtained by compressing uniform volumes of particles or by another suitable manufacturing technique, such as extrusion, moulding or freeze-drying (lyophilization). […] (p. 937);

Granules: Granules are preparations consisting of solid, dry aggregates of powder particles sufficiently robust to withstand handling. […] (p. 912);

Chewing gums, medicated: Medicated chewing gums are solid, single-dose preparations with a base consisting mainly of gum that are intended to be chewed but not swallowed. […] (p. 907);

Powders, oral: Oral powders are preparations consisting of solid, loose, dry particles of varying degrees of fineness […] (P. 926);

Liquid preparations for oral use: Liquid preparations for oral use are usually solutions, emulsions or suspensions containing one or more active substances in a suitable vehicle; they may, however, consist of liquid active substances used as such (oral liquids). […] (p. 916).

3.2.2 Topical Pharmaceutical Forms

Semi-Solid preparations for cutaneous application: Semi-solid preparations for cutaneous application are intended for local or transdermal delivery of active substances, or for their emollient or protective action. They are of homogeneous appearance. […] (p. 935);

Powders for cutaneous application: Powders for cutaneous application are preparations consisting of solid, loose, dry particles of varying degrees of fineness. […] (p. 925);

Liquid preparations for cutaneous application: Liquid preparations for cutaneous application are preparations of a variety of viscosities intended for local or transdermal delivery of active ingredients. They are solutions, emulsions or suspensions that may contain 1 or more active substances in a suitable vehicle. […] (p. 916);

Medicated foams: Medicated foams are preparations consisting of large volumes of gas dispersed in a liquid generally containing one or more active substances, a surfactant ensuring their formation and various other excipients. […] (p. 911);

Medicated plasters: Medicated plasters are flexible preparations containing 1 or more active substances. They are intended to be applied to the skin. They are designed to maintain the active substance(s) in close contact with the skin such that these may be absorbed slowly, or act as protective or keratolytic agents. […] (p. 936);

Patches, transdermal: Transdermal patches are flexible pharmaceutical preparations of varying sizes, containing one or more active substances. They are intended to be applied to the unbroken skin to deliver the active substance(s) to the systemic circulation after passing through the skin barrier. […] (p. 925).

3.2.3 Parenteral Pharmaceutical Forms

Parenteral preparations: Parenteral preparations are sterile preparations intended for administration by injection, infusion or implantation into the human or animal body […]. (p. 923).

3.2.4 Rectal and Vaginal Pharmaceutical Forms

Preparations for irrigation: Preparations for irrigation are sterile, aqueous, large-volume preparations intended to be used for irrigation of body cavities, wounds, and surfaces, for example during surgical procedures. […] (p. 932);

Vaginal preparations: Vaginal preparations are liquid, semi-solid or solid preparations intended for administration to the vagina usually to obtain a local effect. […] (p. 940);

Rectal preparations: Rectal preparations are intended for rectal use to obtain a systemic or local effect, or they may be intended for diagnostic purposes. […] (p. 933).

3.2.5 Oto-Rhinological Pharmaceutical Forms

Preparations for inhalation: Preparations for inhalation are liquid, semi-solid or solid preparations intended for administration as vapours or aerosols to the lung to obtain a local or systemic effect. […] (p. 927);

Pressurised Pharmaceutical preparations: Pressurised pharmaceutical preparations are usually multidose preparations presented in special containers under pressure of a gas and often fitted with a metering valve and contain one or more active substances. […] (p. 933);

Nasal preparations: Nasal preparations are liquid, semi-solid or solid preparations intended for administration to the nasal cavities to obtain a systemic or local effect. […] (p. 918);

Oromucosal preparations: Oromucosal preparations are solid, semi-solid or liquid preparations, containing one or more active substances intended for administration to the oral cavity and/or the throat to obtain a local or systemic effect […] (p. 920);

Ear preparations: Ear preparations are liquid, semi-solid or solid preparations intended for instillation, for spraying, for insufflation, for application to the auditory meatus or as an ear wash. […] (p. 908).

3.2.6 Ophthalmic Pharmaceutical Forms

Eye preparations: Eye preparations are sterile liquid, semi-solid or solid preparations intended for administration upon the eyeball and/or to the conjunctiva, or for insertion in the conjunctival sac. […] (p. 909).

3.3 The Functions of Primary Pharmaceutical Packaging: Containing, Preserving, and Protecting

The selection of primary packaging is closely related to the pharmaceutical form and the route of administration. For example, an injectable liquid uses the ampoule or a glass vial; a tablet – solid oral form – mainly uses the blister; a cream – semi-solid form – uses the aluminium or plastic tube. Packaging a pharmaceutical product is defined as the set of operations by which the pharmaceutical form is placed in

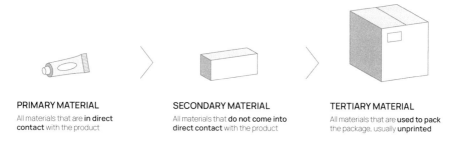

Fig. 3.1 Packaging components

a suitable container (primary packaging) to make it easily identifiable and transportable.

At the same time, proper packaging creates the best conditions for the storage and distribution of the medicine, protecting it from light, dust and, if necessary, moisture (Fig. 3.1). Thus, the packaging system ensures that the pharmaceutical forms have the same qualitative and quantitative characteristics from their preparation to their administration time.

The packaging components are essential to the medicinal product and must be included in the quality assurance system.

3.3.1 Principal Functions of Primary Packaging

Since the packaging comes into direct contact with the medicine, several functions of the primary packaging are essential. These include in particular:

- Containment and protection: the primary packaging must contain the medicine, and must necessarily remain undamaged during transport until the consumer opens it;
- Suitability to the medicine: the primary packaging must safeguard the integrity of the medicine and prevent the possibility of contamination by external agents;
- Non-alteration of the medicine: the primary packaging must ensure the absence of negative interactions and not release foreign substances into the medicine;
- Resistance to external environmental conditions: the primary packaging must ensure the preservation of the product in a given environment, taking into account temperature, humidity, light sources, etc.;
- Ease of use and accessibility of the product: the primary packaging should have suitable characteristics to suit the needs of the consumer;
- Preventing improper use of the product: the primary packaging must prevent the use of the medicine by children, tampering with the product, etc.;
- Ease of transport: primary packaging must facilitate the flow of products in logistical and storage operations;

- Identification and communication: together with the secondary packaging, the primary packaging must allow the medicine to be recognisable as such, avoiding possible misunderstandings with other product categories, and correctly communicate the nature of the contents and the method of administration;
- Sustainability: primary packaging must use eco-friendly materials.

The market daily produces new and different solutions to offer long-term guarantees on the quality of the medicine and make its consumption 'possible' at any time. As simple and partial examples, here are listed:

- strong containers, easy to transport, light, safe, space-saving;
- closures that make it possible to reuse a product that has not been completely consumed;
- dispensing systems that facilitate consumption and simplify product use.

When developing packaging, it is always necessary to balance desired performance and product cost, which impacts the choice of materials and packaging times.

3.3.2 The Choice of Primary Packaging Material According to the Product Contained: Protection and Permeability of the Material to Chemical and Physical Agents

As mentioned above, the type of primary packaging is closely linked to the pharmaceutical form (liquid, solid, semi-solid, spray, pill, powder etc.) and to the characteristics of the substances in the medicine itself, described as follows:

- Solid pharmaceutical forms – medicines for oral use – such as granules, powders, tablets, and capsules are usually packaged in glass or plastic bottles or blisters.
- Semi-solid pharmaceutical forms, such as creams and gels, are usually packaged in aluminium or plastic tubes.
- Liquid pharmaceutical forms, which include medicines for oral use, injectables and medicines that cannot be taken orally, such as lotions, are usually packaged in glass or plastic bottles or ampoules.

When choosing the packaging material, it is essential to consider the product's properties and the protective function of the material against chemical and physical agents such as moisture and light. Medicinal preparations may deteriorate due to chemical incompatibility between formulation components and packaging materials or to moisture, humidity and oxygen, oxygen and light, and temperature variations. Permeability is one of the characteristics of pharmaceutical primary packaging that must be considered when selecting materials. Permeability is the "property of certain bodies to allow liquids or gases to pass through or penetrate them". In chemistry, a semi-permeable membrane is "a membrane between a solution and a pure solvent that can only be permeated by the solvent and not by the solute" (Enciclopedia

Treccani Online 2023c). The gas or vapour moves from an area of high concentration to a place of low concentration to establish an equilibrium. Many types of packaging are made using materials that are semi-permeable to gases. The most common are paper/cardboard; plastic packagings such as High-Density Polyethylene (HDPE), Polyethylene Terephthalate (PET), Low-Density Polyethylene (LDP), Linear Low-Density Polyethylene (LLDPE). Since these materials are semi-permeable, it is necessary to measure their permeability to determine how long the packaging will maintain complete product protection. Glass and aluminium are the only materials used in pharmaceutical packaging that are utterly impermeable to vapour and moisture at room temperature.

Some medicines are sensitive to oxygen and light. These two factors are usually considered together since light often catalyses reactions involving oxygen. The protection from light can be achieved with opaque containers such as coloured plastic or amber glass. For example, glass bottles are available in different colours, the most common being orange or light brown, due to their ability to prevent the degradation of potentially photosensitive contents by ultraviolet light while still allowing sufficient light to pass through for the contents to be easily visible.

Other aspects influence the choice of packaging type, and these are:

- commercial aspects: product image; market trends; product safety (child-proof, tamper-evident); ageing population;
- economic aspects: production costs; logistics costs;
- company policies.

3.3.3 Contamination of the Medicine by Packaging Materials

Raw materials used for primary packaging could contaminate medicinal products due to the interaction between medicinal products and containers. The United States Pharmacopoeia (USP) defines the risk and assessment related to such interactions in chapter: 1663 – Assessment of extractables associated with pharmaceutical packaging/Delivery (2021d, pp. 1–14). This chapter discusses extractables, leachebles, and migrants.

Extractables are organic and inorganic chemical entities that can be released from a pharmaceutical packaging/delivery system, packaging component, or packaging material of construction and into an extraction solvent under laboratory conditions. Depending on the specific purpose of the extraction study (discussed below), these laboratory conditions (e.g., solvent, temperature, stoichiometry, etc.) may accelerate or exaggerate the normal conditions of storage and use for a packaged dosage form. Extractables themselves, or substances derived from extractables, have the potential to leach into a medicine product under normal conditions of storage and use and become leachables […] (pp. 1–14).

Leachables are foreign organic and inorganic chemical entities that are present in a packaged medicine product because they have leached into the packaged medicine product from a packaging/delivery system, packaging component, or packaging material of construction under normal conditions of storage and use or during accelerated medicine product stability studies. Because leachables are derived from the packaging or delivery system, they are not related to either the medicine product itself or its vehicle and ingredients. Leachables are present in a packaged medicine product because of the direct action of the medicine product on the source of the leachable. Thus, leachables are typically derived from primary and secondary packaging, because the primary and secondary packaging can serve as a barrier between the packaged medicine product and other potential sources of foreign chemical entities (e.g., tertiary packaging and ancillary components). In certain circumstances, packaging may directly contact the patient under typical clinical conditions of use (e.g., the mouthpiece of a metered dose inhaler). As a result of this contact, patients may be exposed to leachables from the packaging without the action of the medicine product. Leachables are typically a subset of extractables or are derived from extractables […] (pp. 1–14).

Migrants are also foreign organic and inorganic chemical entities that are present in a packaged medicine product because they have leached into the packaged medicine product from a packaging/delivery system, packaging component, or packaging material of construction under normal conditions of storage and use or during accelerated medicine product stability studies. However, migrants are differentiated from leachables by the circumstance that migrants accumulate in the packaged medicine product after the migrant has crossed a physical barrier, such as that provided by primary and secondary packaging. Because migrants cross a physical barrier, they are not present in the packaged medicine product due to direct action of the medicine product on the source of the migrant because the barrier prevents such direct action. Thus, migrants are derived from secondary and tertiary packaging and ancillary components. Regardless of whether a substance is a leachable or migrant, it is still a foreign substance in the packaged medicine product, and thus its impact must be assessed in the same manner. However, as how a leachable and a migrant become entrained in a packaged medicine product may be different, extractables studies meant to address leachables may be designed and implemented differently than extractables studies meant to address migrants […] (pp. 2–14). Examples of product-packaging interaction include:

- Loss of activity due to absorption or adsorption of the medicine's active ingredient or degradation of the active ingredient induced by a chemical entity diffused by a packaging component. By *absorption*, we intend the process by which a pure gas, brought into contact with a liquid under assigned temperature and pressure conditions, tends to partially dissolve until the conditions of thermodynamic equilibrium are reached (Enciclopedia Treccani Online 2023a). By *adsorption*, we mean the phenomenon whereby the surface of a solid substance, called an adsorbent, fixes molecules from a gaseous or liquid phase with which it is in contact (Enciclopedia Treccani Online 2023b);
- Reduction in the concentration of an excipient due to absorption, adsorption or degradation induced by a packaging component;

- Precipitation. By *precipitation*, we mean the separation from a solution of a substance in the form of an insoluble solid, already dissolved in it or formed as a result of a chemical reaction [...] (Enciclopedia Treccani Online);
- Changes in the pH of the pharmaceutical product;
- Changes in the colour or odour of the product or a component of the packaging;
- Increased fragility of the packaging.

Interactions between the packaging material and the product are evaluated with specific studies at the pre-registration stage or in case of container and/or formulation changes. For example, a plastic container chosen for a particular preparation should ensure that:

- When in contact with the plastic material, the components of the preparation are not appreciably adsorbed on its surface and do not migrate into or through the plastic in any significant way;
- The plastic material does not release substances in a quantity that could influence the stability of the preparation or give rise to a risk of toxicity.

In the last few years, regulatory requirements relating to assessing extractables and leachables from packaging or process or finished product components have grown considerably in the Pharma sector. Substances may migrate from different materials (e.g., polymers, glues, adhesives, and inks, coated and uncoated metal materials, glass, closures, etc.), and patients may therefore be exposed to contaminants through different routes of administration.

As a purely illustrative example, we report an extended extract, among many in the literature, of a study on the damage caused by organic compounds leached from the uncoated rubber caps of pre-filled syringes when taking a medicine administered to patients with chronic kidney disease (Boven et al. 2005, p. 2346).

Background The incidence of pure red cell aplasia (PRCA) in chronic kidney disease patients treated with epoetins increased substantially in 1998, was shown to be antibody mediated, and was associated predominantly with subcutaneous administration of Eprex. A technical investigation identified organic compounds leached from uncoated rubber stoppers in prefilled syringes containing polysorbate 80 as the most probable cause of the increased immunogenicity.

Methods This study investigated whether the incidence of PRCA was higher for exposure to the product form containing leachates than for leachate-free product forms. Antibody-mediated PRCA cases were classified according to indication, product form, and route of administration. Exposure estimates were obtained by country, indication, route of administration, and product form.

Results For 2001 to 2003, the PRCA incidence rate for patients with subcutaneous exposure to Eprex in prefilled syringes with polysorbate 80 and uncoated rubber stoppers (leachates present) was 4.61/10,000 patient years (95% CI 3.88–5.43) versus 0.26/10,000 patient years (95% CI 0.007–1.44) for syringes with coated stoppers (leachates absent). The rate difference was 4.35/10,000 patient years (95% CI

3.44–5.26; P < 0.0001); the rate ratio was 17 (95% CI 3.14–707). A substantial rate difference remained in sensitivity analyses that adjusted for exposure to multiple product forms.

Conclusion The epidemiologic data, together with the chemical and immunologic data, support the hypothesis that leachates from uncoated rubber syringe stoppers caused the increased incidence of PRCA associated with Eprex. Currently, all Eprex prefilled syringes contain fluoro-resin coated stoppers, which has contributed to decreased incidence of PRCA with continued surveillance.

Risk assessment and the consequent toxicological evaluation are factors of absolute importance, necessary to ensure the safety of pharmaceutical products.

3.3.4 Regulatory Compliance. Quality Control on the Production Process and the Final Product: Defects, Contamination, Criticality, and Non-conformity

Primary packaging for pharmaceutical products is heavily regulated during the medicine's testing, registration, and production use.

The registration dossier for medicine must describe the packaging and its materials, as stated by the European Commission (2008):

- 3.2.P.2.4 Container Closure System (name, dosage form) The suitability of the container closure system (described in 3.2.P.7) used for the storage, transportation (shipping) and use of the medicine product should be discussed. This discussion should consider, e.g., choice of materials, protection from moisture and light, compatibility of the materials of construction with the dosage form (including sorption to container and leaching) safety of materials of construction, and performance (such as reproducibility of the dose delivery from the device when presented as part of the medicine product) (p. 17)
- 3.2.P.7 Container Closure System (name, dosage form) A description of the container closure systems should be provided, including the identity of materials of construction of each primary packaging component and its specification. The specifications should include description and identification (and critical dimensions, with drawings where appropriate). Non-compendial methods (with validation) should be included where appropriate. […] (European Commission 2008, p. 21).

Pharmaceutical legislation guarantees the quality and safety of medicines through strict regulations and controls on all stages of production and all materials used. These regulations and controls concern the active substances and the production processes that transform them into a medicine to be placed on the market and the materials used for its packaging.

The quality of pharmaceutical packaging is of paramount importance, not only because of its role in the marketing of the product: primary packaging made from quality materials and according to applicable standards ensures the integrity and durability of the medicinal product.

The pharmaceutical packaging regulation (European Commission 2015b) stipulates that the packaging of medicinal products must meet precise requirements. The quality of the pharmaceutical product cannot only be achieved with controls during and after production. Still, it must be achieved with particular attention to the quality of the packaging materials. It does not matter how much care is taken in preparing a medicine, if inferior or wrong-quality primary packaging components are used. Pharmaceutical production must meet high standards to ensure the purity and quality of its end products. Consumers can receive safe and effective products by adopting and using international standards.

The pharmaceutical industry faces expectations set by both the US Food and Medicine Agency (FDA) and Good Manufacturing Practice (GMP) standards (European Commission 2015b). GMP standards ensure that a medicine is produced, analysed, and released to the market under a quality-controlled and certified regime. Only this allows pharma industries to minimise the danger of unforeseen risks to patient health.

In addition to GMP, packaging and its materials are described and regulated by the Council of Europe, European Pharmacopoeia (2019a) and the United States Pharmacopeia, USP-NF (2021a). ISO Standards also guide the pharmaceutical industry on primary packaging materials with UNI EN ISO 15378 (2011). ISO 15378 stands for primary packaging companies - non-pharmaceutical industries - as they do not necessarily have to apply GMP and ISO 9001 (2008), lacking standards.

In addition to these general standards, there are also specific guidelines for each type of material used (e.g., glass, plastic, etc.).

3.3.5 *Quality Control of Primary Material during the Manufacturing Process of a Medicine*

Volume 4, Chapter 5 of the European Commission, the GMP deals with medicine production (European Commission 2015a). In point 5.45, the GMP states:

> *the selection, qualification, approval, and maintenance of suppliers of primary and printed packaging materials shall be accorded attention similar to that given to starting materials (pag. 9).*

It means that all suppliers of packaging materials must be qualified suppliers, meaning they must have passed a qualification process. The qualification process consists of the pharmaceutical company and the supplier sharing specifications that have been recorded, test batches of the packaging material and an audit of the supplier. Through audits, it is verified that a company complies with the required quality standards and that an effective corrective action plan is established in case of non-compliance. The pharmaceutical company always qualifies at least two suppliers for the same type of primary material to have a backup capable of supplying the material. Depending on the packaging material, the company buys from tube factories, glassworks, plastic material suppliers, etc.

The pharmaceutical company then purchases packaging material from qualified suppliers, who have carried out checks during their production and can certify the quality of the batch. When the batch enters the pharmaceutical company, and before it is used in production, the quality control department performs a statistical sampling of the materials (ISO 2859, 1999) on which it then performs further tests, including:

- Checking the text and graphics of the packaging against the registered text, necessary for the patient;
- Checking the materials used by the supplier against those registered, and those used during pre-marketing trials;
- Checking the measurements on the packaging design drawings, important for the machinability of the material;
- Making pharmacopoeia tests, for glass bottles and for releasing acids or bases.

Text and graphics are checked using software which overlaps the text and graphics registered at the Ministry of Health with those printed on the packaging material delivered by the supplier, highlighting any inconsistencies. This check is of fundamental importance for the safety of the patients, who will have the correct information about the medicine at their disposal. If all tests are positive, the material can be used in production.

The Rules Governing Medicinal Products in the European Union, (2015b, Annex 8, pp. 105-106) lists:

- Principle: Sampling is an important operation in which only a small fraction of a batch is taken. Valid conclusions overall cannot be based on tests which have been carried out on non-representative samples. Correct sampling is thus an essential part of a system of Quality Assurance. (p.105)
- Packaging material: the sampling plan for packaging materials should take account of at least the following: the quantity received, the quality required, the nature of the material (e.g., primary packaging materials and/or printed packaging materials), the production methods, and what is known of the Quality Assurance system of the packaging materials manufacturer based on audits. The number of samples taken should be determined statistically and specified in a sampling plan (pag. 106).

In addition, Chapter 5 of the GMP – Production, describes the behaviour to be adopted when using the materials in production (European Commission 2015a):

- 5.46 Particular attention should be paid to printed materials. They should be stored in adequately secure conditions such as to exclude unauthorised access. Cut labels and other loose printed materials should be stored and transported in separate closed containers so as to avoid mix-ups. Packaging materials should be

issued for use only by authorised personnel following an approved and documented procedure (p. 9);
- 5.47 Each delivery or batch of printed or primary packaging material should be given a specific reference number or identification mark (p. 10);
- 5.48 Outdated or obsolete primary packaging material or printed packaging material should be destroyed and this disposal record (p. 10).

During production, other tests verify the correctness of used materials (to avoid product mix-ups) and the compliance of variable data (e.g., batch number and expiry date).

3.3.6 Defects and Non-conformity of Packaging Material

Defects in packaging materials can be classified into:

- Critical Defects, meaning those that may threaten the life and health of people, violate legal regulations, lead to the damage or alteration of filling material, may seriously affect the reliability of storage, or may impair the efficiency of production, filling or packaging equipment;
- Major Defects, meaning those that may lead to inefficient operation and thus to packaging failures, result in user complaints, cause a reduction in production performance, or impair the efficiency of production tools as well as filling and packaging equipment;
- Minor Defects, meaning those that are minor, do not lead to severe consequences but merely to a general reduction in quality (AKP et al. 2017).

The Pharma industry evaluates all the received claims and, depending on the defect, considers them to improve the use of primary packaging.

In the author experience, the different countries where primary packaging materials are marketed have a very different attitude to reporting non-conformities.

The country with the highest number of reports is Japan, which is particularly attentive to patient needs and to the formal aspects of materials. For example, for the tube presented in Fig. 3.2, it was requested that the corners of the closure fin be bevelled to avoid possible injury by the patient during use.

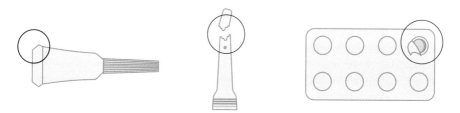

Fig. 3.2 Examples of defects: from left to right, a tube with sharp-edged closure fin; a broken rectal cannulae; some blisters broken before use

Another country with a high number of complaints is Brazil. In this case, more than a sensitivity to the perfection of the packaging, the country's precarious economic situation plays a role. The current brazilian health regulations provide for the reimbursement of the medicine if it is defective. It may happen that the patient uses almost all the medicine and then complains and receives a new pack free of charge.

Mediterranean countries such as Italy, Spain, and Greece hardly resort to complaints. Figures 3.3, 3.4, 3.5 and 3.6 present some examples of packaging material defects collected by the author. In terms of complaints, the USA and Northern European countries are very active, due to the high cost of medicines.

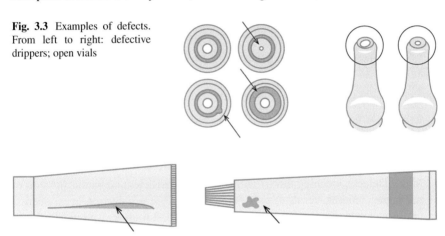

Fig. 3.3 Examples of defects. From left to right: defective drippers; open vials

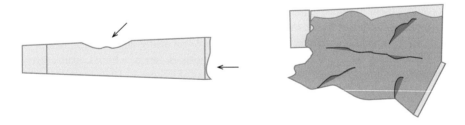

Fig. 3.4 Examples of defects. From left to right: unsealed cream tubes; production-stained cream caps and tubes

Fig. 3.5 Examples of defects. From left to right: production-cut or dented cream tubes

To conclude and to testify how important primary packaging is for protecting and guaranteeing the quality of the pharmaceutical product as well as for providing correct and comprehensible information, we cite an extended summary of one of the many literature texts that point out the potential problems the patient may face if the information on the packaging is not legible (Pazzagli et al. 2009).

Several factors can contribute to medication errors, and packaging may be one cause. For example, a medication can be mistakenly administered either because the

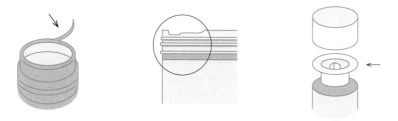

Fig. 3.6 Examples of defects. From left to right: cream tubes with aluminium flake on the spout; jar with broken opening; defective cap that break during use and expose the company to claims

medicine container (e.g., intravenous bag, prefilled syringe, etc.) is similar in appearance to the intended medication's container or because the packages had similar labelling. The Authors describe […] case reports that show how an unclear packaging can be responsible for inappropriate use, and subsequent patient's injuries. Hospital pharmacy staff, prescribing physicians, other healthcare workers, and even patients can play a role in minimizing the occurrence of these types of errors. However also medicine manufacturers have an important role and should provide clear and unique labels and packages for their products, as underlined by pharmaceutical packaging legislation and regulations.

Special food: product and text barely visible. This case concerns a patient undergoing enteral nutrition. The bag containing the liquid for enteral nutrition had been attached to the feeding tube, and the pump had been started. As it had solidified, the food could not flow out, leading to an error in the pump and an acoustic signal that alerted the relatives. In the meantime, a small amount of liquid and air passed through the probe, had caused the patient to become slightly ill. The proper functioning of the enteral nutrition pump made it possible to understand and solve the problem. But why had the nursing staff not noticed the enteral nutrition fluid clotted? The cause lay in the packaging of the product. The product in question, which is intended for gavage feeding (enteral nutrition), is packaged in 500-millilitre bags (primary packaging) that bear indications on the bag number/batch of production, manufacturer, expiry date and composition, clinical indications, method of use, special warnings, and storage. The latter are given in 11 languages for obvious distribution needs in several European countries. Hence, the print almost completely covers the surface area available: one side covered by the lettering, the other with a narrow transparent central column to control the volume of product remaining during infusion. The colour used for the background (perhaps for aesthetic reasons, as the food is hazelnut in colour) would be desirable to make the text more prominent instead of obstructing the product's view. The font size is small, and the distribution of the text compressed to fit the bag's surface. As a result, the essential information that the caregiver or family member/home caregiver should immediately see is difficult to find amidst so many graphics in different languages, which are difficult to read due to the distribution of the text.

In the case described, therefore, the failure to visually display the product contained in the bag and the Special Warnings (e.g., *Do not use if the bag is swollen or if the contents are coagulated*) would have resulted in incorrect administration, which was fortunately blocked by the pump signal [...] (pag.132).

References

AKP – Arbeitskreis Pack Mittel, Gössl R, Horst S (2017) Quality assurance of pharmaceutical packaging materials. In: Principles for the defect evaluation list for packaging materials, vol 12, 5th edn. Editio Cantor, Verlag

Boven K, Stryker S, Knight J, Thomas A, van Regenmortel M, Kemeny DM, Power D, Rossert J, Casadevall N (2005) The increased incidence of pure red cell aplasia with an Eprex formulation in uncoated rubber stopper syringes. National Library of Medicine 67(6):2346–2353. https://doi.org/10.1111/j.1523-1755.2005.00340.x

Council of Europe (2019a) Materials for containers and containers. vol. 1, cap. 3. In: European pharmacopoeia, ed. 10.0. Council of Europe, Strasburgo, pp 419–478. Retrieved from EP 10 (EUROPEAN PHARMACOPOEIA 10th EDITION) pdf free download (webofpharma.com)

Council of Europe (2019b) General texts, monographs on dosage forms, vol. 1, cap. 05. In: European pharmacopoeia, ed. 10.0. Council of Europe, Strasburgo, pp 903–943. Retrieved from EP 10 (EUROPEAN PHARMACOPOEIA 10th EDITION) pdf free download (webofpharma.com)

Enciclopedia Treccani Online (2023a). Absorption - Assorbimento. Retrieved from https://www.treccani.it/enciclopedia/assorbimento

Enciclopedia Treccani Online (2023b). Adsorption - Adsorbimento. Retrieved from https://www.treccani.it/enciclopedia/adsorbimento

Enciclopedia Treccani Online (2023c). Permeability - Permeabilità. Retrieved from: https://www.treccani.it/enciclopedia/permeabilità

European Commission (2008) Presentation and content of the dossier. Notice to applicants medicinal products for human use. Presentation and format of the dossier. Common technical document (CTD). In: Pharmaceutical legislation on notice to applicants and regulatory guidelines for medicinal products for human use, vol. 2B, EudraLex, pp 17–21

European Commission (2015a) Production. In: Good manufacturing practice (GMP), vol 4, cap.5, EudraLex, pp 1–12

European Commission (2015b) The rules governing medicinal products in the European Union. In: Good manufacturing practice (GMP), vol. 4, Annex. 8, EudraLex, pp 105–106

ISO (1999). 2859-1 Sampling procedures for inspection by attributes - Part 1: Sampling schemes indexed by acceptance quality limit (AQL) for lot-by-lot inspection. Retrieved from https://www.iso.org/obp/ui/#iso:std:iso:2859:-1:ed-2:v1:en

ISO (2015) ISO 9001:2015 quality management systems. Requirements. International Organization for Standardization, Geneva

Lai, F. (2023). Progettazione e sviluppo dei medicinali. Principi di biofarmaceutica, Tecnologia, Legislazione Farmaceutica, Modulo di Tecnologia Farmaceutica, Università degli Studi di Cagliari, 1–59, accessed April 2023, retrieved from www.unica.it/static/resources/cms/documents/Lezione2Biodisponibilita1.pdf

Pazzagli L, Ranzani F, Albini E (2009) From packaging to error: exemplary case reports and normative aspects. Pratica Medica & Aspetti Legali 3(3):131–137

UNI EN ISO 15378. (2011). Primary packaging materials for medicinal products. Particular requirements for application of ISO 9001, with reference to Good Manufacturing Practice (GMP). Retrieved from: https://www.iso.org/obp/ui/#iso:std:iso:15378:ed-2:v1:en

United States Pharmacopeia. USP-NF. (2021a). General Chapter, <671> Containers- performance testing, United States Pharmacopeia, Rockville, MD U.S.A.: 1–9, Retrieved from: United States Pharmacopeia 44 - NF 39. webofpharma.com

United States Pharmacopeia. USP-NF. (2021b). General Chapter, <1151> Pharmaceutical dosage forms. United States Pharmacopeia, Rockville, MD U.S.A.: 1–23, Retrieved from: United States Pharmacopeia 44 - NF 39. webofpharma.com

Open Access This chapter is licensed under the terms of the Creative Commons Attribution 4.0 International License (http://creativecommons.org/licenses/by/4.0/), which permits use, sharing, adaptation, distribution and reproduction in any medium or format, as long as you give appropriate credit to the original author(s) and the source, provide a link to the Creative Commons license and indicate if changes were made.

The images or other third party material in this chapter are included in the chapter's Creative Commons license, unless indicated otherwise in a credit line to the material. If material is not included in the chapter's Creative Commons license and your intended use is not permitted by statutory regulation or exceeds the permitted use, you will need to obtain permission directly from the copyright holder.

Chapter 4
Pharmaceutical Forms and Primary Packaging: A Glossary

Elena Piovosi

Abstract Shaped as a glossary, the chapter presents and graphically illustrates the main pharmaceutical forms and the different typologies of primary packaging in direct contact with the medicine, guaranteeing its quality throughout its self-life period.

4.1 Dosage Form

The pharmaceutical form refers to the dosage form in which each type of medicine is presented to be ready for use. The pharmaceutical form is obtained because of a pharmaceutical operation, which combines one or more active ingredient molecules, usually combined, with inactive ingredients (excipients).

It ensures the physical presentation of a medicine and makes the medicine administered by the chosen route (Lai 2021).

The pharmaceutical form can be classified according to:

- physical state: solid, liquid, semi-solid;
- dosage: single dose or multidose;
- mode of release: immediate or modified;
- route of administration.

All the pharmaceutical forms and their description presented in the following paragraphs, follow the guidance provided by the Council of Europe (Council of Europe 2019b).

E. Piovosi (✉)
Scandolara S.p.A, Ascoli Piceno, Italy

4.2 Classification by Route of Administration

Depending on the way of administration, medicines can be categorised according to these main typologies:

- Granules: granules are preparations consisting of solid, dry aggregates of powder particles sufficiently robust to withstand handling […] (p. 912);
- Capsulae: the capsule shells are made of gelatin or other substances, the consistency of which may be adjusted by the addition of substances such as glycerol or sorbitol […] (p. 906);
- Tablets: tablets are solid preparations each containing a single dose of one or more active substances […] (p. 937);
- Chewing gums, medicated: medicated chewing gums are solid, single-dose preparations with a base consisting mainly of gum that are intended to be chewed but not swallowed […] (p. 907);
- Powders, oral: oral powders are preparations consisting of solid, loose, dry particles of varying degrees of fineness […] (p. 926)
- Liquid preparations for oral use: liquid preparations for oral use are usually solutions, emulsions or suspensions containing one or more active substances in a suitable vehicle; they may, however, consist of liquid active substances used as such (oral liquids) […] (p. 916);
- Semi-Solid preparations for cutaneous application: semi-solid preparations for cutaneous application are intended for local or transdermal delivery of active substances, or for their emollient or protective action. They are of homogeneous appearance […] (p. 935);
- Powders for cutaneous application: powders for cutaneous application are preparations consisting of solid, loose, dry particles of varying degrees of fineness […] (p. 925);
- Medicated plasters: medicated plasters are flexible preparations containing 1 or more active substances. They are intended to be applied to the skin. They are designed to maintain the active substance(s) in close contact with the skin such that these may be absorbed slowly […] (p. 936);
- Patches, transdermal: transdermal patches are flexible pharmaceutical preparations of varying sizes, containing one or more active substances. They are intended to be applied to the unbroken skin to deliver the active substance(s) to the systemic circulation after passing through the skin barrier. […] (p. 925);
- Liquid preparations: liquid preparations for cutaneous application are preparations of a variety of viscosities intended for local or transdermal delivery of active ingredients […] (p. 916);
- Medicated foams: medicated foams are preparations consisting of large volumes of gas dispersed in a liquid generally containing one or more active substances, a surfactant ensuring their formation and various other excipients. Medicated foams are usually intended for application to the skin or mucous membranes […] (p. 911);
- Parenteral preparations: parenteral preparations are sterile preparations intended for administration by injection, infusion or implantation into the human or animal body […] (p. 923);

- Preparations for irrigation: preparations for irrigation are sterile, aqueous, large-volume preparations intended to be used for irrigation of body cavities, wounds, and surfaces, for example during surgical procedures […] (p. 932);
- Vaginal preparations: vaginal preparations are liquid, semi-solid or solid preparations intended for administration to the vagina usually to obtain a local effect […] (p. 940);
- Rectal preparations: rectal preparations are intended for rectal use to obtain a systemic or local effect, or they may be intended for diagnostic purposes […] (p. 933);
- Preparations for inhalation: preparations for inhalation are liquid, semi-solid or solid preparations intended for administration as vapours or aerosols to the lung to obtain a local or systemic effect […] (p. 927);
- Pressurised pharmaceutical preparations: pressurised pharmaceutical preparations are usually multidose preparations presented in special containers under pressure of a gas and often fitted with a metering valve and contain one or more active substances […] (p. 933);
- Nasal preparations: nasal preparations are liquid, semi-solid or solid preparations intended for administration to the nasal cavities to obtain a systemic or local effect […] (p. 918);
- Oromucosal preparations: oromucosal preparations are solid, semi-solid or liquid preparations, containing one or more active substances intended for administration to the oral cavity and/or the throat to obtain a local or systemic effect […] (p. 920);
- Ear preparations: ear preparations are liquid, semi-solid or solid preparations intended for instillation, for spraying, for insufflation, for application to the auditory meatus or as an ear wash […] (p. 908);
- Eye preparations: eye preparations are sterile liquid, semi-solid or solid preparations intended for administration upon the eyeball and/or to the conjunctiva, or for insertion in the conjunctival sac […] (p. 909).

The characteristics of these forms will be further defined below.

4.3 Oral Pharmaceutical Forms

4.3.1 Granules

Granules are preparations consisting of solid, dry aggregates of powder particles sufficiently robust to withstand handling (Fig. 4.1). They are intended for oral

Fig. 4.1 Examples of granules

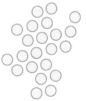

administration. Some are swallowed, some are chewed, and some are dissolved or dispersed in water or another suitable liquid before being administered [...].

Granules contain one or more active substances with or without excipients and, if necessary, colouring matter authorised by the competent authority and flavouring substances.

Granules are presented as single-dose or multidose preparations. Each dose of a multidose preparation is administered by means of a device suitable for measuring the quantity prescribed. For single-dose granules, each dose is enclosed in an individual container, for example a sachet or a vial [...].

Several categories of granules may be distinguished:

- effervescent granules;
- coated granules;
- gastro-resistant granules;
- modified-release granules [...].

4.3.2 Capsules

Capsules are solid preparations with hard or soft shells of various shapes and capacities, containing a single dose of active ingredient(s) (Fig. 4.2). They are usually intended for oral administration. The capsule shells are made of gelatin or other substances, the consistency of which may be adjusted by the addition of substances such as glycerol or sorbitol. Excipients such as surface-active agents, opaque fillers, antimicrobial preservatives, sweeteners, colouring matter authorised by the competent authority and flavouring substances may be added. The capsules may bear surface markings.

The contents of capsules may be solid, semi-solid or liquid. They consist of one or more active substances with or without excipients such as solvents, diluents, lubricants, and disintegrating agents. The contents do not cause deterioration of the shell. However, the shell is attacked by the digestive fluids and the contents are released [...].

Several categories of capsules may be distinguished:

- hard capsules;
- soft capsules;
- gastro-resistant capsules;
- modified-release capsules;
- cachets [...].

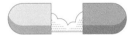

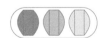

Fig. 4.2 Different typologies of capsules

4.3.3 Tablets

Tablets are solid preparations each containing a single dose of one or more active ingredients. They are obtained by compressing uniform volumes of particles or by another suitable manufacturing technique, such as extrusion, moulding or freeze-drying (lyophilisation). Tablets are intended for oral administration. Some are swallowed whole, some after being chewed, some are dissolved or dispersed in water before being administered and some are retained in the mouth where the active substance is liberated.

The particles consist of one or more active ingredients with or without excipients such as diluents, binders, disintegrating agents, glidants, lubricants, substances capable of modifying the behaviour of the preparation in the digestive tract, colouring matter authorised by the competent authority and flavouring substances.

Tablets are usually straight, solid cylinders, the end surfaces of which are flat or convex and the edges of which may be bevelled. They may have break-marks and may bear a symbol or other markings. Tablets may be coated […].

Several categories of tablets for oral use may be distinguished (Fig. 4.3):

- uncoated tablets;
- coated tablets;
- gastro-resistant tablets;
- modified-release tablets;
- effervescent tablets;
- soluble tablets;
- dispersible tablets;
- orodispersible tablets;
- chewable tablets;
- oral lyophilisates […].

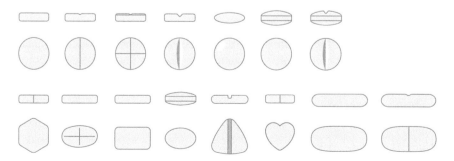

Fig. 4.3 Some examples of the different tablets' form and finishing

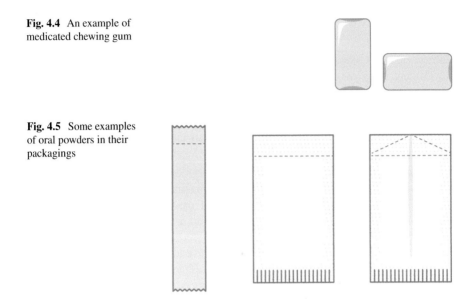

Fig. 4.4 An example of medicated chewing gum

Fig. 4.5 Some examples of oral powders in their packagings

4.3.4 Medicated Chewing Gums

Medicated chewing gums are solid, single-dose preparations with a base consisting mainly of gum that are intended to be chewed but not swallowed (Fig. 4.4).

They contain one or more active ingredients that are released by chewing. After dissolution or dispersion of the active substances in saliva, chewing gums are intended to be used for:

- local treatment of mouth diseases;
- systemic delivery after absorption through the buccal mucosa or from the gastrointestinal tract.

4.3.5 Oral Powders

Oral powders are preparations consisting of solid, loose, dry particles of varying degrees of fineness. They contain one or more active substances, with or without excipients and, if necessary, colouring matter authorised by the competent authority and flavouring substances. They are generally administered in or with water or another suitable liquid. They may also be swallowed directly. They are presented as single-dose or multidose preparations […] (Fig. 4.5).

Multidose oral powders require the provision of a measuring device capable of delivering the quantity prescribed. Each dose of a single-dose powder is enclosed in an individual container, for example a sachet or a vial […].

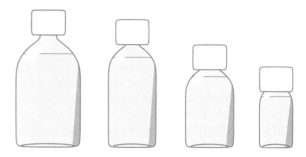

Fig. 4.6 Examples of primary packaging for liquid preparation for oral use

4.3.6 Liquid Preparations for Oral Use

Liquid preparations for oral use are usually solutions, emulsions or suspensions containing one or more active substances in a suitable vehicle; they may, however, consist of liquid active ingredients used as such (e.g., oral liquids) (Fig. 4.6). Some preparations for oral use are prepared by dilution of concentrated liquid preparations, or from powders or granules for the preparation of oral solutions or suspensions, for oral drops or for syrups, using a suitable vehicle […].

Liquid preparations for oral use may contain suitable antimicrobial preservatives, antioxidants, and other excipients such as dispersing, suspending, thickening, emulsifying, buffering, wetting, solubilising, stabilising, flavouring, and sweetening agents and colouring matter, authorised by the competent authority […].

Several categories of preparations may be distinguished:

- oral solutions, emulsions and suspensions;
- powders and granules for oral solutions and suspensions;
- oral drops;
- powders for oral drops;
- syrups;
- powders and granules for syrups […].

4.4 Topical Pharmaceutical Forms

4.4.1 Semi-solid Preparations for Cutaneous Application

Semi-solid preparations for cutaneous application are intended for local or transdermal delivery of active ingredients, or for their emollient or protective action (Fig. 4.7). They are of homogeneous appearance. Semi-solid preparations for

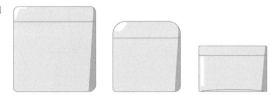

Fig. 4.7 Plastic and glass vases and pots for semi-solid preparations

cutaneous application consist of a simple or compound basis in which, usually, one or more active substances are dissolved or dispersed. According to its composition, the basis may influence the activity of the preparation. The basis may consist of natural or synthetic substances and may be single phase or multiphase. According to the nature of the basis, the preparation may have hydrophilic or hydrophobic properties; it may contain suitable excipients such as antimicrobial preservatives, antioxidants, stabilisers, emulsifiers, thickeners, and penetration enhancers. Semi-solid preparations for cutaneous application intended for use on severely injured skin are sterile […].

Several categories of semi-solid preparations for cutaneous application may be distinguished:

- ointments;
- creams;
- gels;
- pastes;
- poultices.
- medicated plasters;
- cutaneous patches […].

4.4.2 Powders for Cutaneous Application

Powders for cutaneous application are preparations consisting of solid, loose, dry particles of varying degrees of fineness. They contain one or more active substances, with or without excipients and, if necessary, colouring matter authorised by the competent authority. Powders for cutaneous application are presented as single-dose powders or multidose powders (Fig. 4.8).

They are free from grittiness. Powders specifically intended for use on large open wounds or on severely injured skin are sterile. Multidose powders for cutaneous application may be dispensed in sifter-top containers, containers equipped with a mechanical spraying device or in pressurised containers […].

Fig. 4.8 Examples of spray can and mechanical dispensers for powders

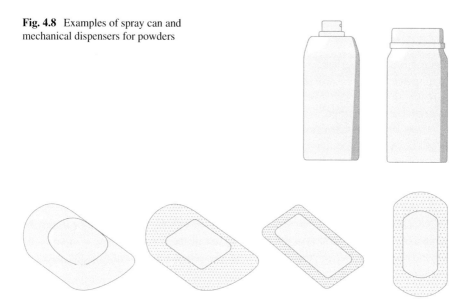

Fig. 4.9 Some examples of medicated plasters

4.4.3 Medicated Plasters

Medicated plasters are flexible preparations containing one or more active substances. They are intended to be applied to the skin. They are designed to maintain the active ingredient(s) in close contact with the skin such that these may be absorbed slowly, or act as protective or keratolytic agents.

Medicated plasters consist of an adhesive basis, which may be coloured, containing one or more active substances, spread as a uniform layer on an appropriate support made of natural or synthetic material (Fig. 4.9). They are not irritant or sensitising to the skin. The adhesive layer is covered by a suitable protective liner, which is removed before applying the plaster to the skin.

When removed, the protective liner does not detach the preparation from the outer, supporting layer.

Medicated plasters are presented in a range of sizes directly adapted to their intended use or as larger sheets to be cut before use. Medicated plasters adhere firmly to the skin when gentle pressure is applied and can be peeled off without causing appreciable injury to the skin or detachment of the preparation from the outer, supporting layer […].

4.4.4 Transdermal Patches

Transdermal patches are flexible pharmaceutical preparations of varying sizes, containing one or more active substances. They are intended to be applied to the unbroken skin to deliver the active ingredient(s) to the systemic circulation after passing through the skin barrier.

Transdermal patches normally consist of an outer covering which supports a preparation which contains the active ingredient(s). The transdermal patches are covered on the site of the release surface of the preparation by a protective liner, which is removed before applying the patch to the skin.

The outer covering is a backing sheet impermeable to the active ingredient(s) and normally impermeable to water, designed to support and protect the preparation. The outer covering may have the same dimensions as the preparation, or it may be larger. In the latter case the overlapping border of the outer covering is covered by pressure-sensitive adhesive substances which assure the adhesion of the patch to the skin.

The preparation contains the active ingredient(s) together with excipients such as stabilisers, solubilisers or substances intended to modify the release rate or to enhance transdermal absorption […]. Transdermal patches are normally individually enclosed in sealed sachets […].

4.4.5 Liquid Preparations for Cutaneous Application

Liquid preparations for cutaneous application are preparations of a variety of viscosities intended for local or transdermal delivery of active ingredients (Fig. 4.10). They are solutions, emulsions or suspensions that may contain one or more active substances in a suitable vehicle. They may contain suitable antimicrobial

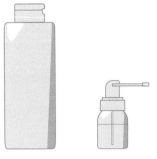

Fig. 4.10 Examples of primary packaging for liquid preparation for cutaneous application

preservatives, antioxidants, and other excipients such as stabilisers, emulsifiers, and thickeners.

Emulsions may show evidence of phase separation but are readily redispersed on shaking. Suspensions may show a sediment that is readily dispersed on shaking to give a suspension that is sufficiently stable to enable a homogeneous preparation to be delivered […]. Preparations specifically intended for use on severely injured skin are sterile.

Several categories of liquid preparations for cutaneous application may be distinguished, for example:

- shampoos;
- cutaneous foams […].

4.4.6 Medicated Foams

Medicated foams are preparations consisting of large volumes of gas dispersed in a liquid generally containing one or more active substances, a surfactant ensuring their formation and various other excipients (Fig. 4.11). Medicated foams are usually intended for application to the skin or mucous membranes.

Medicated foams are usually formed at the time of administration from a liquid preparation in a pressurised container. The container is equipped with a device consisting of a valve and a push button suitable for the delivery of the foam.

Medicated foams intended for use on severely injured skin and on large open wounds are sterile […].

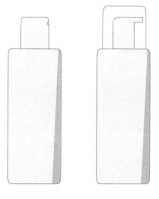

Fig. 4.11 Examples of primary packaging for medicated foams

4.5 Parenteral Pharmaceutical Forms

Parenteral preparations are sterile preparations intended for administration by injection, infusion or implantation into the human or animal body.

Parenteral preparations may require the use of excipients, for example to make the preparation isotonic with respect to blood, to adjust the pH, to increase solubility, to prevent deterioration of the active substances or to provide adequate antimicrobial properties, but not to adversely affect the intended medicinal action of the preparation or, at the concentrations used, to cause toxicity or undue local irritation.

Containers for parenteral preparations are made as far as possible from materials that are sufficiently transparent to permit the visual inspection of the contents, except for implants and in other justified and authorised cases [...]. Parenteral preparations are supplied in glass containers [...] or in other containers such as plastic containers and prefilled syringes (Fig. 4.12).

The tightness of the container is ensured by suitable means. Closures ensure a good seal, prevent the access of micro-organisms and other contaminants, and usually permit the withdrawal of a part or the whole of the contents without removal of the closure. The plastic materials or elastomers [...] used to manufacture the closures are sufficiently firm and elastic to allow the passage of a needle with the least possible shedding of particles. Closures for multidose containers are sufficiently elastic to ensure that the puncture is resealed when the needle is withdrawn.

Several categories of parenteral preparations may be distinguished:

- injections;
- infusions;
- concentrates for injections or infusions;
- powders for injections or infusions;
- gels for injection;
- implants [...].

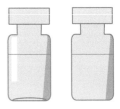

Fig. 4.12 Examples of 2 typologies of primary packaging for parental pharmaceutical forms: from the left, a glass container, a plastic container, and finally a plastic container with a different closure system

4.6 Rectal and Vaginal Pharmaceutical Forms

4.6.1 Preparations for Irrigation

Preparations for irrigation are sterile, aqueous, large-volume preparations intended to be used for irrigation of body cavities, wounds, and surfaces, for example during surgical procedures.

Preparations for irrigation are either solutions prepared by dissolving one or more active substances, electrolytes, or osmotically active substances in water […].

Examined in suitable conditions of visibility, preparations for irrigation are clear and practically free from particles.

Preparations for irrigation are supplied in single-dose containers […].

4.6.2 Vaginal Preparations

Vaginal preparations are liquid, semi-solid or solid preparations intended for administration to the vagina usually to obtain a local effect. They contain one or more active ingredients in a suitable basis […] (Fig. 4.13).

Several categories of vaginal preparations may be distinguished:

- pessaries;
- vaginal tablets;
- vaginal capsules;
- vaginal solutions, emulsions and suspensions;
- tablets for vaginal solutions and suspensions;
- semi-solid vaginal preparations;
- vaginal foams;
- medicated vaginal tampons […].

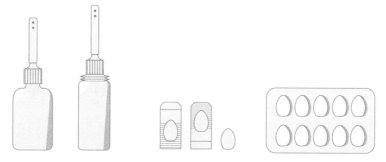

Fig. 4.13 Two examples of primary packaging for vaginal preparation: note the form and length of the dosing nozzle and a single dose ovule and a blister of ovule

Fig. 4.14 Different forms for rectal preparation: on the left, two examples of micro-enema and a single dose suppository

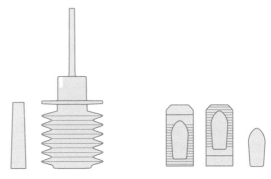

4.6.3 Rectal Preparations

Rectal preparations are intended for rectal use to obtain a systemic or local effect, or they may be intended for diagnostic purposes […] (Fig. 4.14).

Several categories of rectal preparations may be distinguished:

- suppositories;
- rectal capsules;
- rectal solutions, emulsions and suspensions;
- powders and tablets for rectal solutions or suspensions;
- semi-solid rectal preparations;
- rectal foams;
- rectal tampons […].

4.7 Oto-Rhinological Pharmaceutical Forms

4.7.1 Preparations for Inhalation

Preparations for inhalation are liquid, semi-solid or solid preparations intended for administration as vapours or aerosols to the lung to obtain a local or systemic effect. They contain one or more active substances that may be dissolved or dispersed in a suitable vehicle. Depending on the type, preparations for inhalation (Fig. 4.15) may contain propellants, cosolvents, diluents, antimicrobial preservatives, carriers, solubilising and stabilising agents, etc. These excipients do not adversely affect the functions of the mucosa of the respiratory tract or its cilia. Suspensions and emulsions are readily dispersible on shaking and they remain sufficiently stable to enable the correct dose to be delivered. Preparations for inhalation are supplied in multi-dose or single-dose containers […].

Fig. 4.15 An example of an inhaler for oto-rhinological preparations

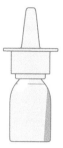

Preparations for inhalation intended to be administered as aerosols (dispersions of solid or liquid particles in a gas) are administered by one of the following devices:

- a nebuliser;
- an inhaler (pressurised metered-dose inhaler, non-pressurised metered-dose inhaler or powder inhaler).

Several categories of preparations for inhalation may be distinguished:

- preparations to be converted into vapour;
- liquid preparations for nebulisation;
- pressurised metered-dose preparations for inhalation;
- non-pressurised metered-dose preparations for inhalation;
- inhalation powders [...].

4.7.2 Pressurised Pharmaceutical Preparations

Pressurised pharmaceutical preparations are usually multidose preparations presented in special containers under pressure of a gas and often fitted with a metering valve and contain one or more active substances. The preparations are released from the container, upon actuation of an appropriate valve, in the form of an aerosol (dispersion of solid or liquid particles in a gas, the size of the particles being adapted to the intended use) or of a liquid or semisolid jet such as a foam. The pressure for the release is generated by suitable propellants.

The preparations are intended for local application to the skin or to mucous membranes of various body orifices, or for inhalation. Pressurised pharmaceutical preparations are provided with a delivery device appropriate for the intended application. Pressurised pharmaceutical preparations intended to be used on severely injured skin or large open wounds are sterile and comply with the test for sterility. Suitable excipients may also be used, for example solvents, solubilisers, emulsifying agents, suspending agents and lubricants for the valve to prevent clogging [...].

Fig. 4.16 An example of nasal spray primary packaging

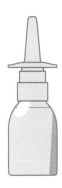

4.7.3 Nasal Preparations

Nasal preparations are liquid, semi-solid or solid preparations intended for administration to the nasal cavities to obtain a systemic or local effect. They contain one or more active substances […].

Aqueous nasal preparations are usually isotonic and may contain excipients, for example, to adjust the viscosity of the preparation, to adjust or stabilise the pH, to increase the solubility of the active substance, or to stabilise the preparation.

Nasal preparations are supplied in multidose or single-dose containers (Fig. 4.16), provided, if necessary, with a suitable administration device which may be designed to avoid the introduction of contaminants [….].

Several categories of nasal preparations may be distinguished:

- nasal drops and nasal sprays;
- nasal powders;
- semi-solid nasal preparations;
- nasal washes;
- nasal sticks […].

4.7.4 Oromucosal Preparations

Oromucosal preparations are solid, semi-solid or liquid preparations, containing one or more active substances intended for administration to the oral cavity and/or the throat to obtain a local or systemic effect. Preparations intended for a local effect may be designed for application to a specific site within the oral cavity such as the gums (e.g., gingival preparations) or the throat (e.g., oropharyngeal preparations). Preparations intended for a systemic effect are designed to be absorbed primarily at one or more sites on the oral mucosa (e.g., sublingual preparations). Mucoadhesive preparations are intended to be retained in the oral cavity by adhesion to the mucosal epithelium and may modify systemic medicine absorption at the site of application. For many oromucosal preparations, it is likely that some proportion of the active substance(s) will be swallowed and may be absorbed via the gastrointestinal tract.

Oromucosal preparations may contain suitable antimicrobial preservatives and other excipients such as dispersing, suspending, thickening, emulsifying, buffering, wetting, solubilising, stabilising, flavouring and sweetening agents. Solid preparations may in addition contain glidants, lubricants and excipients capable of modifying the release of the active substances […].

Several categories of preparations for oromucosal use may be distinguished:

- gargles;
- mouth washes;
- gingival solutions;
- oromucosal solutions and oromucosal suspensions;
- semi-solid oromucosal preparations (including for example gingival gel, gingival paste, oromucosal gel, oromucosal paste);
- oromucosal drops, oromucosal sprays and sublingual sprays (including oropharyngeal sprays);—lozenges and pastilles;
- compressed lozenges;
- sublingual tablets and buccal tablets;
- oromucosal capsules;
- mucoadhesive preparations;
- orodispersible films […].

4.7.5 Ear Preparations

Ear preparations are liquid, semi-solid or solid preparations intended for instillation, for spraying, for insufflation, for application to the auditory meatus or as an ear wash (Fig. 4.17). Ear preparations usually contain one or more active substances in a suitable vehicle. They may contain excipients to adjust tonicity or viscosity, to adjust or stabilise the pH, to increase the solubility of the active substances, to stabilise the preparation or to provide adequate antimicrobial properties. The excipients do not adversely affect the intended medicinal action of the preparation or, at the concentrations used, cause toxicity or undue local irritation […].

Ear preparations are supplied in multidose or single-dose containers, provided, if necessary, with a suitable administration device which may be designed to avoid the introduction of contaminants […].

Several categories of ear preparations may be distinguished:

- ear drops and sprays;
- semi-solid ear preparations;
- ear powders;
- ear washes;
- ear tampons […].

Fig. 4.17 An example of primary packaging for ear preparations: note the form and length of the dosing nozzle, curved to ease the use, management, and intake of the pharmaceutical preparation

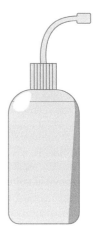

Fig. 4.18 An example of primary packaging for eye drops

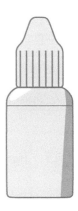

4.8 Ophthalmic Pharmaceutical Forms

4.8.1 Eye Preparations

Eye preparations are sterile liquid, semi-solid or solid preparations intended for administration upon the eyeball and/or to the conjunctiva, or for insertion in the conjunctival sac [...] (Fig. 4.18).

Several categories of eye preparations may be distinguished:

- eye drops;
- eye lotions;
- powders for eye drops and powders for eye lotions;
- semi-solid eye preparations;
- ophthalmic inserts [...].

4.9 Containers

A container for pharmaceutical use is an article that contains or is intended to contain a product and is, or may be, in direct contact with it. The closure is a part of the container. The container is so designed that the contents may be removed in a manner appropriate to the intended use of the preparation. It provides a varying degree of protection depending on the nature of the product and the hazards of the environment and minimises the loss of constituents. The container does not interact physically or chemically with the contents in a way that alters their quality beyond the limits tolerated by official requirements. There are two categories of containers:

- Single-dose container: A single-dose container holds a quantity of the preparation intended for total or partial use on 1 occasion only;
- Multidose container: A multidose container holds a quantity of the preparation suitable for 2 or more doses (Council of Europe 2019a, p. 453).

From USA Department of Health and Human Services Food and Drug Administration (1999), some definitions concerning primary packaging, ranging from materials of construction to components and closure systems:

- Materials of construction refer to the substances (e.g., glass, high density polyethylene 6 (HDPE) resin, metal) used to manufacture a packaging component (p. 2).
- A packaging component means any single part of a container closure system. Typical components are containers (e.g., ampules, vials, bottles), container liners (e.g., tube liners), closures (e.g., screw caps, stoppers), closure liners, stopper over seals, container inner seals, administration ports (e.g., on Large Volume Parenterals (LVPs), overwraps, administration accessories, and container labels (p. 2).
- Primary packaging component: A primary packaging component means a packaging component that is or may be in direct contact with the dosage form (p. 2).
- A container closure system: A container closure system refers to the sum of packaging components that together contain and protect the dosage form. This includes primary packaging components and secondary packaging components if the latter are intended to provide additional protection to the drug product. A packaging system is equivalent to a container closure system (p. 2).

4.10 Primary Packaging Typologies

Several examples of the different typologies of primary packaging and closure systems, categorised according to pharmaceutical form (liquid, solid, semi-solid, spray, etc.), are presented through brief descriptions and meaningful graphic representations.

4.10.1 Primary Packaging for Liquids Intended for Oral Use

In this category, we can comprise:

- bottles, in glass or plastic (Fig. 4.19);
- vials, usually plastic (Fig. 4.20).

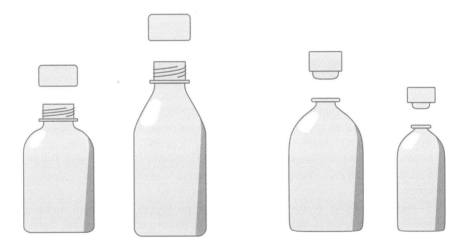

Fig. 4.19 Examples of bottles for liquids, differing for their caps and materials

4 Pharmaceutical Forms and Primary Packaging: A Glossary

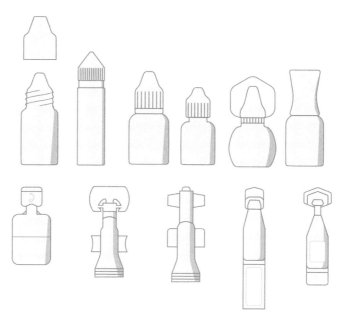

Fig. 4.20 Above, a series of small containers for liquids

4.10.2 *Primary Packaging for Injectable Liquids*

In this category, we can comprise:

- vials, multidose or single dose, usually in glass. It may or may not be sealed; in the latter case, there will be a sealed rubber cap with an aluminium ring (Fig. 4.21);
- pre-filled and ready-to-use syringes, containing the injectable solution (Fig. 4.22);
- infusion bags, made of plastic material in different sizes and ready for parenteral use (Fig. 4.23).

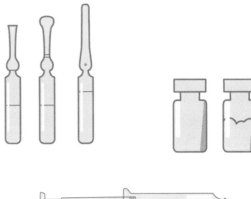

Fig. 4.21 On the left, examples of single-dose glass vials; on the right, examples of multi-dose vials

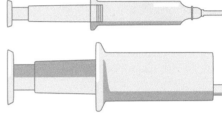

Fig. 4.22 Two typologies of pre-filled syringes

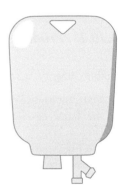

Fig. 4.23 An example of a plastic infusion bag

4.10.3 Primary Packaging for Semi-solids

In this category, we can comprise:

- bottles, jars, and pots, usually in glass or plastic (Fig. 4.24);
- strips, formed by two sealed sheets, usually of aluminium coated on the inside face with a film of thermoplastic material (Fig. 4.25);
- tubes, namely a small cylinder generally in aluminium or plastic, fitted with a lid or stopper (Fig. 4.26).

4 Pharmaceutical Forms and Primary Packaging: A Glossary

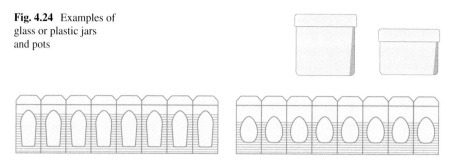

Fig. 4.24 Examples of glass or plastic jars and pots

Fig. 4.25 Examples of aluminium strips for suppositories and ovules

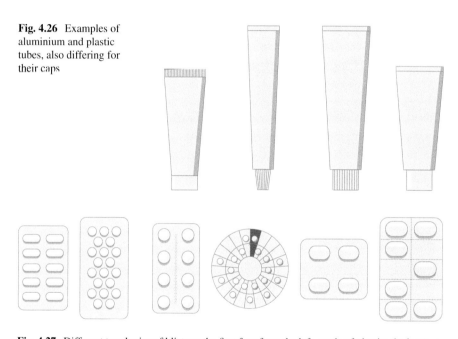

Fig. 4.26 Examples of aluminium and plastic tubes, also differing for their caps

Fig. 4.27 Different typologies of blisters: the first four from the left, made of plastic; the last two, made of aluminium

4.10.4 Primary Packaging for Solids

In this category, we can comprise:

- blister, namely a deep-drawn sheet of plastic material in which the individual solid pharmaceutical forms are placed, and a metal band welded to the plastic part (Fig. 4.27);
- pill bottles, usually in glass or plastic (Fig. 4.28).

Fig. 4.28 On the left, a glass pill-bottle; on the right, a plastic one

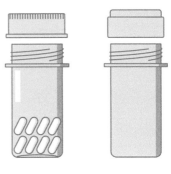

Fig. 4.29 Different typologies of inhaler

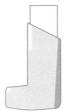 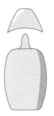 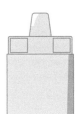

4.10.5 Primary Packaging for Sprays

In this category, we can include inhaler products (Fig. 4.29).

4.10.6 Packaging Closure Systems

In this category, we can comprise:

- screw or press-on caps, plastic or aluminium ferrules (Fig. 4.30);
- sub-caps, usually plastic or aluminium (Fig. 4.31).

4 Pharmaceutical Forms and Primary Packaging: A Glossary

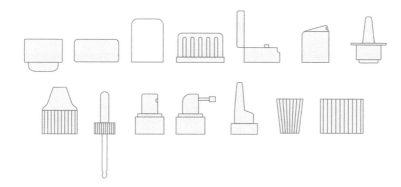

Fig. 4.30 Some typologies of caps, for different usage and pharma management and intake

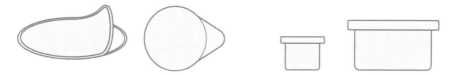

Fig. 4.31 Examples of aluminium (left) and plastic (right) sub-caps

References

Council of Europe (2019a) Materials for containers and containers. In: European pharmacopoeia, vol 1, cap. 3, 10.0 edn. Council of Europe, Strasburgo, pp 419–478. Retrieved from EP 10 (EUROPEAN PHARMACOPOEIA 10th EDITION) (webofpharma.com)

Council of Europe (2019b) General texts, monographs on dosage forms. In: European Pharmacopoeia, vol 1, cap. 05, 10.0 edn. Council of Europe, Strasburgo, pp 903–943. Retrieved from EP 10 (EUROPEAN PHARMACOPOEIA 10th EDITION) (webofpharma.com)

Lai F (2021). Proprietà biofarmaceutiche. In: Tecnologia Farmaceutica Applicata. Università degli Studi di Cagliari. Retrieved from https://web.unica.it/static/resources/cms/documents/Valutazionedelleproprietbiofarmaceutiche_1.pdf

U.S. Department of Health and Human Services Food and Drug Administration (1999) Guidance for industry—container, closure systems for packaging human drugs and biologics. Food and Drug Administration, Rockville

Open Access This chapter is licensed under the terms of the Creative Commons Attribution 4.0 International License (http://creativecommons.org/licenses/by/4.0/), which permits use, sharing, adaptation, distribution and reproduction in any medium or format, as long as you give appropriate credit to the original author(s) and the source, provide a link to the Creative Commons license and indicate if changes were made.

The images or other third party material in this chapter are included in the chapter's Creative Commons license, unless indicated otherwise in a credit line to the material. If material is not included in the chapter's Creative Commons license and your intended use is not permitted by statutory regulation or exceeds the permitted use, you will need to obtain permission directly from the copyright holder.

Chapter 5
Secondary Packaging of Medicines: Design Processes for the Pharmaceutical Industry

Marcello Mariani

Abstract The chapter presents the daily practices of a company producing pharmaceutical cartons and leaflets. It focuses on the complex design processes of these products that play a significant role for pharmaceutical companies. The contribution starts from the author's personal experience within a company that produces secondary packaging and package leaflets for pharmaceutical products. In the chapter, the different phases of the decision-making process are presented, following both the technical and relational aspects. In addition to their description, which brings out the complexity of the relationships between companies, the chapter dwells on the issues of innovation and sustainability linked to the design of secondary packaging and package leaflets, which are indispensable today to remain competitive in the market. In this context, the role of new technologies is included, foreshadowing the possible impact on secondary packaging.

5.1 The Three Pillars of Pharmaceutical Packaging Design

Before describing the main stages of the process, it is worth emphasising a few essential elements for designing pharmaceutical secondary packaging, but more generally for developing a new product or service.

5.1.1 Inter-company Ecosystem

For more than a decade now, the design and innovation of secondary packaging has entailed working and relating within an ecosystem that goes beyond the perimeter of the individual company: in innovation processes, we increasingly speak of an inter-company ecosystem (Fichtner et al. 2005).

M. Mariani (✉)
Renogroup S.r.l., Bologna, Italy
e-mail: marcello.mariani@renogroup.eu

The inter-company work ecosystem is a collection of subjects, individuals and organisations (so-called stakeholders), which interact to satisfy everyday needs or share resources. In this ecosystem, each stakeholder plays a specific role and contributes uniquely. The common goal is to create value for customers and the companies themselves through collaboration and sharing knowledge, resources, and skills.

In the context of a pharmaceutical secondary packaging creation project, the inter-company ecosystem is mainly composed of the customer (i.e., the pharmaceutical company); paper and board, ink and varnish, logistics suppliers; engineering companies; pharmaceutical packaging line manufacturers; regulatory bodies; universities and vocational schools in the area. Due to their need and willingness to collaborate on innovation projects and the creation of new products, it is common for these realities to form complex territorial realities, as is the case with the Packaging Valley Ecosystem in the Bologna area, which exploits all the potential of a district worldwide acknowledged (Andreoni et al. 2017; Andreoni and Lazonick 2020).

5.1.2 Sustainability

A further key element is the sustainability of secondary packaging, in terms of environmental impact and ecological footprint. For example, a new pharmaceutical case design project cannot disregard criteria that characterise the sustainability of a new product, such as:

- Eco-compatibility: the packaging must be made of recyclable materials that are free of substances harmful to the environment and human health;
- Energy efficiency: the packaging production process must be energy efficient and use renewable sources;
- Waste reduction: packaging must be designed to be recycled and minimise waste and waste;
- Accessibility: packaging must be accessible and easily understood by all, including elderly or disabled patients;
- Transparency: packaging must provide complete information on the materials used and the product's sustainability.

5.1.3 Production Efficiency

The sustainability characteristics of packaging can never overshadow the requirements of medicine protection and pharmaceutical line performance: this is the third essential element. Product design is a critical factor in optimising production line performance. If a product is designed efficiently, this can increase production speed, reduce overall costs, and improve the quality of the finished product. In turn, this can increase customer satisfaction and brand loyalty.

Suppose one focuses only on the marketing of the product and not on its optimised design for production performance. In that case, this may lead to inefficiencies in the production lines, increase costs and compromise product quality. Furthermore, a product designed for marketing value alone may not be safe or durable, negatively affecting the company's reputation.

In short, it is essential to design a product that brings added value to pharmaceutical companies based on marketing appeal aspects and production performance aspects (Moschis and Bovell 2013).

5.2 The Conceptual Process of Designing a Product/Service

Entering concretely into the conceptual process of developing and manufacturing a pharmaceutical secondary packaging, we describe the steps that lead a company to design a new case for pharmaceutical companies.

These are:

- start: the beginning of the product design process;
- briefing: a meeting between the pharmaceutical company (customer) and the carton maker (supplier) to discuss the requirements and expectations of the packaging;
- analysis: the study of the requirements and opportunities for the product; study of the materials and technologies to be applied to its production to meet the customer's needs;
- proposal: presentation of solution proposals for the requested product, including drawings, technical specifications and expected costs;
- sampling: realisation of a prototype or sample of the product to verify the quality of the design and automatic processability on the customer's lines, using machine testing;
- commissioning: delivery of the final product to the customer, first commercial order, and market launch.

Before describing each phase, we highlight that each new packaging design project for cartons and pharmaceutical leaflets can start from customer input, meaning a pharmaceutical company, or from an internal requirement of the packaging company. In the following, we will elaborate on the process that starts from a request or need of the pharmaceutical company, as all the steps of this process also have within them all the design steps that start from a design idea of the packaging company, independently of a need expressed by the pharmaceutical company. In the following, we will highlight just a few differences which may be decisive within one or the other design process. Furthermore, in the economy of the paper, we will take as an example the design process of a pharmaceutical case, which is undoubtedly more complex and exhaustive than that of a leaflet.

5.2.1 Start

In the first phase, the pharmaceutical company (from now on, we will refer to it as the customer) submits to the packaging supplier (from now on, we will refer to it as the supplier) an initial input for the design of a new secondary packaging (carton).

The customer may be in one of the following initial situations:

- having available only the pharmaceutical product with its primary packaging (e.g., blister, vial, syringe, etc.), which will be packaged with the carton (secondary packaging);
- have the product and a first idea of secondary packaging available;
- have the product and an existing secondary packaging available, which needs to be improved/modified.

In the first two cases, in addition to the product design part, it may also be necessary to collaborate with the customer on the communication and graphics part; in the third case, the graphic-communication component is almost always present and must only be adapted to the new packaging.

For the type of need we have decided to deal with (i.e., the need to design a new carton originating from the pharmaceutical company), the customer contacts the supplier to submit the request for a new design. The first discussion, necessary to prepare the subsequent phases (especially regarding the company resources to be allocated and the time needed to manage the project) involves (or should always involve) the supplier company figures with both commercial and technical skills.

Compared to this process, here we digress briefly into what can happen if the idea for new packaging originates independently within the supplier company. In this case, namely in the absence of an external client, before starting a design process for a new product—which is intended to be innovative for the market—it is both important and critical to understand the link that exists between the idea, the main trends of the future (e.g. relating to packaging, user lifestyles, materials, technologies, environmental issues, etc.) and the management and development of the company and all the people who work there. A Trend Analysis table is used to understand and envision possible present and future trends (Cook 2015).

The corporate team gives a subjective assessment (numerical vote), on the global and corporate impact of the trend, related to the product, by filling in the table (Table 5.1). The weighted average of the various judgements is inserted into the table itself. These numerical outputs allow the company to assess the different degrees of urgency of the project, providing the evaluation of the strategic importance of the project, which derives from a weighted average of the judgements expressed by the various professional roles and skills involved in developing the idea.

Table 5.1 The table provides an example of the use of the Trend Analysis tool, for a project related to the digitisation of communication in the pharmaceutical sector, involving the introduction of the electronic leaflet (e-leaflet) instead of the paper leaflet

Global impact						Company impact			
Window		Scope		Impact		Plausibility		Urgency	
Evaluation	Scale	Evaluation	Scale	Evaluation	Scale	Evaluation	Scale	Evaluation	Scale
1–4 years	5	Global	5	Important	5	Certain	5	Today	5
5–9 years	4	Wide	4	Significant	4	Probable	4	3–5 years	4
10–14 years	3	Market	3	Medium	3	Possible	3	6–9 years	3
15–20 years	2	Companies	2	Minor	2	Improbable	2	10–14 years	2
>20 years	1	Individual	1	Unimportant	1	Rare	1	16–20 years	1
Never	0	None	0	/	0	/	0	>20 years	0
Score									
20–25 points		Act immediately							
15–19 points		Manage the situation, be ready to respond, prepare action plans to be activated quickly							
10–15 points		Monitor the situation, possible impact, repeat evaluation frequently							
<10 points		Possibly interesting but currently peripheral trend. Keep on radar and reassess on increasing signals							
Result		23							

5.2.2 Briefing

The briefing stage can be divided into two main phases: a customer listening phase and a brainstorming phase.

For the supplier company, the briefing phase involves all the departments that will be included in the incoming design process. In particular: the customer's Sales Representative, the Technical Office Manager, the Production Manager. These figures collect all the information from this phase to bring it to the company for the subsequent Analysis phase.

On the other hand, the customer team is usually composed of representatives of the following company functions: Purchasing Department; Product Management; Packaging Engineering; Production; Marketing.

The *listening phase* opens with the customer explaining the need(s) justifying the request for new secondary packaging.

In principle, the input given to the supplier is already the result of previous consultations, internal to the pharmaceutical company, and therefore known and shared by all participants on the customer side. It is essential to be aware that this does not happen sometimes, and an internal confrontation between colleagues on the client side is generated during this listening phase. At this stage, the supplier must know how to give an authoritative opinion, trying to harmonise any differences of view within the client's team, through the objectivity of his technical knowledge and good interpersonal mediation skills. At this stage, the ability to listen to the client is of great importance, even before the ability to provide answers. A successful outcome of this first meeting, which is fundamental for continuing the project with the customer, very often depends not only on the supplier's technical skills but also on an excellent ability to listen, getting in tune with the customer's needs without making unthought-out judgements, also given the complexity of the problems that the customer company must manage internally and must know how to communicate.

The brainstorming phase follows the listening phase. In it, the customer/supplier confrontation starts: all the players involved are called upon to play an effective and proactive role.

Usually, the main issues on which one is asked to contribute, transversal to each project, are the following:

- the safety of the packaging chosen, depending on the pharmaceutical form (e.g. liquid, solid, mixed) that it must contain and protect. In this respect, it is always necessary to assess whether the materials chosen are correct; whether the type, weight and thickness of the cardboard are adequate for the pharmaceutical form to be packaged; whether the die-cut layout of the carton proposed by the customer is adequate for the product, its size, weight, its logistical handling, and the use that the patient will make of it; whether the solution proposed is the most suitable for guaranteeing the inviolability of the package, anti-counterfeiting, non-accessibility to children, and at the same time easy access for the elderly.
- the industrial reproducibility by the supplier, assessing whether the supplier can produce the die-cut layout chosen by the customer; whether it can be improved to make the supplier's production more efficient and thus contain costs; finally, assessing whether the materials selected are the best in terms of market availability (e.g., certainty of supply), cost, and quality;
- its processability (in jargon "machinability") on the customer's lines, asking whether the packaging will be manual or automatic; whether it is possible to improve the handling of the packaging by the operators (e.g., single-track loaders, packaging boxes); whether used on existing or new packaging lines; whether it will be necessary to involve the manufacturer of the packaging line; and finally—if the product has never been used before—whether it is required to provide for tests of machinability of the same;
- the sustainability and end-of-life management of the product, evaluating the possible type of cardboard chosen (FSC/PEFC, recycled, compostable, etc.); the possibility of dematerialising (at least in part) the product (e.g., by reducing the weight of raw materials, hypothesising the use of e-leaflets as opposed to paper leaflets); the choice of solutions for the graphic design that are as sustainable as possible (e.g., use of vegetable inks, no plastics, no UV varnishes);
- the costs, evaluating the possibility of proposing alternatives to the customer that contain the direct cost of the product (materials, die-cut design, colours, varnishes); the hidden cost that may be hidden behind the production process of making the product at the suppliers premises; any hidden costs due to inefficiencies in the customer's packaging process.

The brainstorming phase ends with defining specific technical characteristics of the packaging to be developed, which represent the first product concept. The supplier undertakes to analyse the elements that define this first concept internally to submit an initial proposal to the customer.

5.2.3 Analysis

In the analysis phase, the supplier brings the concept identified in the briefing phase into the company. At this stage, the supplier may extend the analysis to the main stakeholders it believes can add value to the project. Mainly these are:

- suppliers of raw materials: cardboard, inks, paints;
- die-cut suppliers;
- packaging suppliers;
- packaging line manufacturers.

The concept review must be extensive, with several main objectives:

- ensuring the feasibility of the product to the customer;
- prepare the internal timeline of the project;
- schedule the technical resources needed to implement it;
- schedule the necessary human resources to implement it;
- schedule the time required to implement it;
- create an initial "draft proposal" for the customer.

Especially when dealing with an innovative concept, it is essential to make the best use of the mix of robust technical knowledge in the company, updated to the state of the art regarding materials and production techniques (Fig. 5.1). But it is equally important to incentivise people, especially technicians, to break out of the mould of the already known, of *it has always been done this way* to arrive at an innovative proposal and, above all, according to the customer's specific needs.

To manufacture the packaging in a robotised production process, it is necessary to know all the characteristics of the production line, for example the customer's packaging plant. The type of product to be packaged, its size and weight, greatly influence the design of the carton and the raw materials.

There are many types of machinery in industrial production. Hence, knowledge of the characteristics of the machine is necessary to be able to design packaging that respects in detail all the peculiarities of the production line, such as when and at what point in the process the opening takes place; how filling is determined; the eventual stamping of batch and expiry date; gluing and finally the closing of the pack.

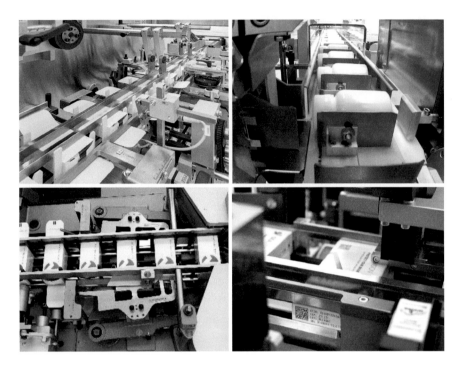

Fig. 5.1 From top-left to bottom-right: packaging opening, filling, closing and stamping. (Source: the author)

5.2.4 Prosposal

As described above, the analysis phase ends with the proposal to the customer, which usually includes the following elements:

- technical drawing of the product;
- die-cut layout;
- technical data sheets of the raw materials considered;
- digital and physical mockup;
- prototype;
- plotter sampling;
- study of packaging graphics.

Here is a detailed description of each of them.

The *technical drawing* of the product must be as complete as possible, indicating all the measurements of the designed packaging and a summary template with the basic information identifying the product/project (Fig. 5.2).

It is usually supplied to the customer in PDF, accompanied by the native format in which it was developed (e.g., .ai, .dwg, etc.).

On the other hand, *the die-cut layout* (Fig. 5.3) is a technical drawing created with a dedicated programme (e.g., Autocad) that precisely defines the structure of

Fig. 5.2 A technical drawing of the packaging

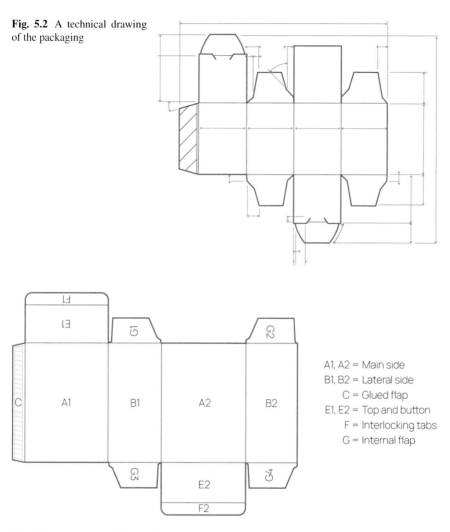

Fig. 5.3 An example of day-cut layout

the packaging, its measurements and provides a guide for the graphic design and creation of the die-cut that will be used in production by the supplier.

In other words, it represents the "cutting and folding outline of the unfolded box, composed of the cutting, abundance and creasing lines". It is the 2D technical drawing of the packaging. Its development is closely linked to the type of material proposed (cardboard), the production machinery and the technical and functional requirements (customer machinability), that it must satisfy.

Below is an example of a drawing of a so-called "linear" carton with alternating interlocking flaps.

The dimensions of the case (the letters on the layout), the cuts and folds (creases) are positioned and sized according to its specific structural aspects, to ensure its correct functioning. The supplier's added value lies in preparing a layout for the customer with all these components in place. The conformity of the die-cut layout also depends on the type of card to be used for the future realisation of the product. Therefore, providing the customer with the technical data sheet of the *raw material* in question is also important. This is a specification in which the cardboard manufacturer indicates a series of values and physical parameters, which are decisive for realising the carton and its industrialisation on the pharmaceutical lines. Among the most important are: weight (g/sqm), thickness (microns), and stiffness (mNm). The whiteness of the carton's outside and inside is also important when designing new packaging for marketing purposes.

At the next stage, an additional element that can make a difference is the *product mock-up* (Fig. 5.4). The mock-up can be digital, such as a 3D rendering of the case, or physical. In this case, it is very important to clarify to the customer the purpose of this intermediate artefact, so that there are no unpleasant misunderstandings with the customer.

As should be well known, the mock-up does not necessarily reproduce all the details of the packaging but reproduces the general formal elements of the case. It is a quick tool to make and serves for initial customer approval, followed by a fine-tuning phase. For example, it can be made from different cardboard than the final one. Mock-ups assume an even more important role with the new opportunities digital printing offers. The latest generation of printers makes it possible to produce entire mock-up series at a meagre cost. Again, it must be made clear to the customer that there is no perfect colour match of a digitally printed sample with an offset

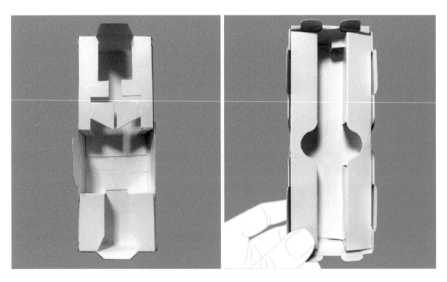

Fig. 5.4 An example of the packaging mock-up

printed one. The colour rendering of the digital model is not the same as during offset production (and vice versa).

The prototype is a *mature* version of the mock-up. It reproduces in detail every line of the finished packaging. It is generally on a 1:1 scale and uses the selected and approved materials.

Producing a prototype directly with the final production process can even be requested by the customer. In such cases, the supplier initiates a real production process (i.e., offset printing, die-cutting, folding/pasting), even if only for a few prototypes. The costs will be much higher, and the time will be longer accordingly.

At this stage, providing the customer with a plotter sample of the packaging may already be necessary. This can serve the customer:

- to make the very first tests of the format in production;
- for product managers to provide to their customers;
- to submit to the regulatory authority.

When this sampling is used for the customer's first preliminary production tests, the cartons are cut with a plotter, folded, and glued by hand by an operator. They will not have the same physical and mechanical characteristics as the exact sampling made by industrial die-cutting and folding/glueing. Their mechanical behaviour will be very different. A classic example is the difficulty in opening the case (splaying), or in closing the interlocking flaps.

In some cases, during the proposal phase, the supplier may also be called upon to study the graphic design of the packaging.

It will then be the responsibility of the supplier's pre-press and artwork department to graphically "dress" the die-cut layout that has been prepared, preparing a digital draft (blueprint), which will then be sent to the customer for approval.

Even in this case, it is always helpful to warn the customer of the difference between the digital colour and the real colour of industrial printing (offset/flexo).

The Proposal phase ends with the supplier presenting the final proposal to the customer.

5.2.5 *Sampling*

The sampling phase cannot be separated from the customer's prior approval of the proposed packaging.

By approval, we mean a formal act of acceptance by the customer, which authorises the supplier to start the actual Sampling phase, which consists of the following:

- industrial sampling;
- customer machine testing.

By industrial sampling, we mean the production of a determined quantity of pieces of the product (in this case, cartons), agreed with the customer, necessary to be used on the customer's automatic packaging line, to verify its production efficiency.

Specific rules guide this phase:

- the first is that the quantity must be congruent with the complexity of the carton to be tested on the line. The more complicated the carton, the higher the amount of sampling industrial must be;
- the second is that the cartons must faithfully reflect the technical characteristics agreed upon with the customer and must be produced by the supplier in exact compliance with all the production steps of future industrial production. The samples are delivered to the customer's production site, where the packaging line is installed and used for the machinability test.

Critical elements of this phase are:

- the compliance with the delivery date set with the customer. Not respecting this deadline for the sample delivery can postpone the test on the line by several weeks, depending on the customer's production schedule. To 'test' the machinability of a new carton, the customer must stop the production lines, suspending the batches of other products.
- the presence of the supplier during the test is strongly recommended, to assist the customer in real-time in case problems arise during the case testing phase.
- in these cases, having an expert in the supplier's team who is familiar with their product and the operation of pharmaceutical packaging lines adds value to the test phase.

The outcome of the test can be positive or negative. If negative, the customer agrees with the supplier on a series of small changes to the carton, correcting any errors for an effective and efficient production cycle. A new date is then agreed upon for a second test, with the new, modified machine trial supply. If the test outcome is positive, we move on to the final production of the packaging in high runs, depending on the customer's commercial requirements.

5.2.6 *Commissioning*

The new packaging is given its final graphic design in this last phase. It is almost always the pharmaceutical company that creates the artwork. The supplier receives the artwork to be contained in the carton and the order with the quantity to be produced. The supplier produces the required number of cartons and delivers them (on time!) to the customer. The pharmaceutical product is packaged in its new 'look' and launched on the market with its packaging.

5.3 New Technologies, Innovation, and Sustainability in Healthcare Secondary Packaging Design

So far, we have presented the complex process leading to producing a new pharmaceutical product packaging in all its details, highlighting its critical aspects. To conclude, we briefly introduce a project called *Ameco, a new Paper Tray* designed by *Renogroup* (Fig. 5.5) It encompasses innovation, the use of new technologies and sustainability as the cornerstones of the design concept.

Most pharmaceutical products, in the form of vials, bottles, syringes, and pens, are packaged inside trays made of thermoformable plastic materials such as: Polypropylene (PP), Polystyrene (PS), Polyethylene Terephthalate (PET), Low-Density Polyethylene (LDPE), High-Density Polyethylene (HDPE), Polyvinyl Chloride (PVC), Polycarbonate (PC), Acrylonitrile Butadiene Styrene (ABS).

Deep thermoforming consists of the vacuum deformation of these materials, which are available in sheet or reel form. Heating through hot air or infrared rays, makes the plastic malleable and moulds it perfectly.

This type of secondary packaging is unsustainable due to the use of plastic materials and the highly energy-intensive process. Packaging companies have recently made it part of their innovative strategies to create products and processes more sustainable.

One of the challenges is to reduce parts or components made of plastics or to replace them with so-called "green" materials. The following example lies precisely within this framework of corporate intent.

It is the first stretched cardboard tray—*Ameco Paper Tray*—with a fully automatic production cycle, which replaces the old, thermoformed tray, guaranteeing enormous advantages in terms of efficiency and reliability.

Its name is a play on words with different meanings: "I'm eco" because it is 100% green and sustainable, but also "AM.ICO", precisely with the meaning of the word friend in the Italian language, thanks to its user-friendly soul.

In the following, we describe the unique features of this tray in terms of sustainability, innovation, and new technologies, linking some of its characteristics to the conception and design process.

Fig. 5.5 An example of the *AMECO Paper Tray*

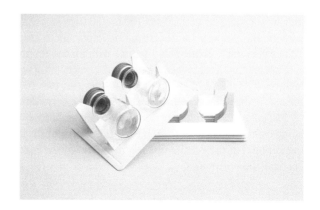

The tray consists of two parts of stretched cardboard: a base with holes and a part that is folded to create cusps and slots intended to receive the product to be packaged (e.g., vials, bottles, syringes, pens, or a mix of them). These two parts, glued together, create the final object.

The pharmaceutical company uses the tray on its packaging lines: the trays' feeding unit picks up the tray with suction cups from a loading surface and places it on a conveyor belt. At this stage, a robotic unit inserts the object (drugs such as ampoules, for example) and then the filled tray is gently handled and inserted into a carton, resulting in a 100% paper-based package.

The three pillars of pharmaceutical packaging design discussed above have been respected in developing this new tray.

The first aspect to emphasise is how *Ameco* is a packaging born from the collaboration of the company that designed it (Renogroup) with its stakeholders, within an inter-company ecosystem (first pillar).

A structured research and analysis phase has been done, involving:

- the raw material suppliers, studying the types of cardboard to be used and the glue to join the two parts of *Ameco*;
- the engineering departments, to analyse the deformation of the cardboard during the cusp creation phase and the design of customised housings for the customer's product;
- the packaging suppliers, to define the best solution in terms of protection and efficiency of the pharmaceutical operators on the packaging line;
- the customer, to ensure maximum security of the product inside the tray;
- the packaging line supplier, with whom we worked in symbiosis to guarantee maximum lines' efficiency.

Ameco is a sustainable solution (second pillar), being composed only of FSC (Forest Stewardship Council) and/or PEFC (Programme for the Endorsement of Forest Certification Schemes) certified tensioned cardboard, which offers the advantage of permanently eliminating thermoformed trays from the packaging system of pharmaceutical companies.

Finally, it has been designed to increase the end pharmaceutical customer's production efficiency (third pillar). *Ameco* can feed an automatic filling line at high industrial process speeds: from 100 to 350 cartons/tray per minute, depending on its configuration (single, multipack). It is important to emphasise that these speeds are higher than those achievable by lines with plastic thermoformed products.

This result was achieved thanks to the partnership work, made by the tray manufacturer with those of the packaging lines, on two fundamental characteristics of *Ameco*: being stackable during delivery and easily removable during use.

The case of *Ameco* confirms how the design of a new healthcare secondary packaging cannot disregard a search for innovation and sustainability that does not chase marketing, but the continuous improvement of the industrial processes of pharmaceutical end customers.

References

Andreoni A, Lazonick W (2020) Local ecosystems and social condition of innovative enterprise. In: The Oxford handbook of industrial hubs and economic development. Oxford University Press, Oxford, pp 77–97

Andreoni A, Frattini F, Prodi G (2017) Structural cycles and industrial policy alignment: the private–public nexus in the Emilian Packaging Valley. Camb J Econ 41(3):881–904. https://doi.org/10.1093/cje/bew048

Cook AG (2015) Forecasting for the pharmaceutical industry. Models for new product and in-market forecasting and how to use them. Routledge, London/New York

Fichtner W, Tietze-Stöckinger I, Frank M, Rentz O (2005) Barriers of interorganisational environmental management: two case studies on industrial symbiosis. Prog Ind Ecol Int J 2(1):73–88. https://doi.org/10.1504/PIE.2005.006778

Moschis P, Bovell L (2013) Marketing pharmaceutical and cosmetic products to the mature market. Int J Pharm Healthc Mark 7(4):357–373. https://doi.org/10.1108/IJPHM-04-2013-0020

Open Access This chapter is licensed under the terms of the Creative Commons Attribution 4.0 International License (http://creativecommons.org/licenses/by/4.0/), which permits use, sharing, adaptation, distribution and reproduction in any medium or format, as long as you give appropriate credit to the original author(s) and the source, provide a link to the Creative Commons license and indicate if changes were made.

The images or other third party material in this chapter are included in the chapter's Creative Commons license, unless indicated otherwise in a credit line to the material. If material is not included in the chapter's Creative Commons license and your intended use is not permitted by statutory regulation or exceeds the permitted use, you will need to obtain permission directly from the copyright holder.

Chapter 6
Secondary Packaging and Leaflets: A Glossary

Marcello Mariani

Abstract Shaped as a glossary, the chapter presents and graphically illustrates the main typologies of pharmaceutical cartons and leaflets. This overview is essential to understand the production manufacturing processes and principal features of cartons and leaflets for the pharmaceutical industry.

6.1 The Main Typologies of Cartons and Secondary Packaging

The principal association of European carton manufacturers (ECMA 2013) has compiled a catalogue containing over 100 different carton formats, recognised at European level. Cartons for the pharmaceutical sector are one part of this ECMA list, but they are still substantial in terms of variety and complexity.

The following paragraphs present some examples of flat cartons and folding cartons. This is not an exhaustive list but represents a review of the main types in use.

M. Mariani (✉)
Renogroup S.r.l., Bologna, Italy
e-mail: marcello.mariani@renogroup.eu

© The Author(s) 2025
A. V. Penati (ed.), *In-Home Medication*, Research for Development,
https://doi.org/10.1007/978-3-031-53294-8_6

These are subject to variations, depending on the requirements of the pharmaceutical industry. Variants may include:

- specific opening features;
- specific use of the packaging;
- anti-fall features (bottom lock cartons);
- single or multi part trays;
- specific requirement from Marketing aiming to promote the product.

Just to give an example, the only feature of the "Specific opening features", in pharmaceutical industry can be expressed as:

- tuck-in cartons (even or odd) -where the flaps are closed and inserted;
- lock-bottom cartons—where one of the edges closes automatically during the carton erection;
- glued flap cartons—where the flaps are glued in line after medicine insertion;
- tray cartons—literally trays holding medicines that in most of the cases require an external carton for packing (unless designed with covering lids).

6.1.1 Rectangular Sleeve

The pre-glued Rectangular Sleeve (Fig. 6.1) has a simple construction. While the Rectangular Sleeve is considered a typology, it is also the underlying structure of most tube-typology cartons. It commonly functions as the slip-on cover in the combination of a tray and sleeve. Additionally, this type is used as the basic structure for many high-end multi-packaging systems. Rectangular Sleeve cartons may feature either locked-side or glued seams.

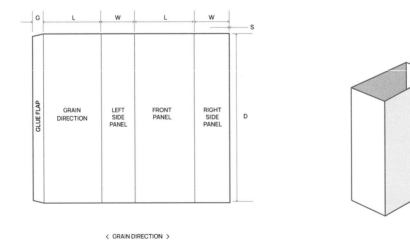

Fig. 6.1 An example of rectangular sleeve carton

6 Secondary Packaging and Leaflets: A Glossary

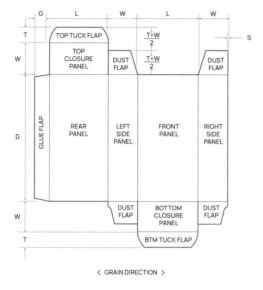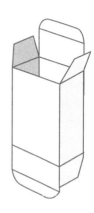

Fig. 6.2 An example of SRT carton

6.1.2 Standard Reverse Tuck (SRT)

The joint on the SRT carton (Fig. 6.2) is located at the seam along the right-side panel, in the rear. The closure panels on top and bottom swing in opposite directions, with the bottom folding in the rear and the top folding in front. This carton can be assembled either manually or by automation. With a friction lock closure on top and a slit lock tuck closure on bottom, as shown here, the carton is easy to open and close, while remaining unlikely to open inadvertently at its base.

6.1.3 Reverse Tuck with Lock Dust Flaps

Generally assembled, filled, and sealed manually, this style allows easy opening and closing while providing considerable reliability, even with weighty contents, against inadvertent unsealing (Fig. 6.3).

6.1.4 Full Overlap Seal End (FOSE)

The FOSE carton (Fig. 6.4) is generally assembled, filled, and sealed on automatic, horizontal or vertical packaging equipment. The usual sequence for closure is dust flaps in first, followed by the inner closure panels (swinging from

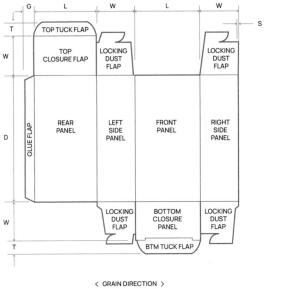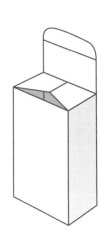

Fig. 6.3 An example of reverse tuck with lock dust flaps carton

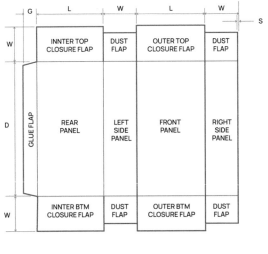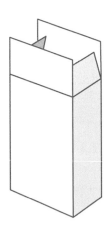

Fig. 6.4 An example of FOSE carton

6 Secondary Packaging and Leaflets: A Glossary

the rear panel) and finally the outer closure panels (swinging from the front panel). Some sift-resistant variations of this style require the inner closure panels to be tucked down first, with the dust flaps next and the outer closure panels last. Partial (POSE) or asymmetric/economy (EOSE) overlapping are also possible.

6.1.5 Tuck and Seal-End with Zipper

This style can be substituted for the FOSE, when having a functional re-closure as well as a secure original closure is important. As indicated Tuck and Seal End Combination with Zipper generally features a zipper.style tear strip in the outer closure panel (Fig. 6.5).

6.1.6 The 1-2-3 Snap-Lock Bottom

Originally known by its inventor's name (Houghland), this style is more generally known today as the 1-2-3 closure (Fig. 6.6). Usually paired with a top tuck closure, the 1-2-3 is almost always employed as a bottom closure and is assembled and sealed manually. This closure style may be applied in a shallow-depth, tube-style counter display carton.

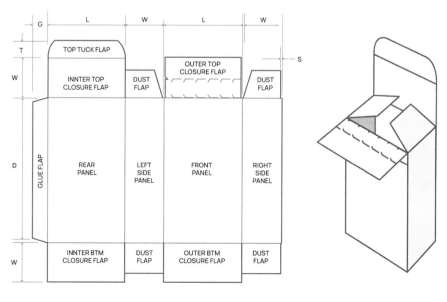

Fig. 6.5 An example of tuck and seal-end carton

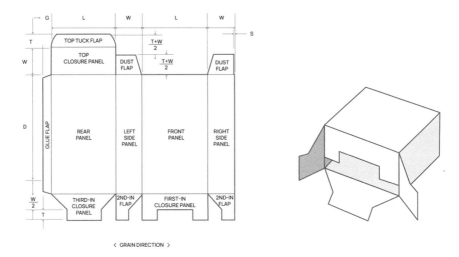

Fig. 6.6 An example of snap-lock bottom carton

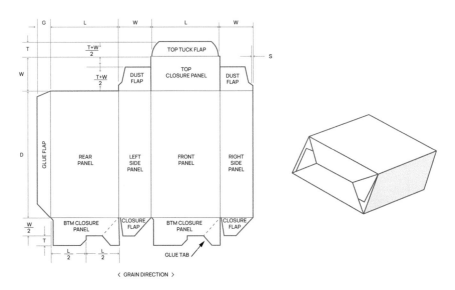

Fig. 6.7 An example of crash-lock carton

6.1.7 Crash-Lock Automatic Bottom

This is a pre-glued and is assembled by hand. It is generally employed when quick setup is required for smaller production volumes that do not warrant investing in automatic packaging equipment (Fig. 6.7).

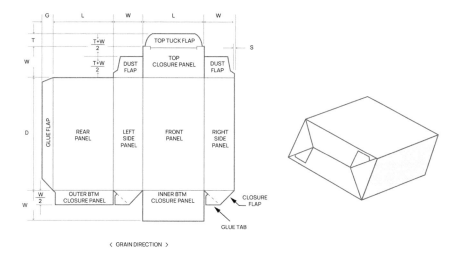

Fig. 6.8 An example of full-flap carton

6.1.8 Full-Flap Automatic Bottom

This is a great solution when the contents are very heavy, or their weight is concentrated on the central axis lengthwise. This style is assembled by hand and is generally employed when quick setup is required for smaller production volumes that do not warrant investing in automatic packaging equipment (Fig. 6.8).

6.2 The Main Typologies of Packaging Leaflets

There are different types of package leaflets. In the following paragraphs, some examples of the most used typologies.

6.2.1 Simple Reel Leaflets

Leaflets are delivered in reel form and then fed to a folding machine in the customer premise before insertion inside the medicine cartons. They contain a limited amount of information compared to other, larger and more complicated flyers. These leaflets are made from mother reels that come off the printing lines and are then cut and rewound. During rewinding, a variable code (flyer numbering) can be printed. The final appearance is a reel of flyers that is packaged in a corrugated cardboard box (Fig. 6.9).

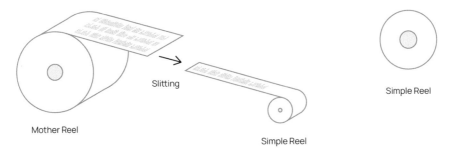

Fig. 6.9 An example of simple reel leaflets

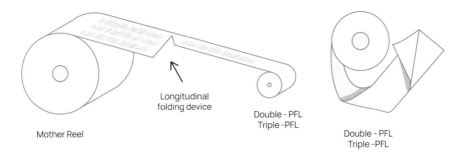

Fig. 6.10 An example of PFL leaflets

6.2.2 Double-Triple Pre-folded Leaflets (PFL)

This product is delivered in reel format. Starting from a mother reel, this is longitudinally half-folded (double-PFL) or three-parts folded (triple-PFL) using a specific machine or tool mounted onto the printing line and re-winded (Fig. 6.10). The final aspect is a reel of leaflets packed in an appropriate corrugated box and contains much more information (double or triple info) than simple reel leaflets. This format is required when Customers have their folding line installed onto a high-speed packing machine. A smaller grammage (37–40 gsm) is preferred for these leaflets resulting in a better longitudinal folding (37 gsm recommended for the triple-PFL formats).

6.2.3 Flat Leaflets

These leaflets require the flat form to be printed on both sides in different dimensions. Before being slit, the printing format is either in sheet form or pile form (e.g., zig-zag) (Fig. 6.11). After slitting in the guillotine, the pile form results in a pre-folded flat leaflet that gives a faster folding performance in the folding machine at the customer premise (due to the initial folding in printing). The pre-folding of this leaflet is obtained by micro-perforation along the whole width. While the width dimension of the sheet compared to the pile can be the same as the length of the sheet format.

Fig. 6.11 An example of flat leaflets

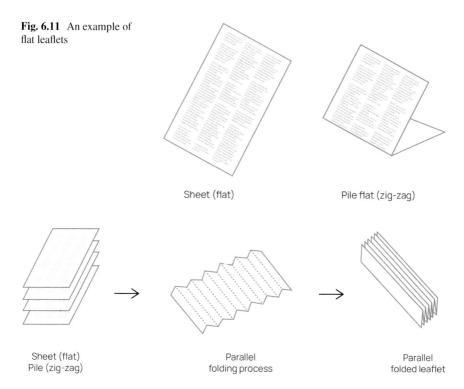

Fig. 6.12 An example of parallel fold leaflets (ECMA—European Carton Makers Association 2013)

6.2.4 Parallel Fold Leaflets (1)

These leaflets (Fig. 6.12) can be produced in different dimensions, according to the customer's needs, starting from a flat leaflet (sheet or pile) or a reel-packed leaflets (e.g., simple rell, 2-PFL or 3-PFL) folded using a specific machine. In the case of reel-fed leaflets, these folding machines are equipped with a cutting station before folding. Usually, customers require this format directly from their leaflet supplier. In this case, the parallel folded leaflets are usually packed in trays and made ready to be fed/inserted into the cartons through leaflets feeder.

6.2.5 Parallel Fold Leaflets (2)

In most cases, feeding these leaflets coincides with feeding the medicine (generally in blister), where the blister engages the leaflet, folds it on the cross-section, and pushes the leaflet inside the carton (Fig. 6.13).

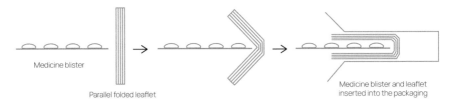

Fig. 6.13 An example of parallel fold leaflets (2)

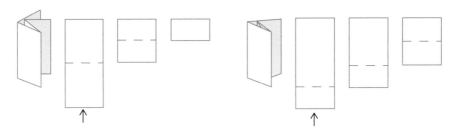

Fig. 6.14 Examples of pure parallel fold (left) and wallet fold (right)

6.2.6 *Parallel Fold Leaflets (3)*

These are the most common parallel fold type for pharmaceutical leaflets, designed in three ways:

- pure parallel fold, namely half-folded each time (Fig. 6.14—left);
- wallet fold, folded over itself each time (Fig. 6.14—right);
- zig-zag fold.

6.2.7 *Cross-Folded Leaflets (1)*

In general, these leaflets are required directly from the leaflets' producer. They are more complicated than the other leaflets, requiring several folding sequences (one or more) in specific machines.

Specifically designed feeders are necessary to insert these leaflets inside the cartons. Depending on the complexity, the additional mechanism and features to hold the leaflets in the cross-folded shape, several families of cross-folded products are available. There are three main categories of cross-folded leaflets:

- open-edge cross-folded, where the two free edges of the folded leaflet are kept free. It is not so used, but in some cases, they are required to simplify the blister insertion as shown in the previous slide;

6 Secondary Packaging and Leaflets: A Glossary

- tagserted cross-folded: the free edged are kept together through a label (tag) that usually is transparent and has a pre-break point to ease the opening of the leaflet;
- outserted cross-folded: same as above but using glue spots instead of a label.

Most complicated tagserted or outserted leaflets foresee the double folding of the free edge (VIJUK technology) to make easy the insertion process avoid that part of the free edge stuck with the cartons making the insertion process more difficult.

6.2.8 Cross-Folded Leaflets (2)

Everything starts from a parallel folded leaflet. Three cross-folded leaflets can be obtained using a specific folding machine (Fig. 6.15):

- Open-edge cross-folded;
- Tagserted cross-folded;
- Outserted cross-folded.

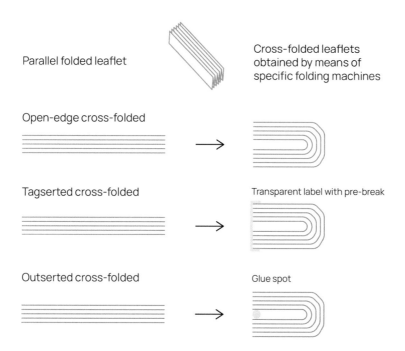

Fig. 6.15 Examples of parallel, open-edge, tagserted, and outserted leaflets

6.2.9 Cross-Folded Leaflets (3)

Folding leaflets can be very complicated and come from a combination of parallel folds and cross folds in various ways, as happens with the combined folds.

6.2.10 Cross-Folded Leaflets (4)

Producers can offer special leaflets that require additional operation to obtain other leaflets. These include up to three outserts folded leaflets (VIJUK type) glued together back-to-back to provide maximum printing space in a compact design and a multi-page folded booklet (e.g., tagserted, outserted and VIJUK type), which offers separate sections for different audiences, marketing purposes and languages.

Reference

ECMA—European Carton Makers Association (2013) Good manufacturing practice guide. V1.1. Retrieved from: https://www.ecma.org/uploads/Bestanden/Publications/GMP/UK%20GMP%20%20Version%201.1%20%2016%2012%202013%20%20-%20FINAL.pdf

Open Access This chapter is licensed under the terms of the Creative Commons Attribution 4.0 International License (http://creativecommons.org/licenses/by/4.0/), which permits use, sharing, adaptation, distribution and reproduction in any medium or format, as long as you give appropriate credit to the original author(s) and the source, provide a link to the Creative Commons license and indicate if changes were made.

The images or other third party material in this chapter are included in the chapter's Creative Commons license, unless indicated otherwise in a credit line to the material. If material is not included in the chapter's Creative Commons license and your intended use is not permitted by statutory regulation or exceeds the permitted use, you will need to obtain permission directly from the copyright holder.

Part II
Prescribing and Dispensing: Accompanying the Patient to the Correct Use of Medicines

Chapter 7
Moving the Care Process in the in-Home Context: The Therapeutic Prescription

Carlo Emilio Standoli, Milena Giovanna Guarinoni, and Enrico Morello

Abstract After a medical consultation or hospitalisation, when the patient returns to everyday life, how is the correct adherence and therapeutic continuity guaranteed according to the indications given by the clinician, especially when it comes to multidimensional therapy (e.g. pharmacological, rehabilitation, etc.)? Do clinicians and hospitals use communication strategies and tools to give indications—through prescriptions—of sometimes complex therapies to be followed effectively? Moreover, what tools does the patient have to tell the general practitioner about the therapies in use or support therapy management at home? In the specific case of medicines, what dialogue is established between doctor and patient to assess the appropriateness of their prescription, considering not only clinical needs but also the patient's lifestyle and preferences? The chapter addresses the process of transitioning care from the hospital to the home setting, presenting the different phases and issues that, on the medical side and the patient side, are experienced from the moment of prescription. The emerging reflections form the basis for formulating perspectives for future models of transition of care and discharge.

7.1 From Hospitalisation to Home: The Discharge Process

Looking at the discharge process without going into the peculiarities of the wards' specialities and the acuity and severity of the patient's condition, the discharge process begins when a patient is considered sufficiently cured to continue care elsewhere, whether in the home setting or another healthcare facility. In the Italian context, in the implementation of the organisational model of the territorial care network (Ministry of Health 2022), home care is to be strengthened, both through

---

C. E. Standoli (✉)
Department of Design, Politecnico di Milano, Milan, Italy
e-mail: carloemilio.standoli@polimi.it

M. G. Guarinoni · E. Morello
ASST Spedali Civili di Brescia, Brescia, Italy

Università degli Studi di Brescia, Brescia, Italy

home-based services and telemedicine, with the support of centres such as the Case di Comunità (Community Centres), in which general practitioners and other specialists are located. With this in mind, hospitals are mainly delegated to intensive care (Ministero della Salute 2024). This structural and organisational change in the health system makes it possible to reduce hospitalisation times by promoting territorial management of the patient: continuity between the hospital, the territory and the home context thus assumes a crucial role. If one then examines the dimension of punctual knowledge of pharmacological therapy, it is necessary to be aware of all the information to manage the patient from the moment of admission, during the period of hospitalisation and at the time of discharge. This precise knowledge represents a guarantee for continuity and adherence to treatment and to avoid any accidental and unintentional discrepancy, which could represent a risk for the patient (Ministry of Health 2014). Precisely to address these risks, the World Health Organisation (WHO) recommends Pharmacological Recognition and Reconciliation interventions aimed at preventing medication errors in the transitions between hospitalisation and return to the home setting (Ministry of Health 2014; WHO 2017).

Pharmacological therapy recognition refers to the process by which information is collected in a systematic, accurate and complete manner on the medicines taken by the patient: this recognition concerns medicines classified by the Italian Medicines Agency (AIFA) subject to restrictive prescription, medicines without prescription (*Senza Obbligo di Prescrizione*—SOP), medicines over the counter (OTC), and even homoeopathic medicines, phytotherapeutic medicines, and possible behaviours such as drug taking, smoking and alcohol consumption. Concerning medicines, the information that is collected is (Ministero della Salute 2014)

- the commercial name and/or active ingredient;
- the pharmaceutical form;
- the dosage;
- the daily dosage;
- the start date and duration of therapy;
- the date and time of the last dose taken (with particular attention to long-acting formulations);
- the route of administration;
- any experimental treatments, including compassionate use and off-label drugs (in particular the therapeutic indication);
- the intake of homoeopathic, phytotherapeutic and supplementary medicines and any other product of non-conventional medicine;
- the presence of known pathologies, allergies or intolerances;
- previous therapies and any undesirable effects;
- intake of foods (high doses of grapefruit, coffee, tea, fruit and vegetables) that may interfere with the therapy;
- the patient's weight and height data;
- lifestyle (possible alcohol intake, smoking and drug use);
- use of medicated medical devices;
- any other data considered significant.

Usually, it is appropriate for the patient to communicate all these data as they are not only therapeutic, but also behavioural and routine in nature; alternatively, in extraordinary cases such as the patient's non-cooperation, demographic factors such as age, or other cases, a family member or caregiver may communicate this information. In the latter case, the doctor must keep track of the source, in case of subsequent changes and additions.

In the ward, before the adoption of a new pharmacological therapy or the integration or substitution of certain medicines (e.g., by active ingredient, dosage, pharmaceutical form, possible drug interactions, etc.), the physician double-checks the Reconciliation document and compares it with what should be the new treatment plan. This phase, called reconciliation, serves to identify any inconsistencies between the treatment plan or critical issues such as interactions, contraindications, possible confusions due to Look Alike Sound Alike Drugs (LASA), and all the information released by AIFA. Regional procedures concerning the *Prontuario Terapeutico* (therapeutic handbook) and territorial continuity management are considered in the Italian context. In the two stages of recognition and reconciliation, the hospital pharmacist always supports the doctor. The person in charge of monitoring and taking charge of the management of the patient's drug therapy on the ward is the ward nursing coordinator.

In these two phases, the physician must communicate effectively with the patient, family members, and caregivers. In the reconciliation phase, dialogue is essential to understand the pharmacological plan and any factors that may influence it; in the reconciliation phase, it is necessary to inform and make the patient, family member and caregiver understand the modification actions that will be implemented. In fact, the patient should be informed about aspects related to the therapy in the strict sense (e.g. possible risks and contraindications, dosages, pharmaceutical form, etc.) that could influence acceptance and adherence to the therapy in the ward context. This first level of communication about the therapy may also form a basis for the establishment of trust and an ongoing relationship between the patient and the ward healthcare staff, another element that may influence acceptance and adherence to the therapy in the hospital setting and subsequently in the home setting (WHO 2017).

As mentioned above, at the end of the hospitalisation period, when the ward staff considers that the patient can be effectively treated elsewhere or is sufficiently healed, the hospital discharge process begins. Usually, this process is divided into two phases: the first one, which is managed by the medical staff, consists of a concluding visit in which all therapeutic activities (e.g. drug therapy management, rehabilitation activities, nutrition management, forthcoming outpatient/ambulatory meetings, etc.) detailed follow-up instructions are also communicated. In addition, the physician should ensure that the patient, family member or caregiver has correctly understood all the information. The doctor is also in charge of updating the pharmacological therapy, with an additional recognition and reconciliation analysis, and completing the discharge letter, which the patient will hand over to the General Practitioner. The second phase, managed by the nursing staff, delivers all the material, from the medical record to the discharge letter. Then, the nursing staff reinforce the pharmacological management with medication boxes and an explanation of the correct medication management (e.g. medication to be kept in the refrigerator). Any deadlines for medication of central venous accesses or wounds are recommended.

The discharge letter is one of the tools allowing continuity of care and assistance because it puts the ward from which the patient is discharged in contact with the general practitioner and the specialists who will take care of the patient. The discharge letter is structured on the basis of regional guidelines and must take into account this information:

- the patient's personal data;
- the reason for admission;
- date of discharge;
- objective examination;
- procedures performed (e.g. laboratory tests, instrumental tests, consultations, reports, etc.);
- diagnosis;
- diagnostic and/or therapeutic programme and follow-up;
- any prescribed therapies at home;
- any new appointments for outpatient examinations or subsequent hospitalisation or inpatient stay, or new examinations to be taken;
- personal data and signature of the doctor.

The discharge letter may include information sheets for nutrition and self-care management. Concerning pharmacological therapy, the specialist doctor reports in the discharge letter both the therapy prescriptions necessary to medicines' dispense, and the discharge therapy proposals, i.e. the indications for the decision of competence addressed to the general practitioner (Emilia-Romagna Region 2024).

When compiling the new therapeutic plan, the doctor must ensure that the selected drugs comply with the prescriptibility and appropriateness rules indicated in the AIFA Notes (AIFA 2023), which define the reimbursability of the drug at the expense of the National Health System (*Sistema Sanitario Nazionale,* SSN); the impossibility of charging the SSN is reported; the active ingredients are present in the *Prontuari Terapeutici Aziendali*, to guarantee greater affordability of the drug (Regione Veneto 2023).

In the therapeutic prescription document, depending on the patient's needs, the doctor may indicate the following types of medicine (Regione Veneto 2023)

- Medicines subject to specialist prescription, namely all those medicines listed by AIFA as subject to prescription and which require a dematerialised or red paper prescription, and class C medicines and not reimbursed by the SSN, which require a white prescription on the doctor's letterhead;
- non-prescription medicines, namely those recommended by the hospital specialist doctor, subject to a repeatable, non-repeatable, or non-prescription prescription. In this case, the hospital specialist doctor will indicate the active ingredient, and then the general practitioner will fill out the dematerialised prescription or red paper prescription. As in the previous case, the hospital specialist will fill out the white prescription on letterhead for class C medicines, and the patient can purchase the medicine at their own expense.

- Medicines used for acute treatment, namely those medicines for which the hospital specialist may directly fill a dematerialised prescription or red paper prescription and which can be dispensed directly from the hospital pharmacy. In this case, the hospital specialist will fill out a white prescription on letterhead for class C medicines, and the patient can purchase the medicine at their own expense.

In specific cases, the hospital dispenses certain medicines to safeguard the continuation of the patient's care outside the hospital setting, guarantee a quick start of the therapy, and support proper adherence (Regione Veneto 2023).

Due to many factors, such as organisational (e.g., the amount of time spent by medical staff on communication with the patient, or the amount of information to be managed and assimilated in a short time by the patient or caregiver), social and cultural (e.g., the degree of medical literacy of the patient, family member or caregiver, or knowledge of the language), emotional (e.g., the vulnerability of the patient, the degree of stress due to admission or discharge), make the moment of care transition and discharge highly critical for the proper passage of information between hospital, territory and patient, and potentially at risk of re-hospitalisation (Forster et al. 2003; Jencks et al. 2009). Especially in the transition from acute to chronic patient, and in the case of patients with multi-morbidity and polypharmacy, it is necessary to understand the leading causes for non-adherence to therapies to develop strategies and implement virtuous mechanisms to support home care and therapy.

7.2 The Discharge Process' Actors

In the discharge letter, the hospital specialist indicates the therapy to be followed at home, having multiple interlocutors. The transition of care from hospital to home is a complex phase involving the specialist, the hospital nurse, the general practitioner, the patient, and, if needed by the patient, the caregiver. The integration of these players, through a greater understanding of the social and health needs and the patient's wishes, through health literacy, leads to improved health outcomes in patients who have to undergo long-term home care.

An ever-present interlocutor is the general practitioner, the professional who takes over the patient's care once discharged. The general practitioner prescribes the person's medication once at home and, therefore, becomes the basic interlocutor. The general practitioner may agree with the hospital specialist and, therefore, continue with the prescription indicated in the discharge letter, or disagree and introduce changes to the hospital's recommendations. The motivations that may lead the general practitioner to make changes in the therapy may be manifold: knowledge of the patient's overall clinical situation (e.g. concomitance of other therapies, lack of efficacy of the molecule in the long term, etc.), but also of the social situation (e.g. impossibility of managing parenteral therapies, etc.).

Another interlocutor of the hospital prescribing specialist is the person responsible for the practical management of the therapy administration. This figure may be the caregiver (for patients such as children, elderly, disabled, etc.), or the patient themselves. The caregiver is a figure who may be a family member or takes care of the person at home for work. Whoever the caregiver is, in the transition between the hospital and the home, they must manage the therapy precisely prescribed by the hospital, respecting the correct medicine, route of administration, dosage, and time.

However, the hospital specialist prescriber's main interlocutor remains the patient, with the burden of experiences, knowledge and education. If, during hospitalisation, the patient can live an experience of "reliance", willingly accepting all that is proposed in terms of therapy, when returning home, the patient experiences a re-appropriation of their life and habits, which may lead them to experience therapy differently from the hospital situation. For this reason, the hospital prescriber should first share the therapeutic pathway with the patient, listening carefully to the needs and wishes of the patient, who is the subject of their own health.

7.2.1 The Acute Patient

Complex patients discharged from ultra-specialist wards (e.g. bone marrow transplantation) represent the borderline information management case between hospital and home. The discharge letter represents the instrument on which therapeutic prescriptions are implemented at the patient's home with the caregiver's contribution and the general practitioner's supervision. In this setting, the general practitioner often does not represent a resource because the specialist department still manages the post-discharge course. Furthermore, the polypharmacological management of therapies, including immunosuppressants, whose plasma monitoring is performed by the hospital, excludes the general practitioner from being an active part of the process. The discharge letter is presented as the first information tool and is explained using an interview as accurately as possible, specifying the indications that emerged from admission, the drugs recommended at home and the subsequent follow-up:

- indications on admission: the discharge letter presents a large body of information structuring the hospital course based on the clinical course and the main events recorded during admission. The final part of this section identifies the main unresolved or ongoing clinical elements that the general practitioner or post-hospitalisation specialists can take care of.
- Pharmacological therapy is usually prescribed in order of importance according to the specialist's treatment principles (e.g. immunosuppressive drugs first, then anti-infectives, then those for any comorbidities or ancillary to the treatments as mentioned above). All drugs are usually indicated with the active ingredient (sometimes with the trade name if the active ingredient is too long or complex), the recommended dosage, and the administration time. If necessary, a section

may be supplemented with nutritional supplements, vitamins, and foods for particular medical purposes.

The last section indicates the recommended behaviour at home under normal conditions and in the event of complications (e.g. fever, respiratory difficulties, diarrhoea, etc.) and the subsequent day hospital or outpatient appointments and the behaviour to be adopted (e.g. do not take immunosuppressive drugs before their plasma dosage is taken).

7.2.2 The Chronic Patient

In oncology, the development of molecular-targeted therapies has enabled the chronic treatment of patients previously only eligible for chemotherapy. The relative manageability of such treatments has made it possible to treat an increasingly elderly population with various comorbidities. In this setting, therefore, elderly patients are forced to handle increasingly complex therapies. A helpful tool for the home management of drugs can be colour coding. According to a specific criterion, therapy sheets with coloured charts are printed, and envelopes of the established colour are prepared to contain the prescribed drugs. In this case, management by the patient and caregiver can be facilitated by referring to certain times of the day and possible therapies as needed. To further reduce errors, a healthcare professional's constant monitoring of the treatment, prescription sheets, envelopes, and any deadlines would be recommended.

7.3 Home Care Between Therapeutic Adherence and Non-adherence

With the progressive increase in life expectancy (WHO 2021) and with the definition of new paradigms of care that tend to empower the patient, one's family, caregivers and community medicine, the correct adherence to therapy—not only pharmacological—becomes crucial for the well-being of the person.

In the case of pharmacological therapy, we can refer to adherence as the extent to which a patient takes medication as indicated and prescribed by their doctor (Osterberg and Blaschke 2005). Pharmacological therapeutic adherence has to consider the achievement of two main goals related to medicine consumption: the prescribed modalities, namely taking into account the type of medicine, the timing, the quantity, and the consumption patterns, and the time, namely taking into account the constancy and continuity in taking medicine (Brown et al. 2016).

It is easy to administer the right drug when there is only one or two to manage. However, if we think that, often, the patient takes a multiplicity of medicines, it becomes complex: at 8 a.m., which medicines do I have to take? Which ones are on a full stomach, and which should be taken between meals? Speaking of administration routes, it is relatively simple if I have tablets to take orally (actually, problems may arise if the patient is unable to swallow a tablet and it is not known whether it can be crushed, dissolved in a liquid, etc.); it gets more complicated if the route is parenteral, rectal, etc. Speaking of dosage, if it is stated 'one tablet in the morning, two in the evening', there should be no problem understanding; it is different if the indication is 2 g × 2, or 150 ml every 12 h.

All this, together with the correct home storage of the medicines (bear in mind that some medicines must always be stored at controlled temperatures, in their original undamaged packaging; some, once reconstituted or diluted, must be consumed in a very short time, etc.), and the control of expiry dates, makes the management of the medicine at home much more complex than in the hospital environment where professionals are trained in these aspects.

In the home setting, it is very challenging to acquire qualitative and quantitative data on therapeutic adherence and, of all the tools to acquire data (e.g., questionnaires, interviews, self-reporting, instrumental analysis), none of them can be considered accurate and precise (Lavsa et al. 2011). Causes that may influence adherence include factors such as the complexity of the therapy or drug interaction, as with LASA (Giannetta et al. 2019), socio-demographic, socio-cultural and socio-economic factors (Napolitano et al. 2016; Sampaio et al. 2020), non-understanding of pharmacological therapy (Napolitano et al. 2016; Pasina et al. 2014) or prescription errors (Dionisi et al. 2022), patient's beliefs and concerns concerning treatment (Hughes 2004; Osterberg and Blaschke 2005), the relationship with one's doctor (Phatak and Thomas III 2006; Gallé et al. 2021), factors related to the physical characteristics of the drug or its management and accessibility (Jansà et al. 2010; Napolitano et al. 2016), or lack of motivation concerning the care pathway (Brown et al. 2016), especially among chronic patients, or the absence of a caregiver.

The data concerning polypharmacy are substantial: in Italy alone, among people over 65 years of age, at least a quarter of them consume at least 10 different medicines daily (AIFA 2024), increasing the risk of error due to forgetfulness, confusion between types of medicine, drug-drug or drug-food interactions, reduced motivation, etc. Voluntary withdrawal or its modification without medical consultation—due to a lack of motivation or a perceived change in health status, for the better or for the worse—are among the most recurrent causes of non-adherence (Pasina et al. 2014). Another phenomenon observed is what is referred to as 'white coat adherence': adherence and compliance vary in the period between two medical visits, as the patient changes his or her drug-taking behaviour just around the time of the visits (Osterberg and Blaschke 2005; Pasina et al. 2014). This behaviour also generates difficulties in defining the actual adherence to therapy with clinical analyses.

Therefore, many concauses influence therapeutic adherence. First and foremost, the human factor, including the patient, family members and caregivers, and general practitioners, hospital specialists and nurses, through to pharmacists. The complexity of communication is seen from the perspective of language and literacy, as well as the ability to empathise. The medicine in its material, formal dimension, how it is consumed and the gestures and rituals it creates. The complexity of the processes, from prescription to dispensing to consumption. Reflection on therapeutic adherence requires a reflection that is not reductionist, linked only to therapy compliance, in other words as that passive behaviour in which the patient follows a list of instructions from the doctor (Mir 2023), but from a transdisciplinary and people-centred perspective, starting from the patient to the medical and healthcare personnel.

7.4 Perspectives to Support a Person-Centred Transition of Care

Prescriptive appropriateness, meaning prescribing the right medicine to the right patient at the right time, requires an accurate quality pathway to ensure patient safety. This pathway is left to the initiative of individual patients. However, it needs to be better structured already in the planning phase of the treatment pathway, integrating the patient's needs according to their requirements (e.g. education, social context, IT skills, etc.) with the needs of professionals. A collaborative process between the different actors involved could support defining the best prescriptive pathway for the individual patient.

In this sense, a first perspective of intervention concerns the patient's discharge process. The patient is truly ready for discharge concerning the time spent communicating and verifying all the necessary information (Facchinetti et al. 2021), to rehearse the care processes that will have to take place in the home context. This training must also involve family members and caregivers, who are very often the ones who take charge and are the custodians of the information of the entire care process (Bragstad et al. 2014; Hagedoorn et al. 2017). A hasty discharge preparation, without the active involvement of family members and caregivers, in the absence of empathy towards what the patient feels, with partial or wrong information, is the first step towards a subsequent re-hospitalisation of the patient.

A perspective of intervention may, therefore concern nursing education and practice, both within the hospital as well as in the territory and at home: the period of transition of care should consider practical and organisational aspects and an increase in the time spent with the patient, to transmit and verify knowledge and skills appropriate to the management of therapy. The nursing staff should be recognised and valued as the guarantor of the transition and continuity of care (Facchinetti et al. 2021). Successful transition of care and discharge also depends on designing interventions and activities that are adapted to the patient's characteristics, skills, and beliefs (McDonald et al. 2002), thus abandoning the reductionist dimension of care to consider the individual's complexity.

The transition of care and the move to the home setting must not represent the end of the relationship between the patient and the staff who cared for the patient. In this, the role of the General Practitioner and their involvement before discharge and during the transition of care becomes paramount (Facchinetti et al. 2021). In addition, the use of different platforms for communication, from telehealth to e-health to more accessible objects and applications adapted to the home context, may represent further levers for increasing motivation and improving therapeutic adherence.

Providing clear and timely instructions and reducing the complexity of pharmacological therapies as much as possible can be further levers towards adherence to medication regimes (Pasina et al. 2014). Recognition and reconciliation therapy actions are necessary to reduce potentially inappropriate prescriptions, to decrease the risk of adverse drug reactions, to simplify and communicate the pharmacological regimen and to keep the person in control and involved in decision-making processes. Active collaboration and networking between patients, relatives, general practitioners, pharmacists, ward doctors and nurses, and pharmacologists is necessary to create and disseminate information for more effective care. Creating, or rather structuring and coordinating, already existing communities of practice, which necessarily share an interest in their own and others' care processes, is a necessary perspective for defining strategies and mechanisms for social innovation in the transition of care.

References

Agenzia Italiana del Farmaco—AIFA (2023) Rapporti Osservatorio Nazionale sull'Impiego dei Medicinali. L'uso dei Farmaci in Italia. Rapporto Nazionale anno 2022. https://www.aifa.gov.it/documents/20142/1967301/Rapporto-OsMed-2022.pdf

Agenzia Italiana del Farmaco—AIFA (2024) Elenco note AIFA. https://www.aifa.gov.it/elenco-note-aifa

Bragstad LK, Kirkevold M, Foss C (2014) The indispensable intermediaries: a qualitative study of informal caregivers' struggle to achieve influence at and after hospital discharge. BMC Health Serv Res 14:1–12

Brown MT, Bussell J, Dutta S, Davis K, Strong S, Mathew S (2016) Medication adherence: truth and consequences. Am J Med Sci 351(4):387–399

Dionisi S, Di Simone E, Liquori G, De Leo A, Di Muzio M, Giannetta N (2022) Medication errors' causes analysis in home care setting: a systematic review. Public Health Nurs 39(4):876–897

Facchinetti G, Albanesi B, Piredda M, Marchetti A, Ausili D, Ianni A, Di Mauro S, De Marinis MG (2021) "The light at the end of the tunnel". Discharge experience of older patients with chronic diseases: a multi-centre qualitative study. J Adv Nurs 77(5):2417–2428

Forster AJ, Murff HJ, Peterson JF, Gandhi TK, Bates DW (2003) The incidence and severity of adverse events affecting patients after discharge from the hospital. Ann Intern Med 138(3):161–167

Gallè F, Sabella EA, Roma P, Da Molin G, Diella G, Montagna MT, Ferracuti S, Liguori G, Orsi GB, Napoli C (2021) Acceptance of COVID-19 vaccination in the elderly: a cross-sectional study in Southern Italy. Vaccine 9(11):1222

Giannetta N, Dionisi S, Ricciardi F, Di Muzio F, Penna G, Diella G, Di Simone E, Di Muzio M (2019) Farmaci LASA: strategie per la prevenzione dell'errore di terapia [Look-alike, sound-alike drugs. Strategies for preventing medication errors]. G Ital Farm Clin 33(3):119–128

Hagedoorn EI, Paans W, Jaarsma T, Keers JC, van der Schans C, Luttik ML (2017) Aspects of family caregiving as addressed in planned discussions between nurses, patients with chronic diseases and family caregivers: a qualitative content analysis. BMC Nurs 16:1–10

Hughes CM (2004) Medication non-adherence in the elderly: how big is the problem? Drugs Aging 21:793–811

Jansà M, Hernández C, Vidal M, Nuñez M, Bertran MJ, Sanz S, Castell C, Sanz G (2010) Multidimensional analysis of treatment adherence in patients with multiple chronic conditions. A cross-sectional study in a tertiary hospital. Patient Educ Couns 81(2):161–168

Jencks SF, Williams MV, Coleman EA (2009) Rehospitalizations among patients in the Medicare fee-for-service program. N Engl J Med 360(14):1418–1428

Lavsa SM, Holzworth A, Ansani NT (2011) Selection of a validated scale for measuring medication adherence. J Am Pharm Assoc 51(1):90–94

McDonald HP, Garg AX, Haynes RB (2002) Interventions to enhance patient adherence to medication prescriptions: scientific review. JAMA 288(22):2868–2879

Ministero della Salute (2014) Raccomandazione n.17. Raccomandazione per la riconciliazione della terapia farmacologica. https://www.salute.gov.it/imgs/C_17_pubblicazioni_2354_allegato.pdf

Ministero della Salute (2022) PNRR—Missione 6 Salute. https://www.pnrr.salute.gov.it/portale/pnrrsalute/homePNRRSalute.jsp

Ministero della Salute (2024) Il nuovo modello di assistenza territoriale in un'ottica One Health. https://www.pnrr.salute.gov.it/portale/pnrrsalute/dettaglioContenutiPNRRSalute.jsp?lingua=italiano&id=5828&area=PNRR-Salute&menu=comecambiassn

Mir TH (2023) Adherence versus compliance. HCA Healthc J Med 4(2):219

Napolitano F, Napolitano P, Angelillo IF, Collaborative Working Group (2016) Medication adherence among patients with chronic conditions in Italy. Eur J Pub Health 26(1):48–52

Osterberg L, Blaschke T (2005) Adherence to medication. N Engl J Med 353(5):487–497

Pasina L, Brucato A L, Falcone C, Cucchi E , Bresciani A, Sottocorno M, Taddei G C, Casati M, Franchi C, Djade C D, Nobili A (2014) Medication non-adherence among elderly patients newly discharged and receiving polypharmacy. Drugs & aging 31:283–289.

Phatak HM, Thomas J III (2006) Relationships between beliefs about medications and nonadherence to prescribed chronic medications. Ann Pharmacother 40(10):1737–1742

Regione Emilia-Romagna (2024). Gestione prescrizioni medicinali inclusi in referti digitali. https://www.ordinefarmacistimo.it/index.php?option=com_content&view=article&id=2923:gestione-prescrizioni-medicinali-incluse-in-referti-digitali&catid=174:circolari-2024&Itemid=129

Regione Veneto (2023) Linee di indirizzo regionale. La continuità terapeutica ospedale-territorio. https://www.sifoweb.it/images/pdf/attivita/sezioni-regionali/veneto/Comunicazione/nota_regionale_124223-23_continuit%C3%A0_terapeutica_Ospedale_Territorio.PDF

Sampaio R, Azevedo LF, Dias CC, Castro Lopes JM (2020) Non-adherence to pharmacotherapy: a prospective multicentre study about its incidence and its causes perceived by chronic pain patients. Patient Prefer Adherence:321–332

World Health Organisation—WHO (2021) Ageing and health. https://www.who.int/news-room/fact-sheets/detail/ageing-and-health

World Health Organization—WHO (2017) Medication without harm. https://www.who.int/initiatives/medication-without-harm

Open Access This chapter is licensed under the terms of the Creative Commons Attribution 4.0 International License (http://creativecommons.org/licenses/by/4.0/), which permits use, sharing, adaptation, distribution and reproduction in any medium or format, as long as you give appropriate credit to the original author(s) and the source, provide a link to the Creative Commons license and indicate if changes were made.

The images or other third party material in this chapter are included in the chapter's Creative Commons license, unless indicated otherwise in a credit line to the material. If material is not included in the chapter's Creative Commons license and your intended use is not permitted by statutory regulation or exceeds the permitted use, you will need to obtain permission directly from the copyright holder.

Chapter 8
Dispensing Medicines: A Necessary Link Between Doctor and Patient

Antonella Valeria Penati

Abstract Based on a broad body of literature, the chapter highlights the plethora of problems surrounding dispensing. These include the information gaps that punctuate the transition between prescription and dispensation, the inadequacy of the documentary supports (medical prescription, therapeutic plan, the patient's pharmacological history, information on current therapies, etc.), a not always transparent allocation of information tasks concerning the medical doctor and the pharmacist. The main insights that have oriented the research on the dispensary context are also presented: the focus on environmental requirements (organisation of space; logistics of pharmaceutical products; lighting, ambient noise), the emphasis on work organisation requirements (allocation of tasks to staff; task overload; task diversification), and the focus on the transformation of the pharmacy's nature from a place for dispensing medicines to a place for selling para pharmaceutical products and providing service). In particular, the chapter focuses on the limitations and problems associated with the prescription and packaging of medicine because of their importance in the dispensing phase.

8.1 Between Prescription and Dispensation: No Man's Land

The prescription of a medicine constitutes the final act in the diagnostic process. It is one of the prerogatives and responsibilities of the medical doctor, who "has autonomy in the planning, choice and application of every […] therapeutic aid. […] The doctor is required to have adequate knowledge of the nature and effects of drugs, their indications, contraindications, interactions, and foreseeable individual reactions, as well as the characteristics of the use of […] therapeutic means […]" (the Italian Code of Medical Deontology, art. 12, pp. 10–12)

The dispensing of medicine "is a medical act to protect the health and psychophysical integrity of the patient. […] It is the exclusive prerogative of the pharmacist who is required to ensure adherence to pharmacological therapies, contributing to a higher level of effectiveness

---

A. V. Penati (✉)
Department of Design, Politecnico di Milano, Milan, Italy
e-mail: antonella.penati@polimi.it

© The Author(s) 2025
A. V. Penati (ed.), *In-Home Medication*, Research for Development,
https://doi.org/10.1007/978-3-031-53294-8_8

of treatment. […] The pharmacist's responsible for "rejecting applications for medicines without the prescribed medical prescription […] or made on prescriptions that do not meet the requirements established by law. […] except in cases of urgency […]. The dispensing of prescription medicines is subject to verification by the pharmacist of the formal and substantive requirements of the prescription to guarantee the protection of the patient's health. […] If necessary, the pharmacist […] shall, before dispensing the medicine, contact the doctor […] for the necessary clarification. The dispensing activity is not only a technical activity but also an activity of professional advice and counselling. In fact, the pharmacist is obliged to "provide clear, correct and complete health information, with particular reference to the appropriate use of medicines, their contraindications and interactions, side effects and their storage" (the Italian Pharmacists' Code of Ethics, 2018, Articles 8; 12; 13; 15).

A reading in sequence of the Italian Code of Medical Deontology and the Italian Pharmacists' Code of Ethics, giving each of the actors involved a specific role, seems to recompose the various stages necessary to make the medicine available to the patient, within a unitary process, guaranteeing its safe and informed use.

And yet, the process that theoretically seems seamless presents, as widely documented in the literature, several 'gaps' and critical situations. These gaps arise above all from a lack of communication and inadequate transmission of information between actors in the system: the pharmaceutical industry, the specialist or hospital doctor, the general practitioner, the pharmacist, and the patient. Despite robust legislation, communication connection tools are scarce.

The dialogue between doctor and patient is partly verbal and partly rendered in documents such as:

- the Medical Record or the Letter of Discharge (after a hospitalisation) showing the treatment carried out, the diagnosis, the therapy carried out at home, the dosage and, not infrequently, during and after the treatment, diagnostic exams necessary to detect values that the therapy might alter;
- the report for the general practitioner (after a specialist examination), giving the diagnosis, therapy, dosage and, not infrequently, during and after treatment, diagnostic exams necessary to detect values that the therapy might alter;
- a brief note, not always present (after a general practitioner's visit), to remind the patient of the dosage of the prescribed medicines;
- the prescription, which acts as a 'witness' in the passage of information between doctor and pharmacist. It is not intended for the patient, who merely transfers the prescription from the prescriber to the dispenser.

As sources of information, the patient has:

- the Package Leaflet, arriving in the patient's hands together with the medicine and formulated to address the doctor, the pharmacist, and the patient simultaneously. Actors with very different information needs;
- the secondary packaging of the medicine, guiding the selection of the medicine at the time of dispensing, with its information apparatus.

A study conducted in Northern Europe on the information needs shown by patients concerning therapies finds that, in addition to the doctor (in first place) and the pharmacist (in third place), the patient reads the package leaflet (in second place) to supplement the information needed to follow the therapy correctly (Mamena et al. 2015). In assessing this attitude towards information, it must be considered that not all patients feel they can turn to the pharmacist for information on how best to manage their therapy.

An observational study based on the transcription of 189 outpatient encounters followed by interviews and carried out 1 week after the visit, found that 49% of the recommendations made by the physicians were remembered accurately without being prompted by the interviewer; 36% were remembered with prompting; 15% were remembered incorrectly or not at all. These percentages decrease significantly if the patient's schooling is low (Barton Laws et al. 2018).

A further study showed that the shortening of hospital stays and the trend towards outpatient care have increased patients' need for specific information even though, as the results of the study show, patients can remember very little of the information they received from the doctor (Kessels 2003). Contributing to this poor result are the patient's memory, the patient's ability to understand the information given by the doctor, whether the information is written down or transmitted verbally, the patient's instruction, and the doctor's use of medical jargon. The study rates the immediate removal of the information supplied by health professionals at between 40% and 80%. It also notes that the greater the amount of information presented, the lower the percentage of remembered correctly. About 50% consists of erroneous or faulty recollections of the information received (Kessels 2003). The lack of a document with a predefined format to help the doctor and pharmacist in giving directions to the patient and the patient in having the information available in a neat and searchable way over time, probably contributes to this.

When the patient comes to the pharmacy for medicine dispensing, pharmacists have the prescription as the only formal information at their disposal. They do not necessarily know the patient to whom they are dispensing the medicine—their medical and pharmacological history. In the case of first-hand familiarity with the patient, they may base their judgement on information 'reported' by the patient or—as we shall see—by tracing back through the laptop to previous medicines purchased from the pharmacy. In both cases, these are unreliable sources.

In this context, to build up an overall picture of helpful information for correctly managing the therapy, the patient must autonomously collect and reconstruct the elements provided fragmentarily by medical documentation, information dispensed by the doctor and pharmacist, and information on the package leaflet.

Information gaps are at the root of the many errors and problems at the dispensing stage.

8.2 Errors in Dispensing

> The National Coordinating Council for Medication Error Reporting and Prevention (NCCMERP) from the United States defines medication error as "any preventable event that may cause or lead to inappropriate medication use or patient harm, while the medica-

tion is in the control of the health-care professional, patient or consumer (Martìnez Sànchez 2013, p. 185)

The chapter stems from the analysis and comparison of the extensive international literature on errors in the dispensing phase and, more generally, on the problems connected with this activity.

The aim is to return the errors most frequently observed when analysing the dispensing activity, the phases in which they occur, and the possible causes, to build a reference framework for the definition of recommendations and design interventions to mitigate errors and encourage better communication between doctor, pharmacist, and patient. As we have already mentioned, many of the errors complained of in the literature originate precisely from the lack of tools to facilitate information exchange between the system's actors (Cohen 1999).

Even though our reflections are based on quantitative data, they avoid referring to statistical data and the formulation of error 'rankings'. This is because, when comparing different studies, it is necessary to address a few methodological issues for the comparison to be rigorous and the data to be meaningful. But also, because errors in healthcare—focusing on medicine dispensing activities—are worthy of attention, because these are common errors that can lead to high morbidity and even fatal outcomes. We refer to the sources analysed in more detail regarding percentage data and refer to the tables in Sect. 8.2 of this book for error statistics. In the following, we will devote ourselves to reconstructing an organic picture of the problems relating to dispensing medicine for the critical aspects detectable in this activity. Due to the point of observation assumed in this book, we will focus on errors that may arise from the doctor's prescription and the medicine's secondary packaging while attempting to give a broad overview of the criticalities of the dispensing moment.

Concerning the comparability of data from different studies, we are interested here to note that, while there is large-scale research relating to errors in the dispensing of medicines in hospital settings, it is more difficult to find a systematic study of a similar nature concerning dispensing in territorial pharmacies (Flynn et al. 2002; Hoxsie et al. 2006; Franklin and O'Grady 2007; Aldhwaihi et al. 2016).

This shortcoming emerges in the literature where it is difficult to find comparable outcomes, lacking a shared approach. The results of the different sources are not easily integrated or recomposable, depending on the research methods, the starting operational definitions, the context of analysis, the delivery system, and the errors' classification criteria (James et al. 2009). Below is a list, as exhaustive as possible, of elements and criteria to be considered to construct the correct premises for making the collected data comparable:

Typological-dimensional characteristics

- Public or municipal pharmacies;
- Private pharmacies;
- Community pharmacies/service pharmacies;
- National single-brand pharmacy chains;
- International single-brand pharmacy chains;

8 Dispensing Medicines: A Necessary Link Between Doctor and Patient

- Online pharmacies;
- Large retailers (for non-prescription medicines);
- Size of the pharmacy concerning the territorial basin served;
- Number and qualification of staff in the pharmacies surveyed.

Methods and size of the survey

- Database consultation;
- Bibliographic collections;
- Direct observation;
- Questionnaires;
- Online questionnaires;
- Interviews;
- Recording of interviews between pharmacists and patients during dispensing activities;
- Recording of pharmacist's thoughts aloud during dispensing;
- Duration of the recording;
- Day of the week;
- Seasonality of the survey;
- Size of the sample of pharmacies involved in the research;
- Peculiarities of the health cultures and regulations on prescribing/dispensing in the different countries.

Research objectives/definition of error

- Objectives of quantitative/qualitative data collection;
- Aims of the observational study;
- Purposes of the data collected;
- Diversity or absence of the definition of error underlying the research.

Presence/absence in the research of peculiar discriminants

- Dispensing of over-the-counter drugs/prescription drugs;
- Repeat prescription/Original prescription;
- Pharmaceutical form;
- Prescriptions made with digital/paper instruments;
- Manual dispensing/Semi-automated dispensing/Automated dispensing;
- Original pack dispensing or Compliance pack;
- Dispensing to regular/occasional patients;
- Dispensing to special categories of patients: infants, children, adolescents, elderly;
- Dispensing to patient/caregiver.

In addition to this long list of issues that can have a significant impact on the collected data, the reluctance to expose the error in the presence of a punitive mentality (Franklin and O'Grady 2007) and in the absence of a culture of problem-sharing that would help to redesign management and logistical activities, physical and digital infrastructures, the drug itself, the prescription and in general the objects that support all the activities that precede the purchase of the drug by the patient. This reticence is a non-secondary factor that contributes to distorting the quantitative data.

To conclude, it is helpful to point out that comparing data on errors at the prescribing and dispensing stage problematic is the unambiguous definition of this type of error, which is sometimes not even prefixed to the study. Based on the comparison of numerous studies on errors in the prescribing and dispensing phases, one research report has revealed differences, even marked ones, between the definitions used (Aldhwaihi et al. 2016), just as distant are the positions in determining whether specific types of events are to be considered errors (Dean et al. 2000). These different positions influence the methods of detection and data collected. For example, concerning prescribing errors, some authors have defined errors as only those recognised by the doctor and the pharmacist. Other studies have included only those that harm the patient in this type of error. Some authors believe that insufficient patient education on the correct use and effects of the medicine should be considered among prescribing errors, giving less importance to bureaucratic-regulatory errors. Other authors, on the other hand, consider the prescription of a medicine by its brand name (instead of its active ingredient) to be one of the errors, namely a type of error that has no implications for the patient's health but contravenes the regulations in force. A similar variety is found in the definition of dispensing errors where, for example, a distinction is introduced between a dispensing error and a near-error, defining by this second term those errors made during dispensing but detected by the pharmacist before the patient left the pharmacy.

8.2.1 Prescription Errors Detected During Dispensing

The first group of errors, widely reported in the literature, consists of those made by the doctor at the prescribing stage. In many cases, the pharmacist detects these errors during dispensing procedures, highlighting a frequent recurrence: the error is not recognised by the person committing it but by those asked to take follow-up action at a later stage (Ferguson et al. 2018).

In this chapter devoted to medicine dispensing, we focus on prescriptive errors limited to those circumstances that allow us to highlight and give meaning to the close interconnections between the different stages preceding the patient's purchase of the medicine. The aim is to delineate the decision-making and management processes, the responsibilities, as well as the information passages and communication exchanges that take place between the different actors in the care system. Our attention lies particularly on verifying the effectiveness of the more traditional tools (paper prescriptions) or the more innovative ones (e-prescribing) in supporting this process and allowing effective and exhaustive communication between doctor, pharmacist, and patient.

Regarding the definition of prescriptive error, we adopt the one proposed by Dean et al. (2000). It emerges from an interdisciplinary group composed of healthcare professionals, clinicians, pharmacologists, and researchers with extensive experience in medication error.

> A clinically meaningful prescribing error occurs when, as a result of a prescribing decision or prescription writing process, there is an unintentional significant (1) reduction in the probability of treatment being timely and effective or (2) increase in the risk of harm when compared with generally accepted practice (Dean et al. 2000, p. 234).

This definition simplifies the framing of prescribing errors detected at the dispensing stage, by directing our attention to the distinction between errors in the prescribing decision and errors in the prescription writing process. This second category also includes errors occurring in the re-writing of therapeutic indications.

The first type refers to errors in medical decision-making: prescriptions that are contraindicated or inappropriate because they do not take into account the patient's overall clinical condition; prescriptions of medicines to which the patient has reported a clinically significant allergy; prescriptions of medicines that do not take into account interactions with other active ingredients in the patient's therapy; prescriptions of medicines in dosages that are inappropriate for the patient; prescriptions of "refills" of a medicine that has given the patient adverse reactions; prescriptions of "refills" of medicine without having carried out the required diagnostic investigations; prescriptions of two different medicines (or two medicines containing the same active ingredient) for the same indication for use; prescriptions of medicines for which there is no indication for the patient's condition, etc. (Dean et al. 2000).

Errors of 'writing', namely errors that occur in the coding phase of the clinical decision and its transposition onto a technical device—the prescription—aimed at translating the therapy into standardised data, include: the failure to communicate or the incorrect communication of information that is essential for correct dispensing (such as the exact, complete and legible name of the medicine; the pharmaceutical form; the dosage—especially in medicines available in several dosages—, the correct unit of measurement, the route of administration). These errors also include omitting the date, the patient's name, and the prescriber's signature.

Writing errors also include 'transcription' errors. These refer to the reading and re-writing of prescriptions previously made by the same doctor or other doctors (e.g., transcriptions by a general practitioner of prescriptions given by a specialist or a hospital doctor). The same type of error can occur when the hospital staff transcribes the patient's home treatment at the start of a hospital stay. This includes transcription automatisms typical of chronic therapies in which a medicine may be renewed without checking for changes (e.g., change of molecule, frequent in chronic therapies, or dosage changes). Finally, all those written directly on a prescription but not formally transcribed in the medical record or the doctor's computer system may give rise to subsequent errors. Failure to transcribe formally may lead to forgetfulness in subsequent prescriptions.

We refer to the tables by Dean et al. (2000, pp. 234 and 235) for an accurate list of the many prescription errors that affect the dispensing act. From the study of these authors, we limit ourselves here to identifying three categories of errors, with different implications on dispensing:

- prescribing errors/problems arising from the decision-making process, namely the clinical decision leading to the prescription;
- errors in prescription writing;
- errors in re-writing.

Each type of error could interfere with correctly dispensing the prescribed medicine. Still, it changes the pharmacist's ability to detect the error and even more so to intervene to correct the error found.

The first type of error—error as the outcome of a clinical decision—is strongly affected by the sharp caesura, established by law, between the activity of the prescriber and that of the dispenser, namely between the activity proper to the doctor and the clinical discretion and expertise, and the activity of health education, control and support of pharmacological treatment that is proper to the pharmacist.

In the absence of a formal passage of information informing the pharmacist of the reasons behind the prescription of a specific active ingredient and the choice of dosage, it is difficult for the dispenser to understand whether the choice made by the doctor is well-considered and intentional, even if outside the guidelines, or the result of an error. Similar doubts may arise from prescriptions potentially harmful to a patient undergoing polypharmacy due to the risk of medicine interactions or adverse reactions related to other diseases the patient is suffering from.

The pharmacist does not always understand the prescriptive decisions of the doctor. But, even when faced with doubts, it is difficult for the pharmacists to intervene: they have no documentation on the diagnostic part. Moreover, the doctor is not obligated to provide information in the prescription to explain the therapeutic choice.

The doubts raised by the doctor's clinical decision make even more sense in the case of prescriptions written by specialist doctors who, especially at the 'first visit', do not know the patient's medical history in depth and must rely on the clinical documentation and the problems 'referred' by the patients themselves. In particular, the therapy has no codified format and is not validated by the general practitioner. When introducing a new medicine into the therapy, the specialist relies on the patient's ability to return therapeutic data in the most complete and correct form possible. For instance, in the elderly patient, these are numerous and complex to return.

The second type of prescriptive error—namely the error occurring in the writing phase is generally caused by forgetfulness, distraction, and haste, leading the physician to write something different from the clinical intention/decision (for a detailed restitution of these different problems we refer to Table 1 of Chen et al. 2005, p. 337).

Even in this case, the literature is rich. It essentially comprises two forms of error: those that result from omitting information necessary to make the object dispensed unambiguous, and those that result from making unintentional errors in filling in the format with the required prescriptive data. In addition, the doctor's incomprehensible handwriting can be equated with an omission of data or lead the dispenser to an interpretative error (Martìnez Sànchez 2013).

Errors at the writing stage (due to absence or inconsistency of information) have been classified as errors of omission or commission. Errors of omission include 'incomplete prescriptions', while errors of commission include uncorrected, illegible prescriptions and indications given through abbreviations or acronyms (Al-Khani et al. 2014) or relating to products no longer available or for hospital use.

These types of errors require proactive intervention by pharmacists to correct them. Differentiating errors of omission (incomplete prescriptions) from unintentional errors of data and information helps highlight the different degrees of risk involved in dispensing. An omission is an evident error and is less likely to cause harm than errors resulting from erroneous data that are not always explicitly apparent and, precisely for this reason, can also be very dangerous. In other words, the absence of a data element that does not allow the identification of the medicine or the patient to whom the treatment is dispensed, produces the suspension of administering until the missing data have been completed. This type of error, unless a medical condition requires immediate administration of the medicine, delays dispensing. In contrast, incorrect medicine entry, such as writing *Metotrexate sodium salt 7.5 mg* 'per day' instead of 'per week' for a patient with rheumatoid arthritis, can lead to severe dispensing errors. This kind of error cannot necessarily be detected by the pharmacist thanks to the prescription because the doctor does not have to justify the treatment concerning the pathology.

The macro-category of writing errors (omission of data and incorrectness of the data entered in the prescription) has given rise to a research interest aimed at verifying to what extent digital prescribing (in use in many countries, and which has also become widespread in Italy, following the Covid-19 pandemic) can mitigate errors. We can here briefly argue that e-prescribing makes it possible to have prescriptions with fewer data gaps, but, at the same time, it produces contradictory results on the error relating to the data entered. Causes of medication errors (Martìnez Sànchez 2013, table 2, p. 185):

- Prescription corrections;
- Illegible prescription (illegible handwriting);
- Prescription of a non-existent medicine, strength, quantity or dosage;
- Missing prescriber information;
- Absent indication of the route of administration;
- Problems with subsidies;
- Medicine no longer in stock;
- Patient wanted to change prescription;
- Medicine not immediately available;
- Prescription is incomplete concerning dose or frequency;
- Medicine is indicated but dose is inappropriate;
- Missing or incorrect patient identification;
- Problems with medicine substitution;
- Medicine duplication.

The list above highlights that any data can be subject to problems of:

- illegibility or distortion of the medicine name;
- illegibility, absence or mistake in the dosage;
- illegibility, lack, or mistake in the number of doses per package;
- illegibility, lack, or mistake of the pharmaceutical form;
- illegibility, or lack of the prescriber's signature;
- illegibility, or lack of name/prescriber's registration number;
- illegibility, or lack of the patient's name.

The third typology refers to the distortion of data that can take place in the rewriting and transcription phase and can be due to causes such as the fast or incomplete reading of the original document; the misinterpretation of some data of the original document; the recombination, in the transcription, of characteristics related to different medicines present in the original prescription; the confusion between dosage and time of intake due to the absence of punctuation that makes the interpretation unambiguous, etc. (for a completeness of examples see Chen et al. 2005).

Suppose a comparison with the source document does not immediately detect them. In that case, the peculiarity of transposition errors is that they risk not remaining occasional but instead setting the tone for subsequent treatment.

The risk of transcription errors is particularly critical in phases of 'therapeutic discontinuity': hospital admission or discharge, specialist visits, and so forth, when new medicines are introduced, substituted, or eliminated.

Frequent transcription errors include those that occur in printing labels or instructions for use that the pharmacist affixes to the packaging prepared by the pharmacist. This type of error can lead to the provision of information that differs from the prescription and/or content (Hoxsie et al. 2006). This type of error refers to those countries where the drug is dosed and packaged by the pharmacist according to the doctor's prescription.

In this review of prescriptive errors that the pharmacist can detect, the literature also includes problems arising from the intrinsic risk of medicine therapy (e.g., side effects, medicine interactions, allergies) and those related to the process of medicine supply and reimbursement. Of these error types, the relevance to the dispensation phase is considered here because, if not recognised and reported, they may recur in subsequent prescriptions.

The literature testifies the presence of prescribing errors on the doctor's side. It rarely depends on a lack of knowledge of the patient's condition and pathology but, by contrast, on a knowledge of the medicines not always appropriate (e.g., side effects, drug interactions, drug manipulability, dosages, pharmaceutical forms available on the market, formal characteristics, and use of the drug). From this knowledge, which is not always adequate, may also depend on 'double prescriptions'. For example, a new medicine whose active ingredient is already present in the patient's therapy under a trade name not recognised by the doctor. Similarly, lack of appropriate knowledge of the shape, size, and surface characteristics (e.g., smooth or rough) of a tablet may lead the doctor to prescribe to elderly or dysphagic patients drugs that they are unable to swallow. The introduction of the legal obligation to place on the market packages equipped with an anti-tampering seal (Directive 62/EU 2011) does not allow the user to know, prior to purchase, the formal characteristics of the medicine and, to date, there is no 'abacus of forms' to help the doctor, pharmacist, and patient in the choice of the medicine, also assessing its formal characteristics. Some of these prescriptive criticalities could be detected at the dispensing stage. But, as we shall see below, in many cases the pharmacist lacks the information, procedures and prerogatives to be able to intervene on behalf of the patient.

8.2.2 Dispensing Errors: Definition

The activity of dispensing a medicine does not end with checking the prescription and the correctness of its information content. As we have seen, verifying prescription data is a fundamental step. But it is not the only one. Dispensing is a complex process consisting of several operations: receipt of the prescription, reading, verification of completeness, interpretation, selection of the prescribed product, removal of the pharmaceutical sticker from the drug packet and its affixing to the doctor's prescription, registration of the dispensing using a numerical code, instructions and advice to the patient, release of the prescribed drug and registration of the sale using a receipt (Weir et al. 2020).

Medicine dispensing consists of a multistage process of technical checks and procedures, operational and organisational activities, mental processes, and dialogical and relational exchanges (James et al. 2009).

Each step in this process is intrinsically linked to the possibility of error. Although there has been increasing research on dispensing errors in recent years, there is no universally accepted taxonomy. One of the most frequently used definitions is the one elaborated by Flynn and Barker in 1999 and subsequently taken up by several authors (Flynn et al. 2002; Hoxsie et al. 2006), adapted and clarified in subsequent studies and which we quote below in its updated form as follows:

> A dispensing error is defined as any unintended deviation from an interpretable written prescription or medication order. Both content and labelling errors are included. Any unintended deviation from professional or regulatory references, or guidelines affecting dispensing procedures, is also considered a dispensing error (Franklin and O'Grady 2007, p. 277).

It is worth introducing a few clarifications here. The literature categorises dispensing errors into two main groups: *content errors* and *labelling errors* (Hoxsie et al. 2006).

Content errors include the dispensing of an incorrect medicine, an incorrect form (e.g., an extended-release product instead of a standard-release tablet), an incorrect pharmaceutical form (e.g., drops instead of tablets), an incorrect quantity (e.g., 12-tablet package instead of 24 tablets), an incorrect dosage (e.g., 10 mg instead of 30 mg), dispensing to the wrong patient, etc.

On the other hand, *labelling errors* are those occurring in non-standard, customised forms of dispensing based on a doctor's prescription. This way of dispensing is prevalent in the United States, the United Kingdom and some European countries adopting galenic preparations. in this case, the pharmacy directly carries out the counting of the doses according to the doctor's prescription, its packaging, the printing of the label containing the identification data (e.g., active ingredient, dosage, quantity to be dispensed, etc.), the dosage and any necessary instructions for use. This can result in incorrect, incomplete, or illegible information, even if only due to the graphic or printing quality of the label (Ashcroft et al. 2005). According to Hoxsie et al. (2006), labelling errors account for the highest percentage of all dispensing errors.

A further clarification concerns the distinction in the literature between "dispensing error"—mentioned above and leading the patient to purchase a medicine that does not comply with the prescription—and "near-miss error".

The latter means any incident detected before the patient receives the medicine. For some authors, this includes all errors detected before the patient leaves the pharmacy (Ashcroft et al. 2005; James et al. 2009).

In the previous section, we gave a qualitative picture of the prescriptive errors detected in the dispensing phase, identifying their types, recurrences, and causes (James et al. 2009; Cheung et al. 2009) without dwelling on the quantitative data.

We follow the same modality in returning the analysis of the different types of errors in the dispensing activities. Here, we face different definitions and extremely diverse practices: from the dispensing of the medicine in the packaging produced by the industry—due to national and/or EU regulations, it cannot be opened at the pharmacy—to forms of dispensing which involve the pharmacist's packaging according to prescription. This process differs in manual, semi-automated or automated packaging (James et al. 2009). The regulations and procedures of the different countries are too different for any data comparison. We will focus on the different types of errors recurrently encountered to highlight the elements that, from a design perspective, could positively influence the process if redesigned.

8.2.3 Dispensing Errors: Methods and Data Retrieved from the Literature

The existing literature reveals the broad interest in dispensing and the related critical issues, with implications to be permanently focused on by various areas of study. Despite the consistency of the available studies and the wide variety of viewpoints, it is still complicated to fully understand the phenomenology of dispensing errors, as so many possible causes contribute to it. Suppose the sources investigated are almost redundant in confirming the types of error and the most recurrent underlying causes. In that case, interweaving the constituent factors and contingencies that converge in favouring a context permeable to error is more problematic. This co-causality is probably why defining the error environment is challenging to analyse, for determining actions to intervene and prevent. These can only arise from a systemic perspective to promote multiple punctual interventions connected in an organic framework.

In the literature, the activities taking place within a pharmacy lie between two polarities: on the one hand, we find "quasi-phenomenological" definitions of the microdynamics in the procedural actions-operations (Ashcroft et al. 2005) and even the mental of the operators, filmed with audio and video while "thinking aloud" (Nusair and Guirguis 2017). On the other hand, we find a division of the context into individual elements separately analysed. In both cases, it is a problem that cannot be evaded when reflecting on the quality of the data collected and the possibility of using it by extending its scope to a broader scale. In the first case, the overemphasis on the peculiarities of the contexts and contingencies affecting pharmacy activity could lead to observations of a local nature.

In the second case, the research focusing on one or a few factors intended as variables capable of influencing error is judged by the authors as insufficient. Indeed, these studies emphasise the need to continue the research to assess the influence of the same factor at the change of context or, the need to supplement the assessment of a given element with subsequent analysis to verify how tight the correlation between the factor considered and the error found is (Weir et al. 2020). Finally, a broad literature concludes with the observation that the research carried out, even in the form of pilot projects, has rarely moved on to the implementation phase, even in the face of promising results, precisely because of the need to correlate individual actions within a broader framework of interventions (Weir et al. 2020). For these reasons, we have chosen to report below the most frequently found evidence in the literature, listed as restitution of a shared basis of recurring elements. These lists presented below, integrate different research sources (James et al. 2009; Ashcroft et al. 2005; Hoxsie et al. 2006; Cheung et al. 2009).

Types of recurrent errors in dispensing process:

- Error in reading the prescription;
- Error selecting medicine from drawer or shelf;
- Error in selecting dosage;
- Error in choosing the packaging with the prescribed number of doses;
- Error in choosing the pharmaceutical form;
- Error in choosing the release mode (e.g., normal/extended);
- Delivery of the medicine to the wrong patient;
- Delivery of an expired medicine;
- Delivery of a deteriorated medicine due to not properly storage;
- Missed assessment of the patient's general health condition (e.g. diabetes, pregnancy status, body pressure, etc.);
- Missed assessment of medicine allergies or intolerances;
- Missed detection of possible interactions with other medicines in the patient's therapy;
- Lack of, inadequate or incorrect instructions to the patient on the use of the medicine;

- Lack of, inadequate, or incorrect instructions to the patient on the storage of the medicine;
- Lack of, inadequate, or incorrect instructions to the patient on the proper disposal of the medicine;
- Filling the packaging with the wrong medicine (for customised dispensing forms);
- Incorrect tablet counting (for customised dispensing forms);
- Inadequate packaging of the medicine (for customised dispensing forms);
- Incorrect labelling/confusing label/label mix-up (for customised dispensing forms);
- Error in choosing the name and/or dosage from the selection lists in the software used to generate the labels.

The factors investigated as error-promoting causes also stem from integrating several sources and have been sorted into categories. Some of them can be placed in more than one category because they have been collected from different points of view. For example, "high workload" may be subjectively perceived and investigated as such (i.e., as a cause of inattention due to fatigue and stress). However, it may also result from poor work organisation (e.g., lack of staff, poor management of work shifts, assignment of tasks not pertinent to the role). A lack of knowledge may be a subjectively perceived weakness but may also result from a work environment that does not train staff. Factors most frequently cited in literature as contributing to dispensation errors:

Human/cultural factors (James et al. 2009):

- Lack of knowledge;
- Incapacity to understand/manage complex prescriptions;
- Poor dexterity;
- Poor predisposition to human interactions;
- Language proficiency;
- Workload;
- Number of prescriptions dispensed per hour;
- Stress;
- Fatigue;
- Hunger;
- Sickness;
- Job dissatisfaction;
- Lack of concentration;
- Patient's state of anxiety;
- Frequency of interruptions;
- Non-compliance with standard operating procedures.

Work organisation (James et al. 2009):

- Multitasking/monotasking;
- Role-based job description;
- Competence-based job description;
- Task-based job description;

- Work shifts;
- Absence of breaks;
- Staff inexperience;
- Quantity and quality of staff;
- Workload management;
- Lack of procedures;
- Failure to check;
- Lack of training;
- Lack of knowledge;
- Poor communication.

Environmental factors (James et al. 2009):

- Insufficient lighting;
- Sound pollution;
- Interruptions/distractions;
- Organisation of work areas;
- Organisation of storage areas;
- Criteria for arranging medicines in drawers and/or shelves;
- Logistics of incoming and outgoing medicine flows;
- Logistics of incoming/outgoing patient-customer flows;
- Presence of privacy areas.

Circumstances (Ashcroft et al. 2005):

- Busier than normal;
- Time of day;
- Not usual pharmacist;
- Not usual dispenser;
- Telephone interruption;
- Staff query;
- Customer/patient query;
- Busy over-the-counter trade.

Artifacts and process infrastructure (Ashcroft et al. 2005):

- Similar drug names;
- Similar packaging;
- Poor doctor's handwriting;
- Ambiguous prescriber's instructions;
- Computer software;
- Complex prescription;
- New prescription;
- Selection of the previous medicine or dosage from the patient's record on the pharmacy computer and not from the prescription.

Checking the appropriateness of prescriptions emerges as a recurring practice, starting with the patient's drug purchase profile, which can be found in the pharmacy's computer history. This behaviour has been attentive because it can be misleading in all cases where the doctor has modified medicine characteristics or dosages with new prescribing indications (Chen et al. 2005).

As mentioned, the pharmaceutical dispensing process is complex and takes place in a working environment with multiple sources of risk, multiple types of errors and various phases in which errors can occur (Abood 1996). This exposure to erroneous actions subjects this environment to the interest of those who observe it as a sociotechnical system (Szeinbach et al. 2007) with a high intensity of interaction between people, between people and objects, instrumental and technological aids, and between people and organisational artefacts necessary for the execution of complex tasks (Phipps et al. 2009). This is why various disciplines are studying it. For example, improving safety conditions is the focus of an area of study that introduces the 'human factor' as an object of interest in healthcare (Stojkovic et al. 2017; Weir et al. 2020). In this area, the interaction between people and the work environment is explored from the point of view of the physical activity involved in work operations; from the cognitive point of view, namely the mental processes involved; from the organisational point of view through the study of methods, tasks, structures, and activities (Harvey et al. 2015); and from the point of view of the sensory and perceptual factors that impact on the environmental quality of work activities. Important in this regard are Buchanan's work on lighting (Buchanan et al. 1991) and Flynn's work on the stresses that workers experience from environmental noise and visual chaos (Flynn et al. 1996), forerunners of this research field (Weir et al. 2020).

Several studies focused on subjective, psychological, motivational, and cultural factors, trying to establish a direct correlation between interpersonal skills, technical skills, specific skills and errors (Grasha and Schell 2001). Others have analysed the relationship between work overload, fatigue, and resistance to work-related stress situations (Flynn et al. 2002). Still, others have focused on the cognitive elements that induce error and the role that routine and work habits can exert in this order of oversights.

Others have focused on workflow management (Angelo and Ferreri 2005), staff organisation, defining and adhering to roles and job descriptions (e.g., adherence to a clear role distinction between pharmacist and pharmacy technician) (Ness et al. 1994; Flynn et al. 2002) or the pharmacist's failure to counsel the patient; failure to follow protocols or a tendency to deviate from codified practices (Jones et al. 2018).

Others have focused on the 'situations' that most expose to error or make dispensing problematic: first prescriptions or complex prescriptions; medicines that require technical advice (e.g., parenteral care, use of devices, dosages that need to be personalised); patients with multimorbidity; time pressure in dispensing; frequency of interruptions in dispensing operations; high number of daily prescriptions filled; multitasking work organisation (Flynn et al. 1999).

Studies and research on the incorporation and integration of new services (Szeinbach et al. 2007) and on the role of technology in streamlining procedures and reducing error (Bates et al. 2001) are equally substantial. Their focus has been on the use of electronic prescriptions and electronic health records, sensing technologies for authentication (e.g., such as barcode reading systems or radio frequency identification tags) (Franklin and O'Grady 2007), barcode scanners to check and match whether the medicine selected from the shelf with the dispensing screen, and automated dispensing systems (Campmans et al. 2018). In detecting the positivity of the use of technology as an element of efficiency in the dispensing system as a whole, many of these studies have problematised the approach to technology as a miracle remedy and, alongside the aspects of positivity, have highlighted its potential adverse effects (Weir et al. 2020; Karsh et al. 2010) if the use of technological tools and infrastructure is not contextualised within the system of established practices and the more complex socio-cultural context.

8.2.4 Spatial Organisation and Environmental Factors

A further group of studies focused on the organisation of the pharmacy, analysed both as a workplace and as the internal environmental factors: all of these can favour a decrease in concentration or an increase in distraction and stress, producing a higher level of error (Weir et al. 2020).

For example, lack of space has been considered a cause of poor interaction between operators and users in dispensing activities, reduced privacy for the patient, and difficulties in recognising distinct operational areas of the work plan for each operator (Harvey et al. 2015).

These are necessary to avoid different operators having small or even partially overlapping or shared workstations and to ensure that the user can attend to dispensing prescribed medication. The literature presents errors in the delivery of therapy to the wrong patient (or the insertion of a medicine intended for one patient in another patient's bag), often made depending on workstations that are too close together or even shared. The identical sequences of technical actions (e.g., detaching the sticker from the drug, attaching it to the prescription, and numbering the prescriptions with progressive codes) would require a space that allows—and indeed prepares for—orderly operation (Lester and Chui 2016). These studies also highlight the usefulness of the patient's presence at dispensing activities (from reading the prescription, taking the drug in the required doses, and bagging it) for the "passive control" they can exert over the dispenser's activities.

One study verified the positive impact on error achieved using dedicated bins/trays for dispensing each patient (Hoxsie et al. 2006). In the absence of an autonomous workspace, sufficient in size to adequately organise the dispensing activity, the use of bins can have a positive effect. Indeed, the bins can be used to collect all prescriptions for an individual patient and all medicines to be dispensed, reducing the error rate detected by pharmacy staff.

Also, in studies on the organisation of space, we find that even the sub-optimal layout of furniture can increase errors and inattentions by generating interference between the daily flow of goods and patients upon entry, waiting and exit. Besides impacting the correct activity of operators, cluttered flows produce visual and acoustic chaos, distractions, and interruptions in staff activities (Lea et al. 2015).

Flynn et al. (1999) identified the interruption of activity (e.g., requests from colleagues, patients, handling of phone calls) as one of the elements capable of significantly influencing the error rate in dispensing activities (on these aspects see also Cheung et al. 2009).

Observational studies on the management of activities within pharmacies have also identified the organisation of work in multitasking mode (Dellve et al. 2018) as a possible source of increased error, suggesting that certain tasks (e.g., answering telephone calls, managing the sale of non-pharmaceutical products or service activities unrelated to dispensing activities) should be entrusted to dedicated figures (Hoxsie et al. 2006). Some authors assume that there is an essential difference between hospital pharmacies and community pharmacies; the staff of the latter are more prone to distractions and interruptions than in the hospital environment by selling a wide variety of non-dispensable items (e.g., devices, healthcare products, cosmetics, service provision) (Hoxsie et al. 2006). Hence, this applies especially to the role that pharmacy assumes in redesigning territorial systems of care. In fact, the new services offered by pharmacy staff include many activities previously the prerogative of other facilities/figures: administering vaccines, taking swabs, supporting health education, booking visits and examinations, providing laboratory tests, and monitoring basic body parameters. Moreover, while several studies have found the pharmacist's work to be characterised by high turnover rates and interruptions and distractions (considered the cultural norm), others have highlighted how commercial pressures create a conflict between the need for pharmacies to be profitable and the need for adequate resources (e.g., from staff to space) to maintain a safe working environment (Garattini and Nobili 2021).

A correct distribution of the different activities within pharmacies can be favoured or hindered by the workspace layout and the design of reserved areas to ensure a protected dialogue between pharmacists and patients.

The layout and organisation of the space are also fundamental in the arrangement of the medicine to be dispensed—both in the display on the shelf and the drawer because the easy accessibility of the medicine and its immediate recognisability depend on this. For the same reasons, importance is recognised in the organisation of stocks (Ruutiainen et al. 2021), which must also ensure the correct rotation of drugs according to expiry date and proper storage. Specific attention is paid to the criteria for ordering/cataloguing pharmaceutical items. The most common arrangement criteria are: the stock arrangement that separates branded and generic drugs, the arrangement that groups stocks according to pharmaceutical form (e.g. tablets, ointments, eye drops), the arrangement in alphabetical order regardless of pharmaceutical form.

8.2.5 The Role of Medicine Packaging in Dispensing

In the context of prescribing and dispensing activities, we have pointed out the incidence played by subjective factors or external environmental contingencies (e.g., noise, frenzy, inadequate workspace, lighting) that can induce or encourage error, especially in a context in which several actors operate under conditions of insufficient communication. Although the result of distraction or superficiality in subjective action, some errors are strongly connected to the artefacts in use. We mainly refer to the 'communicative' ones that serve as tools for the passage of information between actors in a specific operational context—in the case under study, the prescription—and the medicines themselves.

As we shall discuss below, the formal and graphical-informative aspects of pharmaceutical packaging may be at the root of certain specific types of errors in both the prescription and dispensing process. Our attention in this section will focus on the latter. Like other products, the packaging of pharmaceuticals must ensure speed of packaging and low downtime during production, product protection, ease of identification during sale or dispensing, safe storage, ease of use and, at the same time, safety for the user. The quality of packaging must also ensure that the integrity of pharmaceutical products is maintained during storage, shipment, and delivery. At each stage of the product's life cycle—production, transport, sale, use, disposal—packaging must meet specific needs and have precise requirements.

For this chapter, we will analyse secondary packaging for the communicative and formal elements that can contribute to reducing or extending the possibility of error during dispensing in the pharmacy environment.

We will begin with an investigated aspect in the literature and about broad awareness in the medical-pharmaceutical environment. In this section, we will refer to the similar elements between different packaging, first and foremost, and specifically, to the similarity concerning the names of the medicines.

8.2.5.1 Name Similarities: Look-Alike/Sound-Alike Medicines

In the context of prescribing and dispensing activities, we have pointed out the incidence played by subjective factors or external environmental contingencies (e.g., noise, frenzy, inadequate workspace, lighting) that can induce or encourage error, especially in a context in which several actors operate under conditions of insufficient communication. Although the result of distraction or superficiality in subjective action, some errors are strongly connected to the artefacts in use. We mainly refer to the 'communicative' ones that serve as tools for the passage of information between actors in a specific operational context—in the case under study, the prescription—and the medicines themselves.

In the medical realm, the acronym LASA (Look-Alike/Sound-Alike) refers to medicines whose names can be mistaken for others due to their visual or auditory similarity (Bryan et al. 2020). Together with the class of medicines considered to be 'high-risk' or 'high-attention level' (in Italy, known as High Attention Level Medicines, *Farmaci ad alto livello di attenzione Farmaci—FALA*), because their misuse is associated with a high possibility of creating severe health damage for the patient (e.g., Insulins, Narcotics/Opioids, Sedatives, Anticoagulants), LASA medicines are under surveillance by the International Bodies dealing with pharmacovigilance (i.e., WHO, EMA, AIFA, FDA) and the Ministry of Health of the different states (Berman 2004). Due to their similarity, the latter have compiled lists of pairs or triplets of medicines subject to recurrent reports of prescription or dispensing errors.

In Italy, an initial list of similarities was drawn up in 2008 by a working group mandated by the Ministry of Health based on more than a thousand reports collected spontaneously, mainly from hospitals and pharmacies. The working group created a database for statistically analysing data and assessing their recurrence. From this survey, the working group defined a list of LASA drugs (Ministero della Salute 2010a, b), the Ministerial Recommendation No. 12 (Ministero della Salute 2010a, b), and the LASA Medicines Table (Ministero della Salute 2015). In outpatient and inpatient prescribing/dispensing, LASA errors have long been the subject of research extensively documented in the literature (Ciociano and Bagnasco 2014).

Internationally, statistics of the incidence of this type of error and the severity that this exchange can produce are not supported by homogeneous data (Ostini et al. 2012). Still, the evidence that the LASA problem has in the literature is a sign of an issue that cannot be underestimated. Berman (2004) argued that LASA errors are responsible for thousands of deaths and, in the United States alone, result in millions of dollars in costs each year: more than 25% of all drug dispensing errors are attributable to LASA drug mix-ups and, in countries where dispensing involves packaging and labelling the drug at the pharmacy, this percentage rises to 33%. More generally, the rate of LASA errors found in the literature varies between 20% and 25% of dispensing errors in different countries. It poses a significant threat to the safety of patients who risk purchasing inappropriate or harmful medicines. For example, the United States Pharmacopeia recorded 26,604 LASA errors between 2003 and 2006, collected through spontaneous notifications (Lizano-Díez et al. 2020). Confusion between similarly named medicines affects all categories, from those for paediatric use (Basco Jr et al. 2010), to those for oncological use (Emmerton et al. 2020). With LASA drugs, the error can occur due to the similarity of the trade name of a drug pair or the similarity of the name of an active ingredient pair (which, in the case of equivalent drugs, coincides with the drug name), but can also occur between equivalent/speciality drug pairs (van de Vreede et al. 2008).

The error generated by a LASA medicine can occur either during prescription, transcription, or dispensing. In the case of prescribing, the role of the 'drop-down choice' typical of e-prescribing programmes is particularly highlighted. In this selection mode, medicines are listed in alphabetical order and, especially LASA drugs, are at risk of incorrect choice. In the transcription phase, this is mainly a hasty reading error of the original prescription. In the dispensing phase, the error can be generated both in reading the prescription and in selecting and taking the medicine from the drawer or shelf if two LASA medicines are stored next to each other. The error incidence is high when the similarity concerns the prefix of a medicine name because the most common order of arrangement of medicines in the pharmacy drawer is alphabetical (Bryan et al. 2020). LASA errors occur due to lexical elements shared by two or more names. Visually, the error is induced when the names of two medicines have identical parts with identical prefixes, suffixes, or desinences, or when the names are characterised by the presence of similar vowels and consonants even if arranged in a different order (Table 8.1).

8 Dispensing Medicines: A Necessary Link Between Doctor and Patient

Table 8.1 LASA medicines list updated to 2015—extract from Ministero della Salute

		Name similarity		Packaging similarity			
				Different active ingredient		Same active ingredient	
Medicine 1	Medicine 2	Phonetic	Graphic	Different component	Same component	Same component different dosage	Different component same dosage
Adalat 20 mg CPR	Adalat Crono 20 mg CPR		X			X	
Adrenalina 1 mg/1 ml FL	Atropina Solfato 1 mg 1 ml FL		X		X		
Adrenalina 1 mg/1 ml FL	Sodio Citrato 3.8% 1 ml FL				X		
Advagraf 1 mg CPS	Advagraf 0.5 ml CPS		X			X	
Aimafix 1000 UI 1 FL	AT III 1000 UI FL				X		
Aimafix 1000 UI 1 FL	Emoclot 1000 UI FL				X		
Alapril 5 mg CPR	Chiaro 250 mg CPR				X		
Alginor GTT OS Adulti	Alginor GTT OS BB		X		X		
Alfuzosina 10 mg CPR	Oxicodone 40 mg CPR				X		
Alkeran 2 mg CPR	Leukeran 2 mg CPR	X	X		X		
Amplital 1 g FL	Amplital 500 MCG Siringa preriempita		X			X	
Aranesp 20 mcg Siringa preriempita	Aranesp 40 mcg Siringa preriempita		X			X	
AT III 1000 UI FLAC	Uman Complex 500 UI FLAC				X		

(continued)

Table 8.1 (continued)

Medicine 1	Medicine 2	Name similarity		Packaging similarity			
				Different active ingredient		Same active ingredient	
		Phonetic	Graphic	Different component	Same component	Same component different dosage	Different component same dosage
Atenativ 500 UI FL	Atenativ 1000 UI FL		X		X		
Atked 1000 UI/20 ml FL Kedrion	Atked 500 UI/20 ml FL kedrion		X			X	
Atropina Lux 5 mg/ml 10 ml Collirio	Atropina Lux 10 mg/ml 10 ml Collirio		X			X	
Atropina Lux 5 mg/ml 10 ml Collirio	Ciclolux 10 mg/ml Collirio					X	
Atropina Solfato 0.5 mg 1 ml FL (monico)	Atropina Solfato 1 mg 1 ml FL (monico)		X			X	
Atropina Solfato 0.5 mg FL (monico)	Naloxone Cloridato 04 mg FL (produttori vari)			X			

The typeface (i.e., font, character body, colour) also contributes to accentuating the problem, especially in the presence of names with the same length that create a perceptual impact of similarity that overrides the effort of careful reading.

Similarity can also be detected phonetically, in spoken forms (e.g., names with similar lengths and sounds).

Starting from the lists drawn up by the relevant bodies, Berman (2004) proposed some useful examples to define real problematic categories that can occur in LASA designations:

- the names of two medicines differ by a few letters; in this category one can also find medicines used to achieve opposite effects;
- the name of two medicines has the same prefix or suffix;
- the name of two medicines has a common root;
- the sound of the name may be confused with that of another medicine.

LASA errors represent a *lapsus* (Trbovich and Hyland 2017), particularly related to processes of perceptual completion in which the reader's or listener's expectation and the brevity of the perceptual experience have a significant influence.

In addition, especially in the case of Equivalent Medicines where the name coincides with the active ingredient, the medicine names are "artificial" (Lizano-Díez et al. 2020); these names gain meaning only for the community of experts, whereas they are meaningless for end users (in particular, for patients). The difficulty in linking the medicine's name to a pathology precludes the patient from exercising conscious control over the medicines they purchase and, as we shall see later, does not help them better manage home medicine intake.

8.2.5.2 Packaging Similarity and Information Confusability

The interest in the phenomenology of error linked to LASA medicines has contributed to a specific focus on confusion arising from the similarity between names. However, this interest has also extended the focus to the problems of distinguishability of all those "elements" that should unambiguously identify the individual medicine: in addition to the name, the active ingredient(s), the dosage, the unit of measurement, the packaging graphics, and the overall shape of the packaging.

Many medication interchange errors arise from the plurality of information elements which, instead of being read in their individuality (e.g., name of the medicine, active ingredient, pharmaceutical form, dosage, number of doses per pack), are weakened by the "appearance" or graphic/typographical impression of the packaging. The packaging and its graphic elements (e.g., the shape and size of the packaging and the graphic/visual elements that make up the graphic layout) can contribute to accentuating the similarities between packages. It happens in secondary packaging of different medicines produced by the same pharmaceutical company: the visual elements that characterise the brand identity (i.e., font, colour, arrangement of the graphic elements on the page) increases the similarity between packages.

Examples of the difficulty in unambiguously distinguishing the information elements of the packaging due to inappropriate graphic treatment include dosage forms of the same medicine, confusing because they are similar and not sufficiently distinguishable graphically (e.g., 3.75 and 0.375 mg). The graphical appearance may contribute to accentuating or attenuating the possibility of error. However, dosage errors do not depend solely on their graphic treatment. In many cases, they result from interpretation issues related to how the dosage is expressed (Fig. 8.1). For example:

- two dosage forms of the same medicine whose units are expressed using different multiples (e.g., 500 mg and 1 g), thus hampering a rapid comparison of the amount of active ingredient contained;
- different pharmaceutical forms of the same active ingredient have different dosages and different units of measurement in the transition from solid to liquid formulation (e.g., mg, ml). This situation, which, if not properly handled at the prescription or dispensing stage, or using conversion tables included in the package leaflet, is likely to make it difficult for the patient to change the dosage (Lesar 1998; Madlon-Kay and Mosh 2023).

Fig. 8.1 Spoon dispenser of medicines containing acyclovir

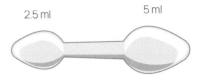

Berman (2004) reports several errors concerning medicines administered intravenously in which the indication of the concentration on the label (40 mg/ml) quickly leads to the use of the entire packet (20 ml equal to 800 mg in total) instead of the correct dose of 40 mg. As well as highlighting the errors that can arise from the concentration of the same medicine expressed with different dilution ratios (e.g., 1:1000 or 1:10,000) or as a percentage (e.g., 1% or 2%). Each of these examples brings reconversion problems that doctors find difficult to deal with.

Medicines are present in the same pharmaceutical form with concentrations expressed in different units. For example, antiviral medicines containing acyclovir are available either as syrup, 8% suspension of 80 mg/ml, or as an oral suspension of 400 mg/5 ml. The presence of the measuring spoon can be helpful, but, since the patient's weight affects the medicine prescription, the conversion to the customised dose is not always easy. To solve this conversion issue and obtain the correct dosages, tips, procedures, and indications can be found on the web: a sign that the problem arises despite the patient receiving instructions from the doctor. For this reason, the Italian *Ministero della Salute* has returned to the issue with several Recommendations: Recommendation No. 7, Recommendation for the prevention of death, coma or serious harm resulting from errors in drug therapy (Ministero della Salute 2008); Recommendation No. 18, Recommendation for the prevention of errors in treatment resulting from the use of abbreviations, acronyms, acronyms, and symbols (Ministero della Salute 2018).

Moreover, in many cases, these are medicines used in emergencies, such as in Emergency and Resuscitation Units (Pérez-Moreno et al. 2017). The researchers have focused heavily on emergency units, believing that these are where the likelihood of error resulting from confusion between the names and packaging of similar medicines is most probable. This occurrence depends on the frequency of verbal orders, crowded storage spaces, and the need to quickly administer high-risk index products and medicine classes in which names are more frequently confused (Fig. 8.2). Add to these circumstances the presence of patients whose medical history is not known in depth nor, necessarily, is there any knowledge of the therapy in use (Hellström et al. 2012).

In addition to the critical points mentioned above, further elements that can make reading the medicine's 'master data' complex are graphic and concern:

- the alteration of the font shape or the use of multiple colours to visually compose the name (Fig. 8.3);
- the name/logo of the company brand which, placed close to the name of the medicine, may lead one to believe that it is part of the name itself;

8 Dispensing Medicines: A Necessary Link Between Doctor and Patient

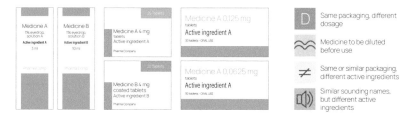

Fig. 8.2 On the left, examples of ambiguity problems in the reading of graphic elements; on the right, examples of symbols used by nursing staff in hospitals indicate LASA medicines

Fig. 8.3 Exemplification of medicine names with changed typography or the use of multi-coloured fonts

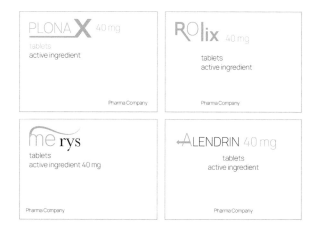

- the information given in the Braille alphabet, which may create optical interference and not allow certain information to be read correctly if overwritten with other visual elements (Fig. 8.4);
- the dosage of the active ingredient is placed next to the name of the medicine or sometimes in an isolated space on the main face of the packaging (Fig. 8.5). It is well known that this complies with current legislation, particularly with Directive 2001/83/EC, which states in Art. 54(a): *"The name of the medicinal product followed by its strength and pharmaceutical form"* (The European Parliament and of the Council 2001). However, we believe that this information element, since it refers to the dosage of the active ingredient, should more appropriately be placed close to it to form a "meaning unit" and make the information on the medicine to be dispensed comprehensible. We will discuss this aspect in Chap. 22.

We have so far addressed some of the problems with the information elements on secondary packaging, which can contribute to errors in dispensing (Fig. 8.6). A final consideration regarding secondary packaging concerns its shape: in addition to optimising the use of shelf or drawer space, this must ensure easy readability of the information. On the first side, we can cite the problems generated by those packages that are too far removed from standard formats (e.g., the cubic pack of D.L-lysine acetylsalicylate sachets, which does not respond well to optimal use of

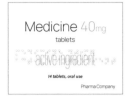
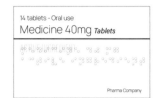

Fig. 8.4 Example of a problem of visual interference generated by overlapping the Braille characters the name of the active ingredient or by using lettering without the necessary visual contrast with the background

Fig. 8.5 Example of a medicine containing two active ingredients. The information indicating the dosage and the two active ingredients are not connected

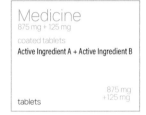

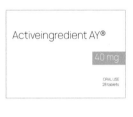

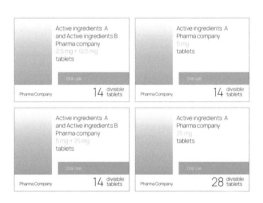

Fig. 8.6 Example of medicine names that cannot be distinguished from the manufacturer's name. On the right, the 'registry' elements identifying different medicines generate significant ambiguity

space in pharmacy drawers; or medicines whose shape does not allow for shelf-stackability). On the second side, we can mention all cylindrical-shaped packs that do not guarantee a rational use of space and do not allow optimal reading of the information on the curved surface. Or again, packs which, due to the size of the base and the base-to-height ratio, risk not guaranteeing the balance of the packaging in the shelf display. The supply chain phase of pharmacies by dispensers should also be carefully considered. For instance, there is a lack of design of the tills used to restock pharmacies to separate heavy medicines (e.g., syrups, vials) from fragile ones (e.g., blister packs). It is common for blister packs to arrive at the pharmacy damaged or crushed due to the random distribution of medicines in the supply case. In addition, medicines that need to be refrigerated represent a significant issue. What is lacking to date is a 'cold chain' system designed to reach the patient. The mode used is that of ice packs that are 'tied' to the medicines by rubber bands or refrigerated bags not explicitly designed for this function. In addition to being logistically problematic systems, they are also environmentally inefficient because many of these ice packs accumulate in the patient's hands and are then thrown away.

8.3 The Role of the Prescription in Dispensing

Prescriptions are the main document with which the doctor prescribes and communicates to the pharmacist the 'identifying' information of the medicine(s) to be dispensed to a specific patient (Al-Khani et al. 2014).

The doctor can write directions manually or by typing on a computer. The prescriptions can have a paper format and be directly given to the patient or have an electronic format and be viewed instantly by the pharmacist in digital format.

In being a prescriptive document, the prescription:

- authorises the patient (not imposes) the use of pharmacological substances;
- defines the active ingredient, the dosage, the pharmaceutical form, the doses of medicine per pack and the number of packs that can be dispensed, as well as indicating the name of the patient, the prescribing doctor, the date of prescription, and the doctor's signature;
- starts a treatment process that must be followed over time to verify—also by specific diagnostic tests—its efficacy and any side effects.

Prescriptions do not contain:

- indications relating to the instructions for the use of the medicine;
- indications relating to the dosage;
- indications specifying the specific medicine prescription;
- indications relating to examinations required before starting or for chronic use of a medicine;
- indications concerning the interval that must be observed before dispensing a subsequent refill.

In the Italian context, prescriptions represent an exclusive dialogue 'tool' between doctors, pharmacists, and the National Health System concerning the administrative part of exemptions. Indeed, the pharmacist collects the prescription and is obliged to keep it for 6 months, except for prescriptions that must be sent to the National Health System for the envisaged refunds. Instructions on use and dosage, as well as why a specific medicine is prescribed, are provided by the doctor to the patient on a separate medium or are sometimes given verbally. This information is not accessible to the pharmacist unless provided directly by the patients. On the other hand, the patient is left with no trace of the information in the prescription unless accessed through the personal electronic health record.

Precisely because of these characteristics, the prescription assumes a limited role that ends with purchasing the medicine. Since it does not contain the information capable of connecting the 'authorisation to purchase' to the acts of treatment, it must be accompanied by other information devices. These are necessary to provide the patient with the information needed to take the medicine correctly and to understand the reasons for prescribing it (among these, we can mention the hospital discharge letter, the document brought to the attention of the treating physician by the specialist after the examination, the indications issued by the general practitioner in written or oral form with the dosage). These indications to the patient could also be helpful to the pharmacist in intercepting possible prescription errors or while dispensing them (Kennedey et al. 2011).

The logistics of the prescription itself increase the potential for error. Especially when it comes to repeated requests for chronically consumed medication, the doctor fills the prescription on the patient's instructions through the intermediary of the outpatient secretarial staff. This request for the medicine(s) is written on paper (sometimes without the patient's full name) and may also be dialled over the phone. After completion, collection by the doctor may be done by the office staff, but the patient frequently picks up the prescription from a special box in the waiting room of the doctor's clinic. These poorly regulated arrangements, while facilitating the user, can, on the other hand, lead to dispensing medicines not explicitly prescribed to a patient (Hoxsie et al. 2006). This occurs also because the pharmacist is not required to verify the relationship between the prescriber and the patient to whom the prescription is addressed.

The automatism with which the prescriptions for chronic intake are issued has the effect of introducing the taking of the medicine itself into a routine procedure, often without the necessary checks on efficacy or side events, which, especially in the initial stages, should be monitored by the doctor. The same automatism also intervenes to the detriment of any diagnostic examinations that should be carried out periodically to continue taking the medicine, whereas, once the therapy has begun, these examinations are not always carried out even though it is the package leaflet itself that indicates the advisability of doing so.

A final remark can be made on placing the medicine sticker on the prescription. This operation, which pharmacists are obliged to do and which serves above all for exemption of the medicine (so that the pharmacy can receive the reimbursement provided for), is still not helpful in matching the prescribed with the dispensed. This type of matching would require a switch to the electronic format of the prescription so that its code can be compared with the identification code of the medicine dispensed (on the potential of the electronic prescription, see Chap. 9 of this text).

In the switch to electronic prescriptions lies the hope of solving many problems connecting prescription and dispensing. E-prescribing has already revealed many potentials that could not be addressed with current paper prescriptions. To be expressed, these potentials require a systemic approach to the prescribing act capable of integrating a set of information that currently resides in different, unconnected documents (Ammenwerth et al. 2008). The actors who must intervene in the several steps of the process have a fragmented view of the patient and care-related knowledge. Some studies demonstrate how the redesign of the prescription, especially in electronic format, can reduce errors in prescribing and dispensing but also influence the physician's choices regarding treatment options. Malhotra et al. (2016) show how the redesign of the prescription interface, in providing predefined opportunities in the selection of medicines, strongly influences physician behaviour (Odukoya et al. 2014). The hierarchical order given to the information, in fact, implicitly acts as a recommendation.

Studying the effect of warnings on medicine interactions, Luna et al. (2007) report a high tendency to underestimate these signals due to the large number of warnings concerning clinically irrelevant interactions.

These are only a few examples, but they are adequate to show how the transition to technological prescription forms must result from careful planning.

Studies that have specifically examined the use of electronic prescribing technology (Weir et al. 2020) have pointed to an increase in the cognitive load on staff when storing information, an increase in inappropriate interpretations of prescriber information by pharmacy staff (e.g. for text boxes that cannot contain the full range of medicine indications), improper use of the 'drop-down' system in the prescriber's choice of medicine and patient, automatic selection of the medicine and/or dose based on the patient's previous purchases (Odukoya et al. 2003, 2014; Franklin and O'Grady 2007; Odukoyn and Chui 2012).

In conclusion, we report some indications emerging from a study aimed at detecting prescription errors at the dispensing stage and how they effectively prevented or intercepted them. In hospital pharmacies where the pharmacist could access patient data (Al-Khani et al. 2014), the research found the opportunity to dispense the required medication more consciously and safely and prevent some prescription errors. The factors that contributed to the identification of prescription errors, before the dispensing of the medicine were:

- the verification of the prescription indication of the medicine;
- the examination of the patient's medical history;
- examination of the patient's pharmacological history;
- an interview with the prescribing doctor;
- counselling the patient during dispensing.

8.4 Towards a Proper Dispensing

Prescribing a medicine, with the assessment of its necessity, the selection of the correct active ingredient, the personalisation of therapy, and the definition of the expected therapeutic response represents the completion of the complex activity of clinical assessment. However, prescribing a medicine is not a matter of closing but of starting a process that must be followed over time, monitoring the patient's response, identifying, and reporting any adverse events, re-evaluating the choice of medicine, the regimen, and the frequency and duration of treatment. It is a process in which collaboration and communication between healthcare professionals is essential, as well as the involvement of the patient, who must be educated about pharmacological care and trained in medicines.

Especially when the patient is faced with complex therapies—this is the case, for example, of the elderly patient or, in general, of the multi-disease patient—an activity of direction, review, and reorganisation of the patient's complete therapeutic regimen is also necessary.

The doctor, the pharmacist, and the pharma industry—through the package leaflet—play relevant but, at the same time, poorly connected and, therefore, deficient roles. For the patient, it is also unclear who to address for information about the treatment and its management, and the fragmentation of information, in addition to the ambiguous role played by the various actors involved in the process, means that the pharmacist's role is also not correctly understood. To some extent, the goal of improving communication and information sharing between general practitioners and pharmacists rests on the expectations of improvement entrusted to the use of technology (e.g. e-prescribing systems, electronic medical records, electronic patient drug history). However, the incentives for increasing services within the pharmacy activities should be carefully observed. This push towards a service pharmacy could take a commercial drift, effectively taking time away from patient counselling. Counselling constitutes a fundamental support for proper dispensing, as defined by Article 12 of the pharmacist's Code of Ethics.

References

Abood RR (1996) Errors in pharmacy practice. U.S. Pharmacist 21:122–132

Aldhwaihi K, Schifano F, Pezzolesi C, Umaru N (2016) A systematic review of the nature of dispensing errors in hospital pharmacies. Integr Pharm Res Pract 5:1–10

Al-Khani S, Moharram A, Aljadhey H (2014) Factors contributing to the identification and prevention of incorrect drug prescribing errors in outpatient setting. Saudi Pharm J 22:429–432

Ammenwerth E, Schnell-Inderst P, Machan C, Siebert U (2008) The effect of electronic prescribing on medication errors and adverse drug events: a systematic review. J Am Med Inform Assoc 15(5):585–600

Angelo LB, Ferreri SP (2005) Assessment of workflow redesign in community pharmacy. J Am Pharm Assoc 45(2):145–150

Ashcroft DM, Quinlan P, Blenkinsopp A (2005) Prospective study of the incidence, nature and causes of dispensing errors in community pharmacies. Pharmacoepidemiol Drug Saf 14:327–332

Barton Laws M, Yoojin L, Taubin T, Rogers WH, Wilson IB (2018) Factors associated with patient recall of key information in ambulatory specialty care visits: results of an innovative methodology. PLoS One 13:e0191940. https://doi.org/10.1371/journal.pone.0191940

Basco WT Jr, Ebeling M, Hulsey TC, Simpson K (2010) Using pharmacy data to screen for Look-Alike, Sound-Alike substitution errors in pediatric. Acad Pediatr 10:233–237

Bates DW, Cohen M, Leape LL (2001) Reducing the frequency of errors in medicine using information technology. J Am Med Inform Assoc 8:299–308

Berman A (2004) Reducing medication errors through naming, labeling, and packaging. J Med Syst 28(1):1–29

Bryan R, Aronson GK, Williams A, Jordan S (2020) The problem of look-alike, sound-alike name errors: drivers and solutions. Br J Clin Pharmacol 87:386–394

Buchanan T, Barker K, Gibson J, Jiang B, Pearson R (1991) Illumination and errors in dispensing. Am J Hosp Pharm 48(10):2131–2145

Campmans Z, van Rhijn A, Dull RM, Santen-Reestman J, Taxis K, Borgsteede SD (2018) Preventing dispensing errors by alerting for drug confusions in the pharmacy information system. A survey of users. PLoS One 13(5):e0197469. https://doi.org/10.1371/journal.pone.0197469

Chen Y-F, Neil KE, Avery AJ, Dewey ME, Johnson C (2005) Prescribing errors and other problems reported by community pharmacists. Ther Clin Risk Manag 1(4):333–342

Cheung K, Bouvy ML, De Smet P (2009) Medication errors: the importance of safe dispensing. Br J Clin Pharmacol 67(6):676–680

Ciociano N, Bagnasco L (2014) Look alike/sound alike drugs: a literature review on causes and solutions. Int J Clin Pharm 36:233–242. https://doi.org/10.1007/s11096-013-9885-6

Cohen MR (ed) (1999) Medication errors: causes, prevention and risk management, 2nd edn. American Pharmaceutical Association, Washington

Dean B, Barber N, Schachter M (2000) What is a prescribing error? Qual Health Care 9:232–237

Dellve L, Strömgren M, Williamsson A, Holden RJ, Eriksson A (2018) Health care clinicians' engagement in organizational redesign of care processes: the importance of work and organizational conditions. Appl Ergon 68:249–257

Emmerton L, Curtain C, Swaminathan G, Dowling H (2020) Development and exploratory analysis of software to detect look-alike, sound-alike medicine names. Int J Med Inform 137:104–119

European Parliament and of the Council (2011) Directive 2011/62/EU of the European Parliament and of the council, amending Directive 2001/83/EC on the community code relating to medicinal products for human use, as regards the prevention of the entry into the legal supply chain of falsified medicinal products. Off J Eur Union:74–87

Ferguson J, Keyworth C, Tully MP (2018) If no-one stops me, I'll make the mistake again': changing prescribing behaviours through feedback; a perceptual control theory perspective. Res Soc Adm Pharm 14(3):241–247

Flynn EA, Barker KN (1999) Medication error research. In: Cohen MR (ed) Medication errors: causes, prevention and risk management, 2nd edn. American Pharmaceutical Association, Washington, pp 15–41

Flynn E, Barker K, Gibson J, Pearson R, Smith L, Berger B (1996) Relationships between ambient sounds and the accuracy of pharmacists' prescription-filling performance. Hum Factors 38(4):614–622

Flynn E, Barker KN, Gibson J, Pearson R, Berger B, Smith L (1999) Impact of interruptions and distractions on dispensing errors in an ambulatory care pharmacy. Am J Health Syst Pharm 56:1319–1325

Flynn EA, Dorris NT, Holman GT, Camahan BJ, Barker KN (2002) Medication dispensing errors in community pharmacies: a nationwide study. In: Proceedings of the human factors and ergonomics society, 46th annual meeting, pp 1449–1451

Franklin BD, O'Grady K (2007) Dispensing errors in community pharmacy: frequency, clinical significance and potential impact of authentication at the point of dispensing. Int J Pharm Pract 15:273–281. https://doi.org/10.1211/ijpp.15.4.0004

Garattini L, Nobili A (2021) Farmacie di comunità, il labile confine fra commercio e sanità. Quotidianosanità.it. Retrieved August 24, 2022 from https://www.quotidianosanita.it/studi-e-analisi/articolo.php?articolo_id=98050

Grasha A, Schell K (2001) Psychosocial factors, workload and human error in a simulated pharmacy dispensing task. Percept Mot Skills 92(1):53–71

Harvey J, Avery AJ, Ashcroft D, Boyd M, Phipps DL, Barber N (2015) Exploring safety systems for dispensing in community pharmacies: focusing on how staff relate to organizational components. Res Soc Adm Pharm 11(2):216–227. https://doi.org/10.1016/j.sapharm.2014.06.005

Hellström LM, Bondesson Å, Höglund P, Eriksson T (2012) Errors in medication history at hospital admission: prevalence and predicting factors. BMC Clin Pharmacol 12(9):1–9. https://

doi.org/10.1186/1472-6904-12-9. Retrieved August 4, 2022, from https://link.springer.com/article/10.1186/1472-6904-12-9

Hoxsie DM, Keller AE, Armstrong EP (2006) Analysis of community pharmacy workflow processes in preventing dispensing errors. J Pharm Pract 19(2):124–130. https://doi.org/10.1177/0897190005285602

James LK, Barlow D, McArtney R, Hiom S, Roberts D, Whittlesea C (2009) Incidence, type and causes of dispensing errors: a review of the literature. Int J Pharm Pract 17:9–30. https://doi.org/10.1211/ijpp/17.1.0004

Jones CEL, Phipps DL, Ashcroft DM (2018) Understanding procedural violations using safety-I and safety-II: the case of community pharmacies. Saf Sci 105:114–120

Karsh BT, Weinger MB, Abbott PA, Wears L (2010) Health information technology: fallacies and sober realities. J Am Med Inform Assoc 17:617–623. https://doi.org/10.1136/jamia.2010.005637

Kennedey AG, Littenberg P, Callas PW, Carney JK (2011) Evaluation of a modified prescription form to address prescribing errors. Am J Health Syst Pharm 68:151–157

Kessels R (2003) Patients' memory for medical information. J R Soc Med 96:219–222

Lea VM, Corlett SA, Rodgers RM (2015) Describing interruptions, multi-tasking and tasks witching in community pharmacy: a qualitative study in England. Int J Clin Pharm 37:1086–1094

Lesar TS (1998) Errors in the use of medication dosage equations. Arch Pediatr Adolesc Med 152(4):340–344. https://doi.org/10.1001/archpedi.152.4.340

Lester CA, Chui MA (2016) Using link analysis to explore the impact of the physical environment on pharmacist tasks. Res Soc Adm Pharm 12:627–632

Lizano-Díez I, Figueiredo-Escribá C, Piñero-López MA, Lastra CF, Mariño EL, Modamio P (2020) Prevention strategies to identify LASA errors: building and sustaining a culture of patient safety. BMB Health Serv Res 20(63):1–5

Luna D, Otero V, Canosa D, Montenegro S, Otero P, de Quirós FGB (2007) Analysis and redesign of a knowledge database for a drug-drug interactions alert system. Stud Health Technol Inform 129:885–889

Madlon-Kay DJ, Mosch FS (2023) Liquid medication dosing errors. J Fam Pract 49(8):741

Malhotra S, Cheriff AD, Gossey JT, Cole CL, Kaushal R, Ancker JS (2016) Effects of an e-prescribing interface redesign on rates of generic drug prescribing: exploiting default options. J Am Med Inform Assoc 23(5):891–898. https://doi.org/10.1093/jamia/ocv192

Mamena AK, Håkonsenb H, Kjomea RLS, Gustavsen-Krabbesundb B, Toverudb EL (2015) Norwegian elderly patients' need for drug information and attitudes towards medication use reviews in community pharmacies. Int J Pharm Pract 23:423–428

Martìnez Sànchez A (2013) Medication errors in a Spanish community pharmacy: nature, frequency and potential causes. Int J Clin Pharm 35:185–189. https://doi.org/10.1007/s11096-012-9741-0

Ministero della salute (2008) Raccomandazione Ministeriale n. 7—Raccomandazione per la prevenzione della morte, coma o grave danno derivati da errori in terapia farmacologica. Retrieved from https://www.salute.gov.it/imgs/c_17_pubblicazioni_675_allegato.pdf

Ministero della salute (2010a) Raccomandazione Ministeriale n. 12. Retrieved October 18, 2022, from https://www.salute.gov.it/imgs/C_17_pubblicazioni_1307_allegato.pdf

Ministero della salute (2010b) Sicurezza delle terapie farmacologiche, Farmaci LASA. Retrieved August 7, 2022, from https://www.salute.gov.it/portale/sicurezzaCure/dettaglioContenutiSicurezzaCure.jsp?lingua=italiano&id=2459&area=qualita&menu=sicurezzaterapie

Ministero della salute (2015) Elenco farmaci LASA aggiornato al 2015. Retrieved from https://www.salute.gov.it/imgs/C_17_pubblicazioni_2502_ulterioriallegati_ulterioreallegato_0_alleg.pdf

Ministero della salute (2018) Raccomandazione n. 18—Raccomandazione per la prevenzione degli errori in terapia conseguenti all'uso di abbreviazioni, acronimi, sigle e simboli. Retrieved from https://www.salute.gov.it/imgs/C_17_pubblicazioni_2802_allegato.pdf

Ness JE, Sullivan SD, Stergachis A (1994) Accuracy of technicians and pharmacists in identifying dispensing errors. Am J Hosp Pharm 51(3):354–357

Nusair MB, Guirguis LM (2017) How pharmacists check the appropriateness of drug therapy? Observations in community pharmacy. Res Soc Adm Pharm 13:349–357

Odukoya OK, Chui MA (2012) Retail pharmacy staff perceptions of design strengths and weaknesses of electronic prescribing. J Am Med Inform Assoc 19:1059–1065

Odukoya OK, Stone JA, Chui MA (2003) Barriers and facilitators to recovering from e-prescribing errors in community pharmacies. J Am Pharm Assoc 55(1):52–58

Odukoya OK, Stone JA, Chui MA (2014) E-prescribing errors in community pharmacies: exploring consequences and contributing factors. Int J Med Inform 83(6):427–437

Ostini R, Roughead E, Kirkpatrick C, Monteith R, Tett S (2012) Quality use of medicines: medication safety issues in naming; look-alike, sound-alike medicine names. Int J Pharm Pract 20:349–357

Pérez-Moreno MA, Rodríguez-Camacho JM, Calderón-Hernanz B, Comas-Díaz B, Tarradas-Torras J (2017) Clinical relevance of pharmacist intervention in an emergency department. Emerg Med J 34:492–493. https://doi.org/10.1136/emermed-2016-206470

Phipps DL, Noyce PR, Parker D, Ashcroft DM (2009) Medication safety in community pharmacy: a qualitative study of the sociotechnical context. BMC Health Serv Res 9(158):1–10. https://doi.org/10.1186/1472-6963-9-158. Retrieved September 18, 2022, from https://www.salute.gov.it/portale/documentazione/p6_2_8_1_1.jsp?lingua=italiano&id=18.

Ruutiainen HK, Kallio MM, Kuitunen SK (2021) Identification and safe storage of look-alike, sound-alike medicines in automated dispensing cabinets. Eur J Hosp Pharm 28:e151–e156. https://doi.org/10.1136/ejhpharm-2020-002531

Stojkovic T, Marinkovic V, Manser T (2017) Using prospective risk analysis tools to improve safety in pharmacy settings: a systematic review and critical appraisal. J Patient Saf 17(6):515–523. https://doi.org/10.1097/PTS.0000000000000403

Szeinbach S, Seoane-Vazquez E, Parekh A, Herderick M (2007) Dispensing errors in community pharmacy: perceived influence of sociotechnical factors. Int J Qual Health Care 19(4):203–209

The European Parliament and of the Council (2001) Directive 2001/83/EC of 6 November 2001 on the community code relating to medicinal products for human use. Off J Eur Communities 28(11):2001. Retrieved from https://eur-lex.europa.eu/legal-content/EN/TXT/PDF/?uri=CELEX:32001L0083

Trbovich PL, Hyland S (2017) Responding to the challenge of look-alike, sound-alike drug names. BMJ Qual Saf 26:357–359. https://doi.org/10.1136/bmjqs-2016-005629

van de Vreede M, McRae A, Wiseman M, Dooley MJ (2008) Successful introduction of Tallman letters to reduce medication selection errors in a hospital network. J Pharm Pract Res 38(4):263–266

Weir NM, Newham R, Bennie M (2020) A literature review of human factors and ergonomics within the pharmacy dispensing process. Res Soc Adm Pharm 16(5):637–645. https://doi.org/10.1016/j.sapharm.2019.08.029

Open Access This chapter is licensed under the terms of the Creative Commons Attribution 4.0 International License (http://creativecommons.org/licenses/by/4.0/), which permits use, sharing, adaptation, distribution and reproduction in any medium or format, as long as you give appropriate credit to the original author(s) and the source, provide a link to the Creative Commons license and indicate if changes were made.

The images or other third party material in this chapter are included in the chapter's Creative Commons license, unless indicated otherwise in a credit line to the material. If material is not included in the chapter's Creative Commons license and your intended use is not permitted by statutory regulation or exceeds the permitted use, you will need to obtain permission directly from the copyright holder.

Chapter 9
The Future Digital Pharmacological Prescriptions Between Therapy Adherence and Integrated Healthcare Personal Plans

Giuseppe Andreoni

Abstract The medical prescription is a most used and common tool to deliver clinical instructions for healthcare actions to the patient and among all the clinical actors involved in the process. Today this informative process is implemented by a paper sheet different in each country for format and content. In Italy it contains a limited set of instructions and mainly reports administrative data, so missing the main function to provide information and to act as a *pro-memoria* tool (about therapy parameters like dosage, assumption plan, interactions) for the patients. This is a factor affecting therapeutical adherence and, consequently, efficacy. New digital technologies offer the new e-health services to empower patients, caregivers, and clinical operators in the frame of the 5-P medicine for a more personalized and accurate approach. This process should involve also the first step towards health which is represented by the access to healthcare and the consequent prescription (pharmaceutical or diagnostic or therapeutical). This chapter discusses the current situation of processes driven by medical prescriptions, their formats, and their expected evolution in the frame of the new digital medicine vision.

9.1 Introduction

The medical prescription is a very common tool to deliver clinical instructions for healthcare actions: diagnostic examination, specialistic consultation for diagnosis or rehabilitation, pharmaceutical indication. Its scope is specifically informative, both for the patient and for the final clinical actor: the specialist for the consultation, the pharmacist for the medicine delivery to the patient, the administrative officer and the technical biomedical operator at the hospital for the diagnostic or rehabilitative interventions. The pharmacological therapy represents the most common and diffused healthcare practice in the world, treating both chronic and time-limited

G. Andreoni (✉)
Department of Design, Politecnico di Milano, Milan, Italy

Bioengineering Laboratory, Scientific Institute IRCCS E. Medea, Bosisio Parini, Italy
e-mail: giuseppe.andreoni@polimi.it

pathologies. It is generally driven to the patient through a prescription of the general practitioner (GP) for common and low complexity pathologies or of a specialist doctor (SD): the first one verbally explains the assumption mode and frequency and deliver a standard health recipe which the patient goes to the pharmacy with to buy/receive the medication; the SD provides the report of the visit with the prescription and this is to be asked again to the GP. In some cases, for low complexity and common pathologies a self-medication is also frequent, according to personal experience and symptoms understanding. This common process should be optimized considering the 5P medicine vision (Pravettoni and Triberti 2020), meaning the proposed strategy to improve the clinical efficacy and efficiency in health and economic sense by a Preventive, Predictive, Personalized, Participatory and Pluri-expert approach that leads the process towards the Precision Medicine (Fig. 9.1). In this way we can also try to minimize the impact of the non-adherence to pharmacological therapy thanks to the so-called patient empowerment and her/his active participation to the process (Andreoni et al. 2022).

The correct prescription, at the right time, with the correct medication, for the exact patient, correct dose (personalized vs standard amount in the package), correct dosage (amount per day/week), correct assumption over time (assumption typology and distribution of assumption per day/week), correct duration (medication assumption and washout) is the perfect "pathway to health". This process and the patient empowerment towards the full understanding of the pathology, of the therapy and of the correct therapeutical plan, need new and more efficient tools for

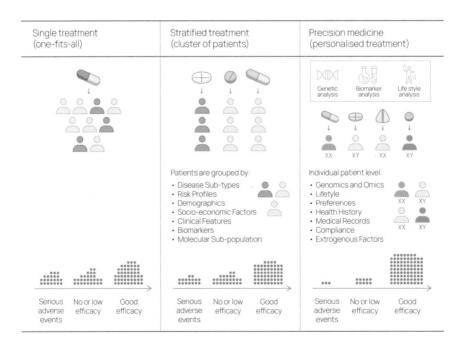

Fig. 9.1 The evolution of the medicine

the complete communication among and the involved actors (e.g., patient, doctor, pharmacist, nurse, therapist, familiar caregiver, etc.) in the very different paths that could be activated.

9.2 The Medical Prescription

9.2.1 The Communication in the Medical Prescription

In pharmaceutical therapies the most common tool is the medical prescription. This process is done by a verbal and written transmission of information from the medical doctor to the patient and or eventually her/his familiar caregiver. Indeed, the correct and complete communication is the first step toward therapy adherence. But Kessels (2003) demonstrated that the verbal component of the process is not sufficient: memory for medical information is often poor and inaccurate, especially when the patient is old or anxious (Kessels 2003) Patients tend to focus on diagnosis-related information and fail to register instructions on treatment. Sinbukhova et al. (2021) recently recorded that patients were able to remember correctly 24.8% of medical information on the next day after consultation by a neurosurgeon on average (Sinbukhova et al. 2021) The main factors affecting the correct communication were anxiety and depression with negative correlation to the level of information assimilated by patients: the higher level of anxiety and depression before surgery led to decrease remembering of medical information by the patients. Their conclusion was that is necessary to increase remembering of medical information by patients because of it is allowing to improve the results of treatment.

Simple and specific instructions are better recalled than general statements (Kessels 2003). The written prescription should complement this process. In fact, patients can be helped to remember medical information by use of explicit categorization techniques. In addition, spoken information should be supported with written or visual material. Visual communication aids are especially effective in low-literacy patients, but again Kessels (2003) found that video or multimedia techniques do not improve memory performance or adherence to therapy. Laws et al. (2018) studied the factors associated with patient recall of key information in ambulatory specialty care visits; their findings showed forty-nine percent of decisions and recommendations were recalled accurately without prompting; 36% recalled with a prompt; 15% recalled erroneously or not at all (Laws et al. 2018) Provider behaviours hypothesized to be associated with patient recall, such as open-questioning and "teach back", were rare. Findings suggest that patient recall could be enhanced if providers were to use more of the techniques to encourage patient engagement, such as open questioning, agenda setting, and teach-back; and limit the amount of information to be remembered in a single visit based on an assessment of patients' ability to recall.

9.2.2 The Format of the Medical Prescription

The medical prescription has no common international standard format. Each country has a different situation for information that this medical document shall contain and provide.

For example, in the USA it is a very informative module (Fig. 9.2a) that must include several items (Kenny and Preuss 2022). In the USA there are five different levels of scheduling for medications (I–V), with schedule I, having the tightest controls, and V, being the least restrictive. Schedule II medicines are the highest level of misuse potential medications that may be prescribed by a clinician; these medicines

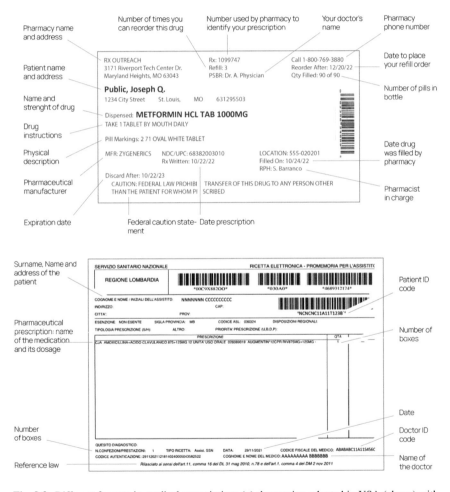

Fig. 9.2 Different formats in medical prescription: (**a**) the version adopted in USA (above) with very detailed contents; (**b**) the Italian format (below) as simple indication of the pharmaceutical treatment

traditionally were only allowed to be filled by paper prescription but today they are prescribable via electronic prescribing of controlled substances (EPCS). Schedule III-V medications may be prescribed by a clinician via traditional paper prescription, by a verbal order over the phone, or using the EPCS system. Practitioners may still write and sign prescriptions for schedule II–V medications if they choose; verbal orders to the pharmacist are only permitted for schedule III–V medications. In case of EPCS, it should also record the following information in the prescription: name of the pharmacy who is receiving the prescription, its telephone number and address.

In Italy, the medical prescription is a more and administrative ticket (Fig. 9.2b), namely standardized sheet where only simple information is given about the medication to be given to the patient by the pharmacist as prescribed by the doctor (usually the GP or sometimes directly the SD), so missing most of the relevant information. This communication problem is exacerbated in case of polypharmaceutical prescription at the same time. With the increase of aging population this condition is becoming quite common. In Italy, in 2017, Valent (2019) recorded that 63.7% of the general population received at least one medicine prescription, and 25,218 persons were co-prescribed ≥5 medications at least once (Valent 2019). The prevalence of co-prescriptions among persons ≥65 years was 31.7%. 20,793 persons used ≥60 defined daily doses of ≥5 medications. The prevalence of all these phenomena was much higher in the elderly than in children and adults. The number of comorbidities significantly affected all types of polypharmacy. We can assume that this situation could be similar in most of the European and western countries with a similar social structure: from this the prevalence of polypharmacy is high, particularly among the elderly.

In the US, the implementation of electronic prescribing has significantly reduced the number of medication errors from a prescription standpoint (legibility, dosage, frequency, etc.) (Kaldy 2016; Volpe et al. 2016). The definition of a set of requirements for the prescriptions was a standpoint. For a pharmacist to dispense a controlled substance, the prescription must include specific information to be considered valid: Date of issue, Patient's name and address, Patient's date of birth, Clinician name, address, DEA number, Medicine name, Medicine strength, Dosage form, Quantity prescribed, Directions for use, Number of refills, Signature of prescriber.

9.2.3 Adherence to Medical Prescription

Polypharmacy is one of the most important risk factors for the onset of adverse medicine reactions, with a consequent impact in terms of increased hospital admissions, increased costs, and mortality. The management and the therapy for chronic diseases is a typical example of polypharmacy and poor adherence. Therapy management is even more difficult when the condition is chronic and therefore implies a constant relationship with the disease throughout one's life.

In a specific report of WHO (2003a), the estimate of adherence in patients suffering from chronic diseases is only 50%, in developed countries; while the impact of low adherence in developing countries was assumed to be even higher, given the scarcity of health resources and inequalities in access to health care (Quaderni SIF 2017). For adhesion or adherence to therapy it is meant the active compliance of the patient at doctor's recommendations regarding times, doses, and frequency of intake of the medicine for the entire course of therapy. More adherence means reduced risk of hospitalization, reduced complications associated with the disease and with lower entity, greater safety, and efficacy of treatments and even reduction of costs for therapies.

Even today, data from studies and literature confirm that adherence to chronic therapies remains an emerging and current problem. 80% of people over 65 suffer from heart failure, respiratory insufficiency, sleep disorders, diabetes, obesity, depression, dementia, hypertension, which often occur simultaneously in the same individual (Ministero della Salute 2017). By 2020, chronic diseases will represent about 80% of all diseases in the world, for the management of which about 70–80% of global resources will be committed.

The National Institute for Health and Care Excellence (NICE) with respect to adherence in chronicity, underlines that there is a high risk of error in taking treatments, especially in the presence of polypharmacotherapy and multimorbidity. WHO estimates indicate that between 30% and 50% of prescribed medicines are not taken as they should (WHO 2003a). Additionally, between 30% and 70% of patients make a mistake or inadvertently switch medications, especially when switching from one regimen or treatment area to another. In the guide, NICE underlines the importance of shared decision and the involvement of the person, as an essential component of evidence-based medicine.

A report commissioned by the Department of Health has revealed that in UK between 5% and 8% of unplanned hospital admissions are due to problems related to the use of medicines and, on preventable adverse events that can be attributed to one or more specific errors (Frontier Economics 2014). Therapeutical adherence is also affected by poor communication. Adherence is more detailed defined as:

> The degree to which a person's behaviour—in taking medications, following a diet and/or making changes to one's lifestyle—corresponds to the recommendations agreed with health care providers.

This definition considers the attitude of the person to comply with the recommendations of the healthcare professional, in all those behaviours that contribute to full adherence to the treatment path, from pharmacological or follow-up prescriptions, to dietary indications, to suggestions for a change in lifestyle (WHO 2003b). When the communication between the clinician and the patient is imperfect, the latter is exposed to adherence error. Poor adherence produces important impacts both from a clinical point of view, and therefore from the health of the community, but also from the point of view of the sustainability of health systems, a growing problem in many countries. It is in fact the main cause of non-effectiveness of pharmacological therapies and is associated with an increase in healthcare interventions, morbidity, and mortality, representing damage both for patients and for the healthcare system and for society. Some studies revealed that 30–50% of adults in America do not adequately follow the prescriptions of long-lasting medicines, with waste of about 100 billion dollars a year and the patient at greatest risk of non-adherence is represented by the elderly in polytherapy (Marcum et al. 2013; Iuga and McGuire 2014). The pharmacological prescription for acute problems (antibiotic therapy) is followed by 3/4 of the patients while if the therapy lasts 10 days, only 1/4 of the patients completes the cycle.

Furthermore, these studies confirm that therapeutic non-adherence is particularly critical in patients with long-term therapies and polytherapy, with all the consequences that may derive from a discontinuity of the treatment (compromised efficacy of the therapy) (WHO 2003b). This is very often due to the psychological and emotional condition of the chronic patient which translates into discomfort, loss of trust, demotivation with respect to the efficacy/benefits of the treatment or due to the complexity of managing the therapy.

9.3 The New Model: Towards Territorial and Personalized Healthcare

To achieve Precision Medicine a structural reform of the healthcare system and its services is needed. The pandemic period demonstrated the need of the exploitation of two main elements.

- The Precision Medicine is targeted to the individual patient and for this it requires the deep knowledge of this patient; data are essential but not exhaustive. The prolonged and comprehensive knowledge about the patient's health and history and about the social environment where she/he lives is needed for a global and efficient approach. Only a clinical operator close to the patient can engage with her/him this kind of trusted relationship to have a full diagnostic, therapeutical or rehabilitation adherence. On this the new concept of Clinical Pathways are rapidly being adopted.
- The territorial medicine is the near presence of services and resources available to the patient in her/his own environment or town (Andreoni 2023). These services need a proper management tool to be activated. The medical prescription should evolve to a service enabling tool, integrating all the necessary information to identify all the actions and their parameters for the best delivery of the proper, personalized care intervention. At the same time, a comprehensive and intuitive Electronic Health Record should be developed and available for the recording and the integration of these data, actions, and outcomes, not for administrative purposes but as factors, parameters, and indexes of an individual health model (Kamel Boulos and Zhang 2021).

The Clinical Pathways define the best diagnostic, treatment or rehabilitative process for a specific pathology, or a clinical problem based on the best technical-scientific knowledge and in relation to the available resources. They allow the Healthcare System to outline, the best practicable approach for the best result for the patient and for the optimization of resources within the healthcare organization. The purpose of the clinical pathways is to define a homogeneous, structured, integrated, and multidisciplinary pathway for the management of the pathology/condition being treated, optimize the network of services and trying to meet the needs of patients, ensure during all stages the continuity of care, promote communication and discussion between the professionals involved. They can describe the entire patient care pathway (Diagnostic Therapeutic Assistance Pathway—PDTA) or one or more phases of the path itself (Diagnostic Therapeutic Pathway—PDT; Integrated Care Pathway—PIC), but always providing the integration between hospital and territorial services (Ministero della Salute 2017). Through this structured protocol the healthcare system aims to guarantee: the reproducibility of actions but in a personalized care plan, the indicators needed to monitor the outcomes and clinical and management level, the uniformity of services provided to all patients, the reduction of the extraordinary events; the integration of the clinical service to the patient with shared communication among all the involved actors, the definition of patient management plan with well identified and clear roles for the actors involved in the process and creating awareness and trust in the patient. And awareness and trust mean empowerment of the patient and the adoption of an active role in co-managing her/his own health, the increase the adherence to the clinical actions by the patient and her/his best achievement of therapeutic targets (with lower expenditure). This patient empowerment strategy is struggling to establish itself because it is linked to the relationship with the treating doctor and with health professionals, which should evolve towards a less asymmetrical model, with the patient called to be an increasingly active part in decisions relating to your health. For this reason, in the next future the education of the patient and her/his caregivers represents one of the most important products of the empowerment process.

In this light, and with these premises, the medical prescription sheet should evolve from an administrative document to a service-enabling document, to a tool describing in a complete, comprehensive, and intuitive format the personal Clinical Pathway for a unique and identified subject in a well-defined health environment with its players (GP, SD, other clinical operators, familiar caregivers, etc.).

9.4 The New Health E-Prescription

This process needs to be integrated into the continuous technological evolution of products and services. Today the technology offers connected devices and mobile terminals, multimodal communication, apps and webapps providing several and different services. Also in medicine, this revolution has opened new perspectives to be fully exploited: smartphone and related apps allows access and consultation of the

Electronic Health Record (and of health digital twins which is the new frontier of health data integration), tele-visit, ubiquitous monitoring of health parameters, up to e-administration of clinical events (Kamel Boulos and Zhang 2021).

In this perspective, also the medical prescription must evolve towards a more mature and evolute format. It has the potentiality to become an active service tool not simply a static administrative ticket. The e-prescription should be co-designed to implement the explicit and implicit needs for a multimodal system for communication, education, reminder, adherence monitoring and other functionalities.

This new e-prescription should be a shared, cloud resident e-document connecting and to be updated by all the actors, each one with the own proper role and different authorization levels: the patient, the GP, the SD, the pharmacist, the rehabilitation operator or the technical for the imaging examination. In other word it should become a single common tool for many services. It is not to be confused with the Electronics Health Record: this is the complete personal health database, while the e-prescription is related and could drive a single, even complex, process. In this way the traditional step-by-step procedure or transfer of the material medical prescription (from the GP to the patient, from the patient to the hospital for the examination or to the pharmacist for the collection of the medicines or to the SD and other options) is translated into a new process, integrated and processed in the cloud and managed by the mobile terminals of the patient, the GP, the pharmacist and so on in relation to the service. To provide a personalized, aware, trusted, and clear process to the patient and her/his familiar caregiver, all the actors should be involved in the co-design process to integrate in this new format the proper information and needed service description with its parameters (for instance, from a simple pharmaceutical prescription to a complex technological examination).

Some possible services that the new e-prescription could enable or embed can be the following suggestions:

- link to multi-media instructions for supporting the correct assumption even for simple situations (even simple but frequent questions like: *can I break the pill before intake? Should I drink only water, or can I drink other liquids?* etc.);
- link to the national pharmaceutical agency and specific webpage, to retrieve all the information about the prescribed medicine, such as active principle, the other ingredients, the possible interactions with other medicines, the different dosages available and any other important recommendations, to maximize adherence and efficacy;
- link to the clinical studies and their full outcomes, pre- and post-market registries of efficacy or adverse events, for a complete awareness about the treatment;
- the generation of a calendar and its download on the mobile device for the complete treatment plan and related reminder;
- the generation of a calendar and its download on the mobile device for examination or rehabilitation sessions;
- link to e-administration services like the procedures and access to online resources for bookings, payments, and other services (GP or Hospital or territorial points).

In this development UX/UI design methodologies could play a very relevant role, supporting access, usability, content readability, intuitive implementation of complex processes of prescription able to avoid errors or misunderstandings that in medicine are so dangerous or increasing adherence that is so necessary.

9.5 Conclusion

The organization of a new healthcare systems and structure after the pandemic emergency is asking the adoption of more efficient and quick tools in the clinical practice and organization. Not only complex task should be redesigned and improved but even starting from the paper-based, static, and poor of information medical prescription is a great kick-off towards the future of healthcare.

The e-prescription shall be integrated in the health information systems: communication is the cornerstone of integrated management and care networks, an indispensable element between the various operators, between the various services, between the different levels (territory/hospital), as well as a central factor of the patient's relationship of trust and his empowerment process. The new technologies available (audio-visual communication, telemedicine, etc.) seem to be able to help facilitate communication and improve assistance in terms of effectiveness and efficiency. The main technological requirement is the interoperability with respect to the various platform and operative systems and its connectivity. The main user requirements are usability and content intuitiveness so to implement an error-free process among all the actors. The main service requirement is the integration so to have a structured continuous process along with the clinical and the administrative procedures. The development of this new format for the medical prescription could be a strategic choice in improving our healthcare services, in saving time, saving costs, increasing efficiency and, above all, the quality of life and our health.[1]

References

Andreoni G (2023) Capsules of health in the city. In: Anzani A, Scullica F (eds) The city of care, Springer series in design and innovation, vol 26. Springer, Cham. https://doi.org/10.1007/978-3-031-14608-4_10

Andreoni G, Caiani EG, Castaldini N (2022) Digital health services through patient empowerment: classification, current state and preliminary impact assessment by health pod systems. Appl Sci 12:359. https://doi.org/10.3390/app12010359

Frontier Economics (2014) Exploring the costs of unsafe care in the NHS: A Report Prepared for the Department of Health. London. Available online: https://www.frontier-economics.com/

---

[1] The author wants to sincerely thank Dr. Erio Morcelli, for the extensive discussion to understand the evolution of the new territorial health scenario, of the introduction of the PDTA with their expected impact, and of the new roles for prescription in the view of a General Practitioner.

media/2459/exploring-the-costs-of-unsafe-care-in-the-nhs-frontier-report-2-2-2-2.pdf. Last accessed on 15 Jan 2023

Iuga AO, McGuire MJ (2014) Adherence and health care costs. Risk Manag Healthc Policy 7:35–44. https://doi.org/10.2147/RMHP.S19801

Kaldy J (2016) Controlled substances add new layer to E-prescribing. Consult Pharm 31(4):200–206

Kamel Boulos MN, Zhang P (2021) Digital twins: from personalised medicine to precision public health. J Pers Med 11(745). https://doi.org/10.3390/jpm11080745

Kenny BJ, Preuss CV (2022) Pharmacy prescription requirements. [Updated 24 Sep 2022]. In: StatPearls [internet]. StatPearls Publishing, Treasure Island. 2023 January. Available from: https://www.ncbi.nlm.nih.gov/books/NBK538424/?report=classic

Kessels RPC (2003) Patients' memory for medical information. J R Soc Med 96:219–222

Laws MB, Lee Y, Taubin T, Rogers WH, Wilson IB (2018) Factors associated with patient recall of key information in ambulatory specialty care visits: results of an innovative methodology. PLoS One 13(2):e0191940. https://doi.org/10.1371/journal.pone.0191940

Marcum ZA, Sevick MA, Handler SM (2013) Medication nonadherence: a diagnosable and treatable medical condition. JAMA 309(20):2105–2106. https://doi.org/10.1001/jama.2013.4638

Ministero della Salute (2017) Direzione Generale della Programmazione Sanitaria. Piano Nazionale della Cronicità. Available online: https://www.salute.gov.it/imgs/C_17_pubblicazioni_2584_allegato.pdf. Last accessed on 15 Jan 2023

Pravettoni G, Triberti SA (2020) "P5" approach to healthcare and health technology. In: Pravettoni G, Triberti S (eds) P5 eHealth: an agenda for the health technologies of the future. Springer, Cham

Quaderni della SIF—Società Italiana di Farmacologia (gennaio 2017) Anno XIII n. 42. https://www.sifweb.org/pubblicazioni/quaderni-della-sif

Sinbukhova EV, Shimanskiy VN, Tanyashin SV, Shevchenko KV, Poshataev VK, Abdurakhimov FD, Lubnin AY (2021) Remembering what the doctor said: how much of medical information will the patient remember? Russ J Neurosurg 23:50–60. https://doi.org/10.17650/1683-3295-2021-23-4-50-60

Valent F (2019) Polypharmacy in the general population of a Northern Italian area: analysis of administrative data. Annali Istituto Superiore di Sanità 55(3):233–239. https://doi.org/10.4415/ANN_19_03_06

Volpe CR, Melo EM, Aguiar LB, Pinho DL, Stival MM (2016) Risk factors for medication errors in the electronic and manual prescription. Rev Lat Am Enfermagem 24:e2742

World Health Organization (WHO) (2003a) Report on medication adherence, Geneva

World Health Organization (WHO) (2003b) Adherence to long term therapies: evidence for action, Geneva

Open Access This chapter is licensed under the terms of the Creative Commons Attribution 4.0 International License (http://creativecommons.org/licenses/by/4.0/), which permits use, sharing, adaptation, distribution and reproduction in any medium or format, as long as you give appropriate credit to the original author(s) and the source, provide a link to the Creative Commons license and indicate if changes were made.

The images or other third party material in this chapter are included in the chapter's Creative Commons license, unless indicated otherwise in a credit line to the material. If material is not included in the chapter's Creative Commons license and your intended use is not permitted by statutory regulation or exceeds the permitted use, you will need to obtain permission directly from the copyright holder.

Chapter 10
Navigating the Complexities of the OTC Medicine Ecosystem

Elena Caratti

Abstract The previous chapters have analysed the difficulties a patient may face in purchasing a medicine, even though supported by the prescription and the information he or she may receive, in written or verbal form, from the doctor during the examination and from the pharmacist during dispensing of the medicine. However, some medicines do not need to be prescribed by the doctor but can be purchased independently by the patient. In these cases, even more so than in the case of medicines dispensed on prescription, it is necessary for the information accompanying the medicine to be comprehensive, understandable and to make certain information available to the patient before the medicine is purchased. This is the case here with over-the-counter analgesics.

10.1 The Over-the-Counter Analgesics

When we have quite common symptoms as headache, toothache, a few fever lines, we use medicines (as Aspirin) that can reduce inflammation (antiphlogistics), or lowering body temperature in case of fever (antipyretics). Several painkiller medicines are defined as over-the-counter (OTC) or non-prescription (SOP) medicines. OTC drugs, also defined as self-medication drugs, are those medicines that are displayed above the pharmacy counter or in areas to which patients have free access.

They can alleviate many symptoms without the intermediation of a doctor. However, as Lynch suggests,[1] the safe use of these drugs requires knowledge,

---

[1] Shalini S. Lynch, *Panoramica sui farmaci da banco* [*Overview of over-the-counter medicines*], https://www.msdmanuals.com/it-it/casa/farmaci/farmaci-da-banco/panoramica-sui-farmaci-da-banco, (consulted on 21.11.2022).

E. Caratti (✉)
Department of Design, Politecnico di Milano, Milan, Italy
e-mail: elena.caratti@polimi.it

© The Author(s) 2025
A. V. Penati (ed.), *In-Home Medication*, Research for Development,
https://doi.org/10.1007/978-3-031-53294-8_10

common sense, and responsibility, because there may be some contraindications, so it is essential to read the package leaflet.

Patients can access them without the requirement of a prescription, they can buy them autonomously, under the advice of a pharmacist, or on the suggestion of advertising which is permitted for this category of medicines. This differentiates OTC from SOP drugs[2] which, although they do not require a prescription, cannot be advertised.

OTC can be acquired at pharmacies, parapharmacies, at supermarkets in specific dedicated corners with a pharmacist, or online. They belong to band C-bis (a sub-class of band C); therefore, their cost is fully charged to the citizen (they can't be reimbursable by the National Health System).

Analgesics, from Greek $ἀναλγησία$ «insensibility to pain», derivation from $ἀναλγής$ «without pain», made by $ἀν$- privative and $ἄλγος$ «pain»,[3] are medicines that are used in therapy to counteract painful stimuli of varying origin and severity (mild, moderate, or severe).

As stated in the MSD (manual version for patients and professionals)[4] analgesics fall into three categories:

- Non-opioids;
- Opioids (narcotics);
- Adjuvants (drugs usually used to treat other problems, such as convulsions or depression, but which can also relieve pain).

Non-opioid painkillers can be utilized for mild to moderate or sometimes severe pain. They are the medicines of first choice for contrasting pain. They don't create the risk of developing physical dependence and are well tolerated.

Among non-opioid analgesics, ibuprofen, ketoprofen and naproxen, are available over the counter, but higher dosages may require a prescription; on the contrary Aspirina C and Paracetamol (for example, the well-known *Tachipirina*), are non-opioid analgesics, and both are over-the-counter drugs.

Many of the most used non-opioid painkillers are also classified as non-steroidal anti-inflammatory drugs (in Italy FANS,[5] NSAID abroad).

---

[2] Non-prescription medicines—more simply referred to as SOPs—are those medicines that can be dispensed in pharmacies without a prescription, they can be taken for ailments that are considered mild and transient. Unlike OTPs, the law prevents SOPs from being advertised in any way and it's necessary the intermediation with a pharmacist.

[3] See https://www.treccani.it/enciclopedia/analgesici_%28Enciclopedia-Italiana%29/, (consulted on 21.11.2022).

[4] James C. Watson, *Pain Treatment*, on https://www.msdmanuals.com/it-it/casa/disturbi-di-cervello,-midollo-spinale-e-nervi/dolore/trattamento-del-dolore?query = analgesico, (consulted on 22.11.2022).

[5] The most diffused FANS are ibuprofen, naproxen, diclofenac, celecoxib, mefenamic, acid etoricoxib, indomethacin, nimesulide, high-dose aspirin, https://www.issalute.it/index.php/la-salute-dalla-a-alla-z-menu/f/fans-farmaci-antinfiammatori-non-steroidei?highlight=WyJhc3BpcmluYSJd#tipologie-di-fans, (accessed 2022 Nov. 22).

They can be taken for short periods of time, without consequences, but it's fundamental to follow the instructions on the package leaflet and to go to a doctor if the symptoms persist or worsen.

As reported in Italy by *Istituto Superiore di Sanità*,[6] it's important to ask the doctor or pharmacist if there is one of these conditions:

- age over 65;
- supposed or real pregnancy status;
- during breast-feeding;
- the patient suffers from asthma;
- there were allergic reactions to FANS in the past;
- there are stomach ulcer problems;
- the patient suffers from heart, liver, kidney, circulatory, intestinal, or high blood pressure problems;
- the patient is taking other drugs (see interactions with other drugs;
- any medication containing aspirin should be avoided to children under 16 years of age.

Despite the ease of purchasing and assuming these medicines, there are many risks of side effects: stomach pain, nausea and diarrhoea, stomach ulcers, which can cause internal bleeding and anemia; it is often necessary to take gastroprotection drugs, such as proton pump inhibitors, along with FANS perforation of the stomach or intestine, headaches, drowsiness, dizziness, allergic reactions, in rare cases liver, kidney, heart and circulatory problems, including heart failure, stroke and heart attack.[7]

For these reasons it is essential that information on the secondary packaging and package leaflet is accessible and comprehensible to all patients.

Another element of complexity is the large number and variety of these drugs in terms of denomination, dosage, and reference pharmaceutical companies.

If we consider the most common medicines based on paracetamol and acetylsalicylic acid, we can find approximately: 46 different denominations and 57 pharmaceutical companies for paracetamol, and 22 different denominations and 19 pharmaceutical companies for drugs with the active ingredient acetylsalicylic acid. The dosages and types of approved packaging are even more varied and numerous.[8]

---

[6] Istituto Superiore di Sanità, ISS, https://www.issalute.it/index.php/la-salute-dalla-a-alla-z-menu/f/fans-farmaci-antinfiammatori-non-steroidei?highlight=WyJhc3BpcmluYSJd#farmaci-alternativi-ai-fans, (accessed 2022 Nov. 22).

[7] See FANS side effects on https://www.issalute.it/index.php/la-salute-dalla-a-alla-z-menu/f/fans-farmaci-antinfiammatori-non-steroidei?highlight=WyJhc3BpcmluYSJd#farmaci-alternativi-ai-fans, (accessed 2022 Nov. 22).

[8] See the medicines database, prepared by the Italian Medicines Agency (AIFA), is the only official database allowing consultation of the updated Summary of Product Characteristics (RCP) and package leaflets (PIL) of medicines authorized in Italy, https://farmaci.agenziafarmaco.gov.it/bancadatifarmaci/.

From this first overview, a very complex context emerges, an ordinary patient may find it difficult to purchase an OTG drug on his or her own, there is a question of whether the information available to him or her is readily readable, comprehensible, and communicatively consistent.

In this regard, it is important to remember, as reported by Di Pace (2019, p. 28), that before drugs can enter the market, they must obtain Marketing Authorisation (AIC) granted by the EMA (European Medicines Agency) and in Italy by the Italian Medicines Agency in collaboration with the Ministry of Health.

Furthermore, the legal basis for the requirements relating to labels and package leaflets are in Directive 2001/83/EC on the Community code relating to medicinal products for human use as amended by Directive 2004/27 EC. The legal basis for the requirements relating to the safety feature appearing on the packaging of medicinal products is in regulation (EU) 2016/161.

These guidelines bind the member states to achieve the envisaged objectives, they are translated into legislative decrees that may vary between the different states of the European Union.

As reported by Di Pace (2019, p. 28), in Italy, the law that implemented the European directive is Legislative Decree No. 219 of 24 April 2006,[9] among the articles, the decree imposes the obligation to use the package leaflet (Art. 76) and the following are regulated: the contents of the package leaflet (Art. 77), changes to the labelling and package leaflet compatible with the summary of product characteristics (Art. 78), signs or pictograms (Art. 79), the language used (Art. 80), the general characteristics of the information in the package leaflet and labelling (Art. 81), the consequences in the event of non-compliance with the labelling and package leaflet provisions (Art. 82).

10.2 A Matter of Texts, Paratexts and Multiple Translations

In the context of over-the-counter analgesics, in this research work, we have analysed more in detail one of the most sold and well-known OTC medicines, that we will call in this chapter Medicine X.

The goal is to frame it within an ecosystem that includes different communication artefacts surrounding the medicine, to analyse it according to semiotic and translation theories.

More specifically, we focused on the relationship between Medicine X and three types of textuality: primary packaging, secondary packaging and the package insert.

---

[9] Legislative decree No 219 of 24 April 2006. Implementation of Directive 2001/83/EC (and subsequent amending directives) on a Community code relating to medicinal products for human use. Entry into force of the decree: 6-7-2006 (Last update to the act published on 12/08/2022).

For more information see the link https://www.normattiva.it/uri-res/N2Ls?urn:nir:stato:decreto.legislativo:2006-04-24;219!vig= (accessed 2022 Nov. 23).

A medical product can be considered, from a semiotic perspective, as a "text", defined by Marrone as an overall configuration of meaning that, by using an expressive support, ensures the creation, transmission, and interpretation of social and cultural meanings (Marrone 2010, p. 18).

Medicines-texts, influence social behaviours, both are located in a unitary framework in which experiences, texts, models, gestures, codes, communicate with each other and only thus function (Lorusso 2010, p. 76).

This perspective places the medicinal product within a social and communicative dimension, in which the community of experts (doctors, pharma companies, legislative authorities), the patients, the cultural and social context, the languages with their codes and rhetoric, constitute a unitary tissue (the semiosphere).[10]

The medicine doesn't live alone, just as a text, it is supported and accompanied by other texts, several productions, multiple communicative artefacts,[11] «which surround and prolong it, to present it, indeed, in the current sense of the term, but also in its strongest sense: to make it present, to ensure its presence in the world, its reception and its consumption», (Genette 1989, p. 3).

These accompanying texts can be defined in term of *paratexts*,[12] although they are themselves texts.

In our specific sector, paratexts can be represented by the summary of product characteristics (SPC),[13] the primary and secondary packaging,[14] the packaging leaflet, the dedicated website, the formats that vehicle advertising.

According to Genette, they are the privileged place of a pragmatics and strategy, of an action on the audience, (Genette 1989, p. 4).

---

[10] The whole semiotic space can in fact be considered as a single mechanism (if not as an organism). It is then not this or that brick that plays a primary role, but the <<big system>> called the semiosphere. The semiosphere is that semiotic space outside of which the existence of semiosis is not possible (Lotman 1985, p. 58).

[11] «Our initiative, in keeping with the design, fabricative, operational, poietic inclination of our discipline, consists rather in considering the visual communicative phenomenon by seeing it as constituted by the material objects produced that make it up. Indeed, we criticise the very notion of visual communication as a generic abstraction and tend to replace it, as a definition or indication of the object of investigation, with the concept of communicative artefact», (Anceschi 1981, p. 14).

[12] The paratext is nothing more than an auxiliary, an accessory to the text. […] A threshold cannot but be crossed (Genette 1989: 404).

[13] This is the expert-to-expert text which in expert terminology describes contents, side effects etc. It is meant for health professionals such as doctors. Furthermore, the SPC provides the authorization body, EMEA, with information about the medicine for them to assess whether the medicine should be authorized, (Brøgger 2013)

[14] With primary packaging we intend the packaging in direct contact with the medicine aimed at its protection and preservation, with secondary packaging we refer to the external packaging that protect the primary packaging and also convey information about the medicine. Secondary packaging is important because it constitutes a communicative artefact aimed at the 'staging' of the pharmaceutical product within analogue or digital sales spaces. See at this regard, Bucchetti (1999).

From this perspective paratexts of medicines are strictly connected to their context and are subjected to a series of *translation*[15] processes that relate them to their users with specific purposes.

These translation processes can be summarised in terms of *endolinguistic translations* (defined also in term of reformulation or intralinguistic translations), *typographical translations* finalized to the transcription of verbal content, *intersemiotic translations* (for example from the verbal content to the visual or vice versa), *interlinguistic translations* (when we translate one language to another), *inter-format translations* (when we have to search new format solutions), and *inter-media translations* (when we transpose contents in the digital involving multimodal directing practices), (Caratti et al. ii 2021, pp. 1105–1112).

Through translation practices, the medicine-text and its paratexts not only determines its own internal heterogeneity, but also it relates to external contexts, multiple media, several users, produces different behaviours, and it opens itself up to a continuous semiotic exchange with other texts or paratexts.

From this point of view, as Lorusso asserts referring to Lotman, the semiotic space (the semiosphere), appears to us as a multi-layered intersection of various texts, which together form a certain layer, with complex internal correlations, varying degrees of translatability and spaces of untranslatability, (Lorusso 2010, p. 83).

The intersection between texts and paratexts and their continuous interexchange can be explained by the concept of *intertextuality*, which Barthes describes as the opening of the text onto other texts, other codes, other signs (Barthes 1991, p. 184), and Genette defines in term of the effective presence of one text in another (Genette 1989, p. 4), the observation of this phenomenon allows us to consider a very common OTC medicine that we will call in this chapter Medicine X, starting from its connections with other texts and more in detail its paratexts.

This theoretical premise allows us to frame the point of view from which we will analyse and deconstruct the traits of Medicine X, conceived semiotically as a text which relates intertextually with its paratexts and other texts. More in detail, we will focus on the relationship among our case study and three typologies of paratexts: the primary and secondary packaging and the package leaflet.

The first step of the research work was to place Medicine X within the context of over-the-counter analgesics based on acetylsalicyclic acid.

10.3 Multiple Formulations Based on Acetylsalicylic Acid

Our case study, Medicine X, has acetylsalicylic acid as its active ingredient and it is a drug that is used as an analgesic (to relieve mild pain), antipyretic (to reduce fever), anti-inflammatory.

---

[15] According to Peeter Torop (2010) translation consists of a deep and total semiotic process involving a transfer from a source text to a target text.

Medicines with acetylsalicylic acid as an active ingredient are numerous, the AIFA (*Agenzia Italiana Farmaco*) drug database site[16] contains 61 entries of which: 22 correspond literally to the term acetylsalicylic acid, (they differ in the pharmaceutical company of reference), 7 to the term Medicine X (with multiple pharmaceutical companies), 7 retain the name of Medicine X but with the addition of terms specifying its purpose (e.g. Medicine X *dolore e infiammazione),* or with the diminutive of the medicine, or with a prefix specifying its use (e.g. CardioMedicine X), 4 maintain the same suffix but with a different denomination (e.g. Xdol), and the others 21 have a completely different name with a different pharmaceutical company.

On the same database, if we look for information on the Medicine X, we find a list of sixteen entries: ten of them correspond to the item Medicine X but differ by pharmaceutical company. Medicine X is present together with other five related products: with the suffix *Actim* (it has been revoked), in association with the terms flu and stuffy nose, with the suffix Act, with the terms pain and inflammation, and with the further specification ACT Pain and inflammation.

On the Italian web site of the pharmaceutical company, Medicine X is communicated with ten different product declinations: from the core product to other differentiations related to their packaging (e.g., in sachets), or intended use (e.g., flu and stuffy nose).

Given these premises, it is evident that for an ordinary Italian patient who needs a remedy against cold diseases, toothache, or headache, it's quite difficult for him to find his way alone around the many declinations of medicines based on acetylsalicylic acid as its active ingredient.

These medicines are present in the market with different use destinations, dosages, multiple packaging systems, different pharmaceutical companies of reference and sales systems, it's extremely important for the patient that all paratextual elements (as packaging and packaging leaflet) support the patient from an informative point of view.

10.4 Focus on Medicine X Effervescent Tablets 400 mg

As reported on the website dedicated to Medicine X, the formulation in effervescent tablets is a product with antifebrile, anti-inflammatory and analgesic action. It acts from the first symptoms of colds and flu, providing rapid relief. It contains vitamin C which has a positive effect on the immune system.

Medicine X with C vitamin is the product that belongs to the pharmaceutical company historical tradition (since the '50–'60 s) with a very high reputation around the world. It's distributed in the world with the same active ingredient and the main graphical codes, but with small differences in the secondary packaging.

---

[16] See https://farmaci.agenziafarmaco.gov.it/bancadatifarmaci/cerca-farmaco, (accessed 2022 Dec.3).

Before analysing the characteristics of Medicine X with vitamin C, it's important to reaffirm that, in the pharmaceutical sector, primary and secondary packaging responds to regulatory aspects defined by the Directive 2001/83/EC, with its subsequent amendments and supplements and a new transposition in Italy by Legislative Decree 219/2006. This Decree was subsequently amended by Legislative Decree 274/2007.[17] It follows that the design of all elements of the medicine and its paratexts are subjected a numerous constraint and structured content.

The Italian version of Medicine X is represented by white and circular effervescent tablets with a diameter of 250 mm and a thickness of approximately 2 mm. The pharmaceutical logo is engraved on one side of the tablet.

Each tablet is placed in a paper pack in strip (primary packaging) sealed at the sides; the tablets are placed two by two in a cardboard box that constitutes the secondary packaging for a total of 10 tablets, in the commerce there is also the 20 or 40 tablet pack.

The primary packaging is the first paratextual element of the medicine, it is the outcome of an endolinguistic translation, in other words it's a reformulation and simplification of the secondary packaging. Its role is to protect and store the medicinal product by maintaining a close semantic correlation with the secondary packaging. Medicine X primary packaging shows the pharmaceutical company logo in the top left-hand corner, the name of the medicine (Medicine X), the dosage, the format (effervescent tablets with Vitamin C) and the active ingredient (acetylsalicylic acid). The typographic and chromatic codes, and the icon represented by the bubble-encircled shield are the same of the secondary packaging, they vary only in size. Additional signs in white are represented by the pictogram of a small scissor with the lowercase words 'open here' flanked by a numerical code. The reverse side of the primary packaging is totally white and bears the batch number (BT175E1 /2) and the expiry date printed on it.

The secondary packaging of Medicine X is the paratext that more than others performs an appellative function,[18] it is characterized by a seductive potential that lends itself to various expressions of ostensive character[19] (Bucchetti 1999, p. 33).

In the last year the pharmaceutical company updated the secondary packaging with the aim of standardizing its identity at European level, the new elements, compared to the past, are: a more contemporary typography; the presence of a yellow symbol with gradient bordered in silver with 3D transparent little bubbles and the central letter C; one effervescent white tablet with little white 3D bubbles on the left (in an older version there were two tablets). This icon was designed to highlight the role and support of vitamin C as an active ingredient (the bubbles) with a defensive action (the symbolic value of the shield). This is a constant element that we can find on the touch points, in the point of sale and in television advertising.

---

[17] For more details see https://www.aifa.gov.it/sites/default/files/2016-05-18_Ranalli.pdf, (accessed 2022 Dec.12).

[18] The appellative or conative function is aimed at generating a reaction in the patient and influencing his behaviour.

[19] By ostensive character we mean a property that tends to show or demonstrate.

The main color codes of the secondary packaging are green as background (this shade of green has been a constant for many years), white for the tablet on the left and white for the closing flap (where the batch number and expiry date are printed), other colors are yellow and metallic grey.

The company logo, the name of the medicine and the informative text are white, while the dosage, drug formulation and active principle are green on a yellow background, also the letter C in the symbol is green with a little orange shadow on a gradient yellow background.

The front of secondary packaging presents elements that fulfil both communicative-informative and communicative-seductive functions (Bucchetti 1999, p. 112), the upper side of the box bears the logo with the name of the drug and the yellow symbol with a C, while the lower side contains text on the therapeutic indications, the composition with the active ingredients (acetyl salicylic acid and ascorbic acid), and the excipients, the mode of use (oral) and the specification that it is a self-medication medicine. On the right-hand side at the bottom, we find the name of the pharmaceutical company.

The backside of the secondary packaging reports the barcode label in the middle, with two short written texts. Above there is a prescriptive and standardized text suggesting reading the package leaflet before use, keep the medicine out of the sight and reach of children and store the medicine at a temperature below 25 °C, there is also an informative short text that states that the expiry date refers to the intact product, correctly stored. The lower text is informative and reports the AIC number, the AIC holder represented by the pharmaceutical company, on the left side rotated by 90° we find the indication with an arrow that suggests reading the expiry date on the left flap.

The right flap reports again the name of the medicine, the number of effervescent tablet and the central mark specifying that it is a non-prescription medicine.

The name of the Medicine X (also embossed in Braille) with company logo and all details reported on the secondary packaging should orient the patient in the process of selection of the medicine: the front of the package informs the patient about the dosage of the effervescent tablet (400 mg), the active principle of the drug (acetyl salicylic acid), the addition of vitamin C (the letter C is enlarged and surrounded by a symbol), and the number of effervescent tablets (10).

For more details about therapeutical indication and composition the patient needs to rotate downwards the box, the body of typographical text is very small and the contrast of the white lettering on the green background makes the reading difficult, especially for an elderly or visually impaired person.

The therapeutical indications report different kind of manifestations: symptomatic treatment of febrile states and influenza and cold syndromes; symptomatic treatment of headache and toothache, neuralgia, menstrual pain, rheumatic and muscular pain.

It then specifies that Vitamin C participates in the body's defense system. This block of information is followed by the composition of the effervescent tablet with the precise dosage of active principles (acetylsalicylic acid 0.4 g. and ascorbic acid 240 mg. = 0.24 g.), but without the dosage of excipients (there is the short indication that it contains sodium).[20] It's specified that the usage is oral, and this is a self-medication drug.

The back of the box suggests reading the package leaflet before the use, but it's impossible to do it at the time of purchase. This is a quite critical issue, because the patient is not always aware of any contraindications or adverse drug interactions. Another important aspect that is overlooked is the age of the patient, which must be over 16 years, but this information is only given in the package insert.

In this case the presence of a QR code[21] on the box could help the patient in accessing web pages containing detailed information on the drug in multiple languages and different modalities (for example through a vocal or video description of the required information).

10.5 Package Leaflet of Effervescent Tablets 400 mg

The package leaflet, also named in Italian as "*bugiardino*",[22] is the paratext which supports the medicine from an informative and prescriptive point of view.

It's characterized by different registers, in the specific case of Medicine X its content is verbal, but also tactile and to some extent sonorous properties, (for the consistency of the foiled paper), are significant. For this reason, it can be considered a hybrid text.

Package leaflet of Medicine X consists of a sheet of 350 × 315 mm with a 3-mm gluing in the middle part to make it more functional when opened, its dimensions when closed are 175 × 315 mm, and the paper weight is approximately 40/50 g/m2. It is folded to form a strip measuring around 300 × 315 mm, which in turn is folded in half to wrap the tablets inside the box.

From a content perspective, it is an example of "highly binding" textuality (Di Pace 2019, p. 25), modelled on technical texts (such as instruction for use) and standardized at European level according to the directive 2001/83/EC, supplemented by directives of 2003/94/EC, 2004/27 EC, 2008/29.[23]

---

[20] The excipient list is very important it should enable the patient to quickly detect the presence of substances to which he or she is allergic. The Medicine X package leaflet specifies that this medicinal product contains 467 mg of sodium (main component of table salt) per tablet. This is equivalent to 23% of the maximum daily recommended dietary sodium intake for an adult.

[21] For more information on the use of QR code see Use of the QR Code on printed matter (CPR, package leaflet, labelling) medicines: state of the art https://www.aifa.gov.it/sites/default/files/2017-02-23_QR.code_BRAGHIROLI_AFI_febbraio_2017.pdf, (accessed 2022 Dec.15).

[22] The term "bugiardino" means deceitful, as De Pace asserts the most credible interpretation of the origin of this term concerns the medical field and more specifically the recognition of the omission of a series of information concerning the negative aspects of taking a medicinal product (Di Pace 2019: 15).

[23] The latest update in 2022 provides a reference standard for electronic medicinal product information (Epi), the digital version of the package leaflet and pharmaceutical product characteristics (Rcp). The agreement represents a crucial step in the project that aims to complement the paper

A coloured header, recalling the main front of the packaging, and a four-sided written text, (black left-aligned on a white background), constitutes the content. The typeface is linear with a size of 8 points and a line spacing of 1.5.

The content of the package leaflet derives from an endolinguistic translation (interpretation of verbal signs by means of other signs in the same language, Jakobson 1987, p. 429), the source text is represented by RCP (Riassunto delle Caratteristiche del Prodotto), named abroad SPC (Summary of Product Characteristics) and the arrival text is the package leaflet (named also as PIL—Patient Information Leaflets). The RCP/SPC is initially developed by the pharmaceutical company, then it is controlled and approved by the local medicine agency (in Italy AIFA, Italian Medicines Agency) and the European Medicines Agency (EMA), (Jensen 2013, p. 5). RCP/ SPC is an expert-to -expert text that is translated in PIL through a terminological simplification for less experienced readers. The package leaflet in English is then subjected to an interlinguistic translation into the other Member State languages.

In brief the Italian version of Medicine X package leaflet is the result of both endolinguistic and interlinguistic translation, with an evident asymmetry between the highly specialized medical language of the RCP/SPC and the language of the patients.

As De Pace asserts, the leaflets share many linguistic traits of the medical report, starting with the use of impersonal verb forms (confirms, seems to appreciate), continuing with the use of entire nominal sentences (not clear evidence [...]), and the use of proper and collateral technicalities as in the case of the expression appreciate (2019, p. 27).

The text of the package leaflet of Medicine X begins with a paragraph inviting the patient to read the leaflet carefully or follow the advice of the doctor or pharmacist, then illustrates in a bulleted list[24] the contents of the leaflet structured in six main points based on a question/answer method (these six paragraphs are articulated in sub-paragraphs highlighted with the use of bold):

- What Medicine X effervescent tablets with Vitamin C is and what it is used for;
- What you should know before taking Medicine X 400 mg effervescent tablets with Vitamin C;
- How to take Medicine X 400 mg effervescent tablets with Vitamin C;
- Possible side effects;

---

information accompanying each medicine with a dematerialized version that is more manageable for patients and healthcare professionals. The adoption of a common standard will enable faster updating of drug information, its harmonization within the EU, and thus faster and more informed choices by consumers and healthcare professionals. An Epi, in fact, can be updated in real time as soon as a change is approved, or new information becomes available. For more details https://www.fpress.it/estero/ue-approvato-lo-standard-per-i-bugiardini-elettronici-dei-farmaci/(accessed 2022 Dec.18).

[24] This textual structure follows a scheme inspired by the *Guideline on the Readability of the Labelling and Package Leaflet of Medical Products for Human Use,* as reported here https://health.ec.europa.eu/system/files/2016-11/2009_01_12_readability_guideline_final_en_0.pdf

- How to store Medicine X 400 mg effervescent tablets with Vitamin C;
- Package contents and other information.

Overall, the text is very dense over four pages, bold highlighting of paragraphs and sub-paragraphs helps the patient in the reading process and in identifying the most important issues such as warnings, allergic reactions, interactions with other drugs, undesirable effects etc.

It is quite common that when faced with such a dense and lengthy text, the patient limits himself to reading the information on the first page and omits the details on the following pages, for example the list of the interaction with other medicines or undesirable effects.

Some important information, that should be mentioned also on the secondary packaging, risk being overlooked with significant consequences: children and adolescents should not take the medicine if they are under 16 years of age, and people over 70 years of age should consult their doctor before taking this medicine.

The poor comprehensibility of the package leaflet is due both to the presence of technical or over-specialised language (for example the list of medicines that could have harmful interactions with Aspirin C), but also to the use of vague expressions which may determine some ambiguities (for example "the use of the product is reserved for adult patients only" is reported on the first page of the informative leaflet, only in the second page it's specified that the medicine should not be taken by children and young people under 16 years of age and there are risks for people over 70 years of age).

The incipit of the section of undesirable effects itself (point 4) has an impersonal and nebulous tone: "like all medicines, this medicine may cause undesirable effects although not all people experience them. […] most side effects are dependent on both dose and duration of treatment".

In synthesis, the content of the package leaflet has a structure and a lexicon that privileges the referential function to the detriment of the communicative function, centred on the reader.

We must highlight the fact that the package leaflet is not only a prescriptive or informative text, but also a legal document aimed at protecting pharmaceutical companies.

10.6 Conclusion

Medicine X has been defined as "wonder drug" for its long story because it is something that has few equivalents in the annals of medical science and one of the most enduring and successful commercial products of all time (Jeffreys 2005, p. 5). Medicine X with C vitamin is equally prodigious, on the market since the 1950s, is one of the best-selling anti-influenza, anti-inflammatory and analgesic drugs internationally. Around this medicine, different paratextual elements have been designed and updated over time, consolidating the brand and its communicative and informative dimension at systemic level.

These paratexts, the primary and secondary packaging and package leaflet, are the result of a series of translation steps that attempt to find a mediation between a plurality of languages of a prescriptive, technical, informative, expositive, or evocative nature.

This is not an easy task; the issues of readability and comprehension of information is still an open question with multiple risks for the patients.

With reference to our case study we can highlight some fundamental issues:

- in the face of a common headache, the patient must orient himself between multiple medicines with the same active ingredient. He/she generally buys the medicine that has the greatest communicative resonance or that belongs to his/her personal history;
- Medicine X is an OTC medicine and as such can be purchased without a prescription. The patient must be informed in advance about the conditions of use and the risks associated with his/her age or with certain pathologies or interactions with other medicines;
- the information on the packaging is not complete and at the time of purchase the patient does not have access to the information on the package leaflet. There are limitations associated to the instant content access, but also to its translation in multiple languages;
- the content of the paratexts is an asymmetric "highly binding textuality" modelled not on the patient and his/her peculiarities, but according to technical and standardised texts. It should be translated in a language more comprehensible, accessible and inclusive, closer to the informal language of a common patient;
- the graphical components of paratexts are regulated by the European Commission, and as many medicines on the market, the visual design of Medicine X is standardized and unsupportive. There should be a further effort by the pharmaceutical company in maximising the number of people who are able to read and understand the information immediately and unambiguously. It's not only a problem associated to the visual codes or visual hierarchies but it's an issue of content accessibility and comprehension.

In conclusion, we would like to affirm that design and communication design can play an active role in the context of health and pharmaceutical products, also in the case of Medicine X, design can facilitate a series of mediation processes with the perspective of creating a stricter relationship with the patients and his / her differences. This entails different aptitudes and competencies: to have the capability of understanding the nature of a problem in all its components, to have the capacity of involving all stakeholders in the design process, to have the sensitivity of observing and measuring the current state of things, to have the expertise of developing and text prototype solutions and iteratively developing and testing prototypes until an optimum solution is found, to have the ability of implementing and monitoring the solution in use (Sless 1992, p. 9). As observes Swann, design for health is now emerging from the shadows to be recognized as a distinct design discipline in its own right. A new discipline with patient safety at its hearth, an evidence-based practice that necessitates system thinking and collaboration to tackle complex challenges and practice governed by a stringent ethical framework (Swann 2017).

References

Anceschi G (1981) Monogrammi e figure. Teorie e storie della progettazione di artefatti comunicativi [Monograms and figures. Theories and histories of the design of communicative artefacts]. La casa Usher, Firenze

Barthes R (1991) L'avventura semiologica. Einaudi, Torino. Barthes R (1985) L'aventure sémiologique. Seuil, Paris

Brøgger N (2013) Translators of patient information leaflets: translation experts or expert translators? A mixed methods study of lay-friendliness, PhD thesis, available at the link https://www.academia.edu/21814838/Translators_of_Patient_Information_Leaflets_Translation_experts_or_expert_translators_A_mixed_methodm_study_of_lay_friendliness (Accessed 20 Nov 2022)

Bucchetti V (1999) La messa in scena del prodotto. Packaging: identità e consumo [The staging of the product. Packaging identity and consumption]. Franco Angeli, Milano

Caratti E, Penati A, Bucchetti V (2021) Translation design for medicine leaflets. In: Research and innovation, in Design Culture(s). Cumulus Conference Proceedings. Roma, vol 2

Di Pace L (2019) La lingua del bugiardino. Il foglietto illustrativo tra linguaggio specialistico e linguaggio comune [The language of the leaflet. The package leaflet between specialist and everyday language]. Franco Cesati Editore, Firenze

Genette G (1989) Soglie. I dintorni del testo. Einaudi, Torino. Genette G (1987) Seuils. Èditions du Seuil, Paris

Jakobson R (1987) In: Pomorska K, Rudy S (eds) Language in literature. Belknap, Cambridge, MA

Jeffreys D (2005) Aspirina. L'incredibile storia della pillola più famosa del mondo. [Aspirin. The story of a wonder drug]. Donzelli, Roma. Jeffreys D (2004) Aspirin. The story of a wonder drug. Bloomsbury Publishing, London

Jensen N (2013) Medical translation for the lay receiver: who are the experts? Translators of patient information leaflets: translation experts or expert translators? A mixed methods study of lay-friendliness. Aarhus: Aarhus University, Aarhus School of Business and Social Sciences (PhD thesis)

Lorusso A (2010) Semiotica della cultura [The semiotics of culture]. Laterza, Roma-Bari

Lotman JM (1985) La Semiosfera. L'asimmetria e il dialogo nelle strutture pensanti. Marsilio, Venezia. Lotman JM (1984) O semiosfere, in Izbrannye stat'i v trëh tomah,1:11--24. Tallin Aleksandra, 1992

Marrone G (2010) L'invenzione del testo [The invention of the text]. Laterza, Rome

Sless D (1992) What is information design? In: Penman R, Sless D (eds) Designing information for people. Communication Research Press, Canberra, pp 1–16

Swann D (2017) Challenges and opportunities for design. In: Tsekleves E, Cooper R (eds) Design for health. Routledge (Kindle edition), London, pp 1012–1308

Torop P (2010) La traduzione totale. Tipi di processo traduttivo nella cultura. Hoepli, Milano. Torop P (1995) Toytal'nyj perevod. Izd. Tartuskogo Universiteta, Tartu

Open Access This chapter is licensed under the terms of the Creative Commons Attribution 4.0 International License (http://creativecommons.org/licenses/by/4.0/), which permits use, sharing, adaptation, distribution and reproduction in any medium or format, as long as you give appropriate credit to the original author(s) and the source, provide a link to the Creative Commons license and indicate if changes were made.

The images or other third party material in this chapter are included in the chapter's Creative Commons license, unless indicated otherwise in a credit line to the material. If material is not included in the chapter's Creative Commons license and your intended use is not permitted by statutory regulation or exceeds the permitted use, you will need to obtain permission directly from the copyright holder.

Chapter 11
Dealing with Medicines Through Online Platforms and Communities

Carlo Emilio Standoli and Umberto Tolino

Abstract This chapter focuses on the link between social media and human health and well-being, with a peculiar interest in the communication of medicine, understood both as an object for treatment and as a commercial product. After an overview of social media and the extent to which they have changed access to the web, the way we create and disseminate content—personal or professional—and communicate with other people, the chapter analyses their contribution and use in medicine. Through observation of the trends on several social media, such as forums, blogs, and social networks, the chapter presents an analysis of the role of medicine in such environment, starting with the norms that regulate their communication and ending with the identification of platforms, channels, actors involved, modes of interaction, and registers of dialogue. Finally, the chapter proposes some reflections on how design culture can intervene in the relationship between medicines and social media, from the definition of guidelines for communication to research for improving the user experience of medicines.

11.1 The Use of Social Media and the Relationship with Healthcare

Today, around 65% of people worldwide have Internet access (Starri 2023). People spend an average of more than 6 h daily connected between websites, forums, social networks, gaming platforms, and other platforms (Starri 2023). Improved infrastructure and technology are crucial in this global spread and increase of Internet access. For instance, the development and adoption of mobile devices have enabled massive access to the network, both geographically and demographically. In this, the paradigm shift between Web 1.0 and 2.0 has also contributed, meaning the possibility for users with access to the web to create communities and content, share

---

C. E. Standoli (✉) · U. Tolino
Department of Design, Politecnico di Milano, Milan, Italy
e-mail: carloemilio.standoli@polimi.it

information, thoughts, personal messages, images, and videos, and even collaborate in real-time: people are now connected in a web-based world without borders (Farsi et al. 2022). Social media embody this paradigm shift of active and participatory web use.

According to the Merriam-Webster dictionary, *Social Media* can be defined as *"forms of electronic communication (such as websites for social networking and microblogging) through which users create online communities to share information, ideas, personal messages, and other content (such as videos)"* (Merriam-Webster 2023). Thus, social media includes sites, blogs and forums, for content creation and sharing, video creation and sharing, and social networks, etc. In the creation and spreading of content on the web, social media enable the creation of bottom-up content, in other words, by network users without specific programming knowledge, and sometimes without actually being experts in the topic of discussion; content can range from the professional dimension to the expression of personal thought, through micro-blogging, to the sharing of one's own experiences, through forums or social networks, to the creation of encyclopaedic entries, etc.

Social media can thus be grouped into categories according to their purpose (Ventola 2014), that is:

- to aggregate knowledge and information (e.g., Wikipedia, GitHub, etc.);
- to create and share content (e.g., blogs and micro-blogs, such as Reddit, Twitter—X, etc.)
- to create and share media (e.g., YouTube, TikTok, Snapchat, etc.)
- for networking, whether professional (e.g., LinkedIn, etc.) or personal (e.g., Facebook, Instagram, etc.)
- for sending instant messages (e.g., Whatsapp, Messenger, Telegram, etc.)
- to play games in synchronous or asynchronous mode
- to sell, buy or exchange products and objects, etc.

In recent years, among the possible uses, social media tools have been used to promote health, both on one's own and in society. Social Media can enable public information sharing, including in the health field, creating a communicative and collaborative atmosphere between everyday users, patients, medical and health personnel, and health and governmental structures. Social media tools can be useful to shorten the distance between patients and medical and health personnel, increase health literacy, or promote healthy lifestyles among different communities. By 2017, representatives of the World Health Organization (WHO) were already highlighting all the advantages and benefits that the intersection between public health understood in its traditional dimension and electronic and mobile health (e-Health, m-Health) would guarantee shortly (Steffelson et al. 2020).

As an essential tool in the health field, social media involves all the stakeholders, from health care providers to patients, from manufacturers of health care products to national and supranational organisations.

Depending on the different users, social media can find different application areas. For example, for physicians and healthcare institutions, social media can be used to present and share the results of biomedical research, reducing the barriers between professionals through immediate contacts compared to those obtained through scientific dissemination and publication. Or, again, in the case of physicians and national and supranational governmental bodies, to communicate good practices for maintaining or monitoring one's health status to the general public. Or to be used for training young doctors by creating and disseminating content for new forms of formal and informal learning (Farsi 2021). Or offer telemedicine services and direct support to people. Over the years, for example, the WHO has organised structured communication activities through the leading social media and created a webpage (i.e., WHO MythBusters) specifically to counter all the unreliable and sometimes conspiratorial information that crowds the web and social media.

If viewed from the perspective of companies that produce and trade products and services for people's health and wellbeing, social media provides a showcase for connecting with different audiences. For example, social media for professional networking can be used to communicate one's research and product development activities to specialist and industry audiences or for recruitment campaigns. Social media for non-professional networking can be used to communicate one's values and corporate vision to a more generalist audience and promote messages to raise awareness of one's health status. In some cases, depending on country regulations, social media can also be used to market one's product range.

If viewed from the patient's perspective, social media can be used in different dynamics, such as top-down, bottom-up and peer-to-peer directions. In the first case, this includes all telemedicine or counselling services, in which the person can benefit from remote monitoring and dialogue with his or her physician or caregiver, allowing for the spreading of care and a significant reduction in time and costs. From this perspective, telemedicine is not intended to be the only service for personal care. However, rather than support for the traditional medical service, it comprises dialogue and direct contact with the physician—such as visual, auditory, tactile, emotional, and empathic. This also includes all actions and activities by healthcare providers to disseminate messages and information for health literacy, influencing the achievement of better behaviour through social reinforcement (George et al. 2013). The second case includes the use of social media platforms and social media that allow the person to find a health care provider—understood as both medical staff and hospital facility—appropriate to the expectations of care (Nayak and Linkov 2019). Indeed, social media represents the new word of mouth, where people can find all the information, they need to choose their preferred care pathway or doctor. At the same time, a person with low health literacy and the increasingly rapid dissemination of medical information—sometimes produced by sources that are not accurate or precise—can create confusion and produce risky behaviours that can damage health. In the third case, peer-to-peer interaction dynamics through social media are used to share information about therapies and treatments, drugs and dosages, doctors and hospital facilities, or to find support from people with whom one shares a health condition (Farsi et al. 2022). This is the case with portals and blogs such as PatientsLikeMe or DiabetesMine, where people-patients can discuss and find support from those with whom they share the same health condition. For example, in the Italian context, a representative case of the use of social media in a health context and with a peer-to-peer dynamic is the initiative led by Salvatore Iaconesi. In 2012, after he was diagnosed with a brain tumour, Iaconesi started the "*La Cura*" project, making his medical records available online to deal with his illness openly. Over the years, he has been able to engage with doctors, neuroscientists, artists, engineers, designers, and ordinary people, approaching the disease from different points of view (Iaconesi and Persico 2016), not only seeking medical advice for his recovery but also developing new ways of communicating, interacting, accepting and coping with his illness and state of health.

Or, again by way of example, it is worth mentioning the role of social media during the Covid-19 pandemic, which was prominent in the dissemination of information, whether to tell what was happening in different countries around the world, to promote virtuous behaviour or share tools and solutions to support treatment, or simply to work remotely or meet loved ones from one's home context. In this regard, an example of the positive use of social media is the experience of Cristian Fracassi, Dr. Renato Favero and the Isinnova team. At the beginning of the first lockdown, to cope with the shortage of intensive care supplies, through contacts via social networks, they re-designed charlotte valves to be adapted to snorkelling masks in order to use respirators; later on, they disseminated the project files, making their invention free to use, so that it could be produced and modified wherever it was needed (Redazione Open Innovation 2020).

However, there are not only positive cases and experiences in using social media regarding health. Again, during the Covid19 pandemic, it happened that many non-expert users, sometimes with a large following of followers, discussed or commented on medical phenomena, including vaccination, making negative judgments without having any element, suitable or knowledge to do so (Pershad et al. 2018). Or, as in the case of the Zika pandemic, studies have shown that at least 12% of the information on social networks such as Facebook was false, misleading and linked to conspiracy theories (Sharma et al. 2017).

Social networks often turn into an 'echo chamber of ideas', where biased and unsubstantiated opinions or points of view have greater resonance than evidence-based facts—not only scientific ones—due to the ease of sharing and dissemination without understanding the content, critical thinking (Weissmann 2012).

Another very recent example of the use of social media in health, and specifically in the use of drugs, is that of Ozempic. This medicine was developed to support treating people with type 2 diabetes mellitus. Its active ingredient stimulates insulin production and, among other effects, contributes to the feeling of satiety by inhibiting appetite (Couzin-Frankel 2023). This second effect was observed during clinical trials, and the manufacturer has considered the possibility of using the drug to treat obesity (Couzin-Frankel 2023).

Between 2021 and 2022, the medicine was then authorised for treating obesity in the United States and the European Union. Starting in 2023, however, the medicine started to be increasingly present on social networks, as it was used by non-obese people to lose weight without diets or physical activity (Mullin 2023; Menietti and Mautino 2023). Many videos have also circulated on platforms such as TikTok, testifying to the before and after use of the medicine. This strong diffusion and interest in the medicine's 'benefits' has led to a substantial increase in the demand for it, often also outside the official channels, as understood from a prescriptive (i.e., the doctor prescribing the drug to the patient because he or she suffers from the disease) and legislative (e.g., the drug being sold through non-legal channels) point of view (Menietti and Mautino 2023). Therefore, this behaviour caused a decrease in the availability of the medicine for those who needed it, such as people with type 2 diabetes mellitus. Therefore, in all these cases, it is possible to see how the use of social networks can hurt people's health—even at a widespread and global level—due to the creation and sharing of content that, for example, questions medical culture without having a scientific basis and evidence, or that encourages bad behaviour.

Therefore, we must consider that social media allows new forms and dynamics of communication even in the world of health and personal care, where an exchange of information of any nature and structure occurs, from personal opinion to scientific evidence. To understand this phenomenon and to understand precisely how medicines and dialogues around the pharmaceutical world were present in social media, qualitative research was carried out on the main sites, forums and social networks used in different ways by pharmaceutical companies, doctors and health professionals, pharmacists, patients and caregivers. This research mainly examines the Italian context, both from a legislative and regulatory point of view and in content creation.

11.2 Medicines on the Web: From Advertising to Peer-to-Peer Dialogue

As addressed in other chapters of this book, the medicine can be considered as a product system composed of multiple levels, starting from the form (e.g., solid, liquid, etc.) defined to make the medicine more effective or based on business optimisation logics, or even to favour its consumption; to the different packaging (e.g., primary and secondary) to contain, protect, distribute, sell and store the medicine, or to communicate and make it recognisable; to the package leaflet, to support and guide the use process. Over the years, in addition to its role as a tool for preserving and maintaining the health of the person and the patient, the medicine has evolved into a true commodity designed for customers.

Some medicines, namely self-medication (over the counter—OTC) and non-prescription medicines (*senza obbligo di prescrizione*—SOP) are subject to the logic of any other type of commodity, from advertising and promotion in traditional and new media to distribution channels. These medicines have gone from being used exclusively for treatment, therapy or preventive purposes, to products to be consumed. For example, in the Italian context, as well as in pharmacies, the medicine can be sold in parapharmacies and through their own physical outlets or Internet sites. In this case, online sales are only allowed to authorised entities recognised by the Ministry of Health, and using intermediary websites or marketplaces such as Amazon or Ebay is prohibited. Both pharmacies and parapharmacies retain their role as health care providers, where a person/patient can turn to a pharmacist to manage pharmacological therapy (e.g., from choosing the medicine to the interaction between medicines, from adherence support to pharmacovigilance).

However, entering these spaces—physical or virtual—the advertising of OTC and SOP medicines becomes evident, from display banners to promotions and discounts, as is the case for any other merchandise within the logic of large-scale distribution. With legislative decree 219/2006, the Italian Ministry of Health defined the fundamental principles, limits, characteristics, and content—acceptable and not—to manage the commodification and regulate the advertising of OTC and SOP medicines (Ministero della Salute 2006). Through the publication of the guidelines on health advertising of OTC and SOP medicines, the Ministry of Health regulated the presence of medicines in traditional broadcast media (e.g. newspapers, television, radio, websites) and social media, provided that the advertising message is authorised (Ministero della Salute 2023). The Ministry of Health must authorise any form of official presentation of medicines through the different media. This also applies to institutional-company websites if the medicine is presented or advertised.

Regarding advertising medicines in social networks, apart from the platform used, the Ministry of Health defines some essential characteristics of the advertising message. For example:

- the social network must technically enable all features concerning 'comments' and reactions (e.g., public likes, emoticons) to be disabled, and the 'sharing' function must also be disabled; and, where this is not technically possible, all messages disseminated on social channels must contain the following disclaimer: 'The Ministry of Health only authorises the content of the advertising message. Any comments are the sole responsibility of the user, the company disassociates itself from user comments';
- it is permitted to include in authorised advertising messages disseminated via social pages/profiles links that are activated in the following cases
  - links referring to websites and/or social pages/profiles containing promotional material already authorised by the Ministry;
  - links referring to content aimed at the public that does not require ministerial authorisation (e.g. containing health education information, self-medication, etc.).

In both cases, the company in charge of the material on the network will warn the user with the following wording: '*You are leaving the site (insert name) containing promotional material authorised under current health advertising legislation*'.

- links to other content aimed at the public (including in foreign languages), which requires ministerial authorisation and has not been obtained, are not permitted.—In the application for authorisation, the applicant must indicate the sites and social pages/profiles to which reference is made, if they are not explicitly mentioned in the message (e.g., 'Find out more' button) (Ministero della Salute 2023)

For different social networks covered by the guidelines (e.g., Facebook, Instagram, YouTube, TikTok, etc.), the Ministry defines specific rules regarding the use of posts containing text and image galleries, image and video carousels, stories or others. For example, it defines the maximum amount of posts that can be published (e.g., each company can submit to the Ministry for approval a total editorial plan containing a maximum of ten posts, of which a maximum of three are videos), or the length of the texts (e.g., each post cannot contain more than 70 words), or the possibility of sharing (valid only for YouTube).

However, these guidelines only concern companies that carry out specific advertising messages, while the actions of other actors, such as influencers—of various kinds—who use social networks to promote products or services, or patient networks, in which people share their experience with such a doctor or medicine, are not regulated.

For instance, in Italy, there is still no specific regulation regarding communication between doctors or between doctors and patients through social media. In the case of professional sites, such as those providing telemedicine services or where it is possible to book examinations (e.g. MioDottore.it, Medicitalia.it, etc.), the dialogue between doctor and patient falls within the dimension of healthcare practice. In the case of social networks, the situation is different. The scientific community predominantly agrees with considering these channels favourably and their use in communicating with patients and the population to convey correct information, combat misinformation, and promote public health. As there is no common regulation or guidance from the ministries, the different professional orders have tried to define recommendations for using social networks. For example, in July 2023, the Italian National Federation of the Associations of Physicians, Surgeons and Dentists (*Federazione Nazionale degli Ordini dei Medici Chirurghi e degli Odontoiatri*—FNOMCeO) drew up recommendations on the use of social networks, covering topics such as data confidentiality, handling friendship requests from patients, creating multiple profiles (i.e., personal and professional), the declaration of possible conflicts of interest (e.g., reporting whether the content of a post is funded or sponsored by a company), and the fight against disinformation and fake news (Santoro et al. 2023).

The Italian Federation of National Associations of Nursing Professions (*Federazione Nazionale Ordini Professioni Infermieristiche*—FNOPI) has also published recommendations on the use of social networks addressed to Italian nurses—citing the title of Marshall McLuhan's work, the medium is the message—, to sensitise them to reflect on the nature of the content published, the different communication channels used, and the potential impact on the different communities. The fallout of a wrong—or misinterpreted—message can indeed negatively affect the individual and the entire professional community, from an ethical, deontological, cultural level (FNOPI 2019).

On the other hand, the Italian Federation of Pharmacists Orders (*Federazione Ordini dei Farmacisti Italiani*—FOFI) sent a communication to all national pharmacist orders, pointing out the presence of some people who, with profiles on Instagram or TikTok and presenting themselves as pharmacists, express evaluations and dispense recommendations on the use of medicines, whether SOP, OTC or prescription drugs (Mandelli and Pace 2023). FOFI points out that this practice is contrary to the Pharmacists' Code of Ethics, and emphasises that advertising for medicines on social networks must be authorised by the Ministry (Mandelli and Pace 2023).

Conversely, the dialogue and exchange of information among patients is not subject to regulation or standardisation—other than that defined arbitrarily by the managers of the site, forum or blog, according to their own cultural, ethical and moral principles. As mentioned, social media are the new word of mouth of health, where users exchange advice on medicines, therapies, diagnoses, treatments, doctor's skills, sometimes without scientific evidence or objectifying experiences. For example, a phenomenon that occurred during the Covid19 pandemic emergency is that of *infodemia*, or the excessive search for and dissemination of information, including false and misleading information, in digital and physical environments that causes citizen-patients to engage in confusion and risky behaviour that can harm health (WHO 2023). Social media all enable the creation of content and the continuous search for immediate solutions: in the dynamics of information sharing between people/patients, where this is self-produced based on the individual's experiences and beliefs, virtuous cases coexist (e.g., PatientsLikeMe, DiabetesMine, MyPersonalTrainer, etc.) with cases that can contribute in creating misinformation.

11.3 Social Media and Medicines: A Qualitative Observation on Online Pharmaceutical Communication

To really understand how medicines and the dialogues around the pharmaceutical world are present in social media, a qualitative research was structured by identifying the main social media, such as sites, forums and social networks, where pharmaceutical companies, doctors and health professionals, pharmacists, patients and caregivers are present.

The qualitative research was conducted with an observation programme that lasted approximately 2 months, starting from the Italian context in consideration of the legislative and privacy constraints, as well as for a better understanding of the modalities and language adopted by the different users, for opportunities to understand the contents and the audience to which they were really addressed. At a second level, the different types of platforms under observation were identified. Amongst these, some institutional sites were selected (e.g., AIFA website), the sites of some pharmaceutical manufacturers, sites for services or consultancy (e.g., MioDottore, MyPersonalTrainer, etc.), forums and micro-blogging platforms, which group together people with shared interests and which deal with the subject of health, and finally some social networks (e.g., Instagram, TikTok, etc.).

A number of representative profiles of the different categories (e.g. companies, physicians, pharmacists, patients and caregivers) were then isolated, in the guise of content-creators or influencers, and of recipients of the information created (e.g. those who search for drug package leaflets or those who comment on the content-creators' posts). For these, observation summary sheets were produced, and a mapping of the themes, processes, and dynamics of interaction was carried out, which changed both due to the platform used and the directionality of the communication itself. For example, in some cases, it was analysed how communication can go from being one-way and institutional, typical of companies that produce drugs or of sites offering assistance and support for treatment (where brief exchanges may take place in the case of areas intended for communication between doctors and patients), to two-way communication (typical of content creators on social platforms) or peer-to-peer (typical of forums and blogs used by patient networks). Another variable observed is the temporality of the interaction, both in terms of the duration of the exchange or the content produced and the synchronicity or asynchronicity of the dialogue (e.g., likes on Instagram live or comments on posts).

A series of contents/posts were then selected, organised by circulation and popularity, based on the number of visits and interactions with the target audience. For some sites and forums, an analysis was also made concerning accesses and consultations occurring monthly, considering the duration of access, gender and age group of the population.

The objective of this qualitative research was to map the experience that the user, interested in medicines or, more generally, in health, may have while browsing, trying to highlight the modalities, recurrences, good practices and criticalities during interactions. In this way, it is possible to map out areas of interest for future project interventions aimed at communication or process innovation relating to the presence of medicines in social media. By choice, this mapping did not examine the presence of medicines on the dark web.

11.3.1 Top-Down Communication on Social Media: Medicine Communication by Organisations, Institutions and Companies

As mentioned in the previous paragraphs, the Italian Ministry of Health has established guidelines for online communication in the health field, defining recommendations and limitations regarding the presence of medicines on social media, with a specific focus on advertising and marketing actions. Nevertheless, medicines are highly present on the web, considering the frequency of use of the leading search engines to obtain information on specific diseases and related pharmacological therapies, as well as the dosage and effects of medicines. The medical and pharmaceutical-related offers is extremely varied and vast, both in terms of numbers and type of service: from medical-scientific information sites, such as the Ministry of Health or the Italian Medicines Agency (*Agenzia Italiana del Farmaco*—AIFA), to forums for direct online consultation—subject to certified access -, to sites offering databases of package leaflets, to sites and company profiles, blogs, Facebook groups, or profiles on social networks where this issue is addressed from different angles and perspectives (e.g. doctor, pharmacist, patient, caregiver, caregiver, etc.), physician, pharmacist, patient, caregiver, expert or non-expert, etc.).

On the official websites of agencies and institutions such as the Ministry of Health and AIFA, health information is treated in a technical-scientific language, given their regulatory role in managing medicines development, use, adoption and management processes. Above all, AIFA is the national authority responsible for medicines regulatory activity in Italy, in permanent dialogue with all specific stakeholders, from pharmaceutical companies, to the medical-scientific world, to patients' and patients' associations. In parallel to its website, where official reports on medicines, guidelines, scientific articles, etc. are published, AIFA has created several profiles on social networks (e.g., Instagram, Twitter-X), which proposes informative content tailored to the audience of these platforms. The content can range from managing medicines in the home or during the different seasons, to the correct disposal of medicines, the differentiation between branded and equivalent medicines, and the correct use of antibiotics. The intent is informative and educational, not to advertise the use of a given medicine. AIFA has also created a podcast covering the same topics. Unlike the website, in the discourse on medicines through social networks, AIFA adopts a language—verbal and enriched with images, as in the case of Instagram—that is relatively simple but includes medical-scientific terminology, intending to increase medical-pharmaceutical literacy among the population.

However, medicine is present in many different ways, both in various containers and on social media. As mentioned, on some platforms and sites, the package leaflets of different medicines are reproduced. These can then be searched and consulted online, like a medical-pharmacological breviary; these databases and handbooks are accessible both from the web and apps on the main markets. The user can then consult the dosage of the medicine, with all the risks associated with the processes of self-diagnosis and self-medication. It is precisely for this reason that in almost all of these sites and apps, a repeated formula invites one to refer to the physician for a correct definition of pharmaceutical therapy, to avoid the temptation and risks related to self-diagnosis and self-medication.

The medicine is also dealt with on sites and platforms offering medical consultancy services (e.g., MioDottore.it, MedicItalia, ABC Salute, etc.), which can be distinguished between those that propose a divulgative and scientific information action and then arrange a visit at the doctor's office, and those that propose the sale of services and consultancy directly on the platform, without an in-person visit. In the second case, it is easy to witness dialogues between a patient—generally situational and inexperienced, and made anonymous on the platform for other readers—who requests a consultation, and then waits for a response from the various doctors. Within 24 h, one can see replies from medical specialists who answer the question expressed in a clear though not exhaustive manner, referring one to a private—and paid—consultation via the platform itself. The user is then free to refer to one or none of the responding doctors. In these dialogues, the medicine is often quoted, from an already defined therapy, from hearsay therapies, or a prescription is requested. In these forums and especially in public exchanges, it is not permitted to advertise, prescribe or dose a drug without an examination or exchange of medical records or examinations.

Over the last few years, pharmaceutical companies have been using social media for different communication actions, from their mission and vision to their research and testing activities, to promoting healthy lifestyles. While having a website has been the main form of web presence aimed at the general public for years, pharmaceutical companies have only recently adopted their official pages on social networks (e.g. LinkedIn, Facebook, Instagram, Youtube, Twitter—X). The content on these platforms is mainly editorial, such as scientific articles, conference proceedings, participation in events and round tables, and graphic posts celebrating international days for preventing or combating a disease. The aim is to inform and raise awareness among the public through graphic and photographic posts and videos, in which company employees are sometimes present. The presence and use of the employee's testimony is conveyed to bring the company itself closer to the public and users: these are often stories that deal with scientific topics, with a communicative register that the public can use and an emotional character. For example, a company operating in the diabetes pharmaceuticals sector uses its social networks to give the floor to employees/patients, who testify about their relationship and living with the disease, also offering suggestions on how to deal with everyday life, in order to have a healthier life and a better relationship with the treatment processes. Another company, on the other hand, has created a column addressing the theme of 'word of mouth' on the web: starting from a news item or post that has gone viral on the web and which deals with health-related issues or the creation, use or management of a medicine, it attempts to address the theme of false or misleading information, presenting qualitative data and authoritative sources, using popular language and sometimes an ironic tone.

Sometimes, through social networks, companies make use of posts containing questions or surveys to start a series of posts in which the given topic is discussed and users' questions are answered, always within the limits of what is defined by the relevant standards and legislation. Also widespread in the feeds of these companies is the use of stories, such as posts about medicines of the past, stories and anecdotes about the inventors of a given medicine that revolutionised treatment processes, etc. The language used is very often scientific, informative, and explanatory.

11.3.2 Bottom-Up and Peer-to-Peer Communication on Social Media: The Cases of Med-, Pharma-, and Patient-Influencers

In recent years, social media influencers have assumed a significant and impactful strategic communicative role in extremely heterogeneous sectors, such as entertainment, fashion, food, travel, etc., capable of directly reaching and engaging consumers (Willis and Delbaere 2022). Social media influencers can be defined as 'third-party users of social media who have achieved micro-celebrity status in the form of large followings on social media platforms and who have a position of influence in their audience' (Delbaere et al. 2021). In the paradigm shift between selling a product and promoting a lifestyle, for companies, social media influencers represent a channel for communication, positioning and enhancing their offer. In fact, compared to traditional merchandise communication channels, social media influencers can reach consumers more quickly as they can recognise themselves in influencers, aspire to such lifestyles and consumption, or have passions or interests in common. It is precisely in the case of communities with common interests, knowledge, skills, or experiences, which often cannot be artificially replicated, that the spread of health influencers, such as med-, pharma- and patient- influencers, lies.

Med-influencers and pharma-influencers are physicians and pharmacists, trained and experienced personnel with an active presence on social networks, who share content in a structured and conscious manner and are recognised as a reference by a community of followers. Med- and pharma-influencers can vary their language and the way in which their messages are presented, using professional or ironic informative modes: the message is always correctly conveyed, avoiding creating ambiguous or even false and tendentious information. For example, in social networks such as TikTok, med- and pharma-influencers mainly create videos in which the language is light and friendly, using gags and dances. In other cases, like some Instagram posts, a more informative and discursive mode may be adopted, conveyed through image carousels or short reels. In both cases, the aim is to inform using modalities and languages that are accessible to heterogeneous audiences in terms of age, education, pathologies, interests, etc., creating short and easy-to-use content to explain symptoms, dosage, management, storage and interaction of medicines. In some cases, med- and pharma- influencers give space to user insights and requests through direct interaction (Instagram Directs) or through posts and comments.

As indicated by the standard, under no circumstances may med- or pharma-influencers give commercial indications or include drugs of specific companies in their content, limiting themselves to advising on active ingredients of over-the-counter medicines concerning specific diseases.

As far as patient-influencers are concerned, they are actively involved in online communities where they share personal experiences with the disease and the care processes, from therapy management to the relationship with doctors. In the most virtuous cases, this exchange of experiences can help in the literacy and self-management of the care process (Willis and Delbaere 2022). Among the patient-influencers, we can identify patient advocates, third-party users of social media who speak out to raise awareness about diseases and illnesses. They are a specialised social media influencer and, in contexts where this is possible, such as in the United States and for specific types of drugs, are recruited by pharmaceutical companies to participate in developing and promoting pharmaceutical products (Willis and Delbaere 2022). While the presence and dissemination of these influencers may help overcome the stigma of certain diseases (Rosen et al. 2024) or contribute to greater literacy concerning the medicine and the treatment process, the lack of medical education and training concerning witnessing a treatment-disease experience may present the risk of conveying ambiguous information to a broad audience. In this regard, we can cite the already presented case of the abuse of Ozempic (Menietti and Mautino 2023) or Kardashian's experience with the Diclegis: to treat her morning sickness, the influencer used such medicine during her pregnancy and did not hesitate to communicate to her followers the benefits obtained from the use of the drug with a post in which she showed and commented on the drug. In doing so, she violated FDA regulations on drug advertising, conveying possible risky behaviour in using and handling medicines (Hauser 2015).

11.4 Possible Design-Oriented Intervention Scenarios to Enhance the Dialogue on Medicines in Social Media

The opportunity to access the internet, the spread of social media, the possibility to create and share information through different channels and modalities is changing the relationship between people and consumer products, also in the specific case of medicines. The entire pharmaceutical management process—from development to marketing, thanks to data mining and the observation of people's behaviour and preferences on social media—to the choice and use of medicines—advertising and word of mouth influence the orientation and purchase choice of the drug, think of the difference between branded and equivalent medicines -, up to the preservation and disposal processes, is influenced by the advent of social media. Even if from a legislative and regulatory point of view, and here we refer to the Italian context, it is not possible to market OTC and SOP medicines directly through social media there are already websites and apps offering the service, which in turn have institutional profiles in the main social platforms. In this context, what contribution can design culture make?

At a first level, design culture could intervene in redesigning certain elements accompanying the medicine, such as packaging. This is the first real means of contact and access to the medicine and information on the medicine, making it a real node in a connected system of tangible and intangible objects and stakeholders in the process of production, use and disposal of the medicine.

A second level concerns the use of social media as a tool for research and analysis, to understand the real points of view, needs, and requirements of the communities of interest with respect to the medicine, in its dimension as an object for treatment that has not yet fully surpassed the dimension of the sole—albeit indispensable—dimension of functionality: a medicine 'works' because it helps the person, the body, to deal with an adverse situation. But as it becomes an object, it must also relate to other needs and necessities. In its extended form, the medicine is also packaging, designed more to protect and preserve the active ingredient than to facilitate use. The medicine is also form, in its various declinations: it can be ingested, injected, smeared, inhaled, and how many of these forms are designed as much for the functionality of the cure as for the process, the acceptability, the accessibility of the cure. The medicine is also process and management of the different phases of storage, use and disposal. Actions of data mining and observation through social media and the involvement of communities of interest, if also interpreted through the culture of the project, could make medicine evolve from the functional dimension to that of use, acceptance, and autonomy of care.

A third level relates to the definition of new service platforms in which the digitalisation of information and the creation of digital twins is accompanied by information on the purchase and use of the medicine and the data conveyed through social media. It could represent a lever for better profiling of the subject and for the development of personalised, participatory and predictive care, while considering the limits imposed by privacy and the ethics of data use.

At a further level, the design culture could translate and make even more accessible all those communities of interest related to the theme of medicine, care and health: the dynamics of communication, involvement, interaction, dialogue, and imitation, taken from the social media world and translated into more health-oriented media, in which the active and participatory involvement of knowledge and care experiences serve to create structured, faithful and supportive information for interactions between widespread communities.

These are just some of the trajectories that design culture could intercept through social media concerning the evolution of the medicine in its dimension of object and node within the care system.

References

Couzin-Frankel J (2023) Obesity meets its match. Science (New York, NY) 382(6676):1226–1227

Delbaere M, Michael B, Phillips BJ (2021) Social media influencers: a route to brand engagement for their followers. Psychol Mark 38(1):101–112

Farsi D (2021) Social media and health care, part I: literature review of social media use by health care providers. J Med Internet Res 23(4):e23205

Farsi D, Martinez-Menchaca HR, Ahmed M, Farsi N (2022) Social media and health care (part II): narrative review of social media use by patients. J Med Internet Res 24(1):e30379

Fnopi (2019) Uso corretto dei social media nella professione infermieristica. Le indicazioni del consiglio nazionale FNOPI del 13/10/2018. Retrieved at: https://www.fnopi.it/aree-tematiche/social-pronunciamento-consiglio-nazionale-13-ottobre-2018/

George DR, Rovniak LS, Kraschnewski JL (2013) Dangers and opportunities for social media in medicine. Clin Obstet Gynecol 56(3):453–462

Hauser C (2015) F.D.A. warns company over Kardashian Instagram marketing. The New York Times. https://www.nytimes.com/2015/08/13/health/fda-warns-company-over-kardashian-instagram-marketing.html

Iaconesi S, Persico O (2016) La Cura. Codice Edizioni, Torino

Mandelli A, Pace M (2023) Comunicazione sanitaria su social media. Retrieved at: https://www.ordfarmbo.it/multimedia/allegati/14378.pdf

Menietti E, Mautino B (2023) L'anno dell'Ozempic [The year of Ozempic]. Il Post. Retrieved at https://www.ilpost.it/2023/12/19/ozempic/

Merriam-Webster (2023) Social Media. https://www.merriam-webster.com/dictionary/social%20media

Ministero della Salute (2006) Decreto Legislativo 24 aprile 2006, n. 219—Titolo VIII Pubblicità. Retrieved at: https://www.normattiva.it/uri-res/N2Ls?urn:nir:stato:decreto.legislativo:2006-04-24;219!vig=

Ministero della Salute (2023) Linee guida sulla pubblicità sanitaria dei Medicinali di Automedicazione (otc) e dei Medicinali Senza Obbligo di Prescrizione (SOP). Retrieved at: https://www.salute.gov.it/imgs/C_17_pubblicazioni_3344_allegato.pdf

Mullin E (2023) The FDA approves weight loss drug Zepbound, a Wegovy and Ozempic rival. Wired. Retrieved at: https://www.wired.com/story/fda-approves-weight-loss-drug-zepbound-wegovy-and-ozempic-rival/

Nayak LM, Linkov G (2019) Social media marketing in facial plastic surgery: what has worked? Facial Plast Surg Clin 27(3):373–377

Pershad Y, Hangge PT, Albadawi H, Oklu R (2018) Social medicine: Twitter in healthcare. J Clin Med 7(6):121

Redazione Open Innovation (2020) Approfondimenti: Le nostre valvole stampate in 3D e le maschere riadattate per l'emergenza COVID-19. Open Innovation–Regione Lombardia. https://www.openinnovation.regione.lombardia.it/it/news/news/4416/lenostrevalvolestampateindelemaschereriadattateperlemergenzacovid

Rosen R, Vasiloudes V, Mhaskar R (2024) The emergence of MedTok: a qualitative analysis of popular medical TikTok videos. Postgrad Med J qgae021

Santoro E, Marinoni G, Carnevale G, Del Zotti F (2023) Raccomandazioni sull'uso di social media, di sistemi di posta elettronica ed instant messaging nella professione medica e nella comunicazione medico-paziente. Retrieved at: https://portale.fnomceo.it/wp-content/uploads/2023/08/Raccomandazioni-FNOMCeO-uso-social-media-posta-elettronica-whatsapp.pdf

Sharma M, Yadav K, Yadav N, Ferdinand KC (2017) Zika virus pandemic—analysis of Facebook as a social media health information platform. Am J Infect Control 45(3):301–302

Starri M (2023) Digital 2023—i dati globali. WeAreSocial. https://wearesocial.com/it/blog/2023/01/digital-2023-i-dati-globali/

Steffelson M, Paige SR, Chaney BH, Chaney JD (2020) Evolving role of social media in health promotion: updated responsibilities for health education specialists. Int J Environ Res Public Health 17(4):1153

Ventola CL (2014) Social media and health care professionals: benefits, risks, and best practices. Pharm Therap 39(7):491

Weissmann G (2012) Epigenetics in the age of Twitter: pop culture and modern science. Bellevue Literary Press, New York

Willis E, Delbaere M (2022) Patient influencers: the next frontier in direct-to-consumer pharmaceutical marketing. J Med Internet Res 24(3):e29422

World Health Organization (WHO) (2023) Infodemic. Retrieved at: https://www.who.int/health-topics/infodemic#tab=tab_1

Open Access This chapter is licensed under the terms of the Creative Commons Attribution 4.0 International License (http://creativecommons.org/licenses/by/4.0/), which permits use, sharing, adaptation, distribution and reproduction in any medium or format, as long as you give appropriate credit to the original author(s) and the source, provide a link to the Creative Commons license and indicate if changes were made.

The images or other third party material in this chapter are included in the chapter's Creative Commons license, unless indicated otherwise in a credit line to the material. If material is not included in the chapter's Creative Commons license and your intended use is not permitted by statutory regulation or exceeds the permitted use, you will need to obtain permission directly from the copyright holder.

Part III
The Daily Life as a Place of Inaccuracy: The Domesticity of Therapy

Chapter 12
Medicines as Designed Objects

Silvia Pizzocaro and Antonella Valeria Penati

Abstract A large amount of healthcare studies are paying very large attention to patients' behaviour with medicines and to patient-related factors leading to successful or poor medication adherence. Despite that, more diffused design-oriented perspectives grafted onto the *medication-user* relation still deserve attention. Although medicines can be the first (and sometimes unique) remedy a patient can rely on when at home, there is a relative *inertia* in designerly ways of conceiving medicines as 'designed things'. The diffusion and ubiquity of pharmacological treatments—specifically their *pervasiveness*—which today represents a nearly complete reality for many countries with mature economies, are in fact still characterized by the lack of an advanced design-oriented perspective about medications, patients, and their interactions: drugs, despite scientific refinement of its pharmacological principle, may remain quite traditional as technical objects. The opportunities offered by healthcare service systems and enabling technologies, as well as the monitoring of therapies, risk not obtaining their desired effectiveness if there is no intervention at the *ground zero* of the drug's 'shape' itself, as it appears in its commodity elements (galenical forms; delivery, dosage and storage co-products; packaging and informa-

---

This chapter is an expanded version of many reflections already debated by the authors in one's own past published papers, and herein revised and enriched with supplementary notes and integrations for this text edition. Mainly concerned specific paragraphs are *The shape of drugs: a matter of typologies and morphologies; Is a medicine an object?; Medicines and science at the everyday level; Medicines as devices for everyday life; Medicines, auxiliary objects and information endowments*. The original background papers are: Penati, A., Pizzocaro, S., Tonelli, M.C., Standoli, C., Iannilli, V., Bucchetti, V., Rebaglio, A., Riccò, D., Andreoni, G., Caratti, E., & Tolino, U. (2020). *Scienza al quotidiano: farmaci come oggetti/Daily Science: Pharmaceuticals as Objects*. DIID Industrial Design/Industrial Design, 69, 120–127; Penati, A., Pizzocaro, S., Standoli, C. E., & Iannilli, V. M. (2021). *The shape of drugs: a matter of human-centred design*. Design Culture(s) Conference, Cumulus Conference Proceedings Rome, 1364–1375. Pizzocaro, S. & Penati, A. (2021). The In-Home Use of Medications: In Pursuit of Design-Driven Knowledge. *Home Cultures*, 17(3), 153–171.

S. Pizzocaro (✉) · A. V. Penati
Department of Design, Politecnico di Milano, Milan, Italy
e-mail: silvia.pizzocaro@polimi.it; antonella.penati@polimi.it

tive attachments); if it is neglected to investigate patients' everyday lives, their fragility, and the nature of the user interactions, which are not scientific, but instead inaccurate and approximate; if the prosaic side of the therapeutic action is believed to be irrelevant.

12.1 Forewords: Some Working Definitions for Medicines

Medicines are substances that have the capacity to change the condition of a living organism for the better. "The prototype of medicines are the *materia medica* that alleviate ill health" (van der Geest et al. 1996, p. 154), *materia medica* being the old-fashioned term "to remind that medicines are material things" (Reynolds Whyte et al. 2002, p. 3). Although intended as beneficial, medicines can also harm accidentally. The potentially noxious effects of medicines are a key concern in the biomedical tradition (Reynolds Whyte et al. 2002). This is why, even if by definition medicines indicate "any chemical substance or product used to modify or examine physiological functions or disease states for the benefit of the patient" (Caprino 2011, p. 10), in summary, the word drug[1] may better refer to "any substance that determines functional changes in the body" (Caprino 2011, p. 9).

A more extensive definition recalls that "Medicines – industrial pharmaceutical products developed based on scientific references relating to biology, biomedicine and pharmacy – are objects saturated with meaning, and very ambivalent. Concrete objects, sometimes prosaic, integrated into the private space and daily time, which seem justified by a material effectiveness on the bodies largely escaping the consciousness of those who consume them; objects whose materiality is also terribly effective, since hundreds of millions of people owe their (sur)vival only to their consumption. They are also the support of an ideal investment, of interpretations, of symbolic elaborations, in relation to the biomedical scientific culture that produces them and with the multiple cultures and subcultures that (re)interpret them. They are also social objects, conveying more or less unequal roles, knowledge and power relations, legitimizing the organization of institutions, systems, networks" (Desclaux and Lévy 2003, p. 5).

Not only are medicines *things,* but the sense of their attributed power is in their concreteness (van der Geest and Whyte 1989). "Their *thinginess* provides patients and healers with a means to deal with the problem at hand" (van der Geest et al. 1996, p. 154). Medicines are tangible, usable in a concrete way, by applying a *thing* "the state of a patient turns into something concrete, into something to which efforts can be addressed" (van der Geest et al. 1996, p. 155). Medicines have "vigorous commodity careers; […]. At the same time, they are the most

---

[1] The Italian authors of this contribution remind the reader that the English word 'drug' means both medicinal products and medication, and those for narcotic use. On the contrary, in current, non-pharmacological, Italian language, the word 'droga' strictly refers to natural abuse substances (narcotics), or synthesis substances (Caprino 2011, p. 11).

personal of material objects, swallowed, inserted into bodies [...]." (Reynolds Whyte et al. 2002, p. 3). Moreover, medicines are "medicinal forms" saturated with meaning (Akrich 1995; Desclaux and Lévy 2003) and "technical objects" (Akrich 1996). With the latter, it is meant that the product has a set of tangible properties, including the characteristics of the devices that allow medicines to be taken (dispensers, containers and integrated devices of measuring, regulation, conservation, portioning, and supply). As the significance of medicines lies in the curative efficacy, the associated devices, although unrelated to the therapeutic efficacy of the underlying pharmacological principles, become an integral part of therapeutic success.

12.2 Medication Errors in Medicine Consumption

The ambiguity of medicinal potency is evident in the derivation from the old Greek word *pharmakon,* poison, from which *pharmaceutical* derives. Indeed, medicines can be simultaneously noxious and beneficial. The increase in medication errors related to user behaviour—notwithstanding an increasingly educated population—emerges nowadays from a complex of factors including:

- the general expansion of medicalization that shaped the figure of the patient as consumer (Conrad 2007; Williams et al. 2011; Gabe et al. 2015), with the concept of medicalisation first intended (Conrad 1992, 2007) as a process by which problems lying outside medicine begin to be treated and defined as medical;
- the significant trends in the personalization of care. The individualized prescription, because of the specific characteristics of many medicines available today, allows appropriate adjustments with the possible consequence of unprecise dosage alteration of the pharmaceutical integrity;
- the spreading of the informal digital information that contributed to the growth of the do-it-yourself medication practices and self care (Akrich and Méadel 2002; Fainzang 2003, 2012; Vicarelli 2009);
- the diffusion of several forms of non-conventional or alternative medications (as for instance phytopharmacy, homeopathy, natural remedies) that may lack either explicit dosage indications and warnings for use;
- the increase in the elderly population, which tends to be affected by multiple chronic diseases, and therefore likely to use many medicines (European Commission 2018; Lumme-Sandt and Virtane 2002).

As we are interested in patient-related factors from the design angle, we are mainly considering the unsuitable characteristics of the designed properties of medicines *per se,* as well as those unfavourable surrounding conditions—i.e. non adequate domestic environments, absence of dedicated care-givers, social contexts of vulnerability, isolation, weakness, debility, temporary incapacity—where, even in cases of elementary pharmacological treatments, the risks of medication error and care discomfort may be high (World Health Organization 2003).

While the growing consumption of pharmaceutical products has fueled extensive research—mainly conducted in the medical-epidemiological field—on their side effects, interactions, and the factors that may alter therapeutic properties (European Medicine Agency 2015a, b), as well as on the many patient-related factors contributing to medication nonadherence, such investigations still offer considerable margins of exploration about user misbehaviours (ranging from abuse to forgetfulness, non-compliance with methods of handling, incorrect storage methods, dosage mistakes, incorrect use interpretations) conditioned by the inherent designed properties of medications. Moreover, any perceptual, physical, or cognitive difficulty induced by lack of affordance of the medicine itself can hinder or reduce access to care, causing the patient not to take the medication correctly or to discontinue therapy altogether.

As a mere side note, one should consider the long list of indications and warnings contained in the Italian Ministerial Recommendations on the handling of oral solid forms (Ministero della salute 2019 [Ministry of Health 2019]) intended for an audience of experts such as health professionals. It is a demonstration of how many precautions are required when dealing with one of the many technical procedures that arise in the practice of care, that is the elementary act of breaking or powdering oral solid substances. An action that the user (and sometimes even the doctor) tends to banalise, attracted by the easy result it can achieve: personalising the medicine dose. The technical gesture—understood as a gesture that presupposes some technical expertise necessary to act correctly—is impoverished by a 'doing' that lacks knowledge and can easily lead to error.

12.3 The Kaleidoscope of Medicinal Forms

Each drug has, where possible, a different pharmacological form with which it is produced and sold (Anderson 2005). Due to the possible alteration of the active ingredient, not all medicines are available in diversified pharmaceutical forms, because this would compromise their effectiveness. The pharmacological forms with which medicines are usually made and sold are solid, semisolid, liquid and gaseous.[2]

Common solid pharmaceutical forms are usually to be taken orally. They can be pills (preparations containing excipients and medical substances), capsules (where granules, powders or solutions are contained in two interlocking cylinders), tablets (with active ingredient and powdered excipients compressed to obtain a compact medicine with different shapes), *cachets* (with active ingredient and excipients contained between two pods one above the other), granules (with different shapes and sizes, which can be taken by dissolving them in water or enclosed in capsules), dragees (that is tablets coated with a thin sugar film to mask unpleasant odor or taste, as well as protect the drug from humidity and light), powders (resulting of the

---

[2] For more about this, see the chapter *Pharmaceutical forms: a glossary* (Chap. 4), in this volume.

trituration of the active ingredient and of the excipients contained in the pharmaceutical formula).

Main semi-solid medicines include creams, gels (rich in water), or other topical substances such as foams and ointments.

Liquid substances too can be administered for oral use, or through injections by means of a syringe or by rubbing them on the skin: they include syrups (that is sugar solutions dissolved in water and ready for use), solutions (with active ingredients dissolved in a liquid solution such as water, oil, or alcohol), emulsions (when two liquids that cannot be mixed together are kept separate in the package and need to be shaken before use), suspensions/lotions (meaning non-soluble powder preparation, suspended in a liquid that is shaken before use).

Finally, as gaseous substances medicines may be inhaled into the body, as spray (with the active principle dispersed in solutions or suspensions and then inhaled in gaseous form) and aerosol (prepared in liquid form that is inhaled).

12.4 The Shape of Drugs: A Matter of Typologies and Morphologies

Today industrial medicinal products appear in a diversity of pharmaceutical forms. The active ingredient defines the shape for the market. As we have seen, if technically permissible, the same active ingredient can give rise to different 'pharmaceutical shapes' according to the dosage required, the difficulty of intake by the patient, and whether it is a medicine for hospital or home care use (Caprino 2011).

The concreteness of 'medical matter' can be recognized in the term 'pharmaceutical shape', which occupies a central place in the pharmaceutical vocabulary. The shape guarantees an object's individuality, recognizability, and identity, in being the outline and boundary of objects. Identifying is one of the ways of knowing, to recognise again, tracing the perceived sensory characteristics of a new object back to previous experience data.

A shape enables us to give a precise physiognomy to 'formless' matter (Flusser 1999). And this prerogative is very relevant in the case of medicines, whose recognition is prior so to avoid intake mistakes.

In particular, the 'pharmaceutical shape' has always had a significant influence in the world of medicines because of the way and mode of intake associated with it. There is a relationship far from trivial between the pharmaceutical shape, the route of medical intake, and a method of treatment. Moreover, the method of intake constitutes one of the crucial point in the relationship between the user and its medicine.

What in the medical-pharmaceutical field is referred to as 'pharmaceutical form' corresponds to what, in the field of design, we call object typology.

The term typology refers to the stabilised character of the form of objects over time (Penati 2016, p. 52). The typology of an object emphasises the typical salient features of each object family (e.g., tables, chairs, bottles, lamps, etc.).

Similarly, capsules, tablets, vials, suppositories, and syringes for injection are object typologies stabilised over time. They represent the formal structure that remains, despite the multiple morphological declinations that individual objects take on depending on technique, specific functions, style and aesthetic intentionality. Indeed, each typology is enriched by formal contingencies because each object is identifiable and recognisable precisely based on its 'morphological characters' or 'morphological variants'.

In the world of artefacts, we recognise many typologies with a long permanence in time and many formal variants (morphologies) that identify their contingencies regarding material, technology, aesthetics, etc.

Unlike other object categories, in typological terms, the pharmaceutical product seems to have stopped at the stage of its advent, showing indifference to incorporating significant elements of innovation.

Its remoteness from the evolutionary dynamics that, through successive 'generations', lead products to maturity, according to that process that Simondon (1958) defined as progressive concretisation.

Let's suppose the task of an object typology is to facilitate, beyond the specific formal characterisations, the recognition of objects and the attribution of the relative function. In the world of pharmaceuticals, we find ourselves with immediately recognisable strong typologies (e.g., capsules, suppositories, syringes) and weak ones (e.g., powders, drops, liquids, creams) that do not possess the same immediacy in communicating the formal identity of the pharmaceutical substance. For this, these amorphous substances (lacking in form) must rely on their packaging (e.g., bottles, vials, etc.), and sometimes even this is insufficient to give them an identity if an adequate information apparatus does not accompany it. This leads to numerous errors in use.

Moreover, in the world of pharmaceuticals, even the 'strong' types (e.g., tablets, suppositories, ovules), have loosened, over time, the rigour proper to the typological connection between pharmaceutical form and route of intake (e.g., suppositories as well as vaginal tablets) and even this 'betrayal' of the vocation inscribed in the formal tradition of the object (its type) can be the cause of errors on the part of the user.

If we observe medicines from the point of view of their morphological characterization, we deal with an objectified world, mostly constituted by raw forms, weak forms: a sort of 'degree zero' of the form (Barthes 1982), imbued with a relevant complexity of use and meaning.

Ultimately, a medicine form, primarily devoid of modal and identity qualities, struggles to meet the minimum requirements of recognisability, ease of understanding and use, typical of the world of commodities. Indeed, we can argue that contemporary medicine 'gives itself' through packaging and may fall into that category of products that require a prosthetic mediation to take on a form of its own, an identity, and a manageability that enables its use (Anceschi and Bucchetti 1998; Pareek and Kunteta 2014). In this sense, the drug would certainly not represent a particular case. We are aware of how formless substances take on the nature of an object through their packaging.

Even in the case of these products (e.g., flours, oils, creams, detergents, perfumes, deodorants), we find ourselves faced with the use—often abuse—of design stratagems aimed at conferring identity traits on the content through sensorial effects (colours, flavours, aromas, tactile effects) or through forms of differentiation, often pleonastic, which are nevertheless a sign of progressive specialisation (Penati et al. 2020).

Conversely, pharmaceuticals seem unfamiliar with using morphological variation to meet the progressive sharpening of our material needs and as a response to the sophistication of the system of needs. And, above all, as a guarantee of recognisability of identity. In the case of medicines, the proliferation of varieties obtained by adding accessory or auxiliary elements—in the sense of marginal and superfluous—to the product's primary function risks being misleading and harmful. However, we cannot forget the ancillary and auxiliary role, in the etymological sense of the term, of signs such as colour, size, surface texture, touch, and silhouette; in the case of formal characterisation, they would assume the role of identity signals and invitations to facilitate the use of the product (Penati et al. 2020).

12.5 Is a Medicine an Object?

Here we propose a reflection on the medicine—which we treat in its broadest sense as a product, developed on scientific findings in pharmacology. We wonder whether the medicine can be taken on as an 'object'—and whether it can be investigated with the conceptual tools of design.

If observed from the design perspective, the medicine is quite peculiar. Even the very fact of categorising it in the disciplined categories of 'object', 'technical object', and 'object of everyday use' can create more than one perplexity, as its concrete contingency, its morphological, typological, experiential, sensorial vocation, and use, elude the conventional idea of an object in itself.

Even if it becomes a product, the result of industrial production processes, the medicine does not easily allow itself to be read as an object, not even as a technical object, so much so that its 'mode of being' belongs to the world of scientific discoveries and its formal imagery. As an object, the medicine appears to be anchored to the realm of raw materials and far removed from the users' needs for usability (van der Geest et al. 1996), from their everyday experience, from the concrete ways in which people come into contact with objects, from the typical relationships established between subjects and objects.

While the object is increasingly personalised, the medicine lacks any personalisation, even those strictly functional ones related to understanding, remembering, learning through use, making the treatment experience easy and accessible, and responding to the need to adapt to the person's characteristics and the duration of treatment. The object works on processes of recognisability; the medicine has no identity vocation, not even a functional one.

Objects construct use behaviour, especially in their domestic dimension. The medicine and the healing processes lack comparison with the power of customary practices, with the "motor habits" (Bordieu 2003, p. 178) and mental habits and their "structuring structures" (Bordieu, *ibid.*) that often persist even when the context of use changes.

The absence of a process of objectification in the case of the medicine can also be observed in its life cycle. Starting from the purchase: in the case of the object of use, it is always also a phase of choice. On the contrary, the user cannot choose the medicine: it is prescribed by an expert, thanks to whom the pharma-product's seriality acquires the exceptionality proper to the unique specimen, and its use becomes exclusive and individual.

Observing its nature as an object, the medicine and its formal traits pose multiple challenges to design. Among these challenges, its formal translation can:

- emancipate the medicine from the principles of science and the body of technology, to bring it closer to the concreteness of people's experience of use (Bürdek 2008; de Seta 1980; Norman 2013; van Onck 1994);
- embrace the mixture of strict functionality and the mytho-poietic character that is proper to quasi-magical objects (Barthes 1982);
- govern the dynamics of consumption for the implications they have on the individual and social scales.

The meanings we use to focus on the factual, experiential, and symbolic traits that characterise the life of objects are embodied by words such as 'thing', 'object', 'technical object', 'everyday objects', 'device', 'social object'. These terms contribute to re-perimeter the status of any object within some open epistemological and phenomenological frames (Molotch 2003; Bertola and Manzini 2004).

The same words may contribute to our aim to better understand the prosaic nature of medicines as objects.

Terms like thing, object, technical object, device, social object, when qualifying a medicine, may contribute to make it understandable from the peculiar angle of the world of goods.

12.6 Medicines as Things

From dictionaries *thing*[3] can be referred to as an object or entity not precisely designated, an inanimate object distinguished from a living being, or the concrete entity as distinguished from its appearances (Merriam-Webster 2022a). The word *thing*

---

[3] Etymological remark: the thing etymology is rooted in the Old English *þing*, a 'meeting, assembly, council, discussion', and later 'entity, being, matter as subject of deliberation in an assembly', and also 'act, deed, event, material object'. In medieval Germanic languages (Proto-Germanic, Old Frisian, and Middle Dutch) *thing* denoted deliberative and judicial assemblies. This old meaning did not survive. *Things* as personal possessions appear in English around 1300.

denotes a massive generality as well as particularities, it designates the concrete yet ambiguous within the everyday, it functions to overcome the loss of other words or as a place holder, it may even designate an amorphous characteristic (Brown 2001, p. 4).

As in Brown (2001), the term *thing* perpetually poses a problem because of "the specific unspecificity that things denote" (p. 3). For the present aim, we limit ourselves to indicate that things are material entities, tangible, sensitive to the touch and to all five senses. Things can be also goods, commodities, and mostly objects invested intellectually and culturally, framed in systems of relationships, inserted in contexts to which they give emotional and sentimental sense and qualities. Things may be invested by emotional charges because they may not necessarily be useful, in the sense of performing a strictly instrumental function.

As concrete devices or commodities for the benefit of the patient, medicines can be considered things that embody the *materia medica* (van der Geest et al. 1996, p. 154). Medicines are things because the sense of their attributed power is in their concreteness (van der Geest and Whyte 1989, p. 345).

Medicines as 'things' also express their sense of indeterminacy, generality, as if they were by nature lacking any distinctive formal attribute. Even when clearly identified in its concreteness by a label, a trademark, a category, a term, or the principle abridgement, a medicine essence may happen to escape recognition, as something whose real name is not known, or something nameless.

12.7 Medicines as Objects

The word 'object' means something 'thrown against', things existing outside the individuals, things placed in front, with a material character, and affecting the senses. As in Moles (1969), the term is constituted on the one hand on the aspect of resistance to the person, on the other hand on the material, concrete character. In short, an object is a material element of the external world that can be manipulated, something material that may be perceived by the senses (Merriam-Webster 2022b). The object, in most western civilizations, is not natural (Moles 1969, p. 5), it is man made.

In addition to being material entities that can be manipulated, objects do not have a mere passive function but produce active relationships, and they can act as manipulators in turn. This implies many plans for consideration (Deni 2002, p. 82) implying considering objects act as manipulators in relation to the subjects using them; objects that structure the action processes of the user; objects that may create the context in the relationship they have with other objects (this is the interobjective dimension); objects that may modify intersubjective relations.

As functional, concrete entities handled and used by patients medicines (i.e. dispensers, containers, blisters, integrated components of measuring, regulation, conservation, portioning) embody the nature of objects that may activate specialized, hyper-technological, or conversely prosaic techniques of manipulation by and between users.

Medicines as 'objects' may also capture the sensorial dimension of the subject who perceives them and, through their attributes, recongnizes them. Moreover, medicines as objects distinct from subjects, escape the principle of otherness once they are taken, that is, when the object becomes part of and transforms the subject. For the medical doctor who prescribes, for the pharmacist who dispenses, for the care giver who administers the cure, the medicine is and remains something other than itself—an object. For the patient who takes the medicine, the subject/object contraposition changes in content: to the typical prerogatives of the object (instrumental, operational, functional, etc.) are added emotional, sentimental, symbolic, ideological, political, etc.

At last, as far as the attitude of objects to manipulate individuals is concerned, this applies to medicines not only in general but in vertu of the forms of explicit addiction that they are able to induce.

12.8 Medicines as 'Technical' Objects[4]

The concept of 'technical object' was coined by Gilbert Simondon (1958) who, inspired by the research of André Leroi-Gourhan (1943, 1945) which had revealed a technical trend within the morphological evolution in the succession of prehistoric tools, elaborated a theory of the individuality and specificity of technical objects. Simondon achieved an epistemological break with common sense: technical objects are not only serving an end, rather they must be known according to their technical essence. In order to introduce an adequate knowledge of technical objects into our culture, he theorized that it is necessary to become aware of their mode of existence.

For Fainzang (2001) considering medicines as technical objects means trying to highlight the links that exist between its material characteristics and the associated forms of use. As a relatively little studied question, it seems that between the marketing of a new molecule and the biochemical action of this molecule in the patient's body, all the stages of a medicine process of concretization are transparent (p. 135). Instead, the proper functioning of the medicine, even reduced to its basic biochemical program, requires a fairly large number of interventions. The medicine itself is defined by its form and by all the devices that frame a more or less explicit program of actions and summon a certain technical and material environment.

As a technical object, a medicine incorporates forms of knowledge that need to be known in order to correctly activate its potential for use. Further, a medicine requires knowledge of appropriate 'techniques of the body' (Mauss 2017): gestures, postures, rules, manners, behaviours of use, etc. As any technical object, a medicine

---

[4] Etymological remark: the adjective technical means pertaining to the useful or mechanic arts, and it stems from the Latinized *technĭcus,* from Greek τεχνικός, *technikós,* derived from τέχνη, 'art, skill'.

12.9 Medicines as Everyday Objects[5]

A ballpoint pen, a washing machine, a mobile phone are examples of objects that are part of daily life, which have become part of everyday habits. These are objects which under their various aspects (economic, political, social, cultural, functional) may have revolutionized people's daily lives when they first appeared, but which—in their subsequent acquisition of ordinariness—are taken for granted. The adjective 'everyday' emphasizes the nature of things that are encountered or used routinely or typically. Like any object, 'everyday' objects primarily signify their function but secondly can also refer to other meanings, namely assuming symbolic values of a social and cultural nature (Barthes 1966, 1985).

Medicines as everyday objects go with the prosaic nature of commodities many pharmaceuticals have acquired. According to Williams et al. (2011) the process of pharmaceuticalization involves "the transformation of human conditions, capabilities and capacities into opportunities for pharmaceutical intervention" (p. 711) and it motivates both micro and macro level concerns to the role of everyday lifestyles and medicines consumption. The pharmaceuticalisation of everyday life has introduced profitable medicines for a range of daily activities. As a consequence, pharmaceuticals may happen to be seen by consumers as goods to resolve problems of daily life (Fox and Ward 2008).

When analysing a medicine as an object in everyday use, the emphasis may fall on adjectives such as trivial, futile, prosaic, material, obvious, ordinary. These adjectives make a medicine—notwithstanding its being the outcome of the most advanced technology and the embodiment of scientific precision—to be 'lumped together' (literally) with the objects that 'we are accustomed' (literally) to using. Even the practices of use may take on specific accents when related to 'objects of everyday life'. Here too adjectives such as customary, routine, repetitive, or usual, may prevail.

---

[5] Etymological remark: 'Everyday' is from Middle English *everidayes, every daies, every dayes* ('everyday, daily, continual, constant'. As opposed to Sundays or high days, from noun meaning 'a week day'. The extended sense of 'to be met with every day, common' is from 1763 (Merriam-Webster 2022c). The adjective describes something which happens or is used every day, or forms a regular and basic part of life, so it is not especially interesting or unusual.

12.10 Medicines and Science at the Everyday Level

Consistent literature widely analyses the nature of objects belonging to the sphere of domesticity and everyday use. Conversely, not as much attention has been paid to medicines and related use processes (which include activities of supply, organisation, notation, preparation, administration/assumption) and, more generally, to care and treatment activities, taking as a filter for analysis precisely the everyday domestic life and the superficiality and haste that characterise its activities.

This is the point of view we have chosen to use in this volume, particularly in this section of the text.

The behaviour triggered by everyday objects can also be found in the use of medicines.

In the context of the meaning just defined, we are interested in making some reflections on the specificity of the pharma-object. We borrow the stances, well-established in sociology and anthropology, of those who, being interested in everyday life as it is, do not seek to amend it from its coarseness and its lack of knowledge but try to make the most of precisely these peculiarities to give it theoretical form and construct a new epistemology of the everyday (Ferrarotti 1986).

Here, we dwell on an initial observation: once they have entered the domains of everyday life, medicines become pervasive but at the same time invisible, like other household objects (Nacci 1998). Through objects, the instances of techno-science enter our life system, becoming commonplace. In the object, 'technological power is miniaturised' (Gras 1993).

This is especially true for the most common objects that populate our daily lives, where the artefact appears to overpower the techno-scientific content, operating on the interface, constructing formal and informative invitations or affordance signs, and introducing norms, rules, and instructions.

In other words, the artefact relies on an apparatus that, while facilitating the use and the relationship between the user and the product, can conceal the scientific principles of which the objects become mediators.

In the object, the scientific and technical world is made friendly—or domesticated—to integrate it and adapt it to the measure of the everyday (Lie and Sørensen 1996). The rhetorics underpinning this transition are those of simplification, gergalisation, normalisation, trivialisation, understood as framing it in the reassuring frames of the obvious, the usual, and the ordinary. To these are added the automatisms, rituals, acquired rules of behaviour, and expedients of our ways of life that deliver us a tacitly learnt and shared knowledge to mitigate the need for continuous learning. This is achieved by replacing the cognitive efforts required in the face of novel elements with the habit of recurring gestures (Penati et al. 2020).

When mixed with the things and objects that populate everyday practices, the medicine borrows their forms and behaviour of use; it imitates their manners; it adopts rough and coarse modes; it adapts improper means and sets up imprinted modalities, typical of do-it-yourself practices.

The power of the everyday shapes techniques, methods and procedures, enslaving the object to its logic. In this way, the medicine escapes the care and caution that should inform its use. Because of these specific prerogatives, the every day and its ordinariness, as the primary context of use of pharmacological therapies, becomes a fascinating object of study for its capacity to introduce exceptions to the rules; to lower attention levels; to favour the promiscuous use of instruments and objects; to accept a certain carelessness in 'following established procedures'.

Alain Gras (1993) identifies a specific category in the "techniques of everyday life" and in the objects that incorporate them; the author observes how the everyday technical object seems almost to seek "its niche", to construct day by day "its sense" which is "a common sense and at the same time an imaginary" that is shaped between "social systems […] and individual life systems" (p. 168). In constructing a niche of meaning concerning the subject and the context of use, the object personalises itself, enters a network of relationships, generates an etiquette and writes its biography (Fiorani 2001).

We may then derive that one can read the medicine as an object, provided one does not emend it from the prosaic nature of everyday life and does not mythologise its scientific nature, implying a presumed rigour of the processes of use.

12.11 Medicines as Devices for Everyday Life

Here we intend to dwell on a further element which, starting from the project areas, has the potential to open up a broader front for reflection on medicine as an object. The problematic opening we propose concerns the object—and the medicine as object—in its device nature.

Besides responding to a specific function, the object-device takes on, etymologically, the properties of disposition and pre-disposition, in the sense of constructing a succession, of indicating a desired sequence, but also of 'having in one's possession' or of making something available to someone.

Then, it has the sense of ordering, giving a rationale according to a valuable criterion for the purpose […], and causing or allowing someone to do something.

Finally, in 'being disposed', we also find the incentive sense of being inclined or making inclined to do something (Cortellazzo and Zolli 1999, p. 479). In the object, therefore, the instrumental body is accompanied by the normative and prescriptive body (Costa 2016, p. 75) and the exhortative body. Agamben, quoted by Costa, defines the device as "whatever has […] the capacity to capture, direct, determine, intercept, control, and secure the gestures, conducts, opinions, and discourses of living beings" (Costa 2016, *ibid.*).

These assumptions provide a valuable starting point for observing the drug as an explicit device and the system of care as a complex set of objects; of subjects; of relations between objects and subjects; of ordered and pre-ordered actions; of prescriptions and written or verbal dispositions, formal and codified or constructed in the natural lexicon of familiar ways of doing things, imposed and transmitted by an authority (the doctor) or simply self-taught (Penati et al. 2021).

12.12 The Use of Medicines: A Matter of Affordance and Accessibility

For the medicine, the primary and secondary packaging and the leaflet assume the role of prostheses, that is tangible extensions of the object. They are entrusted with facilitating and encouraging access to the product. Together they constitute a complex, physical, and verbal apparatus. They are used to allow or forbid specific actions, explain, make understood, and provide warnings to the user about the use of the product and its possible effects. However, as we have stated, their dispositive effectiveness is limited in the case of medicine.

In most cases, they lack those characteristics which, especially in the world of objects, would be worthy of attention: they lack affordance.

The perceptual psychologist James Gibson (1977) introduced the term *affordance* to designate those perceptual elements which, in the environment, have a functional meaning for the observer. The term was later transferred to the specific field of user-product interaction by Donald Norman (1997). Norman uses the term affordance to refer to the formal characteristics of the object that can signal the ways and possibilities by which the user can interact with the object in performing a given action (de la Fuente et al. 2015a). The concept is closely related to issues of object usability. It is related to the design of formal elements capable of suggesting/inducing or dissuading the user from performing or not performing specific actions to obtain a specific result.

In the world of packaging, there is a well-known focus on designing different ways to indicate to the user where and how to open the pack correctly and the gestures that must be used to achieve this. For example: using colour contrasts to indicate the opening area; using verbal messages such as "press and open here" to suggest where and how to open; drawing die-cuts or pre-cuts to indicate the tear area; using tabs that, through their shape, tell the user what to do without having to resort to further verbal explanations (de la Fuente et al. 2015b).

If affordances are well designed, they incorporate 'instructions for use' into the object's shape, intuitively directing a user's actions. Not only does the form of this 'perceptual information' play a role in enabling someone to do something, but the position of these semantic and operational elements also plays a role. Indeed, the position must have a logical relationship and proximity to the action to be performed to minimise the cognitive demand placed on the user.

The affordances of an object include the cues (e.g., using visual signs, use of symbols, formal or verbal elements) necessary to indicate sequences of actions; to guide the user if the same action is to be carried out differently, in two different stages of the process (discriminating); to repeat the same information several times where necessary (redundancy), etc.

Affordances incorporate mental, conceptual, logical, cultural, and perceptual models into the product.

How a user can achieve a desired action are manifold, but their effectiveness is strictly dependent on the user's experience of an object type; on whether the product is being used for the first time or subsequent uses; the cultural conventions or constraints that must be respected by the designer and known to the user (e.g., turning clockwise to close and counterclockwise to open a cap) (In the various chapters of this text we will see how, on several occasions, the analysis of objects highlights a lack of affordances, in the objects that support the use of the drug. To mention a few: lack of invitations to use enabling the user to distinguish between blisters with an opening obtained by exerting pressure on the alveolus and blisters with 'peelable' aluminium; creation in blisters of clearly recognisable areas of prehensibility; information placed too far away from the point and time at which a given action will be exerted, etc.

12.13 Medicines, Auxiliary Objects and Information Endowments

Due to the hermetic nature of its pharmaceutical form, the medicine must be accompanied by concrete or textual aids to facilitate access to the pharmaceutical product. These are: the package leaflet; the packaging; the medical prescriptions; the proper or improper aids with which the user juggles the therapy.

Every medicine, in fact, is accompanied by a set of physical artefacts and information apparatus that need to be designed together with the medicine itself. A medicine along with its auxiliary kits becomes part of a system: the 'medicine system'. This auxiliary equipment is entrusted with the dispositive functions of persuading (prescribing, ordering sequences of actions, inducing the subject to the correctness of treatment practices) and dissuading (forbidding unsuitable or even dangerous behaviour).

These objects and texts, however, although invested with an 'instructional' function, often prove to be weak in linguistic, semantic and pragmatic terms in fulfilling this role.

The knowledge language, which often expresses itself through slang far from common comprehension, generates rejection; the signs/signals deputed to order sequences of actions, do not seem to possess the necessary prescriptive or persuasive force, nor the necessary ordering clarity.

As a first exploratory hypothesis, it is proposed that it is the medicine itself, in its formal hermeticism, in its functional minimalism, that embodies the truly distinctive element (perhaps because it is dense with ideologies, values, and redeeming powers) and possesses the aptitude to influence the user's behaviour, assuming at times the role of the prodigious object or the object that inspires fear because it is potentially harmful. While the packaging that contains it (blisters, bottles, tubes, sachets, etc.) and the information kits with a prescriptive function do not seem to have the strength to intervene to direct and make the experience of using the drug accessible. Their design seems to ensure product integrity and response to rules and regulations, rather than enhancing the user experience.

Prescriptive forms show no attention to finding correct exhortative expressions capable of 'making one inclined' and generating empathy towards the treatment. They talk to the writer, heedless of the user's culture.

The medicine and its packaging do not present feedback capable of reassuring the user of the correctness of one's actions. Moreover, they lack auxiliary advice addressed to the patient to enable framing the pharmacological treatment in the broader scenario of hygiene, dietary, and appropriate lifestyle practices (Penati et al. 2021). Visually, warnings and instructions do not use any rhetorical artifice capable of attracting the user's attention.

It is above all on communication, understood as information apparatus, that we are still far from finding effective languages and ways to raise awareness, warn, inform, create a culture of 'good use', warn against easy excesses, do-it-yourself practices, promiscuous use and 'hearsay'.

On this, we would like to make some remarks: the extensive system of information on the packaging and the leaflet is entrusted with the task of explaining, through textual descriptions, actions, gestures, sequences, procedures, in which components of tacit knowledge are often present (Polanyi 1966). These prescriptive forms also suffer from the problem of being expressed through language and modes of expression that risk being comprehensible and valuable only to the expert user or user who has already experienced the described procedures (Sennet 2008, pp. 177–178).

Secondly, it is possible to notice a substantial imbalance between the negative propositions describing the numerous side effects the drug could cause, compared to the positive ones concerning the benefits. Only a few lines are reserved for these. There is also a lack of references to data on the drug's efficacy in reducing or curing the symptoms of the disease. Finally, there is a lack of descriptive elements on the signs that should announce the hoped-for well-being to encourage the patient to continue the therapy (Penati et al. 2021).

12.14 Medicines in Between Social Objects[6] and Commodities

The idea of objects having a social life is a conceit Appadurai coined in 1986 in a collection of essays titled *The Social Life of Things*. Since then the idea that persons and things are not radically distinct categories has largely been developed, and that the transactions that surround things are invested with the properties of social

---

[6] Etymological remark: in late Middle English 'social' came from Old French, or from Latin *socialis* 'allied, united, living with others', derived from *socius* 'friend, ally'.

relations. Things alone do not have a social life. At most they form parts of complexes that coproduce effects in particular situations. Things and people both can be seen as actors in that they mutually constitute one another. The study of the social role of objects has been largely influenced by the reflections of anthropologists (Douglas and Isherwood 1979; Miller 1987). The meaning that people attribute to things derives from human transactions and motivations, particularly from how those things are used and circulated. Beneath the infinitude of human wants, and the multiplicity of material forms, there in fact lie complex social and political mechanisms that regulate taste, trade, and desire.

A medicine is not only a medically effective pharmaceutical product: it is also a commodity, and an operator for a set of socio-economic networks, practices, representations, socio-cultural constructions associating the treatment in particular—but not only—with the socially represented disease (Desclaux and Lévy 2003, p. 9).

Medicines may be considered social objects with economic significance and resources with political value (Reynolds Whyte et al. 2002). "As things they can be exchanged between social actors, they objectify meanings, they move from one meaningful setting to another" (Reynolds Whyte et al. 2002, p. 5). Pharmaceuticals are not only products of human culture, but producers of it (van der Geest et al. 1996). They are vehicles of ideology, and they direct people's thoughts and actions. Pharmaceuticals are simultaneously vested with symbolic interpretations, resulting from the biomedical culture and the social culture that interprets and processes them. Pharmaceuticals can therefore considered social objects that may activate processes of knowledge and power that are not necessarily egalitarian (Desclaux and Lévy 2003, p. 5).

Out of the main five stages of the social life of medicines that van der Geest et al. (1996) have outlined (i.e. manufacturing, trading, prescribing, buying, and consuming), we mainly selectively focus on the phase of consumption. This is why we can assume that "Only when it is consumed does the substance become a medicine" (van der Geest et al. 1996, p. 164).

Moreover, each life stage of medicines "is characterized by a specific context and particular actors. In the production and marketing phase, the primary social actors are scientists and businesspeople working for pharmaceutical companies. The prescription phase mainly involves health professionals and their patients in the context of a medical practice. Distribution is carried out mostly by dispensers such as pharmacists, or sellers such as storekeepers, drug pedlars, and their customers in a market-type setting. Use occurs mostly in a household setting, away from medical professionals, as does the final phase: efficacy" (van der Geest et al. 1996, p. 156).

The approach of the anthropology of pharmaceuticals (van der Geest et al. 1996) to the question of medication consumption has directed researchers to trace behaviour patterns that, on the one hand, can be ascribed to different society cultural models and, on the other, testify the spread of universal practices. Whether one decides to ascribe the concept of medicines as social objects to cultural diversity or to the universality of individuals' behaviour, the use of medicines is socially constructed by symbolic logics and guided by mechanisms that may escape medical rationality in its strict sense (Fainzang 2005). Medicines are social objects "with economic significance, and resources with political value. Above all they are potent symbols and tokens of hope for people in distress" (Reynolds Whyte et al. 2002, p. 5).

As powerful technical devices and social objects, medicines acquire a status in society: pharmaceuticals are not only products of human culture, but producers of it (van der Geest et al. 1996). They are vehicles of ideology, self-care agents, and they direct people's thoughts and actions. Therefore, many open questions are meant to invest the patient relation with medicines and one's cultural traits, routines, rituals, ideologies, values, beliefs, and even prosaic consumption behaviours learned *via* consumption habits related to other typologies of everyday goods and commodities.

12.15 Conclusions: To Design the Shape of Medicines, to Conceive Their Use

Industrial medicinal specialties can be solid, semisolid, liquid and gaseous. The same active principle can originate different physical *shapes* ranging from tablets to capsules, powders, gels, vials, syrups, emulsions, liquid solutions, or drinks. By shapes we intend the body of prescribed and designed tangible properties allowing the sequence of actions to fulfill the medication management successfully. The final configuration and identity that a medicine may take, although dependent on the chemical-physical composition of its principle, may provide—or better, should also provide—important information on the intake and use methods all along its life cycle (Overgaard et al. 2001). As every medicine also needs to be exposed, sold, stored, protected and preserved, it not only requires the obvious priority of keeping the active principle stable, but it also implies some affordance priorities such as:

- allowing suitable methods of handle and intake;
- avoiding perceptive difficulties or misunderstandings for the end user;
- expressing clear identity traits such as to be recognizable even when medicines are unpackaged and presented in loose form.

Such an inherent set of basic, almost elementary designed properties of medication affordance is often far from complete, or poor, even neglected entirely in worst cases. Not only the designed properties of medicines may be often unsatisfactory, but they are not necessarily explored by default as commodities requiring positive affordances modelled on users' behaviour (Akrich 1998).

Craig and Chamberlain (2017, p. 3) state that, "In healthcare, design is therefore a given. Hospital buildings and interiors, medical instruments and assistive technologies are all or should all be designed with a focus on ease of use, efficiency, performance, and user experience." In spite of that, medicines *per se* and their paraphernalia still frequently are limited to their "ground zero" of designed properties and use modes (Penati et al. 2020).

While still lacking a robust formalization for our reflections—although provisionally inspired by the studies a number of research traditions have already fully consolidated, especially in the field of social sciences (Kleinman 1980; Chast 1995; Akrich 1995, 1996, 1998; Akrich and Méadel 2002; Wyatt et al. 2004; Borgna 2005; Fainzang 2001, 2003, 2005, 2012; Vicarelli 2009)—we limit ourselves to evoke integrative domains for an inquisitive design for care agenda, where "Design can bring care to presence" (Rodgers et al. 2019, p. 74), as in the wider intention of the design for healthcare advancements (Jones 2013; Tsekleves and Cooper 2016; Groeneveld et al. 2018; Nusem et al. 2020).

This is why we wonder whether individual different sensitivities about hygiene, privacy, modesty, embarrassment, inadequacy, need for autonomy, and objective and subjective abilities in managing medication, may motivate to assign the users' body an autonomous formalized statute—*a statute of the body* (Borgna 2005)—when considering medicines from the design angle. Beside, we advocate the relevance of letting medicines be considered *designed materia*—along with *materia medica*—, so to incorporate person-centered medication requirements into more generalizable design concerns.

With respect to medicines as objects, there is a long-established tendency to accentuate the instrumental dimension of commodities (Penati et al. 2020). If we consider medicines in the typologies of syrups, liquid solutions, pills, tablets, ointments, and powders, we can not avoid observing that it may sound rather singular to identify them as 'technical objects' in a strict sense. Nevertheless, we support the relevance and need for an articulated reflection on the 'thinginess' of medicines, aimed at claiming the correlation between the formal properties of medications (state, shape, dimension, proportions, texture, package, contents, co-products, related devices, and information equipment) and their deficiencies or inadequacies related to self medication, non-management by users, or—in worst cases—explicit user-related misuse and errors.

References

Akrich M (1995) Petite anthropologie du medicament [A little anthropology of drugs]. Techniques et Culture 25-26:129–157. Available from: https://halshs.archives-ouvertes.fr/halshs-00119484. Accessed Oct 2022

Akrich M (1996) Le médicament comme objet technique [Medicines as a technical object]. Revue Internationale de Psychopathologie 21:135–158. Available from: https://halshs.archives-ouvertes.fr/halshs-00081737. Accessed Feb 2021

Akrich M (1998) Les utilizateurs, acteurs de l'innovation [Users, actors of innovation]. Education Permanente 134:79–90. Available from: https://halshs.archives-ouvertes.fr/halshs-00082051. Accessed Oct 2022

Akrich M, Méadel C (2002) Prendre ses médicaments/prendre la parole: Les usages des médicaments par les patients dans les listes de discussion électroniques [Taking medication/speaking out: patient medication uses in electronic discussion lists]. Sciences Sociales et Santé 20(1):89–116. https://doi.org/10.3406/sosan.2002.1546

Anceschi G, Bucchetti V (1998) Il packaging alimentare [Food packaging]. In: Capatti A, De Bernardi A, Varni A (eds) Storia d'Italia. Annali 13. L'alimentazione [History of Italy. Annals 13. Food]. Einaudi, Torino, pp 845–886

Anderson S (ed) (2005) Making medicines: a brief history of pharmacy and pharmaceuticals. Pharmaceutical Press, London

Appadurai A (ed) (1986) The social life of things: commodities in cultural perspective. Cambridge University Press, Cambridge

Barthes R (1966) 1985. Sémantique de l'objet [Sematics of the object]. L'aventure sémiologique. Seuil, Paris

Barthes R (1982) Il grado zero della scrittura [The zero degree of writing]. Torino, Einaudi. [Or. Ed. Le Degré zéro de l'écriture (1953). Èditions du Seuil, Paris]

Bertola P, Manzini E (2004) Design Multiverso. Appunti di fenomenologia del design. Edizioni Polidesign, Milano

Bordieu P (2003) Per una teoria della pratica. Con Tre studi di etnologia cabila. Raffaello Cortina, Milano. (Esquisse d'une théorie de la pratique précédé de Trois études d'ethnologie kabyle (1972) [For a theory of practice. With three studies in kabyle ethnology]. Editions du Seuil, Paris)

Borgna P (2005) Sociologia del corpo [Sociology of the body]. Laterza, Bari

Brown B (2001) Thing theory. Critical Inquiry 28(1) Things (Autumn, 2001):1–22

Bürdek BE (2008) Design. Storia, teoria e pratica del design del prodotto. Gangemi Editore, Napoli

Caprino L (2011) Il farmaco, 7000 anni di storia: Dal rimedio empirico alle biotecnologie. Armando Editore, Roma

Chamberlain P, Craig C (2017) Design for health: reflections from the editors. Des Health 1(1):3–7. https://doi.org/10.1080/24735132.2017.1296273

Chast F (1995) Histoire contemporaine des medicaments [Contemporary history of drugs]. La découverte, Paris

Conrad P (1992) Medicalisation and social control. Annu Rev Sociol 18:209–232

Conrad P (2007) The medicalization of society: on the transformation of human conditions into treatable disorders. Johns Hopkins University Press, Baltimore

Cortellazzo M, Zolli P (eds) (1999) Disporre/Dispositivo [Setting/Device]. In Il Nuovo Etimologico Zanichelli. Zanichelli, Bologna, pp 479–480

Costa A (2016) Oggetti, cose, dispositivi: linee di una ricerca [Objects, things, devices: lines of research]. In: Proverbio P, Riccini R (eds) Design e immaginario. Oggetti, immagini e visioni fra rappresentazione e progetto [Design and imagination. Objects, images and visions between representation and design]. Il Poligrafo, Venezia, pp 51–82

Craig C, Chamberlain P (2017) Behaviours: design and behaviour change in health. In: Tsekleves E, Cooper R (eds) Design for health. Routledge, New York, pp 191–203

de la Fuente J, Gustafson S, Twomey C, Bix L (2015a) An affordance-based methodology for package design. Packag Technol Sci 28:157–171

de la Fuente J, Tachibana D, Leemon K, Liu C, Twomey C, Roy S, Bix L, Bisheff S (2015b) Measuring the effect of affordances on a crash cart medicine packaging. In: 27th IAPRI symposium on packaging. Available from https://digitalcommons.calpoly.edu/cgi/viewcontent.cgi?article=1052&context=grc_fac. Accessed Sept 2020

de Seta C (1980) Oggetto. In: Enciclopedia, vol IX. Einaudi, Torino, pp 997–1019

Deni M (2002) Les objets factitifs. In: Fontanille J, Zinna A (eds) Les objets au quotidien [Everyday objects]. Pulim, Limoges, pp 78–96

Desclaux A, Lévy JJ (2003) Présentation: Culture et médicaments. Ancien objet ou nouveau courant en anthropologie médicale? [Presentation: culture and drugs. Old object or new trend in medical anthropology?]. Anthropologie et Sociétés 27(2):5–21. https://doi.org/10.7202/007443ar

Douglas M, Isherwood B (1979) The world of goods. Basic Books, New York

European Commission (2018) The 2018 ageing report: economic and budgetary projections for the EU member states (2016–2070). Institutional paper no. 79. Publications Office of the European Union, Luxembourg

European Medicine Agency–Pharmacovigilance Risk Assessment Committee (2015a) Good practice guide on recording, coding, reporting and assessment of medication errors

(EMA/762563/2014). Available from: https://www.ema.europa.eu/en/documents/regulatory-procedural-guideline/good-practice-guide-recording-coding-reporting-assessment-medication-errors_en.pdf. Accessed Sept 2020

European Medicine Agency–Pharmacovigilance Risk Assessment Committee (2015b) Good practice guide on risk minimisation and prevention of medication errors (EMA/606103/2014). Available from: https://www.ema.europa.eu/en/documents/regulatory-procedural-guideline/good-practice-guide-risk-minimisation-prevention-medication-errors_en.pdf. Accessed Sept 2020

Fainzang S (2001) Médicaments et société. Le patient, le médecin et l'ordonnance [Medicines and society. The patient, the doctor and the prescription]. Presses Universitaires de France, Paris

Fainzang S (2003) Les médicaments dans l'espace privé. Gestion individuelle ou collective [Medicines in the private area. Individual or collective management]. Anthropologie et Sociétés 27(2):139–154. https://doi.org/10.7202/007450ar

Fainzang S (2005) Société–Le charme discret des medicaments [The discreet charm of drugs]. LeDevoir, 20 Aout 2005. Available from: https://www.ledevoir.com/societe/sante/88432/societe-le-charme-discret-des-medicaments. Accessed Nov 2022

Fainzang S (2012) L'automédication ou les mirages de l'autonomie [Self-medication or the mirages of autonomy]. Presses Universitaires de France, Paris

Ferrarotti F (1986) Prefazione. In: Maffesoli M (ed) La conoscenza ordinaria. Compendio di sociologia comprendente. [Ordinary knowledge. Compendium of sociology including]. Cappelli Editore, Bologna

Fiorani E (2001) Il mondo degli oggetti [The object world]. Lupetti, Milano

Flusser V (1999) A philosophy of design. Reaktion Books Ltd, London. Tr. it (2003) Filosofia del design. Bruno Mondadori, Milano

Fox NJ, Ward KJ (2008) Pharma in the bedroom … and the kitchen …. The pharmaceuticalisation of daily life. Sociol Health Illn 30(6):856–868. https://doi.org/10.1111/j.1467-9566.2008.01114.x

Gabe J, Williams S, Martin P, Coveney C (2015) Pharmaceuticals and society: power, promises and prospects. Soc Sci Med 131:193–198. https://doi.org/10.1016/j.socscimed.2015.02.031

Gibson JJ (1977) The theory of affordances. In: Shaw R, Bransford J (eds) Perceiving, acting, and knowing: toward an ecological psychology. Erlbaum Associates, Hillsdale, pp 67–82

Gras A (1993) Grandeur et dépendance. Presses Universitaires de France, Paris. Tr. it. (1997) Nella rete tecnologica. La società dei macrosistemi. Utet, Torino

Groeneveld B, Dekkers T, Boon B, D'Olivo P (2018) Challenges for design researchers in healthcare. Des Health 2(2):305–326. https://doi.org/10.1080/24735132.2018.1541699

Jones P (2013) Design for care: innovating healthcare experience. Rosenfeld Media, New York

Kleinman A (1980) Patients and healers in the context of culture. University of California Press, Berkeley

Leroi-Gourhan A (1943) L'homme et la matière [Man and matter]. Albin Michel, Paris

Leroi-Gourhan A (1945) Milieu et techniques [Environment and Techniques]. Albin Michel, Paris

Lie M, Sørensen K (1996) Making technology our own, domesticating technology into everyday life. Scandinavian University Press, Oslo

Lumme-Sandt K, Virtane P (2002) Older people in the field of medication. Sociol Health Illn 24(3):285–304. Available from: https://onlinelibrary.wiley.com/doi/pdf/10.1111/1467-9566.00295. Accessed Oct 2022

Mauss M (2017) Le tecniche del corpo. Edizioni ETS, Pisa. (Les Techniques du Corps) (1936) Journal de psychologie, XXXII (3-4)

Merriam-Webster (2022a). Everyday. Retrieved December 2, 2022, from https://www.merriam-webster.com/dictionary/everyday

Merriam-Webster (2022b). Object. Retrieved December 2, 2022, from https://www.merriam-webster.com/dictionary/object

Merriam-Webster (2022c). Thing. Retrieved November 30, 2022, from https://www.merriam-webster.com/dictionary/thing

Miller D (1987) Material culture and mass consumption. Blackwell, Oxford

Ministero della salute—Direzione generale della programmazione sanitaria—Ufficio III (October 2019) Raccomandazione n. 19—Raccomandazione per la manipolazione delle forme farmaceutiche orali solide [Recommendation 19—Recommendation for the handling of solid oral pharmaceutical forms]. Available from https://www.salute.gov.it/imgs/C_17_pubblicazioni_2892_allegato.pdf

Moles A (1969) Objet et communication, "Les objets" [Objects]. Communications, no. 13. Editions du Seuil, Paris. Accessible from https://www.persee.fr/issue/comm_0588-8018_1969_num_13_1

Molotch H (2003) Where stuff comes from. How toasters, toilets, cars, computers, and many other things come to be as they are. Routledge

Nacci M (ed) (1998) Oggetti d'uso quotidiano [Daily use objects]. Marsilio, Venezia

Norman DA (1997) La caffettiera del masochista. Psicopatologia degli oggetti quotidiani. Giunti, Firenze. [The psychology of everyday things (1988). Basic Books, New York]

Norman D (2013) The design of everyday things: revised and expanded edition. Basic books, New York

Nusem E, Straker K, Wrigley C (2020) Design innovation for health and medicine. Palgrave Macmillan, Singapore

Overgaard ABA, Møller-Sonnergaard J, Christrup LL, Højsted J, Hansen R, Sonnergaard J (2001) Patients' evaluation of shape, size and colour of solid dosage forms. Pharm World Sci 23(5):185–188. https://doi.org/10.1023/A:1012050931018

Pareek V, Kunteta A (2014) Pharmaceutical packaging: current trends and future. Int J Pharm Pharm Sci 6(6):480–485. Available from https://innovareacademics.in/journal/ijpps/Vol6Issue6/9730.pdf. Accessed Sept 2019

Penati A (2016) Forma degli oggetti [Object shape]. In: Pizzocaro S (ed) Artefatti concreti. Temi di fondamento per il design di prodotto [Concrete artefacts. Foundation themes for product design]. Edizioni Unicopli, Milano

Penati A, Pizzocaro S, Tonelli MC, Standoli C, Iannilli V, Bucchetti V, Rebaglio A, Riccò D, Andreoni G, Caratti E, Tolino U (2020) Scienza al quotidiano: farmaci come oggetti/Daily science: pharmaceuticals as objects. DIID Disegno Industriale/Industrial Design 69:120–127

Penati A, Pizzocaro S, Standoli CE, Iannilli VM (2021). The shape of drugs: a matter of human-centred design. Design culture(s) conference, cumulus conference proceedings, Rome, pp 1364–1375

Pizzocaro S, Penati A (2021) The in-home use of medications: in pursuit of design-driven knowledge. Home Cultures 17(3):153–171. https://doi.org/10.1080/17406315.2021.1916225

Polanyi M (1966) The tacit dimension. The University of Chicago Press, Chicago. [trad. it. La conoscenza inespressa (1979). Armando Editore, Roma]

Reynolds Whyte S, van der Geest S, Hardon A (2002) Social lives of medicines. Cambridge University Press, Cambridge

Rodgers P et al (2019) The Lancaster care charter. Des Issues 35(1):73–77. https://doi.org/10.1162/desi_a_00522

Sennet R (2008) The craftsman. Yale University Press, New Haven/London. [trad. it. L'uomo artigiano (2009). Feltrinelli, Milano]

Simondon G (1958) Du mode d'existence des objets techniques [On the mode of existence of technical objects]. Aubier, Paris

Tsekleves E, Cooper R (eds) (2016) Design for health. Routledge, London

van der Geest S, Whyte SR (1989) The charm of medicines: metaphors and metonyms. Med Anthropol Q 3(4):345–367

van der Geest S, Reynolds Whyte S, Hardon A (1996) The anthropology of pharmaceuticals: a biographical approach. Annu Rev Anthropol 25:153–178. https://doi.org/10.1146/annurev.anthro.25.1.153. Accessed Nov 2022

van Onck A (1994) Design. Il senso delle forme dei prodotti. Lupetti, Milano

Vicarelli G (2009) La sociologie de la santé et de la médecine en Italie: Une perspective historique et relationnelle. Médicaments et société: Entre automédication et dépendance. Revue Sociologie Santé 30:423–440

Williams SJ, Martin P, Gabe J (2011) The pharmaceuticalisation of society? A framework for analysis. Sociology of Health and Illness 33(5):710–725. https://doi.org/10.1111/j.1467-9566.2011.01320.x

World Health Organization (2003) Adherence to long-term therapies: evidence for action. https://www.who.int/chp/knowledge/publications/adherence_report/en/

Wyatt S, Henwood F, Hart A, Platzer H (2004) L'extension des territoires du patient. Internet et santé au quotidian. [The extension of the patient's territories. Internet and daily health]. Sciences Sociales et Santé 22(1):45–68. https://doi.org/10.3406/sosan.2004.1608

Open Access This chapter is licensed under the terms of the Creative Commons Attribution 4.0 International License (http://creativecommons.org/licenses/by/4.0/), which permits use, sharing, adaptation, distribution and reproduction in any medium or format, as long as you give appropriate credit to the original author(s) and the source, provide a link to the Creative Commons license and indicate if changes were made.

The images or other third party material in this chapter are included in the chapter's Creative Commons license, unless indicated otherwise in a credit line to the material. If material is not included in the chapter's Creative Commons license and your intended use is not permitted by statutory regulation or exceeds the permitted use, you will need to obtain permission directly from the copyright holder.

Chapter 13
The In-Home Place of Medications: Perspectives of Domestication

Silvia Pizzocaro

Abstract Starting from the relevance of observing people's behaviors with common types of medicines, this contribution is intended to pinpoint some notes that revolve around in-home medication. What is proposed is a reflection on medicines as tangible, concrete devices that materialize the meaning of medication in the prosaic in-home dimension. While literature mainly intends the domestication of pharmaceutical consumption as either the pharmaceuticalization of daily life, or the domestication of usage, here we will use the term 'domestication' to mean the latter only. This perspective tries to highlight some traits of the use of medicines within the in-home spaces of everyday life, among ordinary things. It also looks at people's real behaviors with medications to let habits, routines, and even rituals emerge. Against the background of these study interests, the consideration is posed that a substantial percentage of medication non-compliances, inconveniences, even errors and/or difficulties may be caused not only by lack of info-communicative aspects, but by the deficiencies of still ameliorable user-centered qualities of medicines themselves. These are deficiencies that may variably concern the usable properties of medicines as commodities (shape, size, proportions, annex co-products for intake or dosage) and the traits of that peculiar relation between users and medication use which may disorient the user, favoring or—conversely—hindering access or correct use, reducing but also potentially inducing possible errors. The framework within which in-home medication is approached here advocates the relevance of those disciplinary contributions stemming from studies in product design, product affordance, product-user cognition and interaction, accessibility, and usability design. Meant as a theoretical contribution, this reflection partly reviews some consolidated studies conducted in the anthropology of pharmaceuticals, while integrating inputs derived from person-centered care literature.

S. Pizzocaro (✉)
Department of Design, Politecnico di Milano, Milan, Italy
e-mail: silvia.pizzocaro@polimi.it

© The Author(s) 2025
A. V. Penati (ed.), *In-Home Medication*, Research for Development,
https://doi.org/10.1007/978-3-031-53294-8_13

13.1 Introduction

Medicines may be defined as 'things' that allow therapy (van der Geest and Whyte 1989), 'medicinal forms' saturated with meaning (Akrich 1995; Desclaux and Lévy 2003) and 'technical objects' (Akrich 1996).

Medicines are substances with materiality, their 'thinginess' is a property that has been of great analytical importance for anthropology: they objectify meanings, they are commodities that can be exchanged between social actors (Reynolds Whyte et al. 2002, p. 5).

By 'medicinal forms' Akrich (1996) means the material characteristics of the product with which the user is dealing, including the characteristics of the devices as packaging, dose delivery system, measuring instrument. Surveys of patient preferences have proved to focus primarily on the galenic form, i.e. the form of the drug itself, and they may produce results that translate into statements that patients find the tablets difficult to swallow, that men may prefer capsules while women have a strong taste for dragees, and that employees and workers may be in favor of liquid forms (Richard and de Lapouge 1988; Akrich 1996).

Considering medicines as 'technical objects' therefore implies trying to highlight the links that exist between their material characteristics and the associated forms of use. Such a consideration has produced insufficient exploration, as if between the marketing of a new molecule and the biochemical action of this molecule in the patient's body, all the stages would be transparent (Akrich 1996, p. 135).

The everyday in-home management of medicines involves procedures, operational schemes, and technical and manipulative abilities. The adjective 'everyday' emphasizes the nature of things that are encountered or used routinely or typically. Like any object, everyday objects primarily signify their function but secondly can also refer to other meanings, i.e. assume symbolic values of a social and cultural nature (Barthes 1966, 1985). Medicines as 'things' imply an implicit knowledge of organizational, procedural, and lexical models that underlie the repertoires of operations falling within the routine automatisms. Therefore, any drug efficacy depends either on its scientific principle and the refined, sophisticated, hyper-technological, or conversely, on the completely prosaic techniques of its consumption on behalf of end users.

At the core of this contribution, we place the act of pharmacological therapy at home as the primary care modality that the patient can access. We also assume that medicines are the hard core of therapy and that they are set apart from other forms of healing.

13.2 A Prosaic Perspective on In-Home Medication

Medication intake is by far a most common medical action. For the purpose of this chapter's commentary, we started by considering the *naif* scenario of the most ordinary questions revolving around medication intake at home: where to keep medicines handy? How and where to organize the home pharmaceutical dispensary? Where to store the residual drug fragments if a portion of the drug is prescribed? Where to expose—or conversely to hide –, to protect, and to preserve medicines?

These questions outline very common routines almost everyone has experienced when managing medication at home. Fainzang (2003) has reported that "Observing the use of drugs in the context of the home makes it possible to identify differences that are not attributable solely to therapeutic reasons (according to which a given use would depend on a given condition) nor solely to individual variations likely to explain the random and accidental nature of these uses. […] far from being fortuitous, these uses, and the behaviors relating to the storage and consumption of drugs, are the subject of regularities, related to cultural logics" (p. 139).

As we are interested in people's experiences, we will mainly refer to the expression 'medication use' or 'medication management' instead of 'medication adherence, patient compliance, and drug administration', which are the terms that the clinical literature tends to use. This is also motivated by the fact that, as observed by Hirsch et al. (2000, p. 80), 'adherence' and 'compliance' speak to a clinician's perspective of keeping to intake schedules, and the term 'drugs' emphasizes prescription medication."

To address patients' habits and behaviors better (ordinary users, older adults, chronic users, and vulnerable people, especially), we chose to identify more closely with the people themselves, who are more likely to refer to drugs as 'medicines' and 'medications', and to adherence as 'medication management' or 'use of medicines'. More notably, the word 'medicine' usually refers to the finished product, ready for the patient to take (Anderson 2005, p. 5). This motivates our preference against the words 'pharmaceutical', 'drug', 'therapeutic drug', or 'medicinal product'. Such an interest in 'domesticated' medication is also motivated by the significant current shift in paradigms of health, with the reductionist view of health that focuses on illness and treatment being replaced by maintaining well-being, equipping individuals with the knowledge and tools to live well, and by fostering models of health increasingly focused on self-management (Chamberlain and Craig 2017, p. 4). While the growing consumption of pharmaceutical products has fueled much research on their side effects, interactions, and the factors that may alter drug therapeutic properties (European Medicine Agency 2015a, b), such investigations, conducted primarily in the medical-epidemiological field, still offer considerable margins of exploration for patient misbehavior with medicines at home. Users' errors usually range from abuse to forgetfulness, non-compliance with deadlines and methods of handling, incorrect storage methods, dosage mistakes, and incorrect use interpretations. Notwithstanding the fact that errors may occur in any phase of medication management, the most critical moment in most treatment processes is precisely that of drug

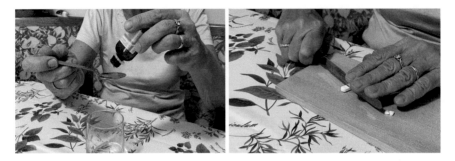

Fig. 13.1 A critical moment in most treatment processes can be precisely that of drug dosing and intake

intake. It is at this step that the patient—either vulnerable or not—must cope with a whole set of procedures; that is, finding where the medication is stored in the home, recognizing the right medication, unboxing medication, reading, and interpreting leaflets or prescriptions, dosing it, performing the intake, and storing the medication properly for successive intakes (Fig. 13.1).

Users' perceptual, physical, or cognitive difficulties in taking medicines can hinder or reduce access to these procedures (Rodriguez-Falcon and Yoxall 2011), by causing the patient not to take in-home medication correctly or to discontinue therapy altogether.

From a clinical point of view, patients as users are the targets medicines aim for. From a general user-centered perspective, users (either patients or not, as it is the case of caregivers) may be the agents of compliance of a critical percentage of non-compliances, inconveniences, user-related errors and/or difficulties or discomfort in medication. Users' perceptual, physical, or cognitive difficulties—especially if related to conditions of vulnerability—can hinder or reduce access to self-medication procedures. The efficacy of medicines may thus be conditioned by the user's executive capacity of care and medication management, along with subjective skills and abilities.

13.3 The Domestication of Medication: The Home Dispensary

While literature mainly intends the domestication of pharmaceutical consumption as the pharmaceuticalization of daily life, implying both the application of pharmaceuticals to normalise specific lifestyle-related activities and the domestication of usage (Fox and Ward 2008), here we will use the term 'domestication' to mean the latter only.

Regardless of any specific category of expected medication users we may consider, any in-home healthcare activity shatters the integrity of the individual,

13 The In-Home Place of Medications: Perspectives of Domestication

familiar, and domestic space. Any treatment activity and its *paraphernalia* tend to adapt to the pre-existing home environment that was not initially designed for that purpose. Medication procedures usually find their room at home according to individual cognitive and sensory patterns. These usually assign a precise location to things and processes that follow people's functional, symbolic, and even moral motivations (Fig. 13.2).

Palen and Aaløkke (2006) remind us that homes are special environments, "The home is its own institution that operates under rules and expectations for privacy, communication, conflict and so on […]. Homes are places where any number of activities take place by different actors throughout the day, from meal preparation, to laundry, to entertainment, childcare, emotional connection and so on" (p. 80). Moving from the relationships that a user may establish with home places during a treatment—here referring largely to Fainzang (2001, 2003, 2005, 2006, 2012), Akrich (1995, 1996) and Akrich and Méadel's (2002) extensive studies—we will limit our attention to some common behaviors and mindsets revolving mainly around the home pharmaceutical dispensary.

The quantity of medicines in the home and their pervasive presence suggest that we should look first at the domestic pharmacy's composition and arrangement. The way in which the home dispensary is set up and placed can reveal recurring patterns. As in Fainzang (2003, p. 145), once the medication has been purchased, it is stored in various places following mechanisms that do not necessarily reveal a utilitarian rationale (Fig. 13.3).

Some individuals have a drawer for medicines, or even multiple drawers for different family members' medication. The medicines may also be placed together randomly, without any specific pharmacological logic. In general, medical storage locations include drawers, bathroom cabinets, cupboard shelves, or even study drawers, where pharmaceuticals may be stored in an archive or among collections of important documents (Fainzang 2003, p. 146). However, a specific logic of organization can be expressed in the separation between medicines in use during ongoing therapies and backup medications (unused medicine, remains and leftovers of previous treatments, medications purchased in anticipation). The latter sometimes are kept in containers, cabinets, and on shelves located in auxiliary or marginal

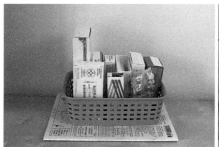 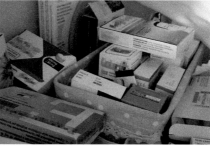

Fig. 13.2 The quantity and variety of medicines in the home motivate the observation of what can be called the home dispensary

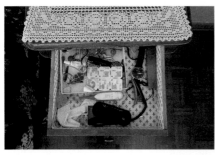
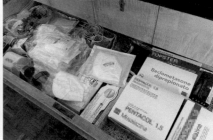

Fig. 13.3 A drawer for medicines may be arranged without any specific logic

Fig. 13.4 Medicines may be placed together randomly on shelves, tables, bedside tables, and stored in cabinets, drawers, without any specific pharmacological logic

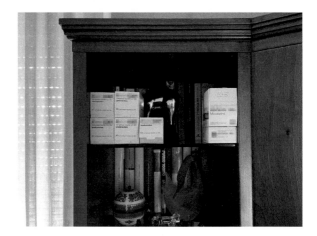

spaces outside the domestic spaces used most. This peripheral spatial location denotes an auxiliary function, identifiable by the category 'it may be useful, sooner or later'. As people often find it difficult to discard these 'remainders', they often expire.

Unlike occasional medicines, those that indicate the relevance of an ongoing therapy can be accommodated in the kitchen (on a shelf, the buffet, or tabletop), in the dining room, in the bedroom (on or in the bedside table), regardless of any link to the time at which the medication needs to be taken (Fainzang 2003, p. 146).

If the family includes several individuals, each may be assigned a different place for their own medicine. If medications are located according to the specialty of their pharmacological principle this may correspond to a more advanced rationale of organization. Finally, the place where a medicine is located by its user may also certainly correspond to its relevance, meaning it has to be ready for use (Fig. 13.4).

13.4 The Kitchen and the Temporal Coincidence with Meals

The question of medication pervasiveness in the home, as well as of their potential use and intake errors, can be addressed by treating medicines as concrete objects that—although in the extraordinary state of therapy—are integrated into the home's private space and temporality, where they serve as vehicles of material effectiveness that address the patient's body.

The fact that medications can occupy a significant presence in the kitchen or dining room leads to remarks on the functional and symbolic nature of the place where medicines are stored (Fig. 13.5—left). The temporal coincidence of taking medicines with meals obviously produces an associative effect and serves as a memory aid. Medicine in full view on the kitchen table, or even next to the dining seat (Palen and Aaløkke 2006, p. 84), indicates the importance of taking that specific medication; furthermore, it reduces the risk of forgetting to take the medication and ensures to some extent that the medicine will be taken as prescribed. At the same time, the kitchen plays the role of a priority social space in which friends are hosted and family members gather. It is the place where other family members, either residents or visitors, can provide informal visual supervision to ensure that the patient is managing his/her treatment (Fainzang 2003, p. 148). Accordingly, placing medicines in the kitchen allows for the active exercise of the family's control and assistance.

Of course, the choice of the kitchen as an elective domestic dispensary also highlights the association between medication, especially if taken by mouth, diet, and nutrition: "Medications have a special status that both brings them closer to and distances them from other products absorbed by the body, and therefore from food" (Fainzang 2003, p. 148). In the kitchen scenario, some specialized pharmaceuticals even tend to hide among foods: this certainly is the case with syrups, food supplements, and medicines that need to be refrigerated (Fig. 13.5—right). Such a

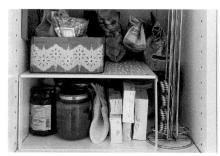 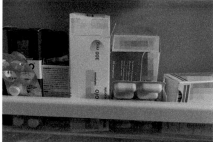

Fig. 13.5 Some pharmaceuticals are often stored among food, as it is the case with syrups, food supplements, and medicines that need to be refrigerated

dissimulation, which on the one hand domesticates pharmaceuticals by classifying them among foods or household items, and thus reduces their sense of extraneousness, on the other leads to potential confusion that can generate misunderstandings and intake errors.

Fainzang (2003) suggested the French, untranslatable neologism *médicaliments*, so to designate those real pharmaceutical specialties for therapeutic purposes whose sometimes casual use reveals the food, sometimes even confectionery, dimension which is conferred, "whose ambivalence is entirely contained in the double motivation of their consumption (medical and gustatory)" (p. 148).

13.5 Where the Sense of Privacy Prevails

Other types of medicines related to the intimate sphere of the body, but dissociated from nutrition, may be kept elsewhere even if they are to be taken at mealtimes. Thus, people tend to place some of their medicines in the kitchen and others in the privacy of their room, or in the bathroom (Fig. 13.6), according to a logic of separation that associates the medication with the body part in need of treatment.

Such a separation can defy any functional logic and responds instead to the constraints the individual's sense of privacy dictate (Fig. 13.7). In fact, the medicine may represent and identify with the organ of the body that receives the pharmacological treatment (Fainzang 2003, p. 150). Thus, a remedy for digestion or blood pressure may be visible on a kitchen shelf, but the anxiolytic, anti-depressant, or medicine related to gynecological or andrological issues will be placed in the bedroom, perhaps in the drawer of the bedside table or in a bathroom cabinet.

Furthermore, all medicines that pertain to private sphere are often found in a personal drawer in the bathroom or bedroom, proving that the perception of the body and women or men's sense of intimacy—the former in particular—affect the

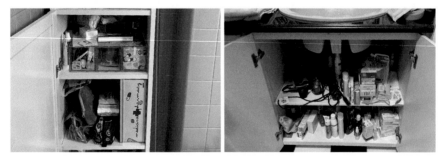

Fig. 13.6 A cabinet in the bathroom can usually perform the task of the in-home medicine dispensary

Fig. 13.7 People tend to place some of their medicines according to a logic of separation that can defy any functional logic and respond instead to an individual's imperfect rationales

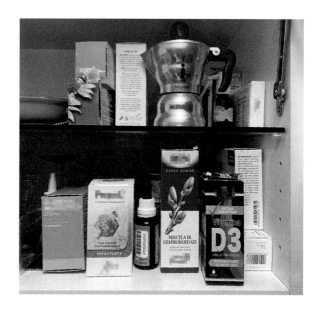

placement of the related medication, which are generally removed from both other family members and strangers' sight when related to individual sensitivities for hygiene, embarrassment, and modesty.

Therefore, the places reserved for medication in the domestic space obey no rational or functional criteria: not only are many medicines kept in the kitchen even if they are not taken with meals, but many medicines taken at meals are elsewhere, depending upon individuals' cognitive perceptions and sense of privacy.

Moreover, as investigated by Palen and Aaløkke (2006), home settings are far from perfect in the ways in which tasks like medication management are accomplished: "Homes and their supporting information systems are tailorable and open to improvement, enabling residents to iteratively perfect placement of medications and steps in their routines, to adapt to the inclusion of new medications, and to optimize the placement of some things vis-à-vis the optimization of others" (p. 85).

13.6 Medication Management as Habit, Routine, or Ritual?

If, on the one hand, people can access medications easily, patients may on the other hand, frequently encounter difficulties in their management. Hundreds of studies have been published about compliance in taking medication and nearly all of them view compliance from a medico-centric perspective (Ryan 1999; van der Geest et al. 1996), along with the consideration of noncompliance as the act of not following professional instructions.

Besides that, there is evidence that noncompliance needs to be further studied from the patient's point of view (Conrad 1985). As Lumme-Sandt and Virtane have observed, "The role of users in the field of medication is often overlooked and ignored, and users themselves tend to be perceived as objects rather than subjects" (Lumme-Sandt and Virtane 2002, p. 299). Conversely, making medication management more sympathetic to patients' needs, incorporating medication into the different in-home contexts, along with respecting patients' lifestyles, habits, and ways of doing things, may highlight all of the actions, knowledge, and tricks that accompany taking new medication. It can also be possible to reconsider them with all of the habits replacing them over time, when the care operations become part of a *routine* (Penati et al. 2020, p. 124). By routine we mainly refer to "sequences of action [that] articulate the spatial and temporal distribution of information around the home" (Crabtree and Rodden 2004, p. 209). Home routines may also help people encode and conceptualize information about their self-medication. As Palen and Aaløkke (2006, p. 84) remind, routines in medication management are usually associated with other activities, including eating meals, bedtimes and naptimes. Routines are also "the means by which people recall or at least *infer* that they have taken their medications. A person might infer—correctly or incorrectly—that if she executed her normal morning routine, for example, then she probably took her medication" (Palen and Aaløkke 2006, p. 85). Moreover, "people manage their medications—with only partial information about what the medication is—through a set of personalized spatio-temporal arrangements and *routines* that they devise in their homes. These physical arrangements and *routines* provide a sense, structure, and rhythm to intake even when people know very little about the medication itself" (Palen and Aaløkke 2006, p. 79). In turn, habits are a constituent part of domesticity. This is the prerogative that, starting with the concept of *habitus* (Bourdieu 1979), injects our actions into a system of perceptual, ethical or aesthetic ways of thinking and actions acquired over time. Habits are an effect of gradual learning of patterns of behavior and associations between the task or its features and the location. To be turned into a habit, a task should be associated with an existing routine task and it also needs to be repeated enough times to become a routine behavior (Stawarz et al. 2014, p. 2270).

To try to hold on a distinct meaning for the two terms habit and routine, here we will simply adopt the sense that "Although routines have a habitual element, not all habits are routines" (Clark 2000, p. 127S). Moreover, "Habits are the relatively automatic things a person thinks or does repeatedly. Routines, in contrast, are a type of higher-order habit that involves sequencing and combining processes, procedures, steps, or occupations. Routines specify what a person will do and in what order and therefore constitute a mechanism for achieving given outcomes and an orderly life" (Clark 2000, p. 128S).

Everyday healthcare habits involve procedures, operational schemes, and technical and manipulative abilities. They refer to an implicit knowledge of organizational, procedural, and lexical models that underlie the repertoires of operations falling within the *routine* automatisms.

However, also the concept of daily ritual (Crespo et al. 2013) may be included in our perspective. Clark (2000) recalls that "Words like *procedure, ritual, ceremony, rite,* and *protocol* typically denote social processes that possess routine" (p. 127S). The strict sense of ritual refers to the established form for a ceremony, and specifically the order of words prescribed for a religious ceremony; or a ritual observance; a ceremonial act or action; an act or series of acts regularly repeated in a set precise manner (Merriam-Webster 2022). The etymology of 'ritual' includes pertaining to or consisting of a rite or rites, from French *ritual* or directly from Latin *ritualis*, 'relating to (religious) rites', derived from *ritus*, 'religious observance or ceremony, custom, usage'. Ritual is something done as or in the manner of a rite. A ritual is a set of actions, often thought to have symbolic value, the performance of which is usually (but not exclusively) prescribed by a religion or by the traditions of a community by religious or political laws because of the expected efficacy of those actions. A ritual may be performed regularly, or on specific occasions, or at discretion. It may be performed by a single individual, group, the entire community; either in public, in private, or before specific people.

In psychology a ritual is a form of compulsion involving a rigid or stereotyped act that is carried out repeatedly and is based on idiosyncratic rules that do not have a rational basis (e.g., having to perform a task in a certain way) (APA Dictionary of Psychology 2022). Rituals may be performed to reduce distress and anxiety. More generally, a ritual may be any habit or custom that is performed routinely. Rituals may be intended as a sequence of symbolic actions often characterised by formality and repetition that lacks direct instrumental purpose.

The attitude that people may show towards chronic medication intake—although repetitiveness and automatisms seem to lead the treatment practices back to recurrent routines—can show the traits of what is out of the ordinary, of what is more significant than simple replication, making a rite out of a routine (Denham 2003).

If routines are operationalized as behaviors linked to daily or regular activities pertinent to health, rituals are better described in terms of celebrations, traditions, religious observances, with their symbolic paraphernalia (Fig. 13.8). This may allow very intimate or family cultural bounds, traditions, values, and memories to emerge.

This may be the case "when the daily dose of pills is contained in a box that bears a sacred image on the lid; or the embroidered delicate white placemat used as the surface on which the medicines have to be placed (even in case of mobility occurrence); or, again, the unpaired cup, a residue from the wedding gift service which, precisely because of its memorable character, is chosen as a container for daily therapy and also a *memento* of an important practice that must not be forgotten.

Fig. 13.8 Any treatment activity and its paraphernalia tend to adapt to the pre-existing home environment

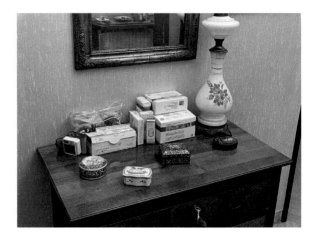

These are mere examples of routines charged with symbolical meaning to such an extent they are closer to an almost magical or religious ritual" (Pizzocaro and Penati 2021, p. 158).

13.7 People Imperfect Rationales: Fast and Frugal

Actions such as rituality, personalization, inaccuracy, hastiness, postponement, do-it-yourself, or tricks solvers, tend to coexist with formalized medication procedures. Such tailored adjustments may also become accepted by individuals to such an extent as to make discretionary medication sometimes "imperfectly perfect" (Palen and Aaløkke 2006, p. 85). Simplified or adjusted procedures—sometimes expressed as "fast and frugal strategies" (Arfini 2016, p. 44)—allow people to reduce individual cognitive effort and relieve the feeling of exhaustion that often accompanies chronic or recurrent self-care.

A vast body of medical literature (among the many, we restricted our investigation to Golant 1984; Martin et al. 1990; Martin 2000; Devlin and Arneill 2003; Mason 2006; Bates 2018) has extensively discussed care in dedicated environments, hospitals in particular, where therapies are codified, regulated, and processed through protocols. Within such contexts, errors are detectable *via* the identified deviations from the foreseen formal procedures: it is thus easier to trace who, where, how, and why an error has occurred (Aronson 2009). Conversely, for the purposes of our attention accorded to in-home care routines, we are strictly referring to in-home self-medication, where no protocols to detect errors are usually developed (Fig. 13.9).

Approaching the matter of in-home medication goes with the close-up consideration of self-medication errors *per se*. Multiple factors leading to poor medication

Fig. 13.9 The dissimulation of pharmaceuticals among household items may lead to potential confusion, misunderstandings, and errors

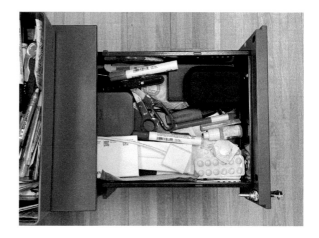

management are normally classified into five categories based on the following factors: socioeconomic, therapy, patient, condition, and health system/healthcare team (HCT) according to Brown and Bussell (2011). Seen from a clinical point of view, the specific patient-related factors usually include a lack of understanding of the disease (Ryan 1999), lack of involvement in the treatment decision-making process (Haynes et al. 2002), or suboptimal medical literacy. The context of self-medication errors is further conditioned by an expanding digital culture and the growth of do-it-yourself medication practices (Akrich and Méadel 2002; Fainzang 2003, 2012), along with the diffusion of several forms of non-conventional medicines that often lack either indication of dosage and leaflets that illustrate the medication's characteristics and use.

On 'self-medication' definition we remind that "Literally speaking, self-medication is the use of medicines based on one's own decision" (Fainzang 2013, p. 493). Moreover, Van der Geest et al. (1996) extremise that, so to imply that to some extent all medication is self-medication, as doctors who administer the medicines cannot be certain they are being taken as prescribed. More precisely, it could be considered that self-medication is the use of a medicine "on one's own initiative, without consulting a doctor for the problem in question, whether the medicine is already in one's possession or whether one procures it to this end" (Fainzang 2013, p. 494).

13.8 People Vulnerability at Home

Palen and Aaløkke (2006) extensively highlighted the management of medication as a prominent activity in the lives of older adults, as it requires a remarkable amount of attention to organize and take medicines. When a patient has to take as many as a dozen pills a day, while self-administering doses of other drugs, the management of medication becomes an all-consuming activity that can become central to a person's daily life (p. 82).

Therapy efficacy—especially in case of long, severe, or chronic therapies—is thus linked to the individual's executive capacity of care, organizing and managing medication, along with individual skills and abilities that, although considered naturally self-learned, indeed must be specifically acquired and refined as if they were effective "techniques of the body" (Mauss 1936). Moreover, it is becoming clearer and clearer that social, emotional, and environmental factors may play a significant role besides physical abilities, particularly in the elder-care experience (Lawton 1982; Lawton et al. 1982; Hirsch et al. 2000). A more extensive definition of care is often needed in the context of aging, exceeding the borders of merely physical conditions (Lorenzini and Olsson 2015, p. 5). Rather, eldercare may be more concerned with maintaining an individual's entire quality of life. As Sudbury-Riley (2014, p. 669) reminds, at least the three concepts of physical, psychological, and social aging are associated with aging itself. Physical aging is obviously about the changes that impact the body, while psychological aging relates to the feelings of physical vulnerability, along with sensations of uselessness, embarrassment, and frustration associated with a failure to carry out daily tasks.

Older adults' perceptions of their own abilities are often out of step with their actual capabilities. According to Hirsch et al. (2000, p. 3), "This can include an elder operating at a level below her capacities, causing her to be fearful of attempting relatively safe tasks. Conversely, the elder may overestimate her own ability, causing her to undertake risky tasks."

The sphere of in-home medication errors may depend highly on the older patient's specific characteristics. Such a sphere is even more relevant when it is expanded to include areas of discomfort, difficulty, embarrassment, and inconvenience, as well as information or support shortcomings, all of which may further affect patients' vulnerability (Brown et al. 2016; Fulop et al. 2010). Moreover, an older patient may often show an inability to codify and verbalize the characteristics of their discomfort or difficulty during treatment.

The performance of the older adult when interacting with the several interfaces along care (with solid, liquid or gaseous substances; drug shapes and colors; medication packaging; containers, blisters and dispensers; dosage tools), may be affected negatively by the decline in cognition and positively, instead, by *familiarity* with a product's features. In line with the above, Micocci and Spinelli (2018, p. 286), along with Hurtienne et al. (2015), point out a dilemma: "whether designers should pursue familiarity, as this enhances the prospects of adoption, or seek innovation through new products that break past molds".

13.9 Conclusions: From *Materia Medica* to Designed *Materia* for Person-Centered Care

While still lacking a robust formalization for our reflections, we have been inspired by the fully consolidated studies in a number of research traditions, especially in the social and anthropological fields (Kleinman 1980; Chast 1995; Akrich 1995, 1996, 1998; Akrich and Méadel 2002; Wyatt et al. 2004; Borgna 2005; Fainzang 2001, 2003, 2005, 2006, 2012).

At the same time, we have been guided by the robust thinking emerging from recent contributions assisting designers to leverage their resources and provided tangible guidelines for those seeking to practice design for health (Jones 2013; Tsekleves and Cooper 2016; Noël 2017; Craig 2017; Schrauwen et al. 2017; Groeneveld et al. 2018; Nusem et al. 2020).

In conclusion we limit ourselves to suggest some open trajectories for paths of enquiry, with the goal of sustaining the relevance of pursuing a design approach for in-home medication management. Being aware of the amount of complex factors invested in the design of pharmaceuticals (drug principles, regulations, stakeholders' involvement, healthcare policies, etc.), we are advocating no more than provisional wayfindings for orientation.

With regards to the problematic context emerging from literature reviews, we limit ourselves to emphasizing the significant role design may play in blending the specialized fields (at least) of product, communication, and experience design that revolve around in-home person-centered care. For Ekman et al. (2013) "Person-Centred Care is the antithesis of reductionistic biomedicine. It asserts that patients are persons and should not be reduced to their disease alone, but rather that their subjectivity and situation within a given environment, their strengths, their future plans and their rights, should be taken fully into account" (p. 134).

As the term "person-centered care" is used to refer to many different principles and activities, and there is no single unique definition of the concept[1] (The Health Foundation 2016, p. 6), we emphasize that if design for medicines is intended to be person-centered, what it may look like may depend on variable complexes of needs and circumstances, and "what is important to one person in their healthcare may be unnecessary, or even undesirable, to another. It may also change over time, as the individual's needs change" (The Health Foundation 2016, p. 6). However, affording people dignity, ensuring coordinated and personalized care, supporting people to

---

[1] As the concept of person-centered care is new and developing, "a range of other terms are also used to refer to similar principles and activities, including patient-centred care, personalisation, and relationship-centred care" (The Health Foundation 2016, p. 9).

recognize and develop their own strengths and abilities when managing in-home medication, are shared principles to start from.

The disciplines and cultures of design may contribute to an improvement of medications to resolve users' difficulties (Jones 2013; Spinelli 2015; Craig 2017; James and Olausson 2018; Spinelli et al. 2019; Karol and Smith 2019), especially when addressing shape recognition, product comprehension, and expected affordance (Norman 2013).

The final shape that medicines may take, although dependent on chemical-physical composition, provides—or better, should also provide—important information on the intake and use methods (Overgaard et al. 2001), especially when performed out of the assisted healthcare places. Furthermore, any medicine also needs to be exposed, stored, protected, and preserved. It requires the active principle be kept stable, the most suitable methods of intake be taken into account, the physical and perceptive difficulties of the user be fully considered. It should possess clear identity traits that would make it recognizable, usable, easy and ready for use.

In terms of a general scale for design strategies that addresses the in-home habits and experiences of self-medication, we hope to highlight the relevance of the exploration and experimentation with ameliorative, in progress design concepts that may be aligned with person-centered *imperfect* rationales.

An agenda of both explorable and viable directions may include either product design improvements that can intervene in the formal, functional, and affordance properties of medicines as objects, or in the integrated devices and auxiliary co-products that may accompany in-home self-care at large, aligned with solutions to ameliorate patients' self-management of medication at large. Without neglecting the almost unavoidable claim for safer, easier, and customizable design solutions to increase in-home medication affordance, what is further evoked is a deeper sensitivity for home spatial features, in-home temporal rhythms, and in-home people habits and rituals, as person-centered priorities to be translated and converted into more generalizable design concerns.

The wide diffusion and ubiquity of pharmacological treatments are partially characterized by the lack of an effectively advanced design-oriented perspective about medication-patient interactions: medicines, despite the scientific very advanced *status* of their pharmacological principle, still remain not necessarily specialized as designed objects (Penati et al. 2020, pp. 123–125). Further, they may remain only partially explored as products characterized by innovative usages driven by users (Spinelli 2015; Spinelli et al. 2019; Manganini 2022) and by the research of quality design standards (Di Carlo 2020), especially when their uptake is performed at home. Neglecting to fully investigate people's daily lives at home, with their fragilities and vulnerabilities, produces a lack of observation and poor knowledge about the nature of the inaccurate and approximate interactions frequently activated by medicines consumers, chronic in particular, when left alone to manage their in-home care.

References

Akrich M (1995) Petite anthropologie du medicament [A little anthropology of drugs]. Techniques et Culture 25-26:129–157. Available from: https://halshs.archives-ouvertes.fr/halshs-00119484. Accessed November 2022

Akrich M (1996) Le médicament comme objet technique [Medicines as a technical object]. Revue Internationale de Psychopathologie 21:135–158. Available from: https://halshs.archives-ouvertes.fr/halshs-00081737. Accessed November 2022

Akrich M (1998) Les utilizateurs, acteurs de l'innovation [Users, actors of innovation]. Education Permanente 134:79–90. Available from: https://halshs.archives-ouvertes.fr/halshs-00082051. Accessed November 2022

Akrich M, Méadel C (2002) Prendre ses médicaments/prendre la parole: Les usages des médicaments par les patients dans les listes de discussion électroniques [Taking medication/speaking out: patient medication uses in electronic discussion lists]. Sciences Sociales et Santé 20(1):89–116. https://doi.org/10.3406/sosan.2002.1546. Accessed November 2022

Anderson S (ed) (2005) Making medicines: a brief history of pharmacy and pharmaceuticals. Pharmaceutical Press, London

APA Dictionary of Psychology. Ritual. Available from https://dictionary.apa.org/ritual. Accessed December 2022

Arfini S (2016) Bolle epistemiche: Scienza e credenza [Epistemic bubbles: science and belief]. In: Magnani L (ed) Introduzione alla new logic. Logica, filosofia, cognizione. [Introduction to new logic. Logic, philosophy, cognition]. Il Melangolo, Genova, pp 43–78. Available from: https://www.researchgate.net/publication/283846599_Bolle_epistemiche_scienza_e_credenza. Accessed November 2022

Aronson JK (2009a) Medication errors: what they are, how they happen and how to avoid them. QJM: Month J Assoc Physic 102(8):513–521. https://doi.org/10.1093/qjmed/hcp052

Barthes R (1966) Sémantique de l'objet [Semantics of the object]. In: Nardi P (ed) Lecture given in September 1964 at the CINI foundation, in Venice, at the conference on art and culture in contemporary civilization. Published in the volume Arte e Cultura nella civiltà contemporanea, [Art and culture in contemporary civilization]. Sansoni, Firenze

Barthes R (1985) L'aventure sémiologique [The semiological adventure]. Seuil, Paris

Bates V (2018) 'Humanizing' healthcare environments: architecture, art and design in modern hospitals. Des Health 2(1):5–19. https://doi.org/10.1080/24735132.2018.1436304

Borgna P (2005) Sociologia del corpo [Sociology of the body]. Laterza, Bari

Bourdieu P (1979) La distinction [The distinction]. Les éditions de Minuit, Paris

Brown MT, Bussell JK (2011) Medication adherence: WHO cares? Mayo Clin Proc 86(4):304–314. https://doi.org/10.4065/mcp.2010.0575

Brown MT, Bussell J, Dutta S, Davis K, Strong S, Mathew S (2016) Medication adherence: truth and consequences. Am J Med Sci 351(4):387–399. https://doi.org/10.1016/j.amjms.2016.01.010

Chamberlain P, Craig C (2017) Design for health: reflections from the editors. Des Health 1(1):3–7. https://doi.org/10.1080/24735132.2017.1296273

Chast F (1995) Histoire contemporaine des medicaments [Contemporary history of drugs]. La découverte, Paris

Clark FA (2000) The concepts of habit and routine: a preliminary theoretical synthesis. Occup Ther J Res 20(1_suppl):123S–137S. https://doi.org/10.1177/15394492000200S114

Conrad P (1985) The meaning of medications: another look at compliance. Soc Sci Med 20(1):29–37. https://doi.org/10.1016/0277-9536(85)90308-9

Crabtree A, Rodden T (2004) Domestic routines and design for the home. Comput Supported Coop Work 13(2):191–220. https://doi.org/10.1023/B:COSU.0000045712.26840.a4

Craig C (2017) Imagined futures: designing future environments for the care of older people. Des J 20(sup1):S2336–S2347. https://doi.org/10.1080/14606925.2017.1352749

Crespo C, Santos S, Canavarro MC, Kielpikowski M, Pryor J, Féres-Carneiro T (2013) Family routines and rituals in the context of chronic conditions: a review. Int J Psychol 48(5):729–746. https://doi.org/10.1080/00207594.2013.806811

Denham SA (2003) Relationships between family rituals, family routines, and health. J Fam Nurs 9(3):305–330. https://doi.org/10.1177/1074840703255447

Desclaux A, Lévy JJ (2003) Présentation: Culture et médicaments. Ancien objet ou nouveau courant en anthropologie médicale? [Presentation: culture and drugs. Old object or new trend in medical anthropology?]. Anthropologie et Sociétés 27(2):5–21. https://doi.org/10.7202/007443ar. Accessed November 2022

Devlin AS, Arneill AB (2003) Healthcare environments and patient outcomes: a review of the literature. Environ Behav 35(5):665–694. https://doi.org/10.1177/0013916503255102

Di Carlo I (2020) Il ruolo della qualità nel prodotto farmaceutico: stato dell'arte e sviluppi auspicabili [The role of quality in the pharmaceutical product: state of the art and desirable developments], supervisor Prof. Antonella Penati, unpublished Master Thesis. Politecnico di Milano, Scuola del Design, academic year 2018/19

Ekman I, Britten N, Bordin J, Codagnone C, Eden S, Forslund D, Swedberg K (2013) The person-centred approach to an ageing society. Eur J Pers Cent Healthc 1(1):132–137

European Medicine Agency-Pharmacovigilance Risk Assessment Committee (2015a) Good practice guide on recording, coding, reporting and assessment of medication errors (EMA/762563/2014). Available from: https://www.ema.europa.eu/en/documents/regulatory-procedural-guideline/good-practice-guide-recording-coding-reporting-assessment-medication-errors_en.pdf. Accessed November 2022

European Medicine Agency-Pharmacovigilance Risk Assessment Committee (2015b) Good practice guide on risk minimisation and prevention of medication errors (EMA/606103/2014). Available from: https://www.ema.europa.eu/en/documents/regulatory-procedural-guideline/good-practice-guide-risk-minimisation-prevention-medication-errors_en.pdf. Accessed September 2022

Fainzang S (2001) Médicaments et société. Le patient, le médecin et l'ordonnance [Medicines and society. The patient, the doctor and the prescription]. Presses Universitaires de France, Paris

Fainzang S (2003) Les médicaments dans l'espace privé. Gestion individuelle ou collective [Medicines in the private area. Individual or collective management]. Anthropologie et Sociétés 27(2):139–154. https://doi.org/10.7202/007450ar. Accessed November 2022

Fainzang S (2005) Société-Le charme discret des medicaments [The discreet charm of drugs]. LeDevoir, 20 Aout 2005. Available from: https://www.ledevoir.com/societe/sante/88432/societe-le-charme-discret-des-medicaments. Accessed November 2022

Fainzang S (2006) La relation médecins-malades: information et mensonge [The doctor-patient relationship: information and lies]. Presses Universitaires de France, Paris

Fainzang S (2012) L'automédication ou les mirages de l'autonomie [Self-medication or the mirages of autonomy]. Presses Universitaires de France, Paris

Fainzang S (2013) The other side of medicalization: self-medicalization and self-medication. Culture, Medicine & Psychiatry 37:488–504. https://doi.org/10.1007/s11013-013-9330-2

Fox N, Ward K (2008) Pharma in the bedroom … and the kitchen…. The pharmaceuticalisation of daily life. Sociol Health Illn 30(6):856–868. https://doi.org/10.1111/j.1467-9566.2008.01114.x

Fulop T, Larbi A, Witkowski JM, McElhaney J, Loeb M, Mitnitski A, Pawelec G (2010) Aging, frailty and age-related diseases. Biogerontology 11(5):547–563. https://doi.org/10.1007/s10522-010-9287-2

Golant SM (1984) A place to grow old: the meaning of environment in old age. Columbia University Press, New York

Groeneveld B, Dekkers T, Boon B, D'Olivo P (2018) Challenges for design researchers in healthcare. Des Health 2(2):305–326. https://doi.org/10.1080/24735132.2018.1541699

Haynes RB, McDonald HP, Garg AX (2002) Helping patients follow prescribed treatment: clinical applications. JAMA: J Am Med Assoc 288(2):2880–2883. https://doi.org/10.1001/jama.288.22.2880

Hirsch T, Forlizzi J, Hyder E, Goetz J, Kurtz C, Stroback J (2000) The ELDer project: social, emotional, and environmental factors in the design of eldercare technologies. In: CUU '00 proceedings on the 2000 conference on universal usability. ACM, New York, pp 72–79. https://doi.org/10.1145/355460.355476

Hurtienne J, Klöckner K, Diefenbach S, Nass C, Maier A (2015) Designing with image schemas: resolving the tension between innovation, inclusion and intuitive use. Interact Comput 27(3):235–255. https://doi.org/10.1093/iwc/iwu049

James F, Olausson S (2018) Designing for care: employing ethnographic design methods at special care homes for young offenders—a pilot study. Des Health 2(1):127–141. https://doi.org/10.1080/24735132.2018.1456783

Jones P (2013) Design for care: innovating healthcare experience. Rosenfeld Media, New York

Karol E, Smith D (2019) Impact of design on emotional, psychological, or social wellbeing for people with cognitive impairment. Health Environ Res Des J 12(3):220–232. https://doi.org/10.1177/1937586718813194

Kleinman A (1980) Patients and healers in the context of culture. University of California Press, Berkeley

Lawton MP (1982) Competence, environmental press, and the adaptation of older people. In: Lawton MP, Windley PG, Byerts TO (eds) Aging and the environment: theoretical approaches. Springer Publishing, New York, pp 33–59

Lawton MP, Windley PG, Byerts TO (eds) (1982) Aging and the environment: theoretical approaches. Springer, New York

Lorenzini G, Olsson A (2015) Design towards better life experiences: closing the gap between pharmaceutical packaging design and elderly people. In: Proceedings of the 20th International Conference on Engineering Design (ICED), 27–30 July, Vol. 9. Politecnico di Milano, Design Society, Milano, pp 65–76

Lumme-Sandt K, Virtane P (2002) Older people in the field of medication. Sociol Health Illn 24(3):285–304. Available from: https://onlinelibrary.wiley.com/doi/pdf/10.1111/1467-9566.00295. Accessed October 2022

Manganini G (2022) Confezione analogica intelligente. Sistema per semplificare i gesti della cura [Smart analogic packaging. A system to simplify the gestures of care], supervisor Prof. Antonella Penati, unpublished Master Thesis. Politecnico di Milano, Scuola del Design, academic year 2021/22

Martin C (2000) Putting patients first: integrating hospital design and care. Lancet 356(9228):518. https://doi.org/10.1016/S0140-6736(05)74196-9

Martin DP, Hunt JR, Conrad DA (1990) The Planetree model hospital project: an example of the patient as partner. Hosp Health Serv Admin 35(4):591–601

Mason T (2006) Designed with care: design and neighbourhood healthcare buildings. CABE, London

Mauss M (1936) Les techniques du corps [Body techniques]. Journal de Psychologie XXXII(3-4):271–293. Available from: http://www.regine-detambel.com/images/30/revue_1844.pdf. Accessed October 2022

Merriam-Webster.com. Ritual. Available from https://www.merriam-webster.com/dictionary/ritual. Accessed December 2022

Micocci M, Spinelli G (2018) Metaphors and analogies through smart materials to mitigate age-related differences in the understanding of technology. J Des Res 16(3/4):282–313. https://doi.org/10.1504/JDR.2018.099536

Noël G (2017) Health design: mapping current situations, envisioning next steps. Des J 20(sup1):S2304–S2314. https://doi.org/10.1080/14606925.2017.1352746

Norman D (2013) The design of everyday things: revised and expanded edition. Basic books, New York

Nusem E, Straker K, Wrigley C (2020) Design innovation for health and medicine. Palgrave Macmillan, Singapore

Overgaard ABA, Møller-Sonnergaard J, Christrup LL, Højsted J, Hansen R, Sonnergaard J (2001) Patients' evaluation of shape, size and colour of solid dosage forms. Pharm World Sci 23(5):185–188. https://doi.org/10.1023/A:1012050931018

Palen L, Aaløkke S (2006) Pill boxes and piano benches: "Home-made" methods for managing medication. In: CSCW '06, November 4–8, 2006, pp. 79–88, Banff, Alberta. https://doi.org/10.1145/1180875.1180888

Penati A, Pizzocaro S, Tonelli MC, Standoli C, Iannilli V, Bucchetti V, Rebaglio A, Riccò D, Andreoni G, Caratti E, Tolino U (2020) Scienza al quotidiano: farmaci come oggetti/Daily science: pharmaceuticals as objects. DIID disegno industriale industrial design 69:120–127

Pizzocaro S, Penati A (2021) The in-home use of medications: in pursuit of design-driven knowledge. Home Culture 17(3):153–171. https://doi.org/10.1080/17406315.2021.1916225

Reynolds Whyte S, van der Geest S, Hardon A (2002) Social lives of medicines. Cambridge University Press, Cambridge

Richard D, de Lapouge D (1988) L'objet médicament, Les formes médicamenteuses par voie orale, L'observance, Le praticien P.P.P. dans Impact Médecin Hebdo, dossier n° 196, 25 juin 1988, 1–14

Rodriguez-Falcon EM, Yoxall A (2011) Beyond a spoonful of syrup: understanding physical barriers to medical packaging. In: Proceedings of the 1st European conference on design 4 health, 13–15 July. Sheffield University, Sheffield, pp 266–286. Available from: https://research.shu.ac.uk/design4health/wp-content/uploads/2012/09/D4H2011_proceedings_v5a.pdf. Accessed October 2022

Ryan AA (1999) Medication compliance and older people: a review of the literature. Int J Nurs Stud 36(2):153–162. https://doi.org/10.1016/s0020-7489(99)00003-6

Schrauwen S, Roberts L, Wright R (eds) (2017) Can graphic design save your life? GraphicDesign&, London

Spinelli G (2015) Innovation is in the eyes of the beholder: the case of the ageing consumers. J Des Bus Soc 1(2):145–161. https://doi.org/10.1386/dbs.1.2.145_1

Spinelli G, Micocci M, Martin W, Wang Y-H (2019) From medical devices to everyday products: exploring cross-cultural perceptions of assistive technology. Des Health 3(2):324–340. https://doi.org/10.1080/24735132.2019.1680065

Stawarz K, Cox AL, Blandford A (2014) Don't forget your pill! Designing effective medication reminder apps that support users' daily routines. In: Proceedings of the SIGCHI conference on human factors in computing systems, CHI 2014, April 26–May 01, Toronto, ON, 2269–2278. Available from: https://doi.org/10.1145/2556288.2557079. Accessed 12 Nov 2022

Sudbury-Riley L (2014) Unwrapping senior consumers' packaging experiences. Mark Intell Plan 32(6):666–686. https://doi.org/10.1108/MIP-02-2013-0027

The Health Foundation (2016) Person-centred care made simple. What everyone should know about person-centred care. The Health Foundation, London. Available at: http://www.health.org.uk/sites/default/files/PersonCentredCareMadeSimple.pdf. Accessed 12 Nov 2022

Tsekleves E, Cooper R (eds) (2016) Design for health. Routledge, London

van der Geest S, Whyte SR (1989) The charm of medicines: metaphors and metonyms. Med Anthropol Q 3(4):345–367

van der Geest S, Reynolds Whyte S, Hardon A (1996) The anthropology of pharmaceuticals: a biographical approach. Annu Rev Anthropol 25:153–178. https://doi.org/10.1146/annurev.anthro.25.1.153

Wyatt S, Henwood F, Hart A, Platzer H (2004) L'extension des territoires du patient. Internet et santé au quotidian. [The extension of the patient's territories. Internet and daily health]. Sciences sociales et santé 22(1):45–68. https://doi.org/10.3406/sosan.2004.1608

Open Access This chapter is licensed under the terms of the Creative Commons Attribution 4.0 International License (http://creativecommons.org/licenses/by/4.0/), which permits use, sharing, adaptation, distribution and reproduction in any medium or format, as long as you give appropriate credit to the original author(s) and the source, provide a link to the Creative Commons license and indicate if changes were made.

The images or other third party material in this chapter are included in the chapter's Creative Commons license, unless indicated otherwise in a credit line to the material. If material is not included in the chapter's Creative Commons license and your intended use is not permitted by statutory regulation or exceeds the permitted use, you will need to obtain permission directly from the copyright holder.

Chapter 14
In-Home. Medicinal Treatment as a Learning Process

Antonella Valeria Penati

Abstract How do patients know what they know about medicines use? And how do they know whether their actions in preparing for treatment are correct? When faced with a new medicine, do patients perceive they must begin a real learning and training process? And, if so, how does this thinking inform their actions? What basic knowledge docs cach patient possess about the use of medicines? How are they formed, and what are the sources of information that educate the patient-user of the medicine? We have noted, in previous chapters (refer to Chap. 8 of this text), the fragmentary way in which the patient is given information about the management of treatment: some of it comes from the doctor, some of it from the pharmacist, and some of it is retrieved from the package leaflet and the indications on the primary and secondary packaging. The medicine itself, its shape and the markings on its surface can give the patient valuable hints on how to take it correctly (on this aspect, see Chap. 16 of this text). How do these different levels of information play out when the patient finds himself, in his own home, 'face to face' with medicines? Through what tools and practices does the patient's knowledge regarding the appropriate and correct medicine use take shape? This chapter attempts to answer these questions by looking at therapy in the home environment as a learning process.

14.1 Medicinal Treatment as a Learning Process

As happens in any learning process, the person's ability to understand, interpret, and apply the instructions they receive is an essential point. This ability is mediated by culture, competencies, previous and direct experience or by observing and sharing the experiences of others, and by the contexts in which the person is. But it also depends on the effectiveness of the information tools used in pharmaceutical products. Does the significant deployment of effort that the pharmaceutical industry devotes to information on the proper use and consumption of medicine produce

---

A. V. Penati (✉)
Department of Design, Politecnico di Milano, Milan, Italy
e-mail: antonella.penati@polimi.it

good and effective information tools, reaching the patient and inducing them not to make mistakes, or persuading them to follow recommended patterns of action? Lastly, how does the everyday context affect in acquiring valuable knowledge for medicine and therapy management? Of this complex intertwining of questions, we present a possible answer in the present contribution, undoubtedly partial. An answer aims to highlight the home context's role in the patient's learning behaviours while using medicines. Within this reflection, it is useful here to point out that by a learning process, we refer to the ability to acquire and interpret information and to the process of acquiring, transforming, using, and reusing knowledge that takes place in practical experience (Kolb 1984; Rosenberg 2001; Roth and Jornet 2014). The use of such a concept, allows us to give importance to the ability to learn and use, in addition to declarative forms of knowledge (*know what*), also modal or procedural forms of knowledge (*know how*) (Polanyi 1979; Berge and Hezewijk 1999; Caron-Flinterman et al. 2005) consisting, for the most part, of knowing "how to do it". This knowledge also requires acquiring the skills to set up organizational schemes, activity systems, procedural and behavioural models. We will reflect on the critical issues of these forms of learning, concerning their replicability and transferability and, thus, their reuse when learned through *familiarization* (Bordieu 2003), a customary way of learning in the domestic domain.

The considerations we propose below take as their premise the Farb Research (University Funds for Basic Research) *Care for Care! Shaping medicines: question of Identity, Use and Communication*. Based on the theoretical premises, this research reflects on the role of design in the world of medicines through direct observation of elderly patients dealing with pharmaceutical therapy in their home settings.

In this chapter, we will propose some considerations that, from this observational activity, are transferred to the level of an initial theorization. In Chap. 15 of this volume, on the other hand, a description of the most recurrent behaviours among users of pharmaceutical therapies in the home context is returned, including through visual notations. Moving from the analysis of user-patient experiences, this contribution shows the distance between prescriptive modalities elaborated elaborates by the pharmaceutical industry (Browall et al. 2013) and adaptive modes that identify a precise learning style in care practices. (Ferrarotti 1986; Palen and Aaløkke 2006; Chanel et al. 2011). These modalities foreground the user's rudimentary inventions, which are far more effective-not least because they are personalized—than sophisticated technological aids that are at least as extraneous to people's lives as the pharmacological products they are supposed to help. Sometimes, on the other hand, it is the hastiness and carelessness of everyday domesticity that mislead the patient, who may go so far as to treat the medicine without due care.

In this observational process, the care process emerges not so much and not only as a physiological or chemical process. Care models embody the relationship between the individual—with their specific needs—and the set of objects necessary for care. Such sets usually include medicines, packages, leaflets and complementary gadgets for handling, manipulation, and storage. The patients themselves often repurpose these sets according to their individual needs.

14.2 Patient Learning Experience in Domestic Contexts

For patients, the domestic healthcare experience represents a set of complex activities and behaviours. It requires real learning processes, such as of: organisational techniques (Carlsson-Wall et al. 2011); techniques of the body (Mauss 2017); techniques of memory; techniques and devices of discipline and self-discipline, etc. To construct an organised process that facilitates therapy management, the patient equips himself with spatialisation logics of therapy and defines real domestic liturgies (Fiese 2007; Pizzocaro and Penati 2021).

The collection of observations conducted on patients makes it possible to advance the hypothesis that an authentic learning style takes place in domestic spaces, in the spaces of our private lives. It is a style of acquiring new knowledge in which specific peculiar characteristics are recognised.

Firstly, it is a form of learning strongly influenced by the 'imprecise', 'improvised', and 'spontaneous', nature that characterises many of the cognitive and problem-solving activities within the home.

Secondly, the learning style in pharmaceutical therapy management seems to follow the pattern of an adaptive process. By the term *adaptive learning*, we generally mean those modes of teaching that are customised based on the learner's learning abilities (Blumberg 2009; Kerr 2016). In this context, on the other hand, we refer to this term to indicate the forms of teaching and learning that the user implements, adapting them to the context's circumstances and resources. Those patients seeking to fulfil each therapy's tasks and circumvent difficulties are cognitive, mnemonic, organisational, postural strategies. Each use what the home environment provides, or practices learnt in other "household matters" and transferred to the therapy setting.

Particularly remarkable here seems to be the concept of *contingency*, which the epistemologist Tagliagambe (1997, p. 48) interprets as an incentive to change a situation one is experiencing through transformative explorations typical of creative activity. It is a type of creativity, the kind generated by contingency, that knows how to choose not only conceivable but also concretely realisable alternatives.

Thirdly, in learning the modes of using medicines, we notice a learning style very close to the processes of autodidactism. One is not a patient. One becomes patient in the absence of a teacher, a guide, or a manual; in short, in the lack of all those tools that have been developed precisely to transmit knowledge from an expert (in the sense of one who has had experience) to the neophyte.

In the case of the body techniques necessary to learn the correct 'manoeuvres' of the body dealing with care processes, the same *body techniques* (Mauss 2017), profoundly studied by sociological and ethno-anthropological sciences as an essential part of the socialisation processes that affect our bodies (Crossley 2007), do not have explicit forms of training.

Knowledge, in this domain, seems more to derive from implicit forms of training: some of it is acquired through *familiarization* processes (Bordieu 2003); some of it is real forms of self-learning and do-it-yourself, often improvised by the patient and remaining on the level of personal knowledge, at most familiar.

Fourth and lastly, let us not underestimate the forms of learning practices that take place within the domestic context—as the caregiving practices—are affected by the spontaneity, the obviousness of the relations between subjects and between subjects and objects proper to the family environment. "Primary knowledge, practical and tacit, of the familiar world" […], Bordieu argues, possesses a "content of obviousness and naturalness" (Bordieu 2003, p. 185) that does not prompt us to question the assumptions, conditions, constraints, and 'truth' of knowledge acquired in such a context.

In this regard, Tagliagambe refers to behavioural genre, behavioural contexts, and situational behaviours as a kind of catalogue or repertoire of ways of doing things, of relatively stable verbal customs and habits that constitute what may be called the "genre of the everyday" (Tagliagambe, p. 95). These "little scripts" belong to the "phenomenology of everyday experience" (ibid.); they clear it from the need to engage in continuous decision-making concerning common and repetitive situations. They are the result of 'typical situations', of 'habitual conditions' that generate 'stereotypes of behaviour' and allow us to act according to semi-automatic operational, organisational, cognitive, affective, and motivational patterns because a whole complex of technical, bodily, postural, gestural, psychological skills come into operation spontaneously.

The modes of transmission of these forms of knowledge occur through interiorised rules and prohibitions, often without the need for an explicit transmission. The knowledge, and even praxeological knowledge, that results from these forms of interiorised constructs, again as Bordieu describes it, a *"habitus"* (Bordieu 2003, p. 206), a kind of *forma mentis* that "impregnates" thoughts and actions (Crossley 2001; Lau 2004; Reay 2004). In the concept of *habitus,* the 'efficacy of a behaviour' is enriched with body attitudes, tastes, and preferences characterising mental and operational patterns in terms of "style" of action and thinking (Bordieu 2003).

14.3 Towards a Phenomenological Analysis of Domestic Therapy

The French sociologist Pierre Bourdieu significantly warned against the "objectification effect, that is, the transformation of a familiar relationship into scientific knowledge" (Bordieu 2003, p. 176). And yet Bourdieu himself has contributed much emphasis on "biographical itineraries", "specific circumstances", and the "cogent value of contextual situations" (Bordieu 2003, p. 176).

The examples of spontaneous sociology, able to bring out "the faces behind the statistics", "the special cases, the exceptions, the nuances", "[…] the set of differences", acquires in this theoretical perspective a significance no less relevant than the statistical data (Bordieu 2003, p. 176).

In the case of home care and the difficulties in the patients' actions and operations with medicines, even the error of one or a few people is remarkable. It deserves to be investigated to assess whether the medicine is accessible to the patient and makes available all the information needed to use the medicines properly.

Silent observation of patients in the familiarity of their home environments allows their feelings of discomfort to be detected. A discomfort the observer perceives through facial or body expressions or exclamations but most often remains unexpressed. Only when the observer can bring it out, by pointing it out to the patient, does it open the way to arrive at forms, even if essential, of encoding.

In most cases, awareness of distress is attributed to one's incapabilities and inabilities. It is expressed as "feeling inadequate" (e.g., unable to understand, manipulate, assume, organize) or needing someone's help. It is rare for patients to trace their 'discomfort' and their suffering to an inappropriateness of the product. If this occurs, it is a lament of whining, not criticism of the object. The patient hardly perceives medicine as a physical product with its materiality and formal characteristics. Medicine as a 'necessary disease' seems to place medicinal products in the sphere of 'intangible' goods (Connor 2014). This state of indulgence enjoyed by medicine should be further explored by contextualizing the subject of medicine and its objects within the cultures of the patient's body, illness, physical and cognitive abilities, and inabilities.

But, in this context, we are more concerned with giving space to the effects produced by the home context on the practices of care, the influence that the familiarity, custom, and spontaneity of the actions that take place in the spaces of the home can have on the forms of use and processes of learning to use medicine.

We refer here again to Bourdieu, as the first who explored the phenomenology of familiarity relations established between subjects and objects in a domestic, friendly, habitual context where it is possible to grasp an underlying order, an implicit code of "things to do" or "things not to do" (Bordieu 2003, p. 266) as long as one knows how to emphasize the way of doing things, the choices and actions that lie within the framework of the obvious, the ordinary, the everyday things seemingly devoid of obligations and constraints. On the contrary, Bourdieu and with him de Certeau (2001) find precisely in situations of familiarity, a context pregnant with constraints, able to direct and orient choices, actions, and solutions.

The family context as a place where it is possible to "let go", "take the chance" (Bordieu 2003, p. 225), to do "in one's way" (De Certeau 2001, p. 5) constitutes a space open to the possibility of "improvising", of combining and recombining knowledge and practices, of internalizing and learning implicitly—through familiarization precisely –, instructions, schemes of action, principles, precepts (Bordieu 2003, pp. 235–236). It is also permissible to prevent formal rules; the effectiveness—true or presumed—of the result obtained wins out over the correctness of the tools and methods used.

In these apprenticeship activities that introduce the patient to the medicine and that take place informally and according to uncodified procedures, there are also experiments, trials, and attempts to train the body in postures, gestures (Denham

2003) and operational expedients that, once learned, tested, and perfected become a constitutive part of the routine practices that are the basis of the experience of care.

De Certeau describes the domestic, the everyday, as a place where consumers reveal what they do with products through modes of use and consumption and *common* practices (De Certeau 2001; p. 3).

The culture of the everyday, in other words, produces, through the many microactivities that innervate it, a real projectuality that defines a kind of "creativity of the everyday" (*ivi*, p. 8) where the gap existing between the object, as it has been thought of by those who produced it, and the manipulations, re-functionalizations, and reuse of products operated by users as forms of adaptation that are also forms of reappropriation (*ibidem*, p. 8; Pizzocaro 2015) of the object is revealed.

De Certeau speaks in this regard of *minuscule, silent* techniques (*ivi*, p. 9), of an inventiveness governed by the art of making do that leads to recombining heterogeneous elements and knowledge based on a practical intelligence that, in a witty way, invents procedures, adapts operational schemes, follows "implicit principles and explicit rules" (*ivi*, p. 96).

The everyday turns out to be a territory of promiscuity, of transfers and reuses of objects and techniques that exploit the multiple functional potentials implicit in the object itself and follow, at the same time, the principle that many things are replaceable with others, not necessarily related in function or scope of use. This is also the case with medicines and care practices.

14.4 Medication Therapies: Bricolage and Transfer of Objects and Practices from Other Contexts of Use

Our everyday contexts, particularly the home, lend themselves well to a spontaneous creativity that feeds off the use of what the context makes available to produce innovations of a frugal nature. These have as their sole purpose to achieve 'local' results. That is, results that do not claim to be replicated, to become models, but simply to resolve contingencies. These are processes that evolutionary theories of innovation have well described as bricolage practices (Lévi-Strauss 1966; Ceruti 1995), ingenious practices triggered by the state of necessity, supported by an intuitive and practical sense, able to set in motion that inherent ability of ours to be able to re-functionalise materials and tools available for performance other than those for which they were designed, recombining them or recombining some of their parts or elements, sometimes allowing original results (Joyce and Craig 2011). Results that, while derived from the randomness of the available elements that dictate the logic of their assembly, once realised, appear to be "the most obvious thing" that could be done (Freeman 2007). This 'putting together' what is available, with a view to a result, does not necessarily produce successful outcomes. Even when it does, it cannot necessarily be transferred to large-scale or industrial-type production. The practices of bricolage that lead to acquiring and assembling things, so to speak, 'on hand', follow logic foreign to the more traditional processes of designing an object. In the latter, purpose leads the designer to seek the best solution, and the design dictates the choice of use of materials and components. On the other hand, the bricoleur uses imperfect materials and components, sub-optimal concerning the result he intends to achieve. In this way, the purpose itself, shaped in part by what is available for use, is resolved roughly (Lévi-Strauss 1966).

As Marchis (2017) notes, if the bricoleur's way of proceeding can be categorised in the forms of "wild thinking"—as Lévi-Strauss says—, this does not mean that we are dealing with a primitive form of thinking. It is, if anything, an "uneducated" form of thinking that the professional man possesses instead (Marchis 2017).

This "putting together", transferring, assembling and 'making sense' of 'second-hand' fragments of knowledge and experience, 'borrowed' and taken from contiguous contexts, for creating something new (Freeman 2007), constitutes a form of learning in practice.

In the case of objects related to care and to patients using medicines, it is a reason for interest faced with non-expert users, who often do not have acquired skills and in-depth knowledge of a product derived from prolonged experience of use over time. Instead, in most cases, one is faced with naïve users who introduce innovative effects into therapy use systems by appealing to knowledge derived from other areas in which they have acquired some familiarity. What are enacted by the user are processes of knowledge transfer, gestures, and organisational modes that follow a pattern of learning based on 'memory patterns' and 'action patterns' that contain information peculiar to other contexts (Thorndyke and Haves-Roth 1979).

Various theoretical studies show us how delicate and sometimes fallacious the process of transferring knowledge from one context to another is. Contextual objectives, available resources, usage constraints, the nature of objects and knowledge transferred, must be equated and evaluated in their similarities and differences. While memory patterns, and consequent patterns of behaviour, help us to save cognitive energy in dealing with new situations, on the other hand, they can lead us to wrong actions. And, in the world of pharmaceuticals, while this transfer process can be virtuous, it can also lead to health-risky behaviour if behaviour transferred by analogy with other contexts of use is not consciously re-contextualised (Figs. 14.1, 14.2, 14.3 and 14.4).

What seems to emerge strongly from the set of patient observation experiences, is the created promiscuity—thanks to the sense of security that the normality of life inside the home entails—between the buying, storing, use and consumption behaviours proper to the food sphere and that of medicines (in particular, this observation applies to oral pharmaceutical forms). Similarly, hygiene, and cosmetics use and consumption patterns seem to influence the use and consumption behaviours proper to creams and ointments.

Once introduced into the domestic environment and the frugal activities proper to everyday context, even medicine—the object of science—becomes frugal, becomes banalized. It enters the domain of the obvious, *the object at hand*, the object that, like the others inside the home, can be used *nonchalantly*.

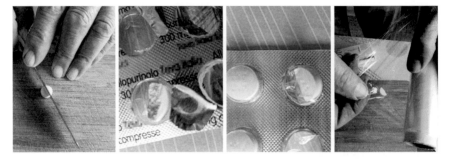

Fig. 14.1 Transfer of gestures, actions and objects from the food context to the pharmaceutical context

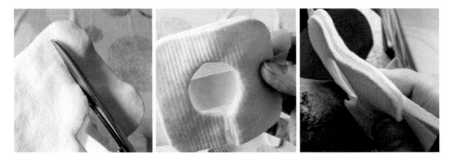

Fig. 14.2 Transfer of objects from the cosmetic context: use of makeup remover discs combined with a strip of plaster. The cotton pads were overlapped to obtain the desired thickness and an empty space was made in the centre to protect the skin ulceration, without compressing it

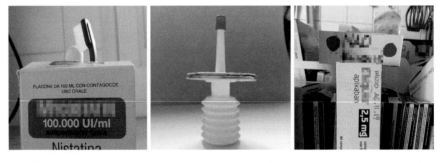

Fig. 14.3 Different approaches and behaviours, product's adjustments and improvements, coming directly from real user experience. From the left side: the secondary pack was cut out at the top because the medicine bottle, once the dropper canula is mounted, is taller than the secondary pack. The patient also inserted a small toothbrush to brush the tongue with the medicine; modifying an enema to ease its handling and use; add signs and symbols to secondary packaging to remind you to take that medicine twice a day

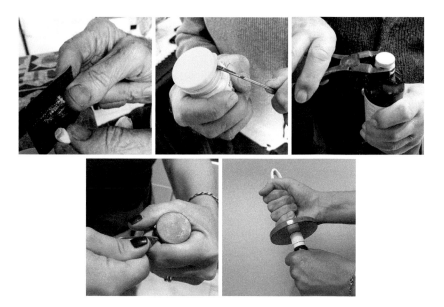

Fig. 14.4 Transfer of gestures, actions and objects from the context of do-it-yourself household. From the top left: sandpapering a pill to ease its swallowing; open a pill bottle with a screwdriver; unscrew the cap of a syrup, when it is sealed, with pliers; breaking the seal of a pill-box with a knife; breaking the seal to mix the active ingredient and excipients using a meat mallet

Sometimes, on the other hand, the patient is aware that the medicine's nature makes it an object to which some attention must be given. But, even in these cases, there is no shortage of transfers of operational or organizational practices and actions, effective in their contexts of origin (e.g., that of domestic techniques of food preparation, handling, and consumption) but wholly inadequate, if not careless, when used with medicines.

Still, real manipulative interventions are implemented in the medicine; proper and improper aids are introduced to facilitate the gestures of care. Tools taken from the domestic context are re-functionalised to the management of therapy (on all these aspects, see Chap. 16 of this text) with the 'adjustments' necessary to make adequate to the support of medicine management, objects born for an entirely different purpose.

In summary, in the case of home therapies, one can frequently observe forms of *do-it-yourself* in medicine use practices and forms of self-alphabetisation around medical objects and languages. The precision with which scientifically sophisticated products, such as medicines, should be treated leaves space for the imprecision of bodily gestures, the promiscuity between objects of care and objects taken from other contexts of everyday life, the manipulation of medicines and their packaging, and the introduction of adaptations of objects of care according to the user's needs.

14.5 Care as a Learned Practice: Domestic Lead Users

These modes of transformative intervention in the sphere of objects find theoretical reference in theories of *learning by using* (Boud et al. 1993) where users play an important role. The literature has paid great attention to product improvement practices by users (Holt 1988), particularly on the processes of improving product performance by so-called 'expert users'. Expert users have special knowledge of specific typologies of objects developed through user experience. A prime example is the world of consumer electronics, which activates its innovation processes precisely based on users' wishes, which have matured during experience. Examples of this are users, such as sportsmen and women, dedicated to extending the performance potential of technical objects. Examples of this are professionals in medical (Katila et al. 2018) and scientific practices (von Hippel 1976, 1986) in general who, along with the specific skills of their profession, develop expertise relating to the devices and tools of the 'craft' (Franke et al. 2006).

In this regard, it should be noted that all virtuous examples of product innovation, resulting from the use by what we have called expert users, have their strength as drivers of innovation, because they occur within what Étienne Wenger (2006) has called "communities of practice".

Informal communities consisting of people who share a common interest concerning, for example, an object and its performance and who share-through through interaction and mutual relationships-experiences, knowledge, skills, and technical abilities (Jeppesen and Laursenb 2009). Communities of practice, based on the sharing of know-how among expert actors, have the prerogative of constructing meaning, giving meaning, and validating the innovations that are produced within them (Franke and Shah 2003), thus paving the way for their social diffusion and the scalability of results from local experience to industrial production. (Amin and Roberts 2008; Hao et al. 2017).

On the other hand, the industry has long since stopped considering those involved in intermediate processes (supply chain suppliers, distributors) as mere performers and the end users themselves as passive adopters. Their involvement is, by now, a pivotal practice of corporate strategies in building the value chain. Even in healthcare industries, user-led innovation has recently begun to play a key role. Indeed, their experience, practical knowledge, and even the judgments are believed able to make about products and processes, to make valuable suggestions in improving healthcare services (Agness et al. 2011); in personalizing forms of care and treatment; in intercepting and thus reducing the reasons for inefficiencies and complaints; in intervening in the prevention of lifestyle-related diseases, such as cardiovascular (Echeverri et al. 2013) etc.

In some specific areas of medicine therapies, there is also increasing patient involvement in drug development. This is the case, for example, in rare diseases and orphan medicines where, since these are very niche markets with no financial incentives, the patients' awareness, concerning the different aspects of the disease and the expertise they demonstrate in the autonomy of therapy control, is precious. Another area where patient experience proves valuable to the company is in chronic diseases characterized by long medication times; times that allow the patient to accumulate a lot of experiential knowledge (Oliveira et al. 2015; Trigo 2016).

These examples of patient involvement have proven valuable in bringing about improvements in diagnosis, subsequent treatments, therapies, and care, especially on the clinical and pharmaceutical levels and in defining the same research themes in both these areas: the quality of life of patients undergoing treatment; the causes of non-adherence to therapy; and the feelings of satisfaction or dissatisfaction, well-being or frustration that accompany treatment and can lead to improvement (Grabowski 2003; Smits and Boon 2008).

From several studies emerge the ability of patients to be carriers of innovation and to share their innovation with other patients with similar pathologies, especially concerning the need to solve substantial limitations and constraints brought to daily life by the disease. In these cases, the development of new devices or new instrumentation used for treatment or significant improvements, obtained through knowledge accumulated during the experience of the use of existing devices (Shaw 1998; de Jong and von Hippel 2009). At the same time, we see the emergence of communities of patients thanks to the online sharing of their care-related misadventures. In particular, the fruit of these sharings is represented by smartphone applications or the development of electronic devices aimed at supporting care.

In the world of home-based pharmaceutical therapy, while we witness the many expedients implemented by users to improve their relationship with objects of care, some of the prerequisites that make object improvement experiences through learning-by-using practices so effective are lacking.

The first assumption is what we have termed the "situated character" (Gherardi and Nicolini 2001) of home care experiences.

Our observations of home therapy show strategies of knowledge acquisition that maintain a local value (Bruner 2001), because they are highly dependent on the context and what it makes available.

Reutilizing what has been learned in a "singular" situation constitutes a critical process (Mortari 2003) for which a valid theory on the criteria of analogy and similarity is needed, allowing for the appropriate transfer of learned knowledge to another context. Even more critically, this process is when dealing with spontaneously developed forms of knowledge and experience, prepared according to operational, and organizational aptitudes, but also talents of skill and genius that remain on the plane of personal experience, which do not have the strength to enter broader circuits of knowledge where comparison and thus validation is possible.

Not only that. The processes of product refinement through the user experience are aimed, for the most part, at objects that arouse interest from an iconic, technological and/or performance point of view, able to attract interest, curiosity and even passion of users and to stimulate their ingenuity. The refinements made by patients to pharmaceutical products or to objects that assist therapeutic practices or to the practical-organizational activities that accompany them, act on products that are poor from the iconic point of view and hermetic on the level of technology and performance, thus being unattractive, unexciting and unsuitable, therefore, to become an object of shared knowledge and to create around them a community that operates through the exchange of knowledge. The improvement activity introduced by the user-patient, in the use of medicines, is closer to the practices of adjustment, adaptation than to refinement and improvement to object innovation. Patients, in the use of medicines, have as their reference and the solution to the contingent problem that besets them. This differentiates them from lead users who nevertheless have as the reference of their innovative action the desire to share the outcomes of their innovative activity up to and including the industry's interest.

A final aspect highlighted here is that the medicine is presented as a simple object. Theoretically, this simplicity leads to observing the patient using categories and viewpoints typical of consumer analysis. But if we analyze the medicine from the point of view of the activities that accompany it (prescribing, dispensing, understanding, memory, manipulation, organization, scheduling) we find it immersed in an operational-managerial and cognitive complexity that immediately brings out the aspects of use as well as those of consumption, opening up new perspectives of interest on subject-object interactions. The patient-user perspective is much more effective in highlighting the multiple learning and transformative activities in medicine therapies than a perspective that sees the patient as simply a consumer (McLaughlin 2008). And even in the now increasingly widespread virtual communities that, using the Web, exchange opinions about medicines (on this aspect, see Chap. 11 of this text), it is well evident that the questions and problems that patients share arise from attitudes more typical of the consumer than those peculiar to the user. One must move to the world of devices-even simple ones-to begin to perceive behind the consumer object, the technical object, the object of use and thus the interest in the act of its conscious transformation.

14.6 Learning "Body Techniques" in Pharmaceutical Therapy

As we have seen, observing the acts of care by emphasizing the medicine as an object of use and not only of consumption allows space for considerations regarding the concreteness and materiality of medicines and the objects that accompany them, introducing learning to use also as an action with transformative potential.

The emphasis on use also allows us to bring to the forefront a different level of learning that concerns the "modes of action", the form and even the formality of practices (De Certeau 2001, p. 63) that involve the body in the acts of care. We note, in this regard, that operational postures, gestures, movements, skills and inabilities are nothing but "techniques of the body" that must be known and trained.

The notion of "techniques of the body" first appeared in 1936 in a paper by French anthropologist, sociologist and ethnologist Marcell Mauss (2017). By this expression, Mauss meant to refer to how men in different societies make use of their bodies, conforming to tradition. Mauss expands the traditional concept of technique, commonly associated with using instrumental goods and objects, by extending it to the body's practices, manners, gestures, postures, and attitudes. These, according to Mauss, are learned slowly, require forms of training that generally begin with observation of others and then require periods of trial and error. The ability to use the body and best perform specific tasks, is educated through observation and imitation of "concatenations" and "sequences of actions" performed successfully by others. The body, from childhood, is domesticated and trained to achieve individual performances, whether sports, military or domestic.

There is a process of "trial and error" that leads to the refinement of these technical skills, as can be seen in the child intent on learning the art of eating spaghetti using a tool, the fork, that requires training in its use that is by no means simple (La Cecla 2002).

Those of the body are modal techniques that are profoundly affected by social habits and customs (how to sit, hold an infant, walk, march, run, etc.) and by the way in which they are used. They do not necessarily involve using objects, but in those actions supported by objects, the body's techniques are modified according to the object so that "good manners" of use are learned. In turn, the object in use, refines itself, supporting missing physical skills.

Bodily techniques, as a common experience, also fully invest in caring for the body and its hygiene, so much so that they constitute an important part of training in medical and nursing practice.

In medical professions, body techniques developed for diagnostic and therapeutic purposes are the result of a long learning process. Just think of resuscitation techniques, clinical diagnostics involving manual interventions that can be performed in the presence and the absence of instruments. Similarly, the different forms of massage, finger pressure, reflexology, etc., belong to professionally trained body techniques (Ruffin 2011; Barrientos-Trigo et al. 2018).

Even in the nursing field, there is a long learning and training process to understand the correct use of medical objects, including medicines.

For example, we can refer to certain notions of nursing practice used in correctly administering eye drops, for which specific' body techniques have been developed that are mostly unknown to the patient (Fig. 14.5). Starting with basic hygiene rules: always clean your hands; never touch the eye drops spout and avoid touching the ocular surface with it so as not to injure the eye and/or contaminate the solution.

The vial should be shaken, and the nozzle should be brought closer to the underside of the eye by tilting the head back slightly. The drops must be instilled into the conjunctival sac by lowering the lower eyelid with the fingers. It is essential to observe the position of the fingers, which, by reducing the eyelid, act as a natural spacer for the hand. The latter rests on them, holding the eye drops bottle at the proper distance from the eye. The subsequent blinking of the eyelid allows the instilled drops to spread over the entire ocular surface. When the professional nurse carries out this practice, the lower eyelid is held down with the help of sterile gauze to ensure maximum hygiene.

Knowing these techniques would educate the patient in correct posture and gestures, so as not to tilt the head too far back—a position of severe discomfort,

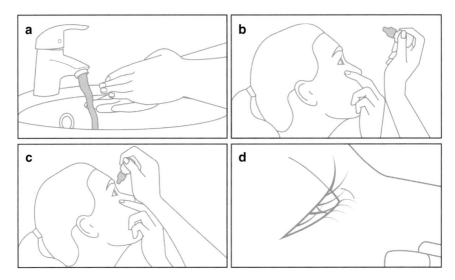

Fig. 14.5 Sequences of action for proper administration of an eye drop: (1) Make sure your hands are washed and dry before applying the product; (2) Sit down and tilt your chin upward. Look up and with two fingers of your nondominant hand gently lower your lower eyelid; (3) Rest your dominant hand (the one you use to write) on the wrist of your nondominant hand to give you more stability. At this point, squeeze the vial and apply a drop to your eye; (4) Close your eyes and blink a few times to distribute the drops all over the eye. (fonte: https://www.visiondirect.it/come-applicare-le-gocce-oculari)

especially for the elderly—, and not to raise the elbow beyond measure to reach with the vial to the eyes, an equally annoying action. Not only that. The erroneous assumption of having to rinse the ocular surface also induces the patient to seek the 'centring' of the eye with the spout exit hole, approaching and sometimes brushing against the ocular surface because the effort that must be exerted on the container and the precision required is difficult to reconcile.

The observation made on the use of eye drops (Fig. 14.6), not only in the elderly patient, showed that, precisely because of ignorance of its primary mode of use, almost all the patients observed are assisted by a third person; that all of them almost recline their heads entirely and, even, some assume the lying position. Conversely, among those who instil eye drops by themselves, some report that they feel safer resting the nozzle on the lower eyelid because, in this way, they can exert a stimulus that they think is more controlled than the impressibility of the drop. They report that this mode makes them more confident that the drops will reach the eye.

This example testifies how medicine administration practices, thought to be complex because of the posture required of the patient and the difficulties in handling the object, but thought to be evident from a 'how-to' point of view, lead to the wrong way of proceeding.

The sequence of actions that must be performed precisely, highlighting the need to know the most suitable body techniques, including prudence, mischief and tricks of the trade that, in the case of professional figures—such as nurses precisely—are

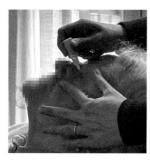 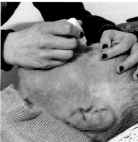 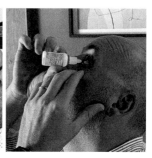

Fig. 14.6 Images of common positions assumed by patients in administration of eye drops and care giver gestures. From left: patient with head reclined backward and care giver behind her; patient lying down; self-administration of eye drops

the outcome of a process of training in use as well as experience gained in the profession in contact with 'masters' or rather with figures of experienced professionals who transmit knowledge validated by institutionalized practice. In the case of the patient, and vice versa, this learning process is the result, often, of forms of self-learning or knowledge learned in a non-professional context where learning through observation does not necessarily evolve the user-patient's knowledge from the *naïve* knowledge stage to the expert knowledge stage (Pizzocaro 2015).

That eye drops administration is just one example. Observation of users reveals that the taking of medicine has, from this point of view, knowledge gaps that do not find any useful reference to guide the patient in the correct positions and gestures. We could add other examples, such as opening glass vials, swallowing capsules, or tablets, injecting oneself, and even basic forms of dressing minor wounds. Actions that we perform in the home environment without a basic culture of care and its technicalities.

We have advanced a first reflection on these that concerns the fallacy of learning notions, modes of operation and forms of knowledge that are not validated because they are imparted and observed in a non-professional context.

We can add a second reflection here. Learning in practice, through the observation of others' gestures, presupposes not only the presence of an expert subject able to transmit knowledge—from the most routine gestures to the virtuosities of practical expertise—but also of a learner able to learn and to grasp, from the master's teaching, the tricks of the trade (Sennet 2009).

For example, awareness of what we learn from simple observation also informs the procedures for testing medicine packaging. Unlike the European ones, the U.S. procedures for testing whether they meet child-proof requirements explicitly require that the children watch the process of opening the pack, making them observe the gestures made by the adult (Code of Federal Regulations 1995) before placing the pack in their hands. This is done because one knows how silently children learn by observing others.

The transfer of knowledge through the form of familiarization occurs mostly silently. Automatisms, routines, and actions learned in daily life are frequently without explanation; they are built over time as quasi-obligatory acts, dispositions cultivated and become acquired habits. Like many of the activities learned by familiarization, then, also in the case of medicine, we are faced with a repertoire of choices, gestures, thought patterns and even beliefs and ideologies able to structure and shape procedures and sequences of actions that occur in a "quasi-automatic way" (Bordieu 2003, p. 207). In a learning context with these characteristics, the poor formal characterization of medicine does not help. It indeed risks leading the user to believe that the experience gained with one medicine can be reused, as is, with other typologically similar medicines.

14.7 Use Instructions in Pharmacological Therapy

Sennett again suggests language can play a relevant role in the passage of skills that takes place in implicit form through observation (2009). The possibility of accompanying gestures with spoken words, with the introduction of explanations, increases the effectiveness of the learning process (Sennet 2009).

But how much of our knowledge about the use of medicines is transmitted by observing the example and, even more, by keeping the example enriched by explanation? And how much of this knowledge is left instead to forms of transcription and translation of experience into the 'instructions for use' characteristic of the package leaflet that accompanies medicines? Suppose the form of familiarization, of 'getting acquainted' with the medicine through observing the experience of others, exposes us to a knowledge of practices that is not necessarily correct. In that case, translating treatment actions into the written form raises further problematic issues.

To refer again to Bordieu (2003, p. 185) "we can do things with words"; that is, we can make others perform actions through word. The issue, however, is not as peaceful as it may seem.

Sennett has dwelt at length on the problems language encounters when describing actions and giving directions as to how they should be performed.

> *Language is always in trouble when it has to describe physical actions, especially when it wants to give instructions. [...] we realize that a gap can exist between the language of instructions and the body. [...] Oral words seem to be more effective than written instructions. As soon as a procedure becomes difficult, we can immediately ask someone, discuss it, make objections. In contrast, when reading a printed page, we can yes reason about it with ourselves, but without the possibility of receiving confirmation, refutation, or correction from others[...]* (Sennet 2009, p. 174).

However, Sennet still reminds us that: "Oral dialogue tends to be messy and full of digressions" (*ibidem*).

The author concludes that "rather than excluding writing, the real challenge is to make written instructions become communicative: expressive instructions must be created" (*ibidem*).

The shift from descriptive to prescriptive language, just as the change from declarative to procedural language, requires skilful management of rhetorical expedients, verbal and visual, able to make a text expressive.

After all, the complex system of information-peritests (Genette 1997) carried on the primary packaging, secondary packaging, and package leaflet confronts us with forms of communication that have the arduous task of verbally explaining even complicated procedures. These explanations suffer issues relating to the translation process (Nergaard 1995; Osimo 2015; Baule and Caratti 2016) and, specifically, to what they are required to explain by way of text descriptions: actions, gestures, and procedures, often involving components of tacit knowledge (Polanyi 1979). These prescriptive forms also suffer the issue of inert denotation (Sennet 2009), a form of writing in which the language, mode of expression and type of information are only comprehensible and useful to an expert user or one who already has experience with such procedures.

Finally, in these texts, there is a strong unbalance between the negative description of the many adverse effects the medicine might cause versus the benefits, liquidated in a few lines, with few references to data on efficacy in reducing or treating symptoms/disease, and with little attention to providing the descriptive comfort of the signs that should herald the hoped-for well-being-as a counterbalance to the long lists of adverse effects (Penati et al. 2021).

Particularly, anyone who has had even superficial experience with information tools to guide the user in the proper management of medicine knows how much distrust patients show towards the Package Leaflet. It is assigned to convey to the user the "good practices" of medicine use. First and foremost, its effectiveness is measured in its ability to attract the user's attention, entice him to read it, and precisely avoid initiating do-it-yourself practices.

And instead, among the most recurrent feelings detected in our analysis, also supported by literature data (McIntosh and Shaw 2003; Herber et al. 2014; Webster et al. 2017) there is a real aversion to reading the Package Leaflet. Many patients interviewed say the preponderant description of side effects intimates them compared to the illustration of the benefits of taking a medicine. Equally significant, especially among the elderly, is the percentage of those who do not consider it necessary to read the P.L., trusting the information provided by the doctor. Among the reasons why patients do not read the package leaflet, we find reading difficulties due to too small a font; difficulty in tracing the contents deemed necessary; and difficulty in understanding the language used to give the information.

So that careful reading of the package leaflet is typical of patients wary of medicines in general and of multi-drug patients who fear the adverse effects of drug interactions or those caused by taking a medicine on organs affected by other diseases. The package leaflet also presents itself as an overly complex tool because it concentrates, at the same time, information of a different nature: it is partly indications for which use is recommended; partly warnings about possible side effects, about risks to be faced in case of non-use or excessive intake; and partly clues about what to do to store, prepare, take, dispose of, and report adverse events. Added to this layering of information is the plurality of referents to whom the information is addressed: the doctor, the pharmacist, and the patient. The specialized language used, far removed from the patient's knowledge and understanding abilities, tend to favour the first two. This rhetoric remains unchanged and treats information, instructions, and recommendations similarly.

In this complex communicative universe, "explanation"—understood as a communicative helpful mode to justify a fact, to make its reasons understood—is almost entirely omitted.

Even the languages—verbal and nonverbal (texts, legends, captions, sayings, pictograms, illustrations, etc.)—are not very "expressive" (Sennet 2009) for patient learning of proper care practices.

14.8 Observing the User in Care: Openings and Perspectives

The chapter has tried to identify in some theoretical assumptions the references to frame and interpret a set of behaviours observed in users taking medicines in a spontaneous context of action, such as the family context. Chapter 15 describes some concrete experiences that represent, in their prosaicity, common behaviours or singular practices of patients that bring us closer to what we can call a phenomenology of home care. On those pages, we will find many forms of personalization of the pharmaceutical product, through the integration of information added by the user; through manipulations of the medicine and its packaging; through the introduction, in the sphere of care, of domestic practices transferred from contiguous contexts; using repurposed objects to adjuvate the management of therapy, etc.

We conceptualized these various activities as forms of learning, particularly as: learning by using; learning by doing; learning from experience. We have defined the boundary of effectiveness and the critical issues inherent in such practices. We find ourselves here arguing that if the user accesses the medicine directly without bothering to read and follow the information in the package leaflet, it is probably because we are dealing with a communication artefact that is not very accessible and has inappropriate persuasive features. In this, the domestic context, we reiterate, lends itself to informality in use, deviation from rules, and using 'shortcuts' as a form of the domestic economy of time management. With all the limitations most identified above, this is why *do-it-yourself* and *learning from experience* become the mode most followed by the patient. In care processes, one of the most recurring elements in learning from experience is the role that error (Metcalfe 2017) plays in patients' actions. In acquiring knowledge through experience, committing, recognizing, and overcoming error (Rafter et al. 2015a, Rafter et al. b) constitutes a significant aspect. The limits of our past experiences, the limitations and fallacy of the senses, the limits of our physical and intellectual capacities, the rules in recognizing unconsciously made errors, and the inadequacy of our memory processes or cognitive inadequacies, are just some of the elements that intervene in the relationship between user and object, in the act of use, leading us to commit or renew errors in the management and proper intake of therapy. It is interesting to point out how the types of errors in our interaction with objects, change according to our knowledge of the object and the stage of the cycle of use in which we interact with the object. We have:

- errors generated by expectations, pre-judgments, or anticipations that we express concerning the medicine even before the initiation of therapy;
- first-use errors sometimes related to misuse of the object;
- errors associated with the disposal of the object;
- errors that occur when restarting a therapy carried out previously;
- errors of the neophyte who does not read the instructions for use and errors of those who have accumulated experience and take medicines without proper precautions;
- errors that occur in the complex actions of management that require the ability to organize, sequence, and schedule the acts of care, procurement of medicines, etc.

The point of view of those who propose error, failure, and *defaillance*, as a fertile ground of analysis for the project, gives importance to behaviours in a state of discomfort, for example, when we are faced for the first time with a problem or a new object whose ways and purposes of use we struggle to understand, or when we use the object in contexts other than the usual one, or in contexts that do not guarantee proper privacy. Putting the error at the centre of the focus of observation allows us to give evidence to the errors peculiar to the subject, the behaviour, abilities, and previous use experiences. But it also allows us to highlight errors induced by the object, its form, deficiencies that define its identity, its ability to communicate and inform, etc. Trained observation of the user, in direct interaction with the object, is an effective way to detect both types of errors.

The observation testifies to how deficient the patient's education in grappling with the treatment techniques is. Also, it shows that the only interface between a complex knowledge system and the patient remains the Medicine Leaflet, a tool most often underestimated or deliberately avoided by the user.

At the University of Maryland School of Pharmacy's Experiential Learning Program, students were involved in an experiment that followed a group of patients struggling with complex forms of drug therapy. The problem most frequently encountered was the lack of therapeutic adherence due to different causes: some dependent on the patient's organisational inability to procure supplies of the depleting medicine in time, others due to technically inappropriate administration; still others related to a suspension decided autonomously by the patient due to the onset of adverse effects or the remission of symptoms for which treatment had been initiated, etc. Pharmacy students were solicited to find a way to remedy the problems encountered. From this experience, 233 documents were drafted in the form of recommendations to introduce 'care education', emphasising correct habits and lifestyles, techniques of appropriate medicine taking, use of aids and adjuvants, etc. (Agness et al. 2011).

On the part of those who design and produce medicines, the study testifies to the critical realisation of how much knowledge the act of medicine treatment needs and how much the patient is lacking because, to date, there are no information tools whose purpose is to educate the patient about treatment as much as instructions for the use of the medicine.

At the same time, approaching the patient to grasp his areas of discomfort is, for the pharma industry, a signal of the shift toward a user culture; a shift already widely addressed by other industries in other commodity sectors and other markets (Sahlsten et al. 2008). The pharmaceutical industry, which is strongly tied to a model of innovation based on science and technology and thus centred on in-house R&D activities (Hara 2003), is struggling to engage the new paradigm initiated a few decades ago in other manufacturing contexts in which users play an active role as bearers of knowledge derived from experience (Baldwin and von Hippel 2011).

The pharma industry's openness to the outside world and the world of users has a long tradition in pharmaceutical product testing processes, as new products undergo lengthy clinical research processes, in which the cooperation of users is required, helpful in providing the necessary information to regulatory authorities (Fylan et al. 2021).

Conversely, user involvement as an active resource, capable of communicating and making expendable information and knowledge based on their daily experience, is less frequent and, in most cases, needs the intervention of professionals—such as physicians, pharmacists, engineers, and technicians—to act as intermediaries (Caron-Flinterman et al. 2005).

For instance, this is the case in activities aimed at testing the functioning of a device in the phase of making new prototypes or in their further development and refinement, but also in the improvement processes that take place in the stages following development, such as market launch.

However, if in clinical research activities aimed at verifying the efficacy of a new active ingredient, or in those of medical device engineering, the user has found its own space for intervention with codified methodologies and protocols, what is still lacking, on the other hand, is the ability to accommodate the feedback on the processes of drug design and its use, deriving from everyday experiences, from the customisation interventions implemented by patients to adapt the objects of treatment to their physical and cognitive capacities.

Closing the chapter, let us add a dutiful notation on the distinction between the many activities to improve products—and medicinal products—carried out by patients and which find room for reflection in the literature. In them, we find:

- Observations on the interaction between patient and medicine focused on difficulties of use. These are observations often made on a specific product or type and are aimed at highlighting critical aspects of the form-function relationship of the object (one example among all the difficulties of opening by the elderly patient of child proof medicines) (Lorenzini and Hellström 2017);
- Patient-user involvement in new product testing activities (Kaufman et al. 2003; Jaspers 2009);
- Patient involvement in design and R&D activities through co-design practices (Donetto et al. 2014).
- The perspective that, conversely, we have proposed in this section of the book is little found in the literature because it aims to observe the practices of improving care with medicines, choosing as a privileged point of observation the domestic space as a place able to:
- Modifying the nature of medicine by normalising it, bringing it back to the habits of use that one has with other everyday objects;
- Offering objects, processes, and prior experiences drawn from the management of the practices of everyday domestic life and transferred to the relationship of use with medicines;
- Bypassing norms, rules of use, prescriptions, and warnings (formulated not to compromise the patient's health), with the exceptions, liberties, and personal manners with which we do things in the 'free zone' that is our home.

As we wait for the pharma industry to fully accomplish the shift to open innovation as well, fully involving patients in the process of designing, testing, and verifying new products after their use in the home dimension, a new sensibility needs to be cultivated, restoring importance to direct observation of the daily reality of care, with the apparent simplicity of objects generating complex processes and procedures. In an industry where economies of production dominate, as medicine packaging is, more significant contact with processes of use could become the spring of innovation in a field that, on the surface, seems to have nothing new to invent.

References

Agness CF, Huynh D, Brandt N (2011) Instructional design and assessment: an introductory pharmacy practice experience based on a medication therapy management service model. Am J Pharm Educ 75(5):1–9. Retrieved February, 15, 2023 from https://www.ajpe.org/content/75/5/82

Amin A, Roberts J (2008) Knowing in action: beyond communities of practice. Res Policy 37(2):353–369

Baldwin CY, von Hippel E (2011) Modeling a paradigm shift: from producer innovation to user and open collaborative innovation. Organ Sci 22(6):1399–1417

Barrientos-Trigo S, Vega-Vázquez L, De Diego-Cordero R, Badanta-Romero B, Porcel-Gálvez AM (2018) Interventions to improve working conditions of nursing staff in acute care hospitals: scoping review. J Nurs Manag 26:94–107

Baule G, Caratti E (2016) Design è traduzione. Il paradigma traduttivo per la cultura del progetto [Design is translation. The translation paradigm for the culture of design. "Design and translation": a manifesto]. FrancoAngeli, Milano

Berge TT, Hezewijk R (1999) Procedural and declarative knowledge. An evolutionary perspective. Theor Psychol 9(5):605–624

Blumberg P (2009) Maximizing learning through course alignment and experience with different types of knowledge. Innov High Educ 34(2):93–103

Bordieu P (2003) Per una teoria della pratica. Con Tre studi di etnologia cabila. Raffaello Cortina, Milano. (Esquisse d'une théorie de la pratique précédé de Trois études d'ethnologie kabyle (1972). Paris: Editions du Seuil)

Boud D, Cohen R, Walker D (eds) (1993) Using experience for learning. Open University Press, Bristol

Browall M, Koinberg I, Falk H, Wijk H (2013) Patients' experience of important factors in the healthcare environment in oncology care. Int J Qual Stud Health Well-being 6(8) Retrieved January, 7, 2023 from https://doi.org/10.3402/qhw.v8i0.20870

Bruner J (2001) Language, culture and self. Sage Publication, California

Carlsson-Wall M, Kraus K, Lind J (2011) The interdependencies of intra- and inter-organisational controls and work practices-the case of domestic care of the elderly. Manag Account Res 22:313–329

Caron-Flinterman JF, Broerse JE, Bunders JF (2005) The experiential knowledge of patients: a new resource for biomedical research? Soc Sci Med J 60(11):2575–2584. https://doi.org/10.1016/j.socscimed.2004.11.023

Ceruti M (1995) Evoluzione senza fondamenti [Evolution without foundation]. Laterza, Roma-Bari

Chanel FA, Huynh D, Brandt N (2011) An introductory pharmacy practice experience based on a medication therapy management service model. Am J Pharm Educ 75(5):1–8

Code of Federal Regulations (1995) Part 1700—Poison prevention packaging. Retrieved April 14, 2023 from https://www.ecfr.gov/current/title-16/chapter-II/subchapter-E/part-1700

Connor S (2014) Effetti personali. Vite curiose di oggetti quotidiani. Raffaello Cortina Editore, Milano. (Paraphernalia: the curious lives of magical things. 2011. London: Profile Books)

Crossley N (2001) The phenomenological habitus and its construction. Theory Soc 30(1):81–120

Crossley N (2007) Researching embodiment by way of 'body techniques'. Sociol Rev 55(s1):80–94. Retrieved by https://journals.sagepub.com/doi/10.1111/j.1467-954X.2007.00694.x

De Certeau M (2001) L'invenzione del quotidiano. EdizioniLavoro, Roma. (L'invention du quotidien. Arts de faire (1990). Paris: Èditions Gallimard)

de Jong JPJ, von Hippel E (2009) Transfers of user process innovations to process equipment producers: a study of Dutch high-tech firms. Res Policy 38(7):1181–1191

Denham SA (2003) Relationships between family rituals, family routines, and health. J Fam Nurs 9(3):305–330

Donetto S, Tsianakas V, Robert G (2014) Using experience-based co-design to improve the quality of healthcare: mapping where we are now and establishing future directions. King's College London, London. Retrieved March, 8, 2023 from https://www.researchgate.net/publication/262198403_Using_Experience-based_Co-design_EBCD_to_improve_the_quality_of_healthcare_mapping_where_we_are_now_and_establishing_future_directions

Echeverri P, Skålén P, Hjalmarson H, Gäre BA, Svensson H, Henriks G, Hellström A, Elg M (2013). Patient involvement for service innovation - An agenda for research and innovation in healthcare and social service. Service Research Center, Karlstad University. Retrieved from https://www.kau.se/ctf/involve

Ferrarotti F (1986) La storia e il quotidiano. Laterza, Bari

Fiese BH (2007) Routines and rituals: opportunities for participation in family health. Occup Ther J Res 27(Supplement):41S–49S

Franke N, Shah S (2003) How communities support innovative activities: an exploration of assistance and sharing among end-users. Res Policy 32(1):157–178

Franke N, von Hippel E, Schreier M (2006) Finding commercially attractive user innovations: A test of lead user theory. J Prod Innov Manag 23(4):301–315

Freeman R (2007) Epistemological bricolage. How practitioners make sense of learning. Admin Soc 39(4):476–496

Fylan B, Tomlinson J, Raynor DK, Silcock J (2021) Using experience-based co-design with patients, carers and healthcare professionals to develop theory-based interventions for safer medicines use. Res Soc Adm Pharm 17:2127–2135

Genette G (1997) Soglie. I dintorni del testo. Einaudi, Torino. (Paratexts. Thresholds of interpretation). (1989). Cambridge NY: Cambridge University Press)

Gherardi S, Nicolini D (2001) Il pensiero pratico. Un'etnografia dell'apprendimento. Rassegna Italiana di Sociologia XLII(2):231–256

Grabowski H (2003) Patents and new product development in the pharmaceutical and biotechnology industries. Georget Pub Pol Rev 8(2):7–23

Hao J, Ya-ting S, Ling-ling S (2017) Understanding innovation mechanism through the lens of communities of practice. Technol Forecast Soc Chang 118:205–212

Hara T (2003) Innovation in the pharmaceutical industry: the process of drug discovery and development. Edward Elgar Publications, Northampton

Herber OR, Gies V, Schwappach D, Thürmann P, Wilm S (2014) Patient information leaflets: informing or frightening? A focus group study exploring patients' emotional reactions and subsequent behavior towards package leaflets of commonly prescribed medications in family practices. BMC Fam Pract 15(163):1–8. Retrieved April 2, 2023 from http://www.biomedcentral.com/1471-2296/15/163

Holt K (1988) The role of the user in product innovation. Technovation 7(3):249–258

Jaspers MW (2009) A comparison of usability methods for testing interactive health technologies: methodological aspects and empirical evidence. Int J Med Inform 78(5):340–353

Jeppesen LB, Laursenb K (2009) The role of lead users in knowledge sharing. Res Policy 38(10):1582–1589

Joyce SR, Craig B (2011) Methodological bricolage–what does it tell us about design? Northumbria University Press, New Castle. Retrieved April, 3, 2023 from Northumbria Research Link: http://nrl.northumbria.ac.uk/id/eprint/8822/

Katila R, Thatchenkery S, Christensen MQ, Zenios S (2018) Is there a doctor in the house? Expert product users, organizational roles, and innovation. Acad Manag J 60(6):1–51. retrieved from https://www.researchgate.net/publication/312508713_Is_There_a_Doctor_in_the_House_Expert_Product_Users_Organizational_Roles_and_Innovation

Kaufman DR, Patel VL, Hilliman C, Morin PC, Pevzner J, Weinstock RS, Goland R, Shea S, Starren J (2003) Usability in the real world: assessing medical information technologies in patients' homes. J Biomed Inform 36(1–2):45–60

Kerr P (2016) Adaptive learning. ELT J 70(1):88–93

Kolb DA (1984) Experience as the source of learning and development. Prentice Hall, Upper Sadle River

La Cecla F (2002) La pasta e la pizza [Pasta and Pizza]. Il Mulino, Bologna

Lau RWK (2004) Habitus and the practical logic of practice: an interpretation. Open Univ Hong Kong Sociol 38(2):369–387

Lévi-Strauss C (1966) The savage mind. University of Chicago Press, Chicago

Marchis V (2017) Storia delle cose—history of things. Retrieved April, 26, 2023 from http://storiadellecose.blogspot.com/2017/11/il-pensieroselvaggio-e-il-bricolage.html

Mauss M (2017) Le tecniche del corpo. Edizioni ETS, Pisa. (Les Techniques du Corps). (1936). *Journal de psychologie, XXXII*(3-4)

McIntosh A, Shaw C (2003) Barriers to patient information provision in primary care: patients' and general practitioners' experiences and expectations of information for low back pain. Health Expect 6:19–29

McLaughlin H (2008) What's in a name: 'client', 'patient', 'customer', 'consumer', 'expert by experience', 'service user'. What's next? Br J Soc Work 39:1101–1117

Metcalfe J (2017) Learning from errors. Annu Rev Psychol 68:465–489

Mortari L (2003) Apprendere dall'esperienza: il pensare riflessivo nella formazione. Carocci editore, Milano

Nergaard S (ed) (1995) Teorie contemporanee della traduzione [Contemporary theories of translation]. Bompiani, Milano

Oliveira P, Zejnilovic L, Canhão H, von Hippel E (2015) Innovation by patients with rare diseases and chronic needs. Orphanet J Rare Dis 10(41):e1–e9. https://doi.org/10.1186/s13023-015-0257-2

Osimo B (2015) Manuale del traduttore, 3rd edn. Hoepli. (Manual for the interpreter), Milano

Palen L, Aaløkke S (2006) Pill boxes and piano benches: "home-made" methods for managing medication. Comput Supported Coop Work 6:79–88. https://doi.org/10.1145/1180875.1180888

Penati A, Pizzocaro S, Standoli CE, Iannilli VM (2021) The shape of drugs: a matter of human-centred design. Design culture(s) conference, cumulus conference proceedings, Rome, pp 1364–1375

Pizzocaro S (2015) Introduzione agli studi sull'utente. Conoscere gli utenti tra ricerca e design dei prodotti. Edizioni Unicopli, Milano

Pizzocaro S, Penati A (2021) The in-home use of medications: in pursuit of design-driven knowledge. Home Cult 17(3):153–171

Polanyi M (1979) La conoscenza inespressa. Armando Editore, Roma. (The tacit dimension. (1966). Chicago: The University of Chicago Press)

Rafter N, Hickey A, Condell S, Conroy R, o'Connor P, Vaughan D, Williams D (2015a) Adverse events in healthcare: learning from mistakes. Q J Med 108(4):273–277. https://doi.org/10.1093/qjmed/hcu145

Rafter N, Hickey A, Condell S, Conroy R, O'Connor P, Vaughan D, Williams D (2015b) Adverse events in healthcare: learning from mistakes. Int J Med 108:273–277. https://doi.org/10.1093/qjmed/hcu145. Advance Access Publication 30 July 2014

Reay D (2004) It's all becoming a habitus': beyond the habitual use of habitus in educational research. Br J Sociol Educ 25(4):431–444

Rosenberg N (2001) Dentro la scatola nera. il Mulino, Bologna. (Inside the black box (1983). Cambridge: Cambridge University Press)

Roth WM, Jornet A (2014) Toward a theory of experience. Sci Educ 98(1):106–126

Ruffin PT (2011) A history of massage in nurse training school curricula (1860–1945). J Holist Nurs 29(1):61–67

Sahlsten MJ, Larsson IE, Sjostrom B, Plos KA (2008) An analysis of the concept of patient participation. Nurs Forum 43(1):2–11

Sennet R (2009) L'uomo artigiano, 3rd edn. Feltrinelli, Milano. (The craftsman. (2009). New Haven & London: Yale University press)

Shaw B (1998) Innovation and new product development in the UK medical equipment industry. Int J Technol Manag 15(3–5):433–445

Smits R, Boon W (2008) The role of users in innovation in the pharmaceutical industry. Drug Discov Today 13(7–8):353–359

Tagliagambe S (1997) Epistemologia del confine. Il Saggiatore, Milano. (Epistemology of the border)

Thomdyke PW, Haves-Roth B (1979) The use of schemata in the acquisition and transfer of knowledge. Cogn Psychol 11(1):82–106

Trigo A (2016) Innovation in the era of experience: the changing role of users in healthcare innovation. J Entrep Manag Innov 12(2):29–52

von Hippel E (1976) The dominant role of users in the scientific instrument innovation process. Res Policy 5:212–239

von Hippel E (1986) Lead users: a source of novel product concepts. Manag Sci 32:791–805

Webster RK, Weinman J, Rubin JG (2017) People's understanding of verbal risk descriptors in patient information leaflets: a cross-sectional national survey of 18-to 65-year-olds in England. Drug Saf J 40:743–754

Wenger E (2006) Comunità di pratica. Apprendimento, significato e identità. Raffaello Cortina, Milano. (Communities of practice: learning, meaning and identity. (1998). Cambridge, NY: Cambridge University Press)

Open Access This chapter is licensed under the terms of the Creative Commons Attribution 4.0 International License (http://creativecommons.org/licenses/by/4.0/), which permits use, sharing, adaptation, distribution and reproduction in any medium or format, as long as you give appropriate credit to the original author(s) and the source, provide a link to the Creative Commons license and indicate if changes were made.

The images or other third party material in this chapter are included in the chapter's Creative Commons license, unless indicated otherwise in a credit line to the material. If material is not included in the chapter's Creative Commons license and your intended use is not permitted by statutory regulation or exceeds the permitted use, you will need to obtain permission directly from the copyright holder.

Chapter 15
Use Phenomenologies. Observing the User While Taking Pharmaceutical Therapies

Antonella Valeria Penati

Abstract As introduced in Chap. 14, the notes below take the Farb Research (University Funds for Basic Research) *Care for Care—Shaping medicines: a question of Identity, Use and Communication* as their starting point. In the previous chapters, we have presented some points of view in which the discipline of design can contribute through a theoretical-critical analysis of the culture of medicine use. In this chapter, we present the outcomes of the observational activity. For three consecutive years, in addition to the research team, it involved classes from the *Metadesign* and *Visual Elements Studios* of the School of Design at Politecnico di Milano. Students were trained to detect the behaviour of patients—their grandparents—while dealing with drug therapy in their home contexts. These outcomes provided an initial basis for corroborating theoretical reflection and were supplemented by an analysis of the research group activities from a design perspective. A perspective that focuses on the formal aspects of objects, on the relationships established between subjects and objects—namely between patient and medicine—, and on the role that the context of use plays in shaping this relationship. The chapter reports reflections derived from observation activities.

15.1 Methodological Notes

Approximately 250 patients were observed in the naturalness of gestures done within the home and in the use of medicines, as it happens in the normality of their daily lives. In the first phase, observers—students as grandchildren—were asked to spend a day with their grandparents without using notation tools or asking questions, but just observing and participating/collaborating in the action where required. The non-intrusive observation made it possible to verify the patients' genuine behaviours and to informally collect the feelings, discomforts, and difficulties that—especially the elderly—encounter in the daily management of therapy.

A. V. Penati (✉)
Department of Design, Politecnico di Milano, Milan, Italy
e-mail: antonella.penati@polimi.it

© The Author(s) 2025
A. V. Penati (ed.), *In-Home Medication*, Research for Development,
https://doi.org/10.1007/978-3-031-53294-8_15

In a second moment, observation continued through the collection of photographic images, videos, questionnaires, and interviews to capture the habits of grandparents' habits in sometimes managing complex therapies. The student's familiarity with the daily life of the grandparent—the object of observation—facilitated the study, making it possible to avoid those states of subjection that can sometimes condition the observed user, causing them to change their behaviour patterns. Analyzing the behavioural customs used in managing care in detail was possible.

From the methodological point of view, the domestic space was defined as the research context, noting how this milieu explicitly influences the construction of behaviours, habits, and rituals. In other words, the domestic, familiar milieu brings out, more than places where formal action is required, some peculiarities of people's natural behaviours in their everyday relationship with medicines (Denham 2003) (on this aspect, see Chap. 14).

The focus was confined to the world of elderly people, both because of the greater physical, manipulative, cognitive, and sensory difficulties that are peculiar to patients in this age group because it is more common in the elderly patient to have to attend to complex therapy for a long time, and because frequently being alone makes the task of care more complex (Gellad et al. 2011; Lonsdale and Baker 2013; Lu et al. 2020). The information gathered through this analysis has fostered reflection on how the process of understanding and interpreting information related to medicine and its intake occurs, and on the processes of adapting the system of objects, which contribute to medicine care, carried out by people also to remedy the lack of indications, their difficulty in understanding or in making an object more familiar to the home context, or again, to personalize standardized information by adapting it to the user's information needs.

Below, we show the outcomes of this observational activity, with the support of visual notations: these are mainly photographic shots that describe the behaviours of users who, within their homes, interact with medicines in their different typologies, caught in the performance of therapy management activities. The images are not intended to capture characteristics of individual medicines, but simply the use that users make of them once the medicine enters the sphere of everyday actions. Difficulties in use are highlighted, noting how common it is for medicines to be taken based on users' customs and beliefs rather than on the directions provided by pharmaceutical companies. The observational activity was supplemented by reading the formal characters of some typologies of medicines, chosen from those that were most frequently found to be in use among the sample of people surveyed. An analysis that, in part, brings to bear the object-the medicine, its packaging and the informational texts that are supposed to facilitate its understanding and proper intake-some of the critical issues detected.

Although we have encountered many different pharmaceutical forms in this survey activity, we limit our interest in the next two chapters (Chaps. 16 and 17) to the elements that appeared to us to be most relevant:

- secondary packaging, which is present in all pharmaceutical packaging;

- blister tablets, which are the most widely used pharmaceutical form in the treatment of elderly patients observed in the present study.

To these we preface this opening chapter, which focuses on the reading of the behaviour of use and interaction with the medicine-object, concentrating on the techniques of organisation, preparation and the techniques used to remember the deadlines for therapy.

15.2 Methodological Notes

Approximately 250 patients were observed in the naturalness of gestures done within the home and in the use of medicines, as it happens in the normality of their daily lives. In the first phase, observers—students as grandchildren—were asked to spend a day with their grandparents without using notation tools or asking questions, but just observing and participating/collaborating in the action where required.

Direct observation, collected through written notations, photo, interviews, etc., reconstructs the wide repertoire of organizational techniques, ways of preparing for therapy, and expedients that each user prepares to "make room" for medication and welcome it among the normal activities of daily life; to prepare doses and prepare for daily intake; to "have memory" of times, dates, and deadlines for therapy. We have tried to separate these three different activities for expository convenience, even though unravelling the interweaving that governs them may sometimes be a necessary stretch for narrative purposes alone.

15.2.1 Organization

This observation's first element of interest concerns the medicines' disposal in the home environment. Different logics can be detected, governing how medicines are arranged/placed. Logics overlap and find, in some cases, novel solutions, even if they are not always adequate to guarantee the safety that therapy management requires.

The restitution of individual solutions, presented as case studies, confirms to a large extent, and complements with the vividness typical of primary sources, what we have found from the literature (see Chap. 13 of this text). They confirm that, in the home setting, there is no real place designated for medicines. Therefore, the adopted solutions result from very personal arrangements and logic. Despite this, it is possible to observe the recurrence of specific behaviours of use of the home's environments, spaces, and furniture.

The first organizational mode, which we find mainly in managing elderlies' home therapies, can be traced back to the situation in which only one person of the couple is autonomous (and thus is also responsible for the spouse's therapy). It is a mode that gives rise to different organizational behaviours than when both can independently control their therapy. In the first case, the sharing of a single space under the direction of the person administering it is prevalent: it may be a drawer allocated for this use, a cabinet, or a shelf, with internal divisions sometimes improvised, sometimes studied instead even managed with dedicated containers (Fig. 15.1). We can find there improper and imperfect partitions, in some cases occasioned by a fortuitous initial occasion that later became a formalized orderly structure: a pen (an example of an object lent to the use of a partition) marks the space intended for the medicines taken by the husband from that intended for the wife's medicines; simple rubber bands group the medicines of two different patients; small re-sealable transparent bags, in some cases with the patient's name indicated; containers discarded from their primary use (ice cream boxes, shoe boxes, wicker baskets, etc.) or containers acquired ad hoc to divide the medicines of different patients (Figs. 15.2 and 15.3). In many cases, the simple right/left (or under/over) convention perimeters the therapy space of two distinct subjects.

In this case, probably also because of a sense of responsibility to others, one can read an order in the use of the space devoted to therapy that is unlikely to be found when each person organizes their own home dispensary.

When people manage therapy independently, they tend to organize their own distinct space, the order of which reflects the individual's personality, their needs, the importance they assign to treatment and, in many cases, the severity of the pathology. Neat forms of organization accompanied by notations on daily dosage are generally used by patients with severe pathology who must pay some attention to compliance with dosages, schedules, and intake frequencies (Fig. 15.4). In the case of individual spaces, however, disorder and lack of dispositional logic prevail (Fig. 15.5).

In self-organization, especially when therapy is not particularly demanding, there is a recurrent practice of identifying places in the house where to place medicines with a tendency to take advantage of residual spaces that are "colonized" with medicines (Fig. 15.6).

Just as worthy of interest is how user-patients derive in the home context, spaces reserved for medicines and therapy. These spaces, sometimes resorting to the

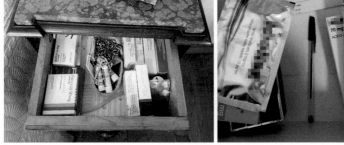
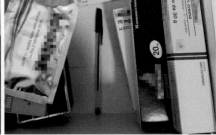

Fig. 15.1 Medicines from two different patients (husband and wife) stored neatly in drawers. Internal division is achieved with improper objects (pen, rosary beads, etc.) 'lent for use'

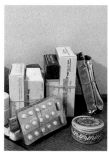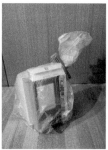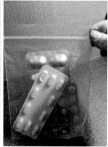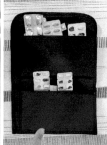

Fig. 15.2 Medicines of different patients separated by simple rubber bands or placed in individual bags or in document holders with multiple pockets

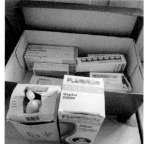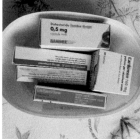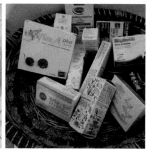

Fig. 15.3 Containers disused from their original function used for medicines: shoe boxes, ice cream boxes, Christmas wicker baskets, etc

'rhetoric' conveyed by expedients such as the use of placemats, doilies, and trays, are framed to conventionally separate the space of care from that intended for other practices (Fig. 15.7). These physical frames are also frames of meaning. They draw a cognitive and behavioural threshold of access to the moment of care.

The medicines' disposal in the home setting can also follow the logic of connection with different rooms (kitchen, bathroom, bedroom) where, generally, a relationship can be detected between where medicines are kept and the room in which they are consumed. An equally used principle in the arrangement of medicines is to keep them close to specific activities that need to be performed. This is a popular 'memory technique', as we will analyze later.

A second organizational level overlaps with the previous one, making it more articulated. This second level is related to the timing of medicine intake throughout the day. In complex therapies, consisting of many medicines, the tendency, unless specific prescriptions related to medicine characteristics, is to ingest the medicines at the same time as the three main meals: breakfast, lunch, and dinner. Although contemporary lifestyles no longer cadence, so categorically, the day around meals—particularly the noon meal—it is also true that the association between food and drug therapy has more than one reason. Not only are meals spaced by regular intervals that make the distribution of therapy throughout the day rational but there is

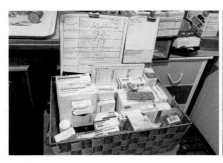
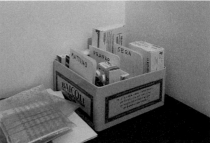

Fig. 15.4 Multifunctional generic containers used by the patient for orderly storage of therapy. In the photo on the left, the patient adapted the container for use by equipping it with a 'bulletin board' containing information necessary for the correct intake of therapy. On the right, the container space was divided by the user to distinguish morning medicines from noon medicines from evening medicines

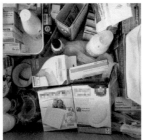
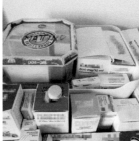
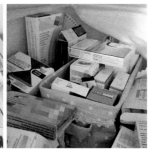

Fig. 15.5 Direct observation of different behaviour and ways to store medicines at home. In the prevailing clutter, it is possible to identify 'dedicated spaces' for individual therapy, separated from the 'overall population' of medicines using containers that 'cut out' even visually, a 'place' for autonomous management. In the left figure, we also notice, the intermingling of medicines; "small medication" products (e.g., bandages, gauze, disinfectants, band-aids); rolls of scotch tape enclosed in bags. In the central figure, next to the container with individual morning therapy, we find medicines, for occasional use (for joint pain, sore throat etc.) used by the whole family. However, there are also medicines that complement the individual therapy (eye drops, medicines in sachets, medicines in bottles etc.) that are separated from the rest of the daily therapy because their bulkiness, the obligatory vertical direction for liquid containers, do not allow them to fit inside the container (a former ice cream box) of the individual therapy. Finally, in the picture on the right, we again notice in the disorderly way the medicines are kept a basket that neatly isolates the group of medicines that make up the patient's daily therapy

also a close connection between the intake of a given active ingredient and the need for it to occur on a full or empty stomach. There is also an incentive in connecting therapy with meals and it is related to the activation of associative memory mechanisms, which, as is well known, make it possible to remember to accomplish specific actions if they are associated with others that, regardless of their importance, occur because they are part of daily habits. The distribution of medicines, according to the times they are taken, is often indicated by notations on the main package,

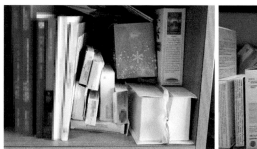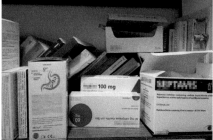

Fig. 15.6 Individual therapies arranged by exploiting interstitial spaces in the home context

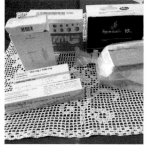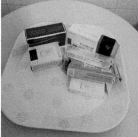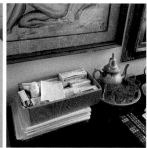

Fig. 15.7 A doily used as a placemat to welcome therapy but also as a frame of meaning for a space 'other' than the context. Similarly, trays and containers accommodate the objects of care, domesticating them to the spaces of everyday life

sub-groupings obtained with signs of the same colour, or internal partitions in drawers, cabinets, etc. From the point of view of "organizational techniques", it is interesting to note that where a medicine is to be taken several times during the day, several users arrange multiple packages of the same medicine, one for each scheduled intake. Indeed, this mode seems more effective than the equally used mode of keeping a single pack with a notation of the different intake times. In many cases, daily calendars can be found next to the therapies. In some cases, these calendars are designed for weekly use of the therapy so that the patient can 'visit' the boxes with a pen to indicate (sometimes to their children) that they have taken medicine.

A further distinction in the arrangement of medicines relates to those "in use" versus stocks, which are generally kept separate (Fig. 15.8).

Medicines in use tend to be located close to the user, accessible or even in visible places. At the same time, supplies are most often stored elsewhere, including in secondary or inaccessible places in the home, such as closets and storerooms (Fig. 15.9). The placement of occasional-use medicines (cough syrups, antibiotics, painkillers, medicines for constipation or diarrhoea, etc.), which tend not to be kept together with medicines that are part of stable therapies nor, once the need for taking them is over, do they end up together with the stock medicines, deserves a note.

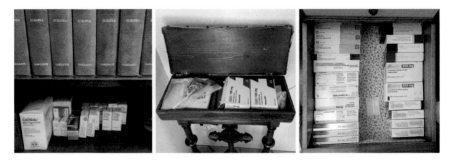

Fig. 15.8 Medicine stocks are kept in separate spaces from those in use

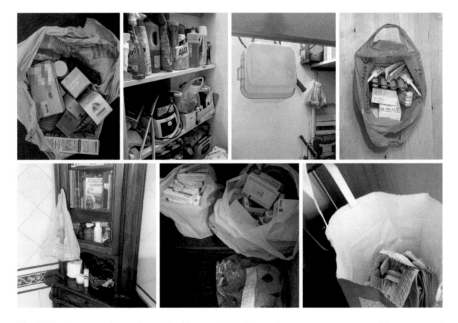

Fig. 15.9 Pharmacy bags play a significant role in home pharmacy management. They are used both to bring together individual therapy medicines and to hold stocks by separating them from medicines in use; to hold Package Leaflets that are removed from packages (but not thrown away); and to hold expired or no longer in use medicines until they are returned to the pharmacy or disposed of. The visual connotations of the bag (e.g., the clear green color, the presence of the cross symbol of the pharmacy) make it a strong identifying element that allows for immediate identification of the place in the home where pharmaceutical products are kept

Occasional-use medicines are destined for non-places (Augé 1996) both at the time of use and when they fall into disuse. Temporariness of use is their characteristic, affecting their spatial location. In interviews with patients, it emerges that, among the medicines purchased, occasional-use medicines are those whose reason for use is most frequently forgotten even a short time later. More than the others, they end up among the out-of-date medicines. The lack of a reference place takes them away from the usual checking procedures that patients do on stocks to ensure they have refills, no expired medicines, etc.

A further consideration of how the home pharmacy is organised concerns the form of the medicine and its packaging. The solid-oral forms in blister packs—e.g., pills, capsules, tablets, etc.—represent a world apart from other pharmaceutical forms: this is so both in the way they are organised and prepared (we will discuss this second aspect later). The blister pack is considered safe packaging and therefore induces more quickly than other types of packaging to get away from the secondary pack and package leaflet. Freed of the packaging parts considered secondary by the patient, blister packs are stuffed without special care other than to take up as little space as possible.

And this is true even when they are left intact in all parts of the original packaging because, unlike other medicines, those contained in blister packs do not have a prevailing direction: they can be placed vertically, horizontally, and even lie on the coast sides of the package. Bottles, vials, and eye drops are not as easy in rational space utilisation. The necessity to maintain vertical direction to prevent spillage of liquids, weight, and bulk are all factors that tend to build separateness in the disposition of medicines. Blister packs tend to develop a system of their own compared to other types of packaging.

From this point of view, the disposal in drawers is the most problematic because particularly bulky packages, such as those of syrups, vials, and sachets, do not always find it easy to place in the same position. This 'not having an eye on' the overall set of medicines is one of the causes of forgetting to take the medication regularly. Separation of medicine from the main place where daily medicines are kept, when it is not a user need but a necessity related to, for example, storage in a refrigerated environment, is likely to affect proper intake.

On the disposal of medicines in the home environment, a final observation concerns the contiguous goods with which medicines share the use of space (Fig. 15.10). Again, despite the variety that characterises the different situations observed, one

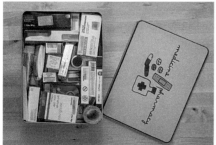 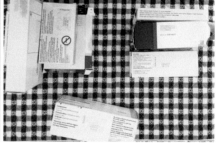

Fig. 15.10 The image on the left highlights the inclination of certain medicine packages to be stuffed into containers simply following the logic of space occupation. The patient does not seem to attach any importance to having the main side of the medicine in the foreground. On the right, the spatial order, obtained by grouping the medicines and giving them a different orientation, becomes, for the user, a 'device' used to indicate a temporal logic of intake

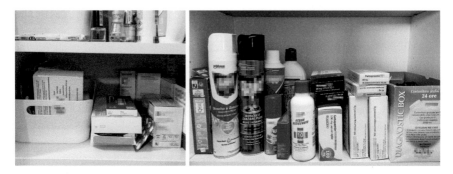

Fig. 15.11 Medicines near products for cosmetics and personal care; medicines and medications near 'poisons' or dangerous products

can detect a prevailing mixing of medicines and cosmetic products driven by a pronounced merchandise contiguity that pharmacies have exploited in their sales locations by playing on the ambiguity between health, wellness, fitness, and aesthetics. In the home environment, it is the proximity between pharmaceutical and cosmetic products (think of products such as creams and ointments); the contexts of use, and the gestures, reinforce this contiguity (Fig. 15.11—left).

There is at least a second contiguity that exploration has brought to the forefront: that with the world of 'poisonous' substances (Fig. 15.11—right). It is not uncommon to find medicines in cabinets that also contain acids, antibacterial substances or insecticides (these are usually dangerous substances, such as bleach, muriatic acid, or substances used as disinfestants at the environmental level (sprays and powders for mosquitoes, cockroaches ants, etc.) or repellents used on the body (disinfectants, mosquito repellents, lice repellents, etc.).

Our observation has revealed that mixing human and animal medicines is less common because, when pets are present, there is a tendency to store pet medicines along with pet food or in inaccessible places in the house, such as basements or garages.

15.2.2 Preparation

This observation's first element of interest concerns the medicines' disposal in the home environment. Different logics can be detected, governing how medicines are arranged/placed. Logics overlap and find, in some cases, novel solutions, even if they are not always adequate to guarantee the safety that therapy management requires (Figs. 15.12, 15.13 and 15.14).

Preparation processes call into question real rituals and can activate dynamics involving the sick person and other family members (sons, in the case of the elderly, or even professional caregivers).

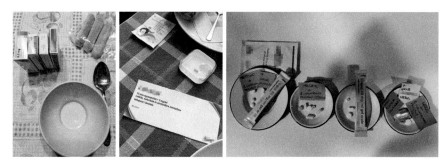

Fig. 15.12 Typical example of preparing a daily breakfast, including morning medicines on the table. In the middle, a trick used to remind one to 'put' a medicine on the table that must remain in the refrigerator until it is taken. On the right, daily therapy preparation with additional memos for medicine that cannot be placed in the small plates

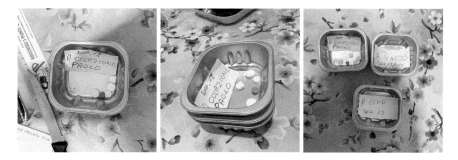

Fig. 15.13 Preparation of daily therapy, splitted according to main meals

For the elderly unable to manage therapy on their own, Saturdays and Sundays become the days when family members, usually sons, check for missing medicines and the need to request new prescriptions and, where patients are unable, arrange for weekly therapy. Here we capture the difference, referred to above, between blister medicines and others. It is a widespread tendency to unblister tablets, capsules and confections in blister packs and subdivide them according to daily use and/or the entire week. Sometimes, this operation is carried out by patients who can manage the therapy independently. Even, it may be the patients who perform this preparation to free themselves from having to, day by day, manage an operation often considered complicated because of the manual but also organizational (and therefore concentration) effort required.

We have observed how this activity, entered in the most usual household routines, is often performed without the necessary attention and indeed with a good deal of carelessness: (a) the different tablets are placed in small containers (cups, saucers) one for each day of the week, thus remaining unprotected for several days and bringing different active ingredients into contact (all the more so when the medicines have been fractionated to obtain the required personal dose); (b) the same medicine, once unblistered, is placed in a single container (e.g., a coffee cup)

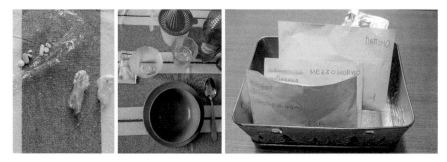

Fig. 15.14 Preparation of weekly therapy with medicines wrapped in transparent film that brings together whole tablets and tablets already fractionated according to the dosage prescribed by the doctor. On the right, envelops used to divide the medicines to be taken during the day

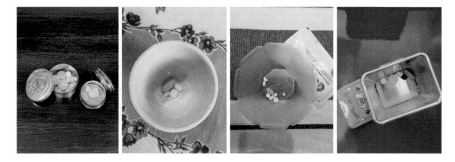

Fig. 15.15 Wedding favors, cups without handles and no longer usable for their original function, ice cream boxes, candy boxes: these are all examples of small containers re-functionalized to contain unblistered medicines for one or more days

containing the weekly dose. We have noted in this organizational mode two dangerous occurrences. The first is determined because, with this modality, the patient is induced to unblister several medicines that do not always correspond to the days of therapy (sometimes even the whole package) and, the next time, repeats the same procedure, not bothering to finish the remaining ones first. In this case, tablets can be found inside small containers, even from quite a long time ago, which usually remain at the bottom. The second is related to the fact that some tablets are very similar to each other. Once the weekly containers are filled with two different but similar medicines, the possibility of an exchange in the intake is high; (c) in one case, we have even found the reduction into powder, by the patient, of the tablets that are to be taken at the same time of the day and, the containers for weekly use, have inside them a powder preparation that is the whole of all the tablets and the patient takes that by dissolving it in a glass of water.

Special attention deserves the objects involved in care (e.g., saucers, cups, containers), which are most often objects disused from other contexts of use and dedicated to the process of taking medicines (Fig. 15.15).

Similar problems also occur when tablets are contained in bottles with child-proof type closure caps. Again, the difficulty of opening, found in most elderly people, induces the preparation of weekly therapy.

Powder pharmaceutical forms contained in sachets, drops, syrups, etc., do not have these same preparation dynamics and are generally prepared at the time of intake. It should be mentioned, however, that solid oral forms generally constitute the predominant part of a therapy.

One inconvenience noted in many patients, regarding the preparation of medicines, is the loss of the tablet because it is easy for it to fall on the floor when opening the blister pack or when bringing it to the mouth. The patient is not always able to notice, which causes a lack of adherence to the treatment plan (as well as making possible the risk—a risk reported to us by more than one patient—of pets taking a medicine found on the ground). Observation also made it possible to note that, frequently, in the elderly or visually impaired patient, the loss of the medicine, once removed from the blister pack, depends on the inability to locate the tablet on the tablecloths because they very often have floral patterns or otherwise unevenly coloured designs (Fig. 15.16).

A separate chapter is needed to focus on the activities to prepare medicines for those taking them outside the home. Still, this order of problems has not been addressed in this text, having focused our attention on all the dynamics that take place within domestic places. It is certain, however, that new lifestyles are leading people to stay away from home for a long time for study or work purposes. These, combined with an increased propensity to travel, place medicine within new dynamics that are by no means commonplace and deserve further design attention. Certainly, one of the outcomes of these changes in the outdoor way of life we observe in the changes in pharmaceutical forms that are moving, in recent years, toward the pharmaceutical form of single-dose liquid sachets, orosoluble tablets, in short, forms that help the patient to take the therapy even in situations that do not make available all the supports (glasses, saucers, water, etc.) that are available inside the home.

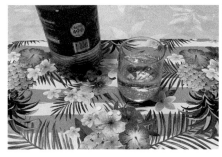
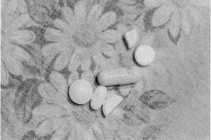

Fig. 15.16 For the elderly patients, it is hard to identify medicines once they have been unblistered

15.2.3 Remember

Among the memory techniques implemented by users, a distinction should be made between those used to remember that they must perform an action—taking the medicines—and those used to remember that they have performed an action—medicine already taken. In both cases, organisational techniques often help the patient remember. In the first case, as anticipated above, associative logics are frequently used, which may be related to places or activities.

In the following figures (Figs. 15.17, 15.18, 15.19, 15.20, 15.21 and 15.22), there are some examples collected in real environment. Putting the medicine in places where one is accustomed to take, at a specific time, a specific action, such as: placing the morning medicines near the coffee pot if one is accustomed to drinking morning coffee; placing the medicine to be taken after lunch near the kitchen sink,

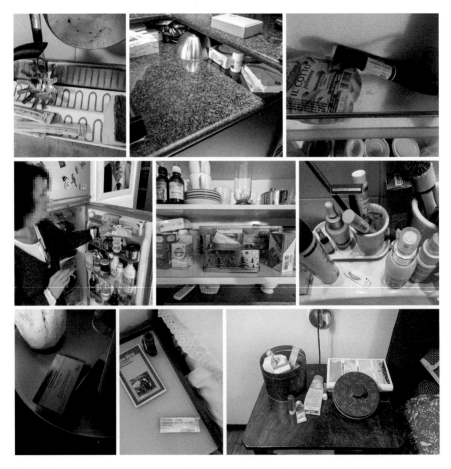

Fig. 15.17 Connection between disposition of medicines and home context of intake

15 Use Phenomenologies. Observing the User While Taking Pharmaceutical Therapies 309

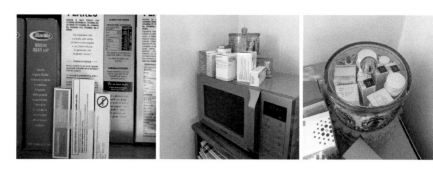

Fig. 15.18 From left to right, it shows a way of activating the memory of taking the medicine, using the concept of a 'parasitic object'. The patient has glued a strip of scotch the morning medicines to the food he usually uses for breakfast so that the indispensable object—the cornflakes—guarantees the memory of the simultaneous medicine intake. The second figure shows the medicines to be taken in the morning, placed over the microwave to prepare breakfast. The third figure echoes the previous one and shows the division of the morning medicines placed in a container from the others. The fourth figure presents a breadbox used to hold medicines, placed on the cooktop in the evening to remember to take the medicines with breakfast in the morning

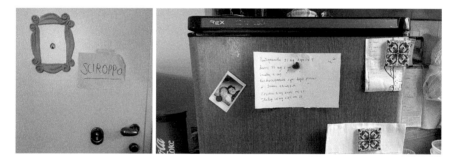

Fig. 15.19 Examples of memory techniques in use by users: messages placed on places of obligatory passage or on furniture and appliances most in use

if one is accustomed to washing the dishes after the midday meal; placing the medicine to be taken in the evening before bedtime on the bedside table near the bed, etc.Preparing the table for the meal, placing at the table, along with plates, glasses and cutlery, also saucers or cups with the medicines already prepared for taking; placing near or even physically attaching, using scotch tape, the medicine to the package of morning cookies or cornflakes; in some cases (for example, where the medicine must remain in the fridge until it is taken, or when its preparation cannot be arranged too long before it is taken, or when the medicine is bulky and cannot be placed on the table, in the medicine saucer along with the other medicines), we have observed patients placing on the saucer along with the pills and tablets that are to be taken, also the missing medicine sticker, cut out from the package precisely to aid the user's memory (Fig. 15.18).An additional expedient is to put a sign or a post-it notes in places of forced passage, such as the front door, to prompt the user to check whether the medicines have been taken before leaving in the morning (Fig. 15.19).

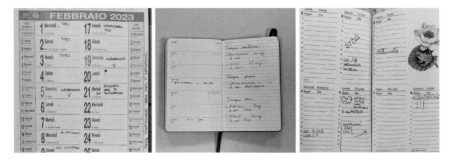

Fig. 15.20 Diaries, calendars, care plans: how the user keeps track of medicine intake, even making use of objects not expressly intended for this purpose

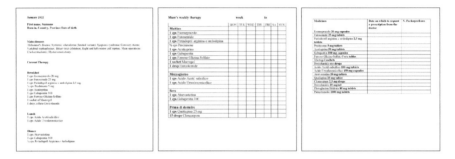

Fig. 15.21 Example of rewriting the therapy by the patient, with different purposes. In the absence of pre-established formats, the patient rewrites the information required for the multiple activities involved in the therapy in various forms. The patient uses the first sheet for medical examinations. It summarises the patient's data (here omitted), the main pathologies, and current therapy. The second sheet shows the daily therapy divided into intake times. A weekly table allows a marker to testify the medicine intake. The third table transcribes the therapy according to the purchases that must be made once stocks are exhausted. It is possible to note how each re-transcription highlights the elements that the user considers most relevant for the purpose

A different problem is remembering to take medicines when they are used other than daily. In these cases, too, users implement their expedients. In cases of weekly medicines, for example, the elective day is Sunday because the habits of this day, so different from those of other days of the week, make this day "memorable". It is easier for the user to associate the therapy with this day and to remember later that they took it. Some report taking a medicine after Sunday church, others upon returning in the afternoon from lunch taken at their sons' home. By the same logic, some users associated taking with the day of the local market, an activity that identifies a discontinuity from other days and makes remembering the activities done during the day easier. In the case of monthly therapy, the typical association is the first day of the month or the first Sunday of the month. Again, it is the discontinuity constituted by the change of the month, and the ease of remembering something that began that is the hook element for memory (Figs. 15.20 and 15.21).

Then, some modalities work on memory processes *a posteriori* and allow answering the question: *did I take the medicine?*

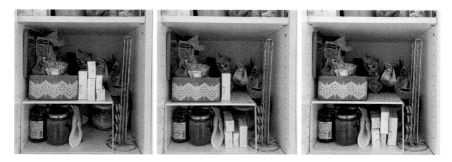

Fig. 15.22 Examples of memory techniques: the patient moves the medicines from the top shelf to the bottom shelf (or from left to right) as taking the medicine. The movement in the space is the way to remember medicine intake

Our observations frequently include organisational techniques that use logic related to spatial order. In these cases, moving from left to right or from top to bottom, the medicines as they are taken becomes the way to verify that the action has been done (Fig. 15.22). The organisational mechanism implemented by users is that at the end of the process, that is, in the evening, all medicines are returned to their original position.

One way, also recalled just above, is to keep charts, usually weekly, showing each day's therapy, broken down by intake times, and patients fill in the chart as they take their medicines.

One indication that comes from the literature (Pullar et al. 1989) is that it proves to be an effective incentive in following the therapy carefully, the prescribing doctor's request to bring back, at the next visit, the used packets of the medicines, keeping the empty blister packs inside and writing on the outer pack the day in which the therapy started.

References

Augé M (1996) Non luoghi, Introduzione a una antropologia della surmodernità. Elèuthera, Milano. [Non-Lieux. Introduction à une anthropologie de la surmodernité (1992). Paris: Seuil]

Denham SA (2003) Relationships between family rituals, family routines, and health. J Fam Nurs 9(3):305–330

Gellad WF, Grenard JL, Marcum ZA (2011) A systematic review of barriers to medication adherence in the elderly: looking beyond cost and regimen complexity. Am J Geriatr Pharmacother 9:11–23

Lonsdale DO, Baker EH (2013) Understanding and managing medication in elderly people. Best Pract Res Clin Obstet Gynaecol 27(5):767–788

Lu J, Zhang N, Mao D, Wang Y, Wang X (2020) How social isolation and loneliness effect medication adherence among elderly with chronic diseases: an integrated theory and validated cross-sectional study. Arch Gerontol Geriatr 90:1–7

Pullar T, Kumar S, Tindall H, Feely M (1989) Time to stop counting tablets? Clin Pharmacol Unit 46(2):163–168

Open Access This chapter is licensed under the terms of the Creative Commons Attribution 4.0 International License (http://creativecommons.org/licenses/by/4.0/), which permits use, sharing, adaptation, distribution and reproduction in any medium or format, as long as you give appropriate credit to the original author(s) and the source, provide a link to the Creative Commons license and indicate if changes were made.

The images or other third party material in this chapter are included in the chapter's Creative Commons license, unless indicated otherwise in a credit line to the material. If material is not included in the chapter's Creative Commons license and your intended use is not permitted by statutory regulation or exceeds the permitted use, you will need to obtain permission directly from the copyright holder.

Chapter 16
Use Phenomenologies: Oral Solid Forms in Blister Packs

Antonella Valeria Penati

Abstract The different pharmaceutical forms and the variety of packaging that make them available to the user generate gestures, interactions, and usage behaviour, which are worthy of interest to those interested in reading the objects' formal attributes and the influence exerted on those using them. In the world of medicines, oral solid blister forms represent an interesting case due to the complex use dynamics dependent on both the 'content'—the medicine—and the 'container'—the blister. Starting from observing how patients use medicines in their home environment, this chapter focuses on how the characteristics of oral solid forms (e.g., tablets, capsules, packets) and those of blister packs can induce incorrect or non-compliant use behaviour. These behaviours are especially characteristic of older people.

16.1 Tablets, Pills, Capsules, and Pearls: Oral Solid Forms

Some brief preliminary issues (Chap. 12 investigates these issues in detail) are necessary to understand recurring modes of action that emerge from observing the patient grappling with daily therapy. In this sampling of observations on the use of blister tablets, it is helpful to start from the wide variety of forms found on the market, all of which fall into the category of drugs sold in solid form and taken orally. The tablet is the generic name given to this class of medicines within which we find:

- the tablet. This name derives from the manufacturing process in which active ingredients and excipients in powder or granule form are held together under the pressure of a compressing machine. The colour is primarily white, but sometimes it has pastel shades such as powder yellow, powder blue, powder green, and powder grey derived from the natural colouring of the active ingredient powder and excipients. The surface is rough;

A. V. Penati (✉)
Department of Design, Politecnico di Milano, Milan, Italy
e-mail: antonella.penati@polimi.it

© The Author(s) 2025
A. V. Penati (ed.), *In-Home Medication*, Research for Development,
https://doi.org/10.1007/978-3-031-53294-8_16

- the pill. It is an umbrella term used as a synonym for tablet. Namely, pills are coated by a process of confectioning—or, more recently, using a film—which gives the surface of the confection a shiny colour and appearance. Sometimes, the pharmaceutical industry may use different surface colours to differentiate the dosages of the same active ingredient. The term pill refers to contraceptive use;
- the capsule. It consists of two cylindrical food-grade gelatin-like shells, contains the active ingredient and excipients mostly in powder or granule form. They may be transparent and allow the colour of the contents to shine through, or they may be opaque and coloured, and the pharmaceutical industry may use different colours to differentiate doses of the same active ingredient;
- the pearl. It is similar to capsules but with an oily content. The colour generally derives from the chromatic properties of the active ingredient contained and the colour of the gelatin used for the casing;
- the effervescent tablet. It is usually larger than tablets due to the need for more active ingredients or excipients. They dissolve in contact with a liquid.

The choice of the most appropriate form to transform the active ingredient into a ready-to-drink format depends exclusively on bio-pharmaceutical constraints, such as the need to mix the active ingredient with the necessary excipients; to obtain gastro-resistant or modified-release tablets; to conceal unpleasant organoleptic characteristics; to guarantee the stability of the active ingredient. On the other hand, ease of use, comprehensibility and recognisability, which can guide the user to the correct use in the daily management of the medicine, have a reduced place in decisions on the pharmaceutical form.

16.2 The Role of Object Typologies

As far as the recognisability of the medicine is concerned, in the case of oral pharmaceutical forms, the different existing types have an archetypal structure fixed in time that unambiguously refers to the route of intake (Caprino 2011). In other words, the link between pharmaceutical form and intake route is unequivocal in the case of solid oral medicines.

Instead, the problem arises when these typological forms, consolidated over time, are attributed to medicines whose intake route is not oral. For example, some medication for vaginal use, which have their formal archetype in the ovum, are now also marketed in the form of the vaginal capsule, tablet or even the vaginal suppository (Fig. 16.1). This transfer of type increases the risk of intake error, not least because users recognise oral solid forms as having the property of acting systemically. Therefore, a capsule or tablet can be taken orally to exert its healing action at the vaginal level is quite normal for the patient.

In our observation, we found at least one further transfer of the capsule's typological form from oral to inhalation use. This concerns the medicine containing the active ingredient glycopyrrolate bromide, used for broncho-obstructive diseases.

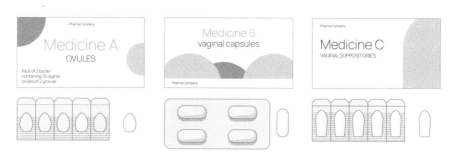

Fig. 16.1 Ovules, capsules and suppositories for vaginal use: changing the way established formal typologies are taken, may lead to confusion in the patient

Fig. 16.2 Capsule for inhalation use

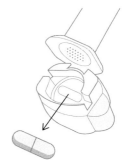

The active ingredient powder is contained in transparent capsules enclosed in blisters. When taken out of the blister, the capsule must be inserted into a device that, by puncturing its surface, releases the powder: then, it can be aspirated (Fig. 16.2). The patient who uses this medicine, and interviewed during our observation of the domestic use of medicines, recounted that they repeatedly swallowed the capsule because, although the process of loading the device seems to move away from the gestures that typically accompany oral medication, the habit inherent in the action of *unblistering* and the shape of the capsule almost automatically and spontaneously recall the gesture of 'bringing to the mouth'.

Focusing on oral preparations and the influence of their form in the overall drug-taking process, the problems with types such as tablets, capsules, granules, pearls, and pills do not manifest themselves in the relationship between pharmaceutical form and route of intake—which, as we have seen, is rooted in the user's experience—but in their poor morphological differentiation that sometimes makes these forms indistinguishable from one another (Fig. 16.3).

Indeed, each tablet can be recognised and distinguished by specific formal details in addition to its colour. First and foremost, its morphological peculiarities include size, base geometry, section profile, and marks on the surface (Fig. 16.4).

Sometimes, these characterisations are minimal, thus increasing the user's difficulty in recognising the medicine, which, once removed from the blister pack, has no distinctive identifying features. Losing the information on the packaging makes medicines challenging to recognise and distinguish (Fig. 16.5). The ability to

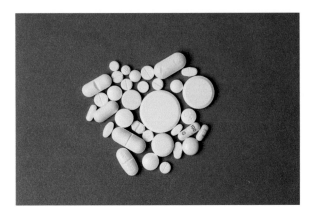

Fig. 16.3 A striking image of the enormous variety of shapes distinguishable by a few formal traits

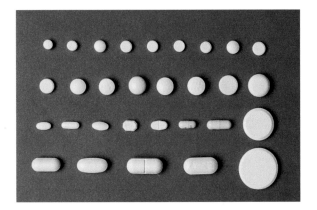

Fig. 16.4 Morphological variety of oral solid forms, traced back to morphograms. We recognise: tablets with a flat circular base and rectangular cross-section; with a flat circular base, rectangular cross-section and bevelled contours; with a convex circular base and lenticular cross-section; with an ovoid, ellipsoidal or teardrop base; with a pentagonal, rhomboidal or hexagonal base; with a figurative base etc

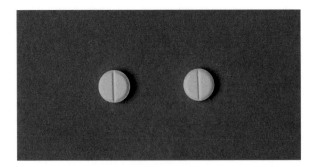

Fig. 16.5 Two very similar pills can be confused with each other: containing the active ingredient *Furosemide* or the active ingredient *Prednisone*, at different dosages. These tablets are frequently found in the treatment of elderly people and can easily be interchanged

identify and distinguish tablets, even from their formal connotations, is particularly useful for patients on polypharmacy who may find it difficult to verify the correctness of the drugs they are taking.

16.2.1 The Role of Colour

One of the elements capable of creating distinction is colour (we focused on colour as a formal attribute of tablets, capsules, and pads in Chap. 21 of this volume). Here, we outline a few considerations drawn from the users' experience we have observed. Colour is a powerful sign of medicine recognition, so much so that several patients call medicines not only by the name of the disorder or organ they are treating (e.g. 'the one for the heart', 'the one for blood pressure') but also by names such as "the yellow one", "the big one", identifying in the formal characteristics, and so in the colour too, the most immediate indicative modality. In the case of colour, we face a feature that, in many cases, is 'not designed' but derives from the natural colouring of the chemical substances used, be they the active ingredient or the excipients. On the other hand, sometimes the colour is chosen and desired by the manufacturer either for marketing reasons (e.g., to make the medicine memorable by creating an association between the brand name and the colour, as is the case with the medicine containing the active ingredient Sildenafil), or to differentiate the dosages of the same medicine. The colour of a tablet or capsule is such an essential attribute in the identity of the medicine that its change, due to the purchase of the same active ingredient of a different brand, is one of the causes of mistrust or even rejection of the therapy by patients—especially the older people—who no longer recognise the medicine they have been taking. This occurs mainly during hospital admissions or, more generally, when there is a discontinuity in the therapy in use, linked either to introducing new medicines or to using generic ones that may have different formal and colour characteristics from those the user is used to taking. It can also occur because the pharmacist dispenses the same active ingredient to the patient, which, in different brands, takes on various formal and chromatic connotations.

Here is a note on the use of colour as a code pharmaceutical companies use to distinguish different dosages of the same medicine. This allows us to make a further point drawn from user observation in homecare. In certain medication classes, it is common for the patient to be prescribed the same medicine to be taken throughout the day in different dosages. In such cases, the tools in the hands of the patient to prevent intake errors lie:

- in careful management of the organisation of therapy;
- in the notations that patients put on the secondary packaging to supplement or amplify certain information that may not be sufficiently distinctive;
- in memorising the chromatic characteristics that change in the case of different dosages, both on the secondary packaging and tablet/capsule.

We refer to Chaps. 12, 17, and 21 for more detailed considerations on using colour as an informative element. We will limit ourselves here to pointing out that, from a perceptual point of view, the increase or decrease of a quantity, such as weight, speed, or length, can be rendered on the visual plane using colour in chromatic 'progression', in other words through chromatic intensities or thickening of signs (e.g. lines, dots, patterns). In representing the increasing transition to different dosages, the colour progression can help make reading the different dosages less confusing. Even in the literature, reading is reported as one of the errors most frequently encountered by patients.

Conversely, the solution most frequently used by companies to differentiate dosages of the same drug is using different colours chosen to emphasise the 'difference' and not the progression. However, the colour variety does not necessarily have a logic that enables the patient to 'attribute' meaning to the different colours. At the same time, the colour progression should ensure that there is such a distance between the colours used that they cannot be confused (we refer to the considerations in the concluding Chap. 22).

16.2.2 *Signs on Surfaces: Recognisability and Manipulability*

Concerning the medicine recognition, besides the shape and the use of colour, sometimes the characterisations that allow the tablet to be recognised are visual marks impressed on its surface.

Among oral solid forms, tablets are those that from a manufacturing point of view can, more than others, be characterised by marks on the surface. Indeed, during the moulding process, the tablet is allowed to be engraved by means of special punches and this possibility is exploited by some manufacturers to imprint the name, dosage and/or logo of the pharmaceutical company on the body of the medicine. This information is very valuable to the user, and is sometimes decisive in helping the patient not to confuse two different doses of the same medicine or two different medicines of identical forms (Fig. 16.6).

Sometimes the surface of the tablet bears an engraved sign (e.g., the tablet of Alendronic Acid, a medicine used for brittle bones, bears a schematic sign of a small bone in some trademarks) that facilitates the recognition process through its connection with the purpose of use (Fig. 16.7).

Some elements are 'indicators of use', including the score-lines impressed on the tablets. In addition to their function, these marks also become implicitly helpful to the patient in recognising and distinguishing one tablet from another.

The score-line, dividing the tablet in two or, when it is in the shape of a cross, dividing it into four parts, is not always capable of guiding the user to follow the correct behaviour or dissuading them from performing specific actions. In some cases, it may induce the user to perform incorrect actions. Indeed, the formal elements of the medicine are not always evaluated for their ability to persuade/discourage use.

Fig. 16.6 Example of medicines with naming or dosage indications

Fig. 16.7 Example of a tablet identifiable by the mark impressed on its surface

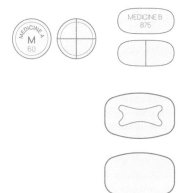

Besides being a clue that helps to distinguish one medicine from another on a formal level, this line represents an explicit permission for the user to proceed in scoring the medicine.

However, as the essential distinction between 'dividing' and 'fragmenting' is not at all clear to the patient, the score-line is interpreted by the user as a possibility to divide the tablet and fragment it.

Adding to this first problem is the reasons why a patient fragments the medicine are different. Mainly there are two:

- to break up the medicine into doses, following the dosage instructions given by the doctor. In this case, the fractioning is related to taking the different parts at different times/days;
- to facilitate the swallowing of large tablets in the case of children, older people, and dysphagia. In this case, the intake of different parts is simultaneous, a short distance apart.

The 'sign' on the tablet acts as a 'signal', a gateway that authorises the patient to 'manipulate' the medicine. However, this sign cannot make the patient act correctly. Indeed, sometimes manipulation can alter the active ingredient. In some cases, tampering is permitted, but only if immediately before intake. In others, tampering is prohibited because the active ingredient may enter the bloodstream too quickly in high doses. In still other cases, the surface of the medicine is coated so that the user does not encounter the active ingredient (Fig. 16.8).

Therefore, different conditions make dividing the medicine equally problematic and worthy of attention. The potential uses evoked by the sign are very complex and nuanced. Without reading the Package Leaflet, which warns the patient to handle the tablet only under specific conditions and in particular ways, through the splitting sign, one risks inducing the patient to perform wrong actions, dangerous to their health. The Italian Ministry of Health has drawn up a Recommendation for Handling Solid Oral Pharmaceutical Forms on this issue (Recommendation No. 19, Ministero della Salute 2019). However, these documents are addressed to healthcare personnel and do not go so far as to educate patient care behaviour at home.

Fig. 16.8 The figure refers to the medicine containing the active ingredient Pyridostigmine bromide extended-release. The Package Leaflet, under Mode of Use, states: "The sustained-release tablet may be divided into equal parts, but should not be divided further as this would compromise the delayed release of the active ingredient". Under the administration mode, the package leaflet of another brand of the same active substance states: "[…] Swallow the tablets without chewing with half a glass or a full glass of water. […] The retard tablet has an incision line, which only serves to break the tablet in two for easier swallowing and not to divide it into two half-doses. Even in difficult swallowing cases, however, the tablet should not be broken into smaller fragments, as this may compromise the sustained release of the active ingredient […]". The second description is significantly more articulate. In both cases, this information 'reaches' the patient, almost at the end of the package insert. In other words, the 'score-line' is presented with an 'immediacy' that needs a very articulate explanatory 'mediation'. It is not sure that the patient will read this information because of the propensity already denounced in the text not to read the package insert and because this information is placed at the end of a long and articulate text

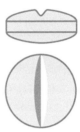

Fig. 16.9 The figure refers to the medicine containing the active ingredient Azathioprine. Under the heading administration method, the package leaflet states: "[…] Swallow the tablets whole, with a little water. The tablet must not be split or broken". And then again at the end: *"The following information is intended for doctors or healthcare professionals only. Instructions for use, handling and disposal.* There are no risks associated with handling the tablets with the coating intact. No special safety precautions are necessary in this case. […]. However, immunosuppressive agents should be handled strictly with instructions when healthcare personnel halve tablets […]. Surplus medicines and contaminated devices must be stored temporarily in clearly labelled containers […]". The line imprinted on the tablet, however, contradicts what is written in the package insert, comforting the user who decides to break the tablet

Sometimes, this line is marked and becomes more than an interpretable index. In some medicines, it is not merely a superficial trace but erodes the tablet with a deep 'wedge-shaped' section, leaving it weakly united in the central part (Fig. 16.9). The action of breaking, in this way, is not only communicated visually but is also facilitated in terms of the leverage effort the user has to make, thus constituting an unequivocal message of permission. Yet forms so characterised on the indicative level can then be contradicted by the prohibitions in the leaflet.

In addition to the precautions mentioned above, under how to store Azathioprine, another pharmaceutical company's leaflet states: "If it is necessary to halve the film-coated tablet of Azathioprine 50 mg, skin contact with the powder or split part of the tablet should be avoided". This passage is illuminating in explaining the shape given to the tablet: once the medicine has been broken, the wedge-shaped section imprinted in the tablet's body allows the smallest surface area for contact with the active ingredient. And yet, if the medicine is broken on the doctor's instructions, the patient could touch a potentially harmful fragment to put it back into the blister pack or other container or pick it up again for the following intake (Fig. 16.10).

In our observation, we encountered two cases of patients taking this medicine at the dose of half a tablet per day on the doctor's recommendation.

Through observation, we noted how much of the broken medication remains in the environment through the crumbs and dust dispersed in the cut and found on kitchen utensils such as knives and cutting boards, with the effect of reducing the dose taken by the patient and increasing environmental contamination by chemical agents.

Concerning the manipulation of tablets and how the shape can take on indicative value, starting from observations, we can point out that the elongated shape of the tablet (oblong tablets) makes it easier to grasp the medicine between the fingers, increasing the possibility of the user carrying out manipulative manoeuvres. We also find this type of shape used in powerful slow-release painkillers for which altering the unit dose is highly inadvisable and even dangerous (Fig. 16.11).

Among the tablets, the shape that best avoids manipulation where this is dangerous to the patient's health is the lenticular shape with a higher thickness in the centre and gradually decreasing towards the edges. This shape makes it difficult to grip the tablet and more challenging to cut, as a knife blade can never rest on the entire surface (Fig. 16.12).

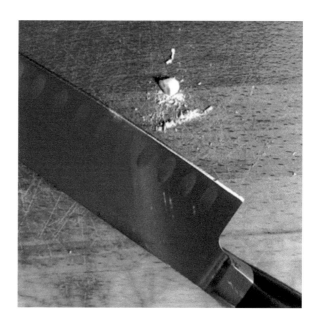

Fig. 16.10 The picture represents the typical situation that arises after tablet crushing: not only is there a loss of active ingredient that reduces the dose taken by the patient, but there is also contamination of the instruments and planes on which the tablet was cut

Fig. 16.11 The picture refers to the medicine containing the active substances Oxycodone hydrochloride and Naloxone hydrochloride, used in pain therapy. These are slow-release painkillers that do not have to be broken. However, the shape of the tablet makes it easier to break it

Fig. 16.12 Shape of the most suitable tablet for not being manipulated

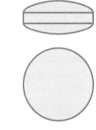

Fig. 16.13 The shape of the capsule can easily induce the patient to open it to dissolve the powder in water

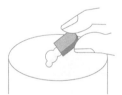

Regarding the manipulability of oral pharmaceutical forms, a different discussion deserves the capsules, which lend themselves to being opened by the user because they have two parts that are close by sliding over each other, without any seal. The small 'goblet' shape of each of the two halves does not discourage misuse, consisting of pouring the powder into a glass to be dissolved in water (Fig. 16.13). On the other hand, dissolving a powdered active ingredient within a liquid is a procedure not alien to the world of pharmaceuticals and constitutes a formalised mode of use. And this, for most patients who lack the basic rudiments of pharmacological culture, is sufficient to extend, by contiguity, behaviours legitimised by the fact that they occur within the same cognitive and operational 'context of action'.

Observing the medication's shape can help us to understand which elements may lead the patient to perform incorrect operations. As mentioned above, difficulty in swallowing leads the patient to fragment tablets. This motivation often has psychological roots; in the older people's world, this problem is widespread, primarily due to physiological difficulties. In part, the shape, size and surface characteristics affect this difficulty. In contrast, we face an underestimation of how much the body's techniques can help in making the correct administration of tablets easier (on this aspect, see Chap. 14). Those working in the healthcare sector know the proper ways to alleviate this discomfort for which suitable procedures, expedients and body postures have been defined, such as: taking a few small sips of water beforehand or chewing a small piece of bread to draw saliva to the mouth and moisten it; placing the tablet on the tongue by moving it as far back as possible towards the throat; taking a few sips of water, preferably from a small bottle, to direct the flow of the liquid; keeping the head upright slightly bent forward (to avoid sucking in air). If the medicine has an unpleasant taste, it is better to swallow it with cold water, as this attenuates the taste perception.

Again, from the patients' actions, one can see how much the medicine's shape contributes to making swallowing harder or softer, as shown by several studies on this issue (Drumond and Stegemann 2020; Hummler et al. 2023; Overgaard et al. 2001).

16.3 The Blister

Among the several classifications in literature, delving into indispensable aspects for the correct knowledge and management of pharmaceutical forms, here we choose to deepen the one referring to the route of administration. We believe this is the description closest to the end user's experience. Since the topic is the result of consolidated manuals to which all pharmaceutical companies refer, we will include extensive excerpts from scientific references describing the various pharmaceutical forms. All the following pharmaceutical forms and their description follow the guidance provided by the Council of Europe (2019).

In some countries, such as the United States, tablets, capsules, granules, and pearls are sold in special plastic vials and dispensed by the pharmacist in the exact number of doses prescribed by the doctor. In most European countries, these pharmaceutical forms are packaged in blisters, named for the characteristic pre-formed 'bubbles' used to contain the pharmaceutical product. Data from the Italian Ministry of Health indicate that in 2018 in Italy, oral solid forms sold in blister packs accounted for 92%.

Blister packs are packages made from a thin plastic sheet into which a predefined number of alveoli are moulded by thermoforming to contain the individual solid pharmaceutical forms (Fig. 16.14). It is a multi-dose packaging system that conceptually derives from the juxtaposition of individual doses of medicine preserved, one by one, from environmental contamination, shock, and pressure. The blister makes it impossible to encounter the contained drug without irreparably tampering with the aluminium film, the integrity of which guarantees that the product is intact. On the back page, the plastic foil—primarily PolyVinyl Chloride (PVC) or PolyEthylene Terephthalate (PET)—is heat-sealed to an aluminium film that serves as a closure. The plastic film is densely textured to give the blister more rigidity and facilitate its adherence to the underlying aluminium foil.

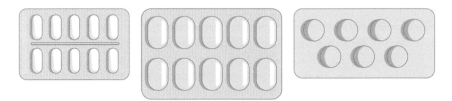

Fig. 16.14 Blisters in plastic and aluminium film (on the left); blisters with the upper part in rigid aluminium foil and the lower part in breakable aluminium foil (centre); Blister with 'peelable' aluminium/aluminium film (on the right)

The plastic foil can be transparent and allow a glimpse of the medicine, its presence or absence, and its morphological characteristics. Alternatively, this foil is opaque for those medicines that need to be preserved from the offence of light. In the case of the plastic-aluminium film, the opening is done by finger pressure on the part of the plastic bubble containing the pill, capsule or tablet until the underlying aluminium film is 'broken through' and released.

A second type of blister is one in which both the upper film containing the cavities for the medicines and the lower film acting as 'closure' in aluminium. As in the case of the plastic-aluminium blister, it can be opened by pressing the medicine in such a way as to cause the underlying aluminium film to tear. However, 'peelable' aluminium-aluminium blisters, with a type of opening that uncovers the pill compartment by 'dragging' small free aluminium flaps, are increasingly popular. The aluminium-aluminium blisters do not allow a glimpse of the medicine contained. Sometimes, they do not even allow a glimpse of its shape and size.

In all the cases described above, the lower aluminium foil constitutes the closure and the page on which all the information about the medicine, the manufacturer and the expiry date.

As seen so far, all the elements characterising the blister on a formal level are the result of production logic. However, when they encounter the user, their shape acts as a sign of recognition and direction of the user experience. Their arrangement can become the object of interpretation by the user, who projects meanings onto them that go beyond their strictly functional role.

Some signs have a visual imprint with a strong impact on the recognisability of the content, such as reinforcing ribs, surface textures, the shape and pitch of the housings, and full and empty spaces drawn by present and missing tablets (Fig. 16.15).

In other words, all of these define a gestalt, a perceptual, formal, structural, and functional configuration. Unlike other forms of packaging for drugs, which hardly ever aim to create a 'visual order', blister packs have the appearance of actual 'units of measurement' of the drug. The primarily linear order of the blisters recalls the idea of 'doses arranged in succession', going some way towards the temporal logic that oversees the treatment process (Fig. 16.16).

16 Use Phenomenologies: Oral Solid Forms in Blister Packs

Fig. 16.15 The figure illustrates blisters (taken from existing ones) with alveolus arrangements without functional sense. In some cases, these are arrangements derived from standard formats adapted to different medicines to optimise production economies

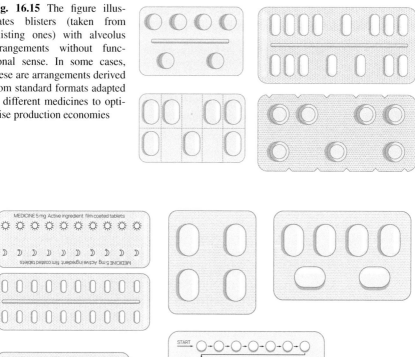

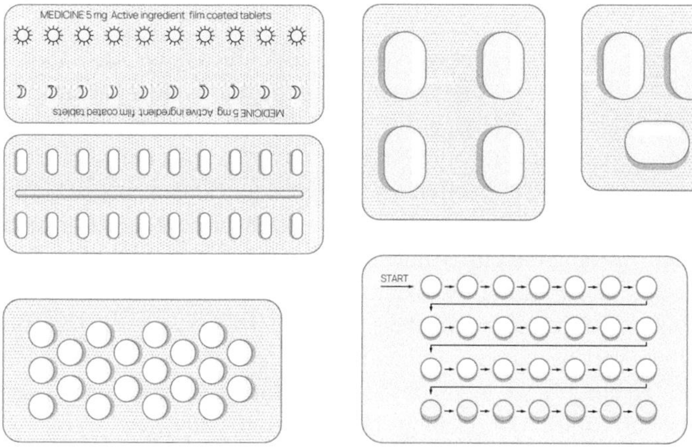

Fig. 16.16 Top left: Illustration of the blister of an anticoagulant drug with a fixed dosage of two tablets per day (one in the morning and one in the evening). The tablets are arranged in two rows; on the back of the blister, the graphic representation of the sun and moon helps the patient manage the intake. Top centre: blister containing four Alendronate tablets. The medicine must be taken weekly and the blister is for 1 month. The well-spaced tablets visually support taking them at intervals over time. Top right: blister containing an antiviral drug with two active ingredients in different tablets. The daily dosage schedule is three tablets arranged vertically and horizontally. Patients should not take the horizontal tablet with particular diseases. The other arrangement helps the doctor at the prescribing stage in giving the correct information to the patient about the intake pattern by referring precisely to the horizontal and vertical direction of the tablets (the explanations in the package leaflet would be much more effective if they similarly used the blister configuration to give the patient the intake information. Viceversa, the PIL refers to the colour of the tablets—pink and white—which the patient cannot see because the blister is in aluminium). Bottom left: arrangement of the alveoli functional in the case of medicines for which the patient should never split the blister into single doses. Bottom right: example of a contraceptive pill blister with a timetable for taking, lines indicating the correct sequence to follow, and insertion of placebo pills indicated by a different colour

Despite the complex phenomenology of use that it intends to govern, the blister presents itself as a simple object. A promise of simplicity, in which it is:

- Simple, easy, and quick to open and get the medicine out;
- Simple, easy, and fast to trace all the information on the primary packaging close to the medicine;
- Simple, easy, and quick to view and check the doses taken and those still in the package.

16.3.1 Simple, Easy, and Quick to Open and Get the Medicine Out

The fact that the alveolus is quick and easy to open is contradicted by observation of what users do when taking tablets or capsules in blister packs. In older patients, this activity is carried out 1 day a week (e.g., at the weekend) by the patient themselves, who prefers to devote concentrated time to removing from the blister instead of performing it every day. Sometimes, this activity is delegated to children, grandchildren or professional caregivers. Especially for those who no longer have intact grasping and pressing gestures, opening the blister may not be such an easy task. Apart from the observation made in the world of the older people, where this difficulty is also found in subjects without impaired use of their hands, there is data in the literature referring specifically to patients with inflammatory arthritis of the hands. Among the packaging methods, the blister pack is one of the most difficult, in a ranking that sees it right behind vials with child-proof openings (Hughes et al. 2009).

The blister is opened by pressing with a finger on the plastic housing, deforming the cavity containing the tablet with the pressure necessary to 'breakthrough' the underlying aluminium foil using the contained product, thus allowing it to escape. Difficulties may arise concerning the size of the product, its consistency, the pitch of the matrix created by the housings, the presence or absence of 'prehension areas' on the blister, the elasticity of the aluminium foil, and the pressure resistance of the cavity containing the medicine. Any of these factors can contribute to the failure of the opening process:

- a large, soft or fragile medicine is likely to bend or break;
- a medicine that is too tiny risks not breaking easily;
- the blister cavities too close to each other may result in multiple openings even if the strain is directed on a single alveolus.

The user can't recognise even the different types of opening (e.g., 'pressure' and 'peelable') and may use the wrong gestures, altering the medicine's integrity or even returning to the pharmacy, failing to open the blister and believing it to be defective. Blister packs often lack the correct affordance signs to guide users to the right action (Fig. 16.17).

Regardless of what one might think, it should also be noted that blister packs are exclusively for storing the medicine before use and that the only interaction the user

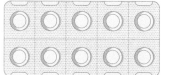 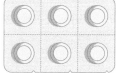

Fig. 16.17 Examples of blisters with affordance signs. On the left, it facilitates the opening of the pharmaceutical dose and a clear indication that it is a 'peelable' blister; on the right, a hint enables the separation of the dose from the blister

Fig. 16.18 Fragments of medicine placed in the blister

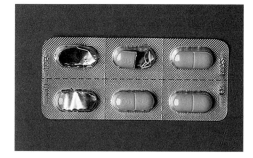

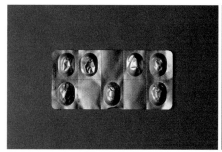 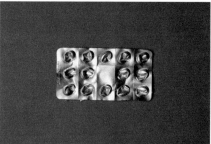

Fig. 16.19 Here is an example of aluminium-aluminium blister deformation making a challenging use due to interference with the secondary packaging and the leaflet when reinserting the blister after use

has with this form of packaging is to 'pop' the tablet out of the blister. What happens instead—and not occasionally—is that users use portions of the medicine according to the doctor's prescription and store the leftover fragments inside the empty cavities (Fig. 16.18).

The observation revealed the many contrivances that users use to keep these 'leftovers': among the most common is the attempt to reseal the alveolus containing the leftover tablet by rejoining the flaps of aluminium foil resulting from the break or the use of transparent kitchen foil wrapped around the blister (see Chap. 15).

A side note concerns aluminium-aluminium blisters when the upper and lower sheets are thin. In this case, it is easy to observe how the excessive elasticity of the material produces a greater difficulty in opening and an overall deformation of the blister, which can bend in several places, making it challenging to handle but also to store in the secondary pack (Fig. 16.19).

16.3.2 Simple, Easy, and Fast to Trace All the Information on the Primary Packaging Close to the Medicine

Even the information system placed on the aluminium surface sealing the blister pack does not always make all the necessary information available to the patient. Consider in this connection that the integrity of this information page is very short. It ends as soon as the use of the drug begins, and the tearing of the aluminium foil is necessary for tablet removal (Fig. 16.20). In allowing access to the medicine, the tear removes any information. Information about the name of the medicine, its dosage, the proprietary pharmaceutical company, and the expiry date are sometimes present on the surface sporadically and, in most cases, are not present on each dose (Fig. 16.21). In this respect, one must consider how much patients' lifestyles have changed over time: for study or work reasons, they spend much time out of home.

Although the pharmaceutical industry recommends never separating the pharmaceutical contents from the primary and secondary packaging and the package leaflet, patients who spend time away from home do not carry the entire package with them, especially if it is bulky.

Typical outdoor medicine management behaviour is to separate the blister portion containing the required dose of medicine. This separation of the dose from the blister pack is made easy in pre-cut blister packs; where this 'invitation to portion out' was not arranged at the production stage, the user cuts the dose to be taken outside the home with scissors. This separation can result in much information being lost. The problem of loss of information arises especially with occasional-use medicines that may remain in the purse, wallet, pockets, of jackets and coats for a long time and, at the time of need, are not necessarily fully recognisable. Only in a limited number of medicines is the expiry date affixed to the individual dose. In most cases, it is stamped on the edge of the packaging. This may be ink-printed (like the other information on the back of the blister pack) or may be stamped into the material when the packaging is closed.

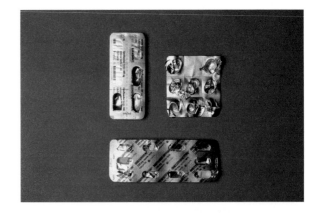

Fig. 16.20 Blister before and after use. The opening of the alveoli alters the information on the tablet housings. When the information is distributed on the closure sheet, even in the part anchored to the blister, it continues to be visible after use

Fig. 16.21 Example of an expiry date on the edge of the packet: on the top, the expiry date embossed in the material (which is much less legible); on the bottom, the printed date in ink

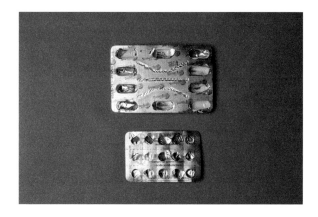

As we have seen with the example shown in Fig. 16.20, in addition to the individual dose, the information must also remain available on the blister pack: even with advanced use of the packaging, the user always has the information identifying the medicine being taken available.

The pharmaceutical industry has not carefully considered the issue of taking medicine outside the home. Indeed, there is a strong effort to make more accessible those medicines presenting more significant difficulties in intake in an environment lacking the necessary accompanying aids (e.g., the transformation of tablets into oral suspensions contained in single-dose sachets). However, a focus on redesigning the packaging system to meet the needs of new consumers and new lifestyles is not yet fully mature.

The blister pack has not yet been redesigned to ensure the separability and autonomy of the single dose of medicine for needs such as taking it outside the home. In this regard, it is worth pointing out that blister packs come in a wide variety (Fig. 16.22), such as:

- single doses separable from the blister by pre-cuts;
- doses that can be separated from the blister two by two;
- doses that can only be separated by cutting the blister with scissors because pre-cuts are missing;
- blister alveoli arranged in dense succession or according to geometries that do not permit separation of the single dose even using scissors. In fact, cutting would affect the integrity of the housing.

These different opportunities offered by the blister, do not seem to have a coherent connection with the 'conditions' and 'constraints' of use that the packaging should guarantee and govern simultaneously. In other words, there is a lack of reflection on the flexibility of use behaviour that the blister pack and its conformation allows or hinders concerning the risks and/or potential harm that a medicine may generate if taken non-compliantly for lack of the necessary information.

In the case of medicines with a high risk of side effects, not only should one not allow the blister pack to be split up—e.g., through the arrangement of the alveoli—but the entire packaging design should be designed so as not to allow the primary,

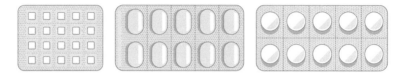

Fig. 16.22 Examples of a blister: complete (on the left) and pre-cut (on the centre and right) to be divided into individual doses

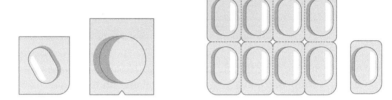

Fig. 16.23 On the left, some portion of the blister with sharp corners. On the right, the blister with rounded outer corners and rounded inner corners formed when separating the dose from the blister

secondary and package leaflet to be broken up. A different matter is the case of over-the-counter medicines or medicines for occasional use, for which the possibility of reducing the traditional blister into single-dose packs should be designed, if necessary, while still guaranteeing that the user can carry all the information needed to recognise the medicine even at a distance.

One final note on this subject. The possibility of obtaining individual doses from the whole blister pack, either by pre-cutting the blister during production, or by cutting the blister with suitable tools such as scissors, has to reckon with certain shrewdnesses typical of the design of products designed for use. Among non-pharmaceutical commodities, in any product that is permitted to divide the initial unit into sub-doses, these are designed to maintain the quality and accuracy inherent in the original format (Fig. 16.23). The single dose may not be a sub-product, the gross outcome of manipulative user interventions. Each part, where subdivision of the packet is permitted, must retain the completeness of data that the entire blister pack possesses; the single dose template, where it is separated, may not have sharp sides; the portion of the blister pack inserted into the pocket or bag must not be able to be opened by accidental breakage of the foil.

16.3.3 Simple, Easy, and Quick to View and Check the Doses Taken and Those Still in the Package

This third point is the one that brings the complexity of the relationship between contents and container into action. At least in the transparent plastic/aluminium version, the blister allows a glimpse of the contents and thus the full/empty, indicating how close you are to the end of your doses. However, this reading is not so safe and proper for blisters with alveoli made of opaque material, either plastic or aluminium. Both of these materials (aluminium to a greater extent) warp by absorbing and retaining the gesture of finger pressure in their shape. But their deformation can also occur due to pressure received accidentally. These material deformations can mislead users regarding the number of drugs still available.

Furthermore, the blister reveals itself to be more fallacious and less able to respond to the expectations placed on its form when it is used as a unit of measurement, as a calendar, as an indicator of the fulfilment or non-fulfilment of the correct management of therapy. This happens for different reasons:

- hardly any blister is designed from the idea that the week can be the unit of measurement of time on which we are used to make checks of our daily fulfilments/non-fulfilments. The alveoli that make up the blister rows rarely correspond to the number seven (i.e., the number of days in the week);
- the start of therapy can take place on any day of the week. The blisters cannot insert a 'start', making it correspond to the day of the start of treatment. There is a lack of a simple recommendation that the physician could suggest to the patient at the prescription stage, such as starting therapy on Mondays in the case of medication that is not of an acute nature;
- there is no space on the secondary packaging or on the blister, where the user can note the day of the start of therapy, which would enable them to make a quick check that the treatment is being taken correctly;
- a sequence order is rarely indicated on the blister to make it easier to check the correspondence between days since the start of therapy (or since the beginning of the pack) and medicines taken. Without this indicator, the patient does not follow a sequence and, if there are two or more blister packs in the pack, does not necessarily take the drugs in an orderly fashion from the same blister pack until it is exhausted.

Most of the above criteria can be found in the packaging of contraceptive pills equipped with a schedule of therapy, a timeline (indicating to the patient the direction to take the drugs), a starting day, and, to prevent the patient from confusing the day of restarting therapy after the withdrawal pause, placebo doses have been included in the blister.

The case of the contraceptive pill pack is an example of a good packaging design that considers many of the memory problems that every user encounters in managing therapy through some formal and communicative shrewdness. These shrewdnesses could easily be extended to all packaging of medicine taken with a fixed dosage (e.g., one tablet per day).

To conclude, these certainly are not exhaustive notes on "blister tablet phenomenologies", with two observations from which some design recommendations can be derived.

A first observation concerns those types of medicine whose intake follows dosage patterns that vary radically according to the pathology to be treated. An example relies on tablets based on the active ingredient methotrexate (Fig. 16.24).

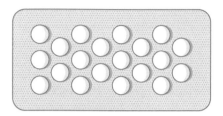

Fig. 16.24 The blister contains tablets based on the active ingredient Methotrexate

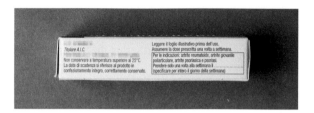

Fig. 16.25 The warning about the medication regimen is written on the smaller side of the packet. The guidelines suggest the use of the main sides of the pack for warnings to users. The warnings are written in small letters, without appropriate interlineations between the different contents. The most prominent warning concerns the storage instructions (written in red)

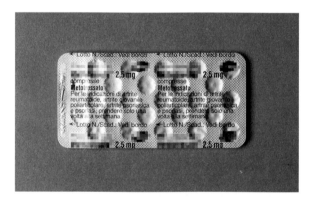

Fig. 16.26 Methotrexate: aluminium foil of blister pack closure with barely legible indications

This medicine, an antineoplastic, is used as a chemotherapeutic agent in treating certain forms of cancer and is taken daily for short, concentrated intervals. Conversely, it is taken weekly or in even longer intervals in patients suffering from rheumatic diseases such as certain forms of arthritis.

The literature reports many intake errors, which usually consist of following the daily intake pattern in patients with rheumatic diseases. A low dosage taken daily and continuously over time generates serious, even fatal, side effects (Moore et al. 2004). To tackle this severe problem, pharmaceutical companies have revisited the communication apparatus accompanying this medicine, which comes from tablets in blister packs.

In the first instance, we overlook the considerations regarding the effectiveness of the notes inserted by the pharmaceutical companies either on the secondary pack

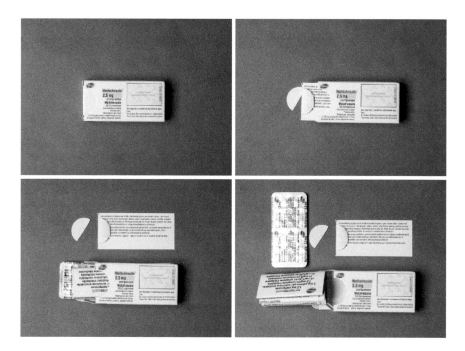

Fig. 16.27 Sequence of actions when opening the packaging to encounter the information card

(Fig. 16.25), the blister (Fig. 16.26) or by adding a card to supplement the leaflet with some notes for the patient (Figs. 16.27 and 16.28).

We consider the positioning of the tablets in the blister and their suitability to attract the user's attention to the dual treatment regimen managed by a single pack. In the arrangement of the tablets, finding any element capable of directing the two types of user towards the correct intake is problematic.

In our observations, we met a patient who uses this medicine to treat rheumatoid arthritis. We interviewed him, asking if he had any doubts about his intake, mainly its weekly frequency. The user replied that the great number of tablets in the blister pack, prompted him to look carefully at the instructions provided by the doctor at the time of the prescription because the blister had no different and distinctive connotation from those containing tablets for daily use. Indeed, the high number of tablets contained in the blister had led him to think of a frequency of intake.

Therefore, we checked whether effective communication could attract attention and inform the patient without uncertainty. We identified this information in several places on the packaging.

We wondered if the user had noticed this information. We observed him interacting with the packaging, inviting him to look for this information.

Although there was a specific posology warning for patients with rheumatoid arthritis enclosed in a frame, we noticed that the user did not superficially dwell on reading the information written on the secondary packaging. The first source where the user looked for information was the package leaflet (which was still sealed). The

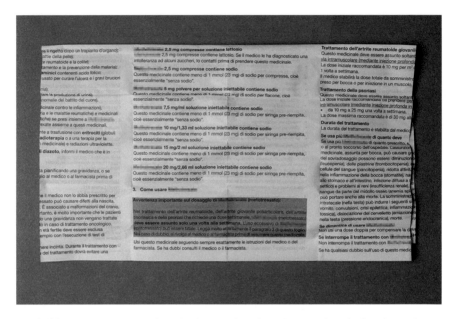

Fig. 16.28 Important warning about the therapeutic regimen in the package leaflet: the text has an inadequate contrast to the background and the warning is not at the beginning of the package leaflet

information on how to take it for patients with rheumatoid arthritis is not immediately at the beginning, as one would expect, but on the fourth side. Moreover, the warnings are written on a dark grey background and are almost illegible. We then asked the user if he had noticed an additional card inserted by the company as a warning for patients following the indicated treatment regimen for rheumatoid arthritis. The patient did not notice the card because it was placed under the blister pack, and glued to the case wall. When the user was asked to tear off the opening/closing flap, through which the card with the warnings can be removed, he froze because the flaps of paper being pulled away from the packet and dragged by the flap led the patient to believe that he was doing an incorrect operation, tampering with the package.

This information is presented on the blister with a text that is not centred on the blister itself but falls in line with the compositional logic of the aluminium coil. The ability to attract the user's attention is not very effective due to the presence of text without visual accents, the reflection of the aluminium foil, and the concavities generated by the aluminium foil in adhering to the blister at the alveoli.

The observation of an individual user, stimulated to interact with the packaging and search for the information necessary for a correct intake of the medicine, has no value as a guide in redesigning the packaging and information in medicines with these peculiarities of use. However, the observation only confirms what the literature has already amply observed concerning this drug. It induces one to rethink the design of dual-regimen blister packs according to more explicit guidelines or, better still, to think of two packs, each dedicated to the individual pathology treated.

A second note, brief and conclusive, concerns the blister pack as a form of packaging that predetermines the number of doses dispensed. The number of doses in the blister pack rarely coincides with the number prescribed by the doctor. Herein lies one of the crucial issues destined to divide supporters and detractors of the blister pack.

The problem arises not so much for therapies to be taken for conditions requiring continuity of treatment, such as chronic diseases, but for occasional ailments requiring the temporary use of drugs. In these cases, predetermined doses have the inherent limitation of never being 'in measure'. They may exceed the doctor's prescription, generating waste or inducing the patient to continue therapy until the contents of the packet are exhausted. Compared to the medical prescription, they may be insufficient, causing the patient not to complete the treatment or forcing him to repurchase a second packet, which will almost certainly have surplus doses. In both cases, the non-adherence to the quantity of medicine concerning the need for treatment risks producing effects on the patient's health and on the environment where, in most cases, the surplus tablets are dumped without adequate care for disposal. Even when kept by the patient because of future needs, surplus is almost never reused because the necessary information is lacking to enable the user to make appropriate use of it when needed. In the case of certain medicines, think of antibiotics (on which there is tiny culture on their specificity of service, on the effects of antibiotic resistance linked to misuse or dispersion in the environment and the animal and plant life cycle), the redesign of the blister according to the logic of the 'multiple' dose or the standard pack to which the modules necessary to complete the treatment according to medical indications should be added, should be part of future industrial strategies.

References

Caprino L (2011) Il farmaco. Settemila anni di storia. Dal rimedio empirico alle biotecnologie [The drug. Seven thousand years of history. From the empirical remedy to biotechnology]. Armando, Roma

Drumond N, Stegemann S (2020) Better medicines for older patients: considerations between patient characteristics and solid oral dosage form designs to improve swallowing experience. Pharmaceutics 13(1):32

Hughes M, Carr W, Carr A (2009) Improving patient safety: reducing medication errors through use of acceptable, accessible medicines packaging. Patient Saf. Online. https://doi.org/10.1211/PJ.2009.10967943

Hummler H, Stillhart C, Meilicke L, Grimm M, Krause E, Mannaa M, Gollasch M, Weitschies W (2023) Impact of tablet size and shape on the swallowability in older adults. Pharmaceutics 15(4):1042. https://doi.org/10.3390/pharmaceutics15041042

Ministero della salute—Direzione generale della programmazione sanitaria—Ufficio III (2019) Raccomandazione n. 19- Raccomandazione per la manipolazione delle forme farmaceutiche orali solide. Retrieved from https://www.salute.gov.it/imgs/C_17_pubblicazioni_2892_allegato.pdf

Moore TJ, Walsh CS, Cohen MC (2004) Reported medication errors associated with methotrexate. Am J Health Syst Pharm 61(13):1380–1384. https://doi.org/10.1093/ajhp/61.13.1380

Overgaard ABA, Møller-Sonnergaard J, Christrup LL, Højsted J, Hansen R (2001) Patients' evaluation of shape, size and colour of solid dosage forms. Pharm World Sci 23:185–188

Open Access This chapter is licensed under the terms of the Creative Commons Attribution 4.0 International License (http://creativecommons.org/licenses/by/4.0/), which permits use, sharing, adaptation, distribution and reproduction in any medium or format, as long as you give appropriate credit to the original author(s) and the source, provide a link to the Creative Commons license and indicate if changes were made.

The images or other third party material in this chapter are included in the chapter's Creative Commons license, unless indicated otherwise in a credit line to the material. If material is not included in the chapter's Creative Commons license and your intended use is not permitted by statutory regulation or exceeds the permitted use, you will need to obtain permission directly from the copyright holder.

Chapter 17
Use Phenomenologies: What Does the User Do with the Secondary Medicine Packaging and Package Leaflet?

Antonella Valeria Penati

Abstract This chapter supplements the remarks contained in the paragraph *The role of medicine packaging in dispensing* of this text. In that context, we addressed the important role that secondary packaging plays in the dispensing process, especially in terms of its informational connotations. In this chapter, we look instead at the dynamics of patient use, once the medicine has entered the context of everyday use. In addition to the informational aspects, functional aspects such as opening, closing, containing, storing etc. come into play. It is in the relationship with the patient that the secondary pack demonstrates its informational and usage effectiveness. The medicines under analysis were 'taken' from the contexts of use under observation. To return the problems observed, the mode of illustration was chosen, eliminating the medicine's identifying marks, while leaving the description of the problematic elements, from our point of view, relating to information and form, which were returned in 'anonymous' form.

17.1 Secondary Medicine Packaging in Use

In the paragraph *The role of medicine packaging in dispensing* of this volume, we began our reading of the secondary packaging of medicines, starting with the studies that have had the pharmacist as the reference user for all those activities that involve high interaction with the medicine at the time of dispensing.

In the context of dispensing, the external packaging of the medicine-the secondary packaging in fact-takes, to all intents and purposes, the role of an object in and of itself, with a strong autonomy concerning the contents, which no one can access, not even the pharmacist, because of the seals imposed by the anti-tampering regulations (European Parliament (the), Directive 62/EU 2011).

A. V. Penati (✉)
Department of Design, Politecnico di Milano, Milan, Italy
e-mail: antonella.penati@polimi.it

At the dispensing stage, as we highlighted in the part of the text mentioned above, the clarity of the multiple information elements that cover the entire surface of the packaging is especially relevant. Each of these is of fundamental importance in the process that leads to the unambiguous identification of the medicine to be dispensed, distinguishing it from others by name, the dosage of the active ingredient, number of doses contained, pharmaceutical form, etc. In the pharmacy, the packaging certainly does not lose its value as a container. Still, this function becomes, as to say, secondary to the visual component because it is in the design of the information elements that the functional effectiveness of the secondary packaging is expressed.

As soon as the medicine enters the patient's sphere of use, not only does the packaging fully manifest and tangibly acquire all its functional prerogatives (containing, preserving, shaping, facilitating access to the contents, dosing, informing, etc.), but the information apparatus itself and even the way it is 'put on the page', in the patient's sphere of use, assume a different utility concerning the specific needs of those who dispense the medicine.

As is well known, the information necessary to correctly identify a medicine is regulated, as well as specific principles of a hierarchical arrangement of information on the page are recommended, and also what information must necessarily be on the main page of the packaging and, according to what logic, some of it must be close to each other, to create connections of meaning (European Parliament, Directive 2001/83/EC, art 54).

Similarly, specific Guidelines are now well-established that suggest the most appropriate ways for the informational use of images and pictograms that can supplement, but not replace, verbal information (European Parliament, Directive 2001/83/EC, art 62).

Yet even though the repertoire of recommendations has grown over time, primarily due to user experience and its incorporation and transformation into precept for proper design, there remain many gaps in the effectiveness of the information elements accompanying the medicine in appropriate use.

For example, our observations show that, for the user, the name of the medicine and its active ingredient, so crucial to the pharmacist, have little effectiveness to remember the pathology, the organ, and the reason why that medicine is taken. Even more so, in occasional-use medicines—such as an antibiotic—a long time after its use, patients are not even able to remember why that medicine was prescribed, by what doctor, and under what circumstances. This is precisely why, on the secondary packaging, the patient is used to making notes (Fig. 17.1), especially at the beginning of the therapy and before becoming familiar with it. These are annotations related to the patient's name (in case two or more patients are taking medicine in the house); the reason why the medicine was prescribed (translating into familiar language abstract designations and ineffective in reconnecting the name to the reasons for its assumption, for example: *Warfarin Sodico*, 'anticoagulant'; or *Amiodarone Cloridrato*, 'for the heart'; *Perindopril Arginina e Amlodipina*, 'for blood pressure'; *Sodio Alginato e Sodio Bicarbonato*, 'for digestion'; to the dose of medicine that is to be taken (this is especially the case when several doses are taken within the day or fractions of the single dose or different doses on different days); to the date of

17 Use Phenomenologies: What Does the User Do with the Secondary Medicine...

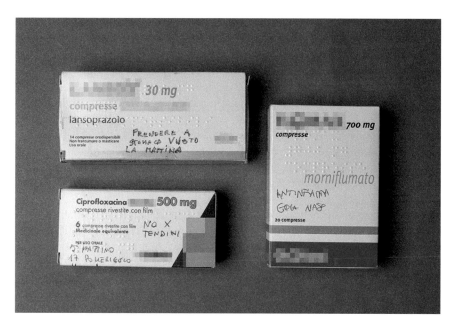

Fig. 17.1 Example of notations written by patients on medicine packages to customise them according to medical prescriptions

Fig. 17.2 Examples of medicine packaging in which there is a space inviting customisation through user information

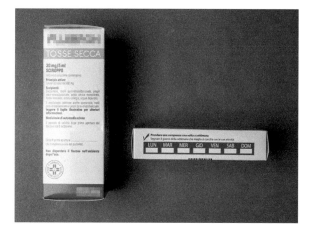

opening the pack or starting therapy to verify compliance with shelf life or adherence to the prescribed dosage. In other words, the secondary pack becomes, for the patient, 'the blackboard', the 'calendar', the 'post-it' on which to note information able to personalize its use.

Some pharmaceutical companies, having picked up on this need of the patient to integrate general information with information related to personal therapy, have begun to expressly provide in secondary packaging, spaces dedicated to user notes (Fig. 17.2).

Again, from the interviews conducted with patients, it emerges that, in the custom that accompanies the daily intake of medicine, it is not so much the "registry" elements that the patient refers to distinguish one medicine from another-as is the case in pharmacies-, but instead it is the overall graphic elements that are grasped by the patient 'at a glance'. In daily practice, the medicines in use are often arranged in a specific order (mainly when the therapy consists of many drugs) and are managed according to intake sequences that, once set, are repeated daily through semi-automatic actions. The order and sequences of gestures regulate the taking practices and not the analytical recognition of the information elements that identify the individual medicine. The patient uses a careful reading of the medicine's master data at crucial moments, such as changing therapy, ending a medicine and replacing it with refills, etc.

Paradigmatic of this behaviour is the story of a patient who, in a moment of inattention, did not put his usual medicine—the active ingredient of which is *Clonazepam*—in the kitchen drawer reserved for his therapy, but left it on a shelf, next to the medicines used by his wife. Among the medicines in his wife's therapy was a medicine whose active ingredient is *Bromazepam*, a medicine with secondary packaging bearing a strong visual similarity to the former (Fig. 17.3). Both medicines, in fact, despite having distinct proprietary names and not belonging to the same corporate brand, have a very similar overall image, especially at the top of the opening. This organisational defaillance is said to have caused a serious intake error, which was fortunately prevented by the different olfactory impression of the two solutions and the speed at which the drops came out, which made the user suspicious of a possible packaging mix-up.

While many patients report that they carefully observe the information related to the 'drug registry' only on particular occasions, even more report that they do not read at all the information on the secondary packaging associated with instructions for use, storage regulations, precautions related to securing the medicine, etc. From the experiences collected, some users even 'get rid' of the secondary pack when they put the

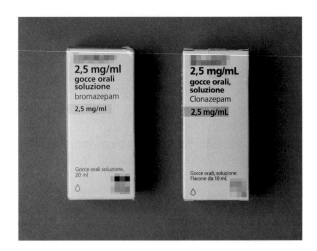

Fig. 17.3 Medicines with a different name and different active ingredient but easily confused by the graphics of the case

medicine in the containers they use to organize home therapy keeping only the primary pack. Even the package leaflets are often thrown away without even being read. Sometimes the secondary pack is thrown away, while the package leaflets are stored separately from the medicines (e.g., in drawers used for collecting medical documents and filed meticulously inside transparent envelopes); sometimes. They are stored in bulk inside bags (Fig. 17.4). But the practice of having 'naked medicine' with only the primary packaging is widespread, especially in the case of blister packaging.

Several hypotheses can be made about why patients do not read the information in the secondary pack of medicines. Indeed, the most plausible, confirmed by the patients interviewed, lies in the belief that all helpful information is contained in the Package Leaflet. Then there is, especially among the elderly, the sense of respect for the doctor's authority and trust in the indications received from him. These would not make further information necessary. There is probably also a behaviour derived from the habits of using packages of other products to which we rarely pay attention except for the little information searched for on first use.

One can suppose that underlying this distracted attitude is also the ambiguity of the addressee to whom the information on the secondary pack is addressed: in fact, it is not very clear which ones pertain to the Pharmacist and which ones are intended for the user-patient.

An additional problem probably needs to be considered: the temporal inconsistency between the time of reading the information and the time of use. Some of the information available on the secondary pack concerns how to conserve the package before use, the possible effects of taking medicine; and the post-use and disposal phases.

Mainly, the user tends to read the information found on the package, at the time of its opening, which often coincides with using the contained product. Utilitarian logic prompts the patient to read only when the need for information emerges. This a condition that, by analogy with most everyday products, may not even arise because custom tends to shape user behaviour. Unfortunately, in the case of medicines, reliance on custom, can produce even serious errors. For this reason, all the indications on secondary packaging, which the user should apprehend before use, should be rethought from the formal point of view to have greater visibility and ability to attract attention.

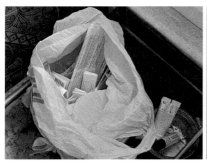
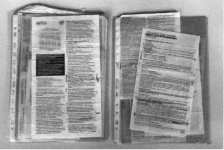

Fig. 17.4 User behaviour when using packaging leaflets

As well as should be present on the secondary pack and have visibility of all those useful information even before the purchase: intolerances; size of solid oral forms when they could create swallowing difficulties; prohibition of use or attention to use in children or pregnant women, or the elderly, etc. This applies, in a particular way, to non-prescription medicines that might have adverse effects for some patients. And these directions are even more necessary because the inner contents of the medicine cannot be inspected, and therefore the content of the information that must be placed on the outside of the product must also be carefully rethought.

We emphasise here the importance of depicting on the secondary packaging the shape and size, in real scale of the medicine contained, especially when it is a solid form for oral use. Indeed, many patients have difficulty swallowing and the impossibility of opening the secondary packaging makes it difficult to assess the ability to take the drug. It is not uncommon that, especially in the elderly patient, precisely because of the size of the medicine, there is a need for manipulation (crushing, splitting, etc.) of the medicine, sometimes improperly. Sometimes there is even a necessity to change medicine, throwing away, in effect, the pack that was mistakenly purchased due to insufficient information.

Currently, on the secondary packaging of medicines, the representation of the shape of the tablet contained is either missing altogether or, as sometimes happens, is represented with a three-dimensional image that does not necessarily refer to the real shape of the medicine contained (Fig. 17.5). Indeed, in many cases, these images generically allude to the fact that the content is an oral solid form, but this image does not necessarily correspond to the content.

In this regard, in addition to adding a realistic representation of the content (correctly representing the actual tablet shape and size), consideration should also be

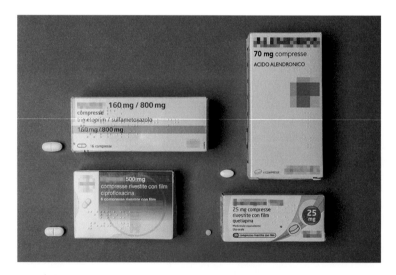

Fig. 17.5 Examples of medicines in which the representation of the medicine on the secondary pack does not correspond to the size of the contained medicine. The illustration is only intended to indicate to the user the type of medicine contained, not its actual characteristics

given to reviewing/prohibiting the use of images, included in the pack for purely advertising purposes, where these may lead the user to misinterpret the pharmaceutical form contained. Two examples are illustrated below (Fig. 17.6), chosen from among many on the secondary packaging of medicines. In the first case, a tablet is represented leaving a trail; in the second case, the name of the medicine is 'decorated' with a cloud of circles of different sizes. The intention is probably to represent the beneficial force released by the medicine. These images, however, may evoke the trail of bubbles typical of effervescent tablets. Whereas the medicines in question are coated tablets that must be swallowed while drinking water.

A final example is those corporate brands that resemble or can be traced back to pharmaceutical forms (Fig. 17.7). These graphic elements risk confusing the user as to the form of the medicine contained and may even be confused with operational indications that the user should/could make on the medicine. We refer here in particular to labels that have great similarities with typical tablet representations. The ambiguity generated by the mark, due to its shape, can be further amplified by the fact that, on the medicine's packaging, the mark is not positioned next to the company's logo, to constitute a communicative unit, but is placed in an isolated position. This makes it difficult to assume that the visual sign of the trademark is part of the corporate image system and the user might instead interpret that sign as an indication of the fractionability of the contained medicine.

We add a reflection here. Medicine does not represent a consumer good that motivates the user to purchase it. Users don't choose the medicine: it is prescribed and represents a necessity for the patient. It is also necessary to consider the "passive

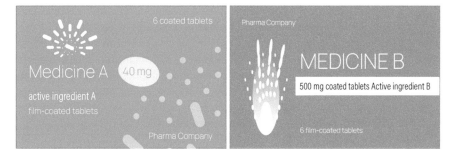

Fig. 17.6 Examples of images that may confuse the user as to how to assume

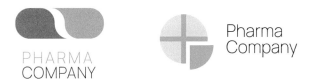

Fig. 17.7 Fictitious examples of company brands (simulating existing brands) that refer to the tablet/capsule form and may therefore confuse the user. It should be noted that these trademarks referring to a solid oral form may also be present on packages containing drops, syrups, etc.

purchase" condition in the lack of 'informational curiosity'. A curiosity that instead the consumer shows for the products he purchases motivated by needs or desires. Even in the case of ordinary consumer products, however, of the information on the packaging, only that which interests the user at first use is sought. If they are goods for continuous use, the information on the packaging is no longer re-read in subsequent uses. In medicine, conversely, we are faced with a wrapper that is as important as the product it contains, constituting, with its information, an integral part of it. For some of these, the patient may need to access it several times during therapy. It is crucial to consider the processual aspects involving the communicative elements. Indeed, one can speak of a kind of "communication life cycle" that follows—or instead should follow—the life cycle of a medicine, emphasizing different information based on the information necessity that may be different at other times during therapy:

- the medicine is being taken for the first time by a neophyte patient who has no information about how to use it, how to store it, how it interacts with other medicines or food and drink, and any adverse effects, and for whom it is necessary to assess what "initiation of therapy" information needs to be accessed as a priority to facilitate the experience of treatment;
- the medicine has been taken for some time because it is part of the daily therapy of a patient who can be defined as an "expert"—in the etymological sense of one who has gained experience and therefore needs unique information generally related to particular situations or eventualities;
- the medicine is taken occasionally or is prescribed sometime after the first intake, a type of use this lends itself to various errors related to the mixture of erroneous memories, forgetfulness, etc.

Precisely because the patient's knowledge about the medicine changes over time, special attention should be given to those information items that, especially at first use, need a didactic level of explanation. One example is the way of taking medicine, which is usually communicated with short formulations (e.g., "Medicine for oral use" or even just "Oral use"). These brief indications are understood not necessarily by everyone. This is further compounded by the fact that the modes of oral intake are different. Usually, this difference is indicated through an additional indication, separate from the previous one, which in the formulas "Film-coated tablets"; "Gastro-resistant tablets"; "Extended-release tablets," etc., subtend different ways of taking a medicine orally. Indeed, in some cases, the medicine does not need to be handled and can only be swallowed with water. In other cases, however, the tablets can be broken, crushed and even dissolved in water. In still other cases, they must be held in the mouth until dissolved. This modality is referred to by terms such as—orosoluble, orodispersible, and sublingual. The user does not always understand the differences between these definitions. This same information should also be found inside in a more articulated form. Thus, attention should be paid to indications related to the use of medicines, such as preparations in drops or powders in sachets, which, not possessing a form that unambiguously associates them with a route of intake, can give rise to even serious errors.

Secondary pack information, additionally, should be grouped into "sense areas" for the user and the actions he needs to take and be positioned at the point closest to the action to be performed (Fig. 17.8).

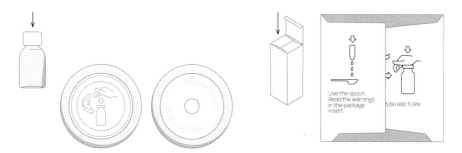

Fig. 17.8 Examples of spatial positioning of information that supports the user's action and precedes the action to be performed in a time-correct manner. The illustrations shown in the second example (on the right) are on the flaps of the packaging. Their purpose is to indicate the sequence of actions that the user must perform: (1) press and rotate the cap to open; (2) pour the drops by counting them. The logical sequence would be more correctly represented by inverting the position of the images and positioning action (1) on the left and action (2) on the right

From a communication perspective, the medicine package is presented as a complex artefact with layered information: partly arranged on the secondary package, partly on the primary package, partly on the package leaflet, and partly on the medicine itself. This layering does not always correspond to the user's information needs, which change depending on the user's experience of use.

And finally, the information on pharmaceutical product packaging does not always follow communicative hierarchies that can facilitate the user's information experience by guiding their reading. This observation applies to the disposition of information both between inside and outside the packaging and on the outside, that is, on the different faces of the secondary packaging.

Secondary packaging, in most cases, is shaped like a rectangle parallelepiped (Fig. 17.9). The dimensions of the different sides of the parallelepiped are, in addition to the graphic layout, essential elements in identifying the front and back of the packaging. In the case of parallelepipeds with two predominantly sized faces, recognition of the 'main page' is intuitive (most horizontally developed packages are included in this typology, characterized by two large-sized faces that serve as the front and back; two intermediate-sized faces that constitute the edge sides of the packaging; and two smaller sized faces that generally correspond to the opening/closing flaps). It is not as intuitive to identify the main face in the case of packages with four faces of the same size. Such are, for example, packages of vertically developed medicines (syrup packs, eye drops, drops, etc.) in which the two smaller faces constitute respectively the base of support (unusable from the communicative point of view) and the top, the part intended for the opening/closing of the package that the user sometimes tends to tear off to hand it over to the doctor or pharmacist when he runs out of medicine, and there is a need to buy a refill.

In the case of solids with the longest side on the horizontal plane (Fig. 17.10), the user knows, by custom, what information he will find on the main page: name of the medicine, active ingredient, dosage, amount of product contained, pharmaceutical form, route of intake, brand logo and brand name. On the back is an area for the

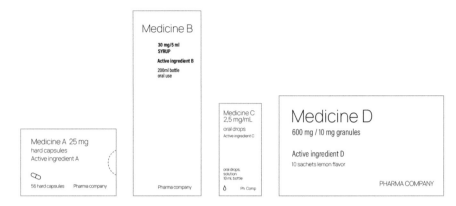

Fig. 17.9 Illustration of the main types of secondary packaging: the first is typical of medicines in blister packs, which, although of different sizes, are characterised by a side opening; the other type (characterised by an opening from the top) is typical of syrups, little bottles containing drops, and packaging of medicines in sachets

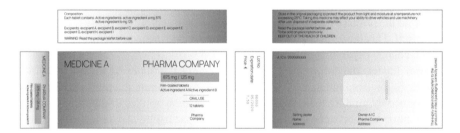

Fig. 17.10 The image, although illustrated by a fictitious medicine, reproduces the layout of a real medicine package on the market. The example demonstrates the irrational placement of information on the outer packaging

pharmacist, where there is the sticker by legal duty. All the information required by law and which the law itself suggests should be placed on the main faces of the packaging (e.g., *To be sold on prescription*; *Keep out of sight and reach of children*; *Read package leaflet before use*; *Do not dispose of container in the environment*, etc.) are not necessarily found on the back page, although, for the user, this is the most intuitive side where to look for them, in terms of size and therefore importance of the page.

In addition to the problematic traceability of the information contents (not always arranged in a hierarchical order and not present in a precise place in the packaging), these are in any case underestimated by patients because they have now entered into everyday use and our daily language to the point that their prescriptive importance is weakened. Many of the prescriptive contents we find in the packaging, for example, are part of advertisements during which they are read, at the close of the spot, at such a speed as to make them almost incomprehensible, thus giving the idea that they are ancillary messages of secondary importance. The graphic way this information is presented in the packaging diminishes its content, with no specific order being present and none of the many artifices that the graphic treatment of a text makes available to create visual hierarchies and points of attention being used. Nor are they necessarily found on the main pages of the packaging but are sometimes placed on the minor sides. In addition, the randomness in the use of capitals, boldface, use of colour; the absence sometimes of interlines that distance the different 'warnings' (Fig. 17.11), making them perceived in their autonomy; the presence of text written vertically on a horizontal page (forcing the patient to rotate the packaging to read the text); the use of a reduced font body that is not sufficiently contrasted by the background colours or illegible because it is on a dark background, are all elements that contribute to weakening the 'appeal' contained in these prescriptive propositions. The perception of certain randomness seems to stem from 'filling' the available space more than from a communication design that is attentive to the reader's reading paths and need for comprehension. The area given to a corporate image, which can come to dominate and take a back seat to informational and prescriptive elements, also plays a significant role in this.

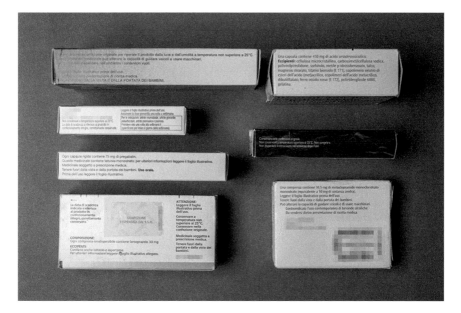

Fig. 17.11 The image illustrates a few examples of the graphic layout of the warnings from which various readability problems may arise: (1) most examples show that the back of the packet is used in few cases to give information to the patient; smaller sides where the body of the character is of necessity reduced are favoured for this purpose; (2) each pharmaceutical company decides autonomously what prominence to give to the different contents (laid down by law), through the use of capital letters, bold type, red colour, frames etc., in order to give a different relevance to the information for the user; (3) the individual warnings are hardly ever perceived independently through the use of appropriate interlineations; (4) in addition to the size of the font, the contrast between text and background also intervenes to reduce the readability of the information; (5) information on the presence of substances that must be well highlighted for certain patient groups (e.g. lactose), indistinct from general warnings such as 'keep out of the sight and reach of children'

Sometimes the language of the indications is also not immediately understandable due to the positioning on the secondary pack. An example is the sentence, "*The expiration date indicated refers to the product in intact, properly stored packaging*," which directs the patient's attention to problems with the integrity of the packaging as a whole and not the integrity of individual doses. And in fact, it is a widespread practice among patients to 'unblister' (a week, sometimes even a fortnight before use) tablets, pills, capsules, etc., interrupting the protection given by the primary pack.

The same warning, carried on the primary pack, may be more effective in influencing user behaviour.

Similarly, the phrase: Store in the original package to protect the product from light and humidity at a temperature not exceeding 25 °C. contains three different indications:

- the product must be protected from light (the secondary pack should provide this, and sometimes the primary pack when it is opaque or dark);
- the product must be protected from humidity (the primary pack should provide this); and
- the product must be protected from temperatures above 25 °C, and for this purpose, the pack proves to be an insufficient device because the only expedient the user can take is to store the medicine in a temperature-controlled place. The fact that the firm has fulfilled its informational obligations does not mean that it has made the user understand what concrete actions the user must take to ensure the integrity of the medicine. Moreover, the fact that this indication appears on a minor side of the package, along with other information that is important to the user but not at all distinguishable from each other, only distances it from the goal that should be a priority: to give adequate information to induce correct behaviour.

From the various reasons listed above, although summarily, it can be understood why so much information reported in the secondary pack is not perceived in its importance or even read.

17.2 Opening and Closing Signs

Observing user behaviour, we also note that, very often, the secondary packaging did not unambiguously indicate the correct side of opening. In a population that is 90% right-handed overall, the natural opening direction of a horizontal pack with side openings should be the right side. And on this side one would expect to find some clear indication for the user. Instead, it is rare for the words 'open here' to appear on medicine packs. Sometimes it is the die-cut mark that generates an invitation to open. Sometimes it is the tamper-evident seal indicating that that is the side to be opened by cutting the seal. it is an implicit indication and, as such, weak. Sometimes it is the die-cutting that tells the user that they have to tear the cardboard in order to open (Figs. 17.12 and 17.13).

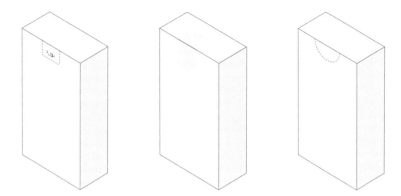

Fig. 17.12 Types of opening with greater or lesser capacity to properly guide the user's gestures

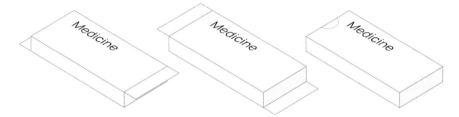

Fig. 17.13 Variety of box openings with different levels of difficulty for the user, because the opening is not visible or because the opening is on the wrong side

Sometimes, it is the shadow line generated at the top of the right side that makes the gap between the upper face and the side closing flap intuitable. When the opening is on the upper side, it not only attracts attention through sight, but also indulges the opening gesture with the thumb. Opening on the left side, on the other hand, is discouraged when the closing flap fits at the bottom of the pack, effectively disappearing and offering no invitation to use, even for the hand. In all these cases, however, these are weak invitations, not even explicitly designed to achieve the required action. Even on these seemingly minor aspects of operation, alternate design attention is devoted by the pharmaceutical industry. In some cases, the packaging design becomes refined, going so far as to produce a double layer of cardboard on the closure flap, so that the top layer, bearing the medicine data, can be removed and handed to the doctor for the next prescription. This is a clever redesign of the closure flap, redesigned to comply with the legal requirement to have tamper-resistant closures, at the same time, panders to the practice in use by patients of tearing/cutting off the opening flap containing the necessary data to be handed over to the doctor for the prescription of the following doses. But the cutting of the secondary pack to pick up a small label containing the master data of the medicine, is also used by the patient to report on the daily therapy sheets the visual elements of the packaging to make it easier to choose the suitable pack, among the many in the therapy (Figs. 17.14, 17.15 and 17.16).

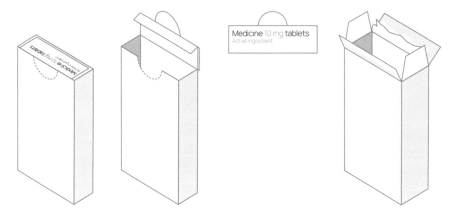

Fig. 17.14 On the left, detail of opening with flap joined to the packet by a die-cut; the flap can be separated from the packet so that it can be used as a tag to be shown to the doctor for subsequent prescriptions. On the right opening flaps closed with a glue stitch. Once opened, the pack cannot be resealed

Fig. 17.15 Packaging designed to be opened on the left side with a die-cut invite

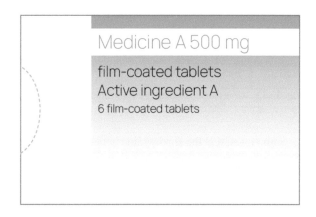

In the face of a few exemplary cases, we find closures obtained with a glue stitch that, once opened, can no longer be closed again, giving a "sloppy" and worthless impression to the container and its role and to the medicine contained. It is closures such as these that do not allow for all the tasks that are sometimes assigned to secondary pharmaceutical packaging: keeping in the dark some medicines that should not be exposed to light for too long; storing any medicine fragments dispersed in the package; making access somewhat less easy for children who might be more attracted to exploring the inside of an open package.

Even the opening from above, which would seem to pose less of a problem by indicating a quasi-obligatory action, nevertheless shows similar inattention to the patient's gestures.

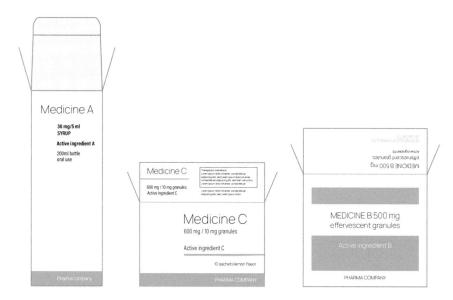

Fig. 17.16 On the left the syrup package with the correct opening of the top. In the centre packaging containing powder in sachets, with the top opening from the back towards the front. In doing so, the user turns the packet over, thus losing information about the pharma they are taking. The third picture even shows the same situation as the pack in the centre, but on opening, the cover graphic appears 'upside down'

If the format of the medicine cases falls within the two case histories, we have seen—parallelepiped with predominantly horizontal development and opening at the side and parallelepiped with predominantly vertical development and opening at the top—some medicines present a certain ambiguity in this respect.

We report below two packs whose graphics and position of the opening follow the behaviour of vertically developed packs, although they have a geometric shape and therefore a mode of placement in drawers and shelves typical of horizontally developed boxes (Fig. 17.17). This generates perplexity in the user on the opening side.

This insistence on designing proper accessibility to the contents, in the case of medicine, is of particular importance not only for the apparent reason of making it easy for people, often the elderly, to access necessary and, in some cases, life-saving products, but also because it is essential to establish, perhaps even to regulate, whether the patient should find the medicine right away or, before accessing the medicine, should 'encounter' the Package Leaflet.

Again, the case is varied and is dictated by the requirements of the packaging system. In fact, at the stage of inserting the medicine and package leaflet inside its primary pack, the packaging machines, after folding the Package Leaflet, give it the characteristic open C shape with a final folding. Inside this "C shape" formed by the Package Leaflet, the blister packs (in the case of tablets) are threaded, and the package leaflet and blister are placed in the secondary packaging together. At this point, the secondary packaging is ready to be sealed.

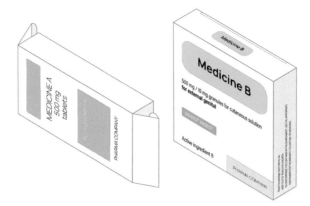

Fig. 17.17 On the left, the packaging shape suggests an opening on the right side. The graphics are designed as if the pack opened from the top. On the right, the pack graphic indicates an opening from the top. Indeed, the packaging opens from the top. Nevertheless, the packaging shape would find a more appropriate opening placement on the right side

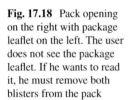 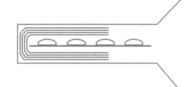

Fig. 17.18 Pack opening on the right with package leaflet on the left. The user does not see the package leaflet. If he wants to read it, he must remove both blisters from the pack

What sequences of action can the user follow when opening the medicine package? The first situation in which the user may find himself is immediately seeing the blister packs, slipping them out of the secondary packaging, and starting therapy without needing to take out the package leaflet that remains at the bottom. In this first situation, the user may not even see the package leaflet and, therefore, may not need to read it before taking medicine (Fig. 17.18).

If interested in reading the information about the medicine, before the start of therapy, the user can open the packaging from the left side and slide out the package leaflet or take out, from the right side, the entire contents, namely both the package leaflet and the blister packs. In this first scheme of element arrangement, the reinsertion of the blisters within the packaging is not easy because the package leaflet obstructs it. It happens when the blister is made of soft, pliable materials (e.g., aluminium-aluminium) that flex easily (Fig. 17.19).

Getting the blister back into its 'natural seat' is not easy in this case. This same difficulty also occurs when the patient has opened the package leaflet. After opened, it is difficult to fold the package leaflet back into the exact same starting shape and compact thickness as before the opening. This discomfort, according to patients, is one of the reasons why there is such a strong tendency to get rid of the leaflet or, if one is scrupulous, to store it in a different place than the secondary packaging. The proposed example concerns blister packs, but the same situation is also found in syrup or eye drops package.

17 Use Phenomenologies: What Does the User Do with the Secondary Medicine… 353

The second pattern of the internal arrangement of blister packs and the related leaflet is when the patient, upon opening, first finds the package leaflet that 'wraps' the medicine blisters (Fig. 17.20). In this scheme, taking out the package leaflet is a necessary step to 'get to' the medicine.

Suppose it does not necessarily involve the patient reading the information. In that case, arranging the different internal elements ensures the right path the user should take to take a medicine correctly. Some patients (especially those who are used to not reading the leaflet) said they were irritated by this 'barrier' to the immediate use of the medicine. And indeed, a small percentage claimed that they felt a real discomfort and therefore eliminated the package leaflet from the secondary container for this very reason (Fig. 17.21).

However, this is the correct arrangement of the elements that compose the package and the one best suited to make the patient perform the correct sequence of actions. Even with this second scheme, in any case, the problems of reinserting the blister packs and package leaflet, remain unchanged.

Similar problems are encountered with upright, top-opening packages: syrups, drops, single-dose sachets (Fig. 17.22). Here too, where the package leaflet is placed underneath the medicine, the patient has to take it out in order to read the package leaflet.

This reflection drawn from the observation of ambivalent user behaviour allows us to highlight how seemingly minor aspects-in the case observed the arrangement

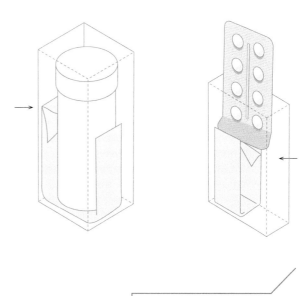

Fig. 17.19 Possible interference of the package leaflet in the removal and reinsertion of the primary pack into the secondary pack

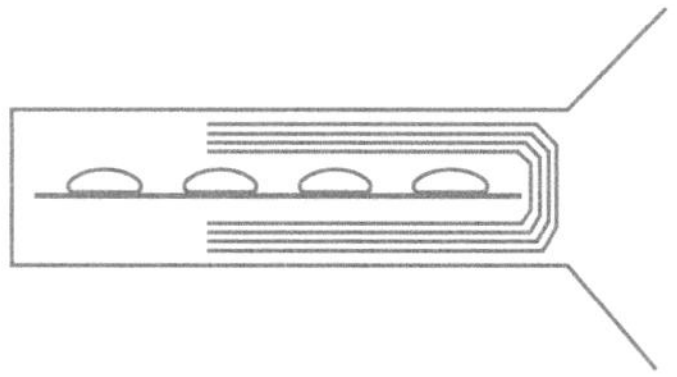

Fig. 17.20 Pack opening on the right with package leaflet on the right. The user has to get in touch with the package leaflet to access the medicine

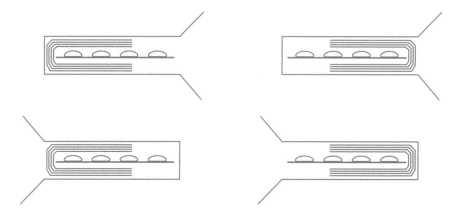

Fig. 17.21 The opening patterns currently on the market show that there is no designed relationship between opening side and package leaflet placement

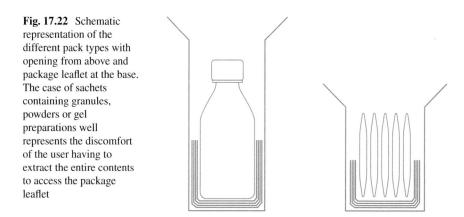

Fig. 17.22 Schematic representation of the different pack types with opening from above and package leaflet at the base. The case of sachets containing granules, powders or gel preparations well represents the discomfort of the user having to extract the entire contents to access the package leaflet

of the different product components within the package-can create obligatory or strongly pre-determined action sequences, thus influencing patient behaviour.

Indeed, as on many other aspects, there is a lack of deep user analysis that could give useful design guidance to make the medicine use experience more effective and easier, perhaps going so far as to change the folding pattern and placement of information content within the package.

17.3 Secondary Packaging and Primary Packaging: Visual Identity

It is good practice, we know, that secondary packaging, primary packaging, package leaflet and medicine are never separated. We know equally well, however, that this does not happen in the user experience. Leaving aside the misbehaviour which, we have seen, punctuates the user experience, there is however a moment when, correctly, medicine, primary pack and secondary pack are separated. This is the moment when the medicine is taken. In complex therapies it may happen that the user, once the primary pack has been removed from its outer packaging, is no longer able to recognise the medicine. As we described in Chap. 12, medicines (especially oral solid forms) have a low degree of morphological differentiation and this is one of the causes that may lead to the medicine not being recognised once it has been removed from the secondary pack and blister. Sometimes, however, it is also the primary packaging that has insufficient identifying features and is poorly differentiated and/or does not carry the information necessary for the correct recognition of the medicine. Single-dose eye drops are an example of how difficult it is to recognise the medicine being taken once it has been taken out of its packaging. But the world of blister tablets itself is not immune to this problem. In fact, it can happen that the information about the medicine is not written on the aluminium foil that closes the blister pack, with sufficient frequency (Fig. 17.23).

Opening the tablets, by tearing the aluminium foil, has the effect of removing the information written on the foil. The Guidelines of the European Community recommend precisely in this regard that the frequency of the written information be carefully considered so that the medicine remains recognisable until the end.

It is therefore necessary that between secondary pack, primary pack and, if possible, medicine there are graphic elements (e.g., colour, graphics of the written parts etc.) that visually connect the different elements of the pack.

A second element which can confuse patients as to the recognisability of the medicine, especially patients taking the same medicine at different dosages throughout the day, is the lack of visual identity between secondary and primary packaging and drug. The use of certain colours on the outer packaging is sometimes not accompanied—or even contradicted—using an identical colour on the medicine as well. The example below, we believe, eloquently illustrates the difficulty in recognising the medicine that the user may encounter (Fig. 17.24). The example illustrates just

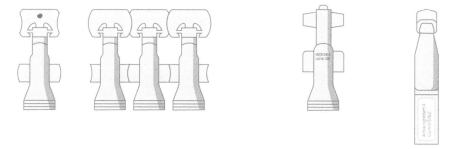

Fig. 17.23 On the left, marks made by the patient to distinguish two eye drops (one of which is a cortisone with limits on daily dosage) with too similar primary packs and with the brand name of the drug almost invisible. The patient covered the cap of one of the two packs with paper scotch on which he drew a small mark. On the right is an ex-ample of a primary pack of an eye drop that not only ensures better prehension, but also provides a space to give the correct information about the medicine's name

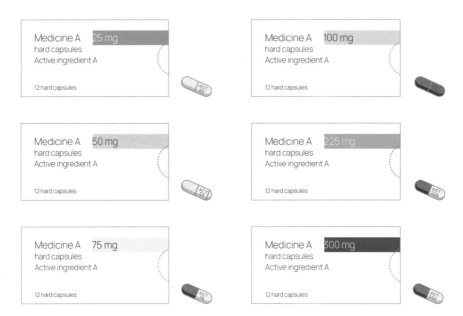

Fig. 17.24 Example of a medicine with multiple dosages. The colour variations indicating the progressive increase in dosage in the secondary pack are not well 'interpreted' using different colours which have little meaning for either the pharmacist or the patient (they are in fact neither colours in chromatic contrast nor colours in chromatic progression). Similarly, the capsules are not able to communicate the progression of the different dosages. In addition, there is no colour relationship between secondary packaging and capsules

as clearly the lack of a criterion for translating the increase/difference in dosages of the same medicine through the use of colour. This applies both to capsules, compared with each other, and to secondary packages, compared with each other. As the dosage of the active ingredient increases, one might expect a 'crescendo' colour transition on the same colour scale (on the use of colour in the world of medicine, see Chap. 17) to emphasise the increase in dosage or, conversely, the use of colour contrast, simply to emphasise the diversity of dosages.

17.4 Secondary Packaging and Package Leaflet. Interferences in Use

In Chap. 17, dealing with the observations made on users, we described the most recurrent usage behaviours of the Package Leaflet: some patients immediately throw it away (literally 'get rid of it') upon opening it; others separate it from the secondary pack and put it away separately, thinking they will read it when needed; some keep it inside the secondary pack, complaining, however, that the presence of the Package Leaflet 'gets in the way' of the medicine's usage operations when it comes to taking it out and putting it back in its secondary pack.

If we try to trace the set of critical issues collected back to a few macro-categories, we observe that the Package Leaflet is weak as an information tool:

- in terms of usability (difficult to take out, open, refold, store in the pack; but also difficult to read because of the grammage of the paper, which produces visual interference between the page being read and the text contained on the remaining page, which is visible in transparency. It is also difficult to read because the folds of the paper fall over the lines of text;
- in terms of accessibility (challenging to track down the information and understand it);
- in terms of education about treatment (a considerable part devoted to side effects doesn't match with an equally important part dedicated to the benefits of taking a medicine, the support that a proper lifestyle can have in enhancing the effectiveness of the medicine; the expedients related to nutrition; and prevention).

Recently, there is a new sensitivity to the problems of information overload. Some pharmaceutical companies are supplementing the package leaflet with a card that summarises the most important information on the usability of the medicine, possible interactions with food and drink, and important warnings for the user (Fig. 17.25).

Similarly, in some medicines, information on the effects of the medicine is supplemented with advice on a correct lifestyle and diet aimed at reinforcing the logic of prevention. Below, we devote it to the Package Leaflet in its nature as an object. We do not dwell here on its usability related to the dynamics of reading: the invitation to read in a specific order; the easy traceability of the content searched for; the redundancy of information when necessary; the distinction between information destined for doctors, pharmacists, and technical personnel and that for the user; and

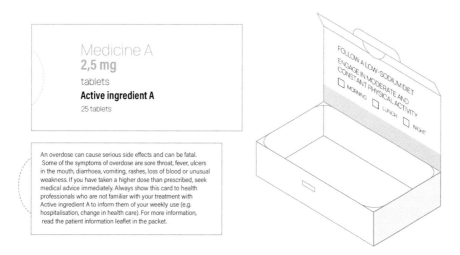

Fig. 17.25 Example of package mini-leaflets supplementing the traditional package leaflet and example of a medicine introducing information aimed at prevention

the need for linguistic forms that users can also understand. Instead, we turn here to its usability as a 'three-dimensional object' whose phenomenologies of use, beyond its communicative function, have much to do with ergonomic issues of manageability. As we have seen, the package leaflet has its placement in the medicine package, and, not necessarily, there is a close connection between its placement and the opening side. This is the case both because there is often no clear indication to the user of what the opening side should be and because there is no definitive opinion in Pharmaceutics as to whether the user, upon opening the medicine package, should find, as the first interface of the medicine, the leaflet.

There is then at least a second reflection concerning using the leaflet as an object and the multiple interactions generated between the leaflet, primary packaging, and secondary packaging.

Folded up in the packaging almost as if to wrap the blister, vial, or bottle, the Package Leaflet must be opened to 'go to work'. And, once it has performed its informational function, it is not easy to follow the folds exactly to return it to its original shape. This leads to the difficulty of reinserting the I.F. into the package and even more so of reinserting the medicine—blister or vial it may be—since interferences are created that hinder the correct repositioning of the medicine in its case.

A concluding note on medicine packaging. We have noted through observations made from the medicines most used by users, the many differing behaviours that run through the patient's experience dealing with drug treatment and the high level of interaction between the different physical and informational components that make up the drug package. We have indicated some of the more usual patient behaviours that can result from inattention, misunderstanding, and lack of basic culture about the role of medicines and their nature, but certainly in part are due to the careless design of the informational and physical features the packaging (Fig. 17.26).

Where the packaging, its shape, and the information given prove particularly ineffective is in getting the patient to perform the right sequence of steps to make the treatment effective and less risky.

We focus here on two elements that could easily be redesigned to increase their effectiveness: giving greater emphasis to visual and verbal information that educates the patient to properly dispose of the primary packaging, the secondary

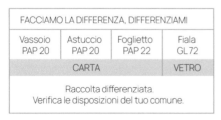
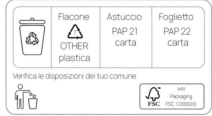

Fig. 17.26 Examples of the recent introduction on the secondary packaging of medicines of complete instructions for proper disposal. Please note the text are in Italian since we're referring to the Italian context

packaging with the package leaflet, and any remaining medicine. The indications on the packaging do not have the strength to attract the user's attention. Even when they do, they risk giving the wrong information by not specifying promptly that the different components of the pharmaceutical pack must follow a separate collection process.

A second piece of information that is too weak concerns the process of reporting possible side effects, product defects, and interactions with other medicines. No user knows what procedure they should follow to report a problem that has arisen using the medicine. In this regard, it would be important for a part of the package leaflet to contain clear instructions, addressed to the patient, on how to report problems encountered in taking a medicine, or issues related to the usability of the medicine with an indication of the recipients and their contact details to whom these reports should be addressed.

We believe that the active involvement of the user in the return of the user experience can be a valuable information asset for the pharmaceutical company and the agencies responsible for regulatory activities and verification of product requirements.

References

European Parliament and of the Council (The) (2001) Directive 2001/83/EC of 6 November 2001 on the Community code relating to medicinal products for human use. Off J Eur Communities 28(11):2001. Retrieved from https://eur-lex.europa.eu/legal-content/EN/TXT/PDF/?uri=CELEX:32001L0083

European Parliament and of the Council (The) (2011) Directive 2011/62/EU of the European Parliament and of the Council, amending Directive 2001/83/EC on the Community code relating to medicinal products for human use, as regards the prevention of the entry into the legal supply chain of falsified medicinal products. Off J Eur Union:74–87

Open Access This chapter is licensed under the terms of the Creative Commons Attribution 4.0 International License (http://creativecommons.org/licenses/by/4.0/), which permits use, sharing, adaptation, distribution and reproduction in any medium or format, as long as you give appropriate credit to the original author(s) and the source, provide a link to the Creative Commons license and indicate if changes were made.

The images or other third party material in this chapter are included in the chapter's Creative Commons license, unless indicated otherwise in a credit line to the material. If material is not included in the chapter's Creative Commons license and your intended use is not permitted by statutory regulation or exceeds the permitted use, you will need to obtain permission directly from the copyright holder.

Part IV
The Pharmaceutical Product System: Premises for the Definition of a Repertory of Good Practices

Chapter 18
How Political and Cultural Situations Are Impacting Pharma Industries

Annabella Amatulli

Abstract The pharmaceutical industry is governed by several rules and requirements defined by Health Authorities across the world: the goal is to develop efficacious and safe medicines, to treat and protect patients. However, more than in the past, pharma industries should take care of changes imposed by cultural and social behaviors. Special attention should be paid on gender-medicine, personalized and individualized drugs/treatments, rare diseases, and development of so called "orphan drugs" and activities designed to support patients and families in need (donation of drugs, patient journey, patient support programs etc.…). But also, initiatives finalized to avoid the waste of good drugs and prescription of the right amount of medicine—this because there is the urgent need to protect the environment, reduce the waste and addressing the requests coming from the new generation of patients. The question is: how the companies can embrace these bottom-up requests in compliance with requirements and rules? How should the companies interact with Health Authorities to spread the voice of the real-world? The industry should be aware that the voice is not only the voice of patients in needs but also the one of healthy citizens that could be patients in the future.

18.1 Society as a Driver of Innovation for the Pharmaceutical Industry

The pharmaceutical industry is governed by several rules and requirements defined by Health Authorities across the world: the goal is to develop efficacious and safe medicines, to treat and protect patients.

For each step of the development process (e.g., research and discovery, non-clinical development, clinical development I, II, III, post-approval life cycle management, and pharmacovigilance) (Eupati 2015), there is a bunch of rules, guidelines, and requirements; the Authors of this book already described some of the guidelines related to packaging of the drug and, usability test in other chapters.

A. Amatulli (✉)
Enterprise Therapeutics S.r.l., Milan, Italy

When are these patient-materials discussed with Health Authorities? For example, the aspects related to packaging of the drug (external carton and patient leaflet) are discussed with Health Authorities during the last phase of the process: Marketing Authorization Application and Phase 4. This means when all the clinical steps are ended, and the Companies described data collected from the clinical studies in a patient friendly way—following specific guidelines released by Health Authorities.

Is it included patients voice in all steps of the development? Short answer: no.

As mentioned above, for each step of the development process there are several rules to be respected and the key role of professionals involved in Regulatory Affairs is managing these rules, apply them and guide other Company's functions (from clinical development, statisticians and manufacturing plants) in conducting their activities following what has been negotiated with Health Authorities.

For this reason, Regulatory Affairs department should monitor not only the regulated environment but also the external one. Regulatory Affairs should start to think about the patients' need beyond the drug: from the improvement of the way of administration, to the need of additional devices combined with the drug and their usability, patient journey, and related support to quality of life, how social behaviors could impact the adherence to the therapy and so on.

Therefore, it is essential for these professionals change the mindset and open an early dialogue with Health Authorities: is the development plan proposed representative of the entire population? Is it inclusive for gender, ethnicity etc....? Since to develop a drug are usually requested more of 10–15 years, looking to the future, the assumptions used for this plan and discussed "now", will still in place?

In this chapter the Author focused the attention about the impact of social behavior or requests from patients/citizens on development plan of the drugs (i.e., gender medicine) and try to predict the future challenges and opportunities for the pharma companies (i.e. AI) based on own professional experience.

Lastly, throughout the text, some actions has been identified in order to improve the development of the drugs, taking into consideration the patients voice or specific needs.

18.2 How the Healthcare Environment Is Impacted— Simply—By the Evolution of the Society

Thinking about all the rules and guideline mandatory for the companies, one of the main challenges for the developers is that the "regulatory rules" applicable today (at the beginning of the development journey), for sure will change at the time of registration of the drug.

Therefore, the developer can launch the drug on the market after 15 years and from those moment starts the Phase 4 of the development plan. What's happen after 15 years? Usually, not only the regulatory rules are changed but is changed the world in general: the behaviors, the attention to social-economic impact of health (is there money to pay medicines?), the improvement of clinical practice for a specific disease (often, accompanied by new technologies for the diagnosis of the disease) and, generally speaking, there is an increase about the knowledge of the patients about the disease itself and the treatments' options.

Especially from 1990s to 2000s there was an extraordinary explosion of new technologies in clinical setting and in parallel patients started to use internet, together with Health Authorities and companies (Douw et al. 2003; OECD 1998).

The acceleration of the exchange of information led to:

- the improvement of clinical practice sharing of best practice, also in critical area such as rare diseases,
- the improvement of communication between Health Authorities and from Health Authorities to companies, patients etc.
- the ability of the companies in reading "in real time" new guidelines released by Health Authorities realizing how should adjust something in the development process of the drug (just to give an example).

Public consultation from institutions, Authorities and other actors in the health spaces became more accessible, also for patients, allowing the possibility to collect the voice of the entire community.

Therefore, more than in the past, pharma industries started to take care of changes imposed by cultural and social behaviors since it was easier intercept the needs earlier, thanks to what has been mentioned above.

In addition, it is essential to keep in mind the final goal of a pharma company: to give a safe and effective drug to patients with the aim to improve not only the clinical status of the diseases but also the quality of life of patients and their caregivers.

In this chapter a special attention is reserved to gender-medicine, rare diseases, and development of so called "orphan drugs" and activities designed to support patients and families in need thanks to the involvement of patients in regulatory process as well. But also, initiatives finalized to avoid the waste of good drugs and prescription of the right amount of medicine. This because there is the urgent need to hear the "voice of patients" on various aspects, protect the environment, reduce the waste and addressing the requests coming from the new generation of patients.

Disclaimer: what is stated in the chapter should be read taking in mind that political situation especially in Europe and in countries like Italy where the National Health Systems pay for the health of all citizens (universal model). Not only companies but *in primis* politicians should take care of the voice of patients because (more than often) they must deal with the economic situation of the country.

For this reason, Companies/Developers are doing their part in fill some gaps, proposing solution to institutions and politicians to find the best journey for the patients.

18.3 A Key Example of Request from the Bottom: Gender Medicine and the Voice of 50% of Entire World Population, Women's Voice

As mentioned, social situations and evolutions can have a significant impact on the pharmaceutical industry, and there are a lot of different factors at play.

Starting with the biological differences, gender medicine is an important area of focus for the pharma industry, as there are many conditions that affect women differently than men. For example, heart disease often presents differently in women and can be misdiagnosed or underdiagnosed as a result (Keteepe-Arachi and Sharma 2017). Additionally, many drugs have different effects on men and women due to differences in metabolism and other physiological factors. By taking these differences into account, pharma companies can develop more effective and personalized treatments for patients.

The World Health Organization (WHO) defines Gender Medicine, or rather Gender-specific Medicine, as the study of how (sex-based) biological and (gender-based) socioeconomic and cultural differences influence people's health. A growing amount of epidemiological, clinical, and experimental data shows significant differences in the development, progression and clinical signs of conditions that are common to men and women, the adverse events associated with therapeutic treatments, the response to such treatments and nutrients, and in lifestyles. Gender also accounts for major differences in access to healthcare (WHO 2021).

The history of medicine spans thousands of years and is influenced by a wide range of social, cultural, and political factors. Throughout history, the role of gender in healthcare has been significant, shaping the way medical professionals have approached diagnosis, treatment, and care.

In the past, medicine was often practiced by women and focused on reproductive health. However, as medicine became more formalized and male-dominated, women's medical knowledge and expertise were marginalized. Women were also often excluded from medical education and training (not only excluded from clinical development of drugs).

In the nineteenth century, significant strides were made in the field of medicine, but women still faced discrimination and barriers to practicing medicine. Despite this, some women were able to make notable contributions to the field. For example, Elizabeth Blackwell became the first woman to earn a medical degree in the United States in Keteepe-Arachi and Sharma 2017, and Florence Nightingale is widely regarded as the founder of modern nursing (Elizabeth Blackwell; Winkelstein Jr 2009).

Regarding the development of tailored drugs, in early 900, medical research predominantly focused on male bodies, and most clinical trials excluded women as participants. The assumption was that the male body was the standard, and findings from studies on male subjects would apply to both genders. However, this perspective began to shift in the mid-twentieth century with the introduction of the birth control pill, which required studies involving women (even because it was a drug only for women) (Verdonk et al. 2009).

The women's health movement in the 1970s and 1980s further highlighted the need for gender-specific research, particularly in areas such as reproductive health and breast cancer. In the 1990s, the National Institutes of Health (NIH) in the United States mandated that women be included in clinical trials, leading to an increase in gender-specific research.

In the twentieth century, the role of gender in medicine became increasingly important, particularly in the areas of reproductive health and the treatment of diseases that affect men and women differently. For example, heart disease, which was long considered a "man's disease", is now recognized as a leading cause of death among women (Long et al. 2008).

Similarly, breast cancer, which primarily affects women, has received increased attention in recent years, leading to improved screening and treatment options. Let us go deeper in the analysis of breast cancer.

Because male breast cancer is rare, there is very limited information on how to treat men diagnosed with the disease. Indeed, each year, about 2000 cases of male breast cancer are diagnosed in the United States, resulting in about 500 deaths, according to the National Cancer Institute. Although it can strike at any age, breast cancer is usually diagnosed in men ages 60–70 (Cancer.gov).

Why does it often take so long to recognize the signs of breast cancer in men? One reason for the late-age (and later-stage) diagnosis may be that men, and their doctors, don't think they are at risk of breast cancer. For this reason, Food and Drug Administration (FDA), one of the main Health Authority in the world, recently released a guideline for the development of drug in male breast cancer (U.S. Department of Health and Human Services et al. 2020).

As stated in the document "Males have historically been excluded from clinical trials of breast cancer drugs because breast cancer in males is rare. This exclusion has resulted in limited FDA-approved treatment options for males with breast cancer. Treatment strategies for males with breast cancer are not based on data from prospective, randomized clinical trials. Rather, clinical management of male breast cancer is generally based on clinical experience with breast cancer in females and data from studies conducted in females with breast cancer".

Thanks to the voice of women (as patients and medical practitioners) now gender medicine is being integrated into medical education and clinical practice.

Research into gender differences in health has been ongoing for several decades and has revealed significant differences in the way that men and women experience and respond to disease. For example, women are more likely than men to develop autoimmune diseases such as lupus and multiple sclerosis, while men are more likely to develop cardiovascular disease at a younger age.

One area of research that has gained particular attention in recent years is the importance of including women in clinical trials. Historically, women have been excluded from clinical trials due to concerns about the potential effects of hormonal changes on study outcomes, as well as a lack of understanding about the biological differences between men and women and the impact on fertility.

However, excluding women from clinical trials has significant implications for our understanding of how drugs and other treatments work in the female body. For example, drugs that have been tested only on men may not be as effective or safe for women, as women may experience different side effects or have different responses to treatment.

As another result, women have been misdiagnosed, underdiagnosed, or not treated optimally for conditions that affect them differently than men.

In parallel, there is the lack of gender sensitivity among healthcare providers. There is a need for greater awareness and training for healthcare professionals to recognize and address gender-based differences in health outcomes. Additionally, gender-based stereotypes and biases can affect medical decision-making and may result in poorer health outcomes for patients.

Fortunately, there has been a push in recent years to increase the representation of women in clinical trials. In the United States, the National Institutes of Health (NIH) has implemented policies to ensure that women are included in all phases of clinical research, and that sex-specific analyses are conducted to identify any differences in treatment outcomes between men and women.

While there is still much work to be done to ensure that women are adequately represented in clinical trials, this research is a critical step towards improving our understanding of gender differences in health and developing more effective treatments for all individuals.

Moving closer to today, in Europe is became effective on 31th January 2023 the new European Clinical Trial Regulation No 536/2014 with the goal to create an environment that is favourable to conducting clinical trials in the EU with the highest standards of ethical and safety protection for participants. In addition, the Regulation requires more transparency of clinical trials data, including the publication of these data, starting from the population groups included in the studies.

"Unless otherwise justified in the protocol, the subjects participating in a clinical trial should represent the population groups, for example gender and age groups, that are likely to use the medicinal product investigated in the clinical trial" and "non-inclusion must be justified. It also contains new rules for including pregnant and breastfeeding women under strict protective measures" (European Institute of Women's Health Policy Brief 2017).

We are living a moment in which the scientific knowledge on sex differences is clear and are available the first supportive legislation, but it is time to move from the theory to the practice and implement the rules/guideline into regulatory and clinical practice in order to improve the healthcare of citizens.

Greater awareness among healthcare providers, more gender-inclusive research, and advances in technology are critical to addressing gender-based health disparities and ensuring that all individuals receive the best possible care, regardless of their gender.

However, to the best of the author knowledge, while sex differences in drug use have been demonstrated in some therapeutic areas, there is a lack of overviews regarding gender differences concerning the use of drugs in an entire population (Orlando et al. 2020).

In addition, a study said that women experience adverse drug reactions (ADRs), nearly twice as often as men, because most drugs currently in use were approved based on clinical trials conducted on men. The common practice of prescribing equal drug doses to women and men neglects sex differences in pharmacokinetics and dimorphisms in body weight, risks overmedication of women, and contributes to female-biased adverse drug reactions (Zucker and Prendergast 2020).

One of "famous" case study happened in 2013, when the US Food and Drug Administration (FDA) intervened to correct the dosage of sleeping medication containing the active ingredient zolpidem for women, because the recommended dose—based on male bodies—impaired alertness, putting patients at risk of accidents when driving to work the next morning.

For the above-mentioned reasons and examples, what companies can do to further develop gender-medicine and engage Health Authorities in the discussion?

The advancement of technology and data science has provided developers with new tools to analyze and interpret data in a way that is more inclusive of gender differences. Furthermore, there is a growing movement towards gender-inclusive research, which seeks to ensure that both men and women are included in clinical trials and other medical research studies.

In parallel to more inclusive clinical trials, thinking about new tools and technologies available that could be used by companies to advance gender medicine, for sure Artificial Intelligence (AI) will potentially play a great role.

Here below a list of potential technologies that based on Author's knowledge should be evaluate and applied on gender medicine but also other areas of drug development:

- Artificial Intelligence (AI): it has the potential to transform healthcare by improving diagnosis, treatment, and disease prevention. AI algorithms can analyze large datasets to identify patterns, make predictions, and generate personalized recommendations for patients—knowing that in Europe the new Clinical Trials Regulation requests more transparency, this means that all data of studies will be available for everyone. AI can be particularly useful in gender medicine, where sex-specific factors can affect disease presentation, diagnosis, and treatment response and therefore can easily identify sex-specific risk factors and develop personalized plans for men and women. In addition, the AI could be used to reduce the number of animal studies that are mandatory for the development of drugs.
- Omic technologies: *Omic* technologies are primarily aimed at the universal detection of genes (genomics), mRNA (transcriptomics), proteins (proteomics) and metabolites (metabolomics) in a specific biological sample (Horgan and Kenny 2011). R&D group of Companies could use omics technologies, such as genomics, transcriptomics, proteomics, and metabolomics, can help identify sex-specific biomarkers that can be used for disease diagnosis, prognosis, and treatment. For example, genomics can help identify genetic variants that increase disease risks in men or women. Proteomics can help identify sex-specific protein

biomarkers that can be used for early disease detection and treatment monitoring and consequently new target for therapies. Companies can discuss the validation of this methods with Health Authorities, improving the development of new drugs due to the availability of new guidelines.
- Precision Medicine: Precision medicine is an approach that considers individual variability in genes, environment, and lifestyle for each person (it is an integration and a continuation of the omics). By tailoring treatments to individuals, precision medicine can improve health outcomes and reduce health disparities. Precision medicine has the potential to advance gender medicine by accounting for differences in sex-specific genetic, environmental, and lifestyle factors that may affect disease risk, prevention, and treatment. This is important because there are differences not only in biological terms but also in the access to care: Gender inequalities and gender norms intersect with socioeconomic, geographic, and cultural factors and create structural barriers when accessing healthcare (WHO 2019). As highlighted in Fig. 18.1, several population groups, such as lone parents, older people, migrants and people with disabilities, and women in particular, stand out as highly vulnerable to unmet healthcare needs. Gender is an important determinant of healthcare access and uptake. Taking in account EU

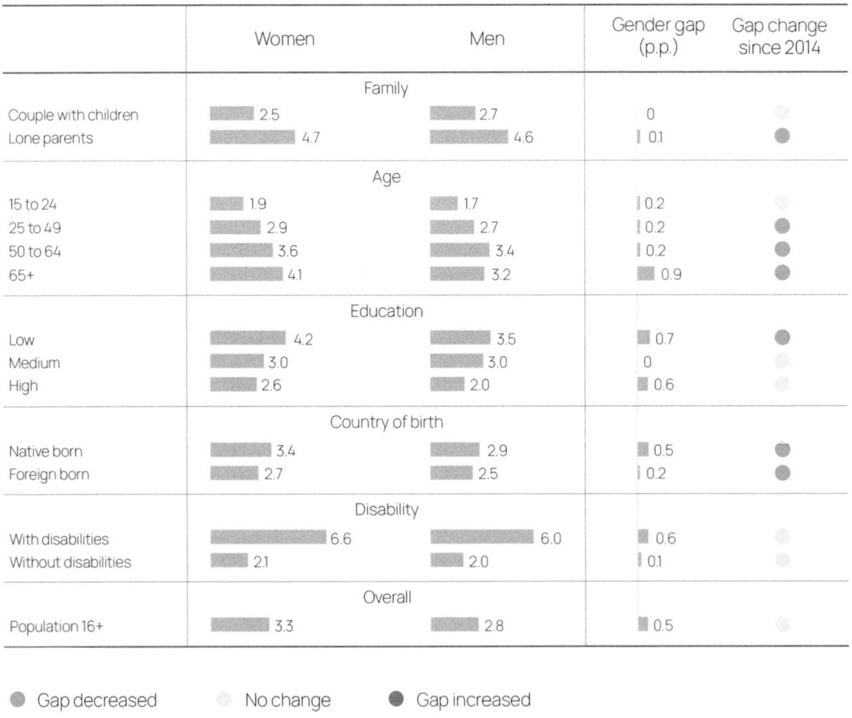

	Women	Men	Gender gap (p.p.)	Gap change since 2014
Family				
Couple with children	2.5	2.7	0	
Lone parents	4.7	4.6	0.1	●
Age				
15 to 24	1.9	1.7	0.2	
25 to 49	2.9	2.7	0.2	●
50 to 64	3.6	3.4	0.2	●
65+	4.1	3.2	0.9	●
Education				
Low	4.2	3.5	0.7	●
Medium	3.0	3.0	0	
High	2.6	2.0	0.6	
Country of birth				
Native born	3.4	2.9	0.5	●
Foreign born	2.7	2.5	0.2	●
Disability				
With disabilities	6.6	6.0	0.6	
Without disabilities	2.1	2.0	0.1	
Overall				
Population 16+	3.3	2.8	0.5	

● Gap decreased   ○ No change   ● Gap increased

Fig. 18.1 Women and men with unmet needs for medical examination, by family composition, age, education level, country of birth and disability. Note the lack of increased gap data in the table (EIGE 2021)

Table 18.1 The table presents the involvement of patients at different stages during the development of a medicine, and their involvement in a wide range of EMA activities

Patients representing their community	Patients representing their organisation	Patients as individual experts
Management board Scientific committee(s)	Patients' and Consumers' Working Party (PCWP) EMA consultations Workshops	Scientific advice/protocol assistance procedures Scientific advisory/ad hoc expert groups Scientific committee consultations Review of documents

countries, which have a completely different healthcare system respect US, the Universal access to health services has not been fully achieved. About 3.3% of women and 2.8% of men report unmet needs for medical examinations. Across different population groups, gender clearly intersects with other social factors to hamper access to health (Table 18.1). Certain groups are more likely to report unmet medical examination needs: women and men with disabilities (women, 6.6%; men, 6%), lone parents (women, 4.7%; men, 4.6%), women with a low level of education (4.2%) and those over 65 years (4.1%). The most common reason cited for unmet healthcare needs is cost. Women are more likely to mention finances as an obstacle to seeking healthcare, with 33% of women and 29% of men saying that they cannot afford it. Women and men with disabilities and women with a low level of education are more likely than others to have little income because they either are not in paid work or are in precarious jobs. Companies can provide Patient Support Programs and/or develop other initiatives to reduce this gap (financial support to have access to approved medicines, support in patient journey etc.).

- Wearable and mobile health technologies: Wearable and mobile health technologies can monitor health in real-time and provide personalized feedback to patients and/or physicians. These technologies can be particularly useful in gender medicine, where sex-specific factors can affect disease risk and prevention. For example, wearable technologies can monitor sign and symptoms of a diseases and detect differences between women and men.

18.4 Orphan Drugs: The Challenge to Give a Cure to Patients Without Hope

Thinking about all the rules and guideline mandatory for the companies, one of the main challenges for the developers is that the "regulatory rules" applicable today (at the beginning of the development journey), for sure will change at the time of registration of the drug.

Another voice is raising from the patient's side. Patients affected by rare disease and waiting for treatment.

Personalized and individualized drugs are also becoming increasingly important, as our understanding of genetics and other factors that influence health continues to advance. With personalized medicine, treatments can be tailored to an individual's specific genetic makeup, leading to more effective and targeted therapies. Similarly, individualized medicine considers a patient's unique medical history, lifestyle, and other factors to develop a treatment plan that is best suited to their needs, as also described above for gender-medicine.

However, in the last decade, rare diseases and orphan drugs became another area of focus for the pharma industry. These conditions often affect small numbers of patients, making them less economically viable for drug companies to develop treatments for. However, there is a growing recognition of the need to support these patients and develop treatments that can improve their quality of life.

Let us start from the definition of orphan drug from regulatory standpoint:

In Europe: a medicine for the diagnosis, prevention, or treatment of a life-threatening or chronically debilitating condition that is rare (affecting not more than 5 in 10,000 people in the European Union) or where the medicine is unlikely to generate sufficient profit to justify research and development costs (EMA, Orphan Medicine).

In USA: a drug intended to treat a condition affecting fewer than 200,000 persons in the United States, or which will not be profitable within 7 years following approval by the FDA (FDA, Orphan Drugs).

It is essential that pharmaceutical companies continue to invest in the development of these drugs, and providing support to patients and families who may not have access to other treatments.

Here plays a central role the politics and who write legislation. In both Europe and US, there are legislations in place to support the development of orphan drugs, giving to developers various incentives, such as:

- Tax credits for qualified clinical trials;
- Exemption from fees;
- Years of market exclusivity after approval;
- Specific regulatory pathways to guarantee approval of the drug in less time.

Despite these incentives, the development of a drug for rare disease remains critical for several reasons from scientific difficulties to ethical considerations:

- No availability of validated clinical endpoints. This means find them and discuss with Health Authorities how validate them;
- Insufficient patients data (due to the difficulties to enroll patients in clinical studies). Usually to achieve the sample size for a clinical study in rare diseases, developers should open clinical centers across the world, but often it is not enough. In order to enroll patients in an acceptable timeframe, costs related to R&D increase a lot;

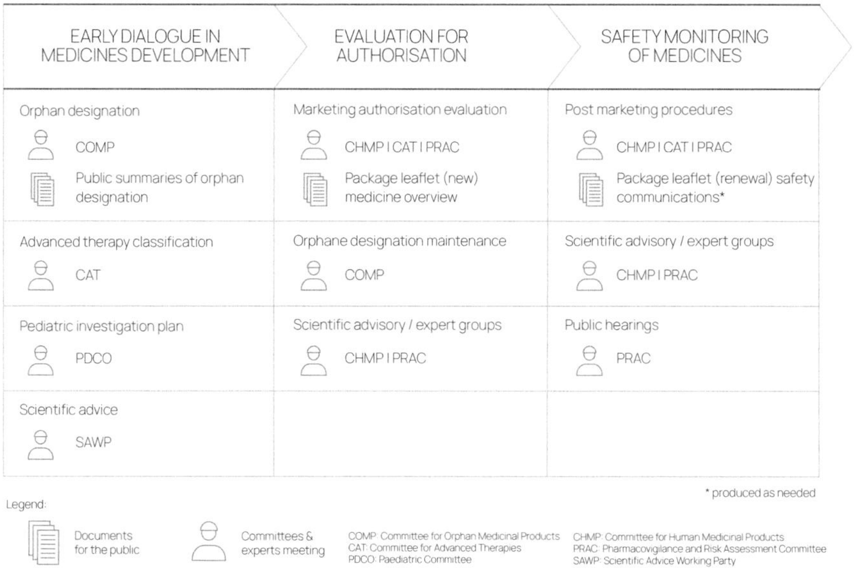

18 How Political and Cultural Situations Are Impacting Pharma Industries

EARLY DIALOGUE IN MEDICINES DEVELOPMENT	EVALUATION FOR AUTHORISATION	SAFETY MONITORING OF MEDICINES
Orphan designation COMP Public summaries of orphan designation	Marketing authorisation evaluation CHMP I CAT I PRAC Package leaflet (new) medicine overview	Post marketing procedures CHMP I CAT I PRAC Package leaflet (renewal) safety communications*
Advanced therapy classification CAT	Orphane designation maintenance COMP	Scientific advisory / expert groups CHMP I PRAC
Pediatric investigation plan PDCO	Scientific advisory / expert groups CHMP I PRAC	Public hearings PRAC
Scientific advice SAWP		

*produced as needed

Legend:
- Documents for the public
- Committees & experts meeting
- COMP: Committee for Orphan Medicinal Products
- CAT: Committee for Advanced Therapies
- PDCO: Paediatric Committee
- CHMP: Committee for Human Medicinal Products
- PRAC: Pharmacovigilance and Risk Assessment Committee
- SAWP: Scientific Advice Working Party

Fig. 18.2 Patient involvement in the regulatory life cycle of a new medicine. (Source: EMA website)

- No control groups or appropriate comparator. This means perform RCT (randomized-clinical trial, which is the gold standard in clinical development) using active ingredient versus placebo. From ethical standpoint, the issue is related about giving placebo to a patient with a life-threating rare diseases;
- New clinical designs should be discussed with Health Authorities and HTA bodies (for the reimbursement of the drug), acceptable also from their standpoints.

Finally, especially for the development of drugs for rare disease, is becoming more important listen the voice of the patients. These diseases, more than another, are the example on how the clinical condition not only impact the patient but also the community in which he/she lives. How a disease can destroy a family from emotional standpoint to the economic one. Indeed, just to give an example, European Medicines Agency (EMA) released guidance about the involvement of patients during the development of the medicine (Table 18.1).

Patients, consumers, and carers are involved in a wide range of EMA activities, as either representatives of European Union (EU) patients' and consumers' organisations, representatives of their own organisation or as individual experts depending on the nature of the activity (Fig. 18.2).

Dealing with the entire development plan of a drug (Eupati 2015), also EMA represents in a graphic way in which processes patients and carers are involved along the medicine's lifecycle at EMA: patients can get involved in every aspect of the regulatory lifecycle of a medicine from pre-submission and evaluation through to post-authorisation. In this way, the Health Authorities can listen the patients' voice and the pharma companies, improving the development of medicines.

18.5 Environment and Drugs

Thinking about all the rules and guideline mandatory for the companies, one of the main challenges for the developers is that the "regulatory rules" applicable today (at the beginning of the development journey), for sure will change at the time of registration of the drug.

The last example about the impact of social behavior on pharma industries is how the sensitivity towards the environment is reducing the wasting of good products (and the shortage of medicines).

This world should need to address the environmental impact of pharmaceuticals. There are concerns about the amount of medication waste that is generated, and the impact this can have on the environment.

Just to give an Italian example, 10 years ago when a pharma companies must change the Patient Leaflet of the drug in the carton box (due to an update of information included) the rules imposed to withdrawn all the drug packages containing the obsolete info available on the market and destroy them as soon as the info is approved, despite the new info didn't have any impact on safety & quality of the drug (AIFA 2014). This situation sometimes created both shortage of the drug and a huge waste of good drug!

The legislation was improved in Europe but in any case, after 6 months from the approval of the updated Patient Leaflet, pharma companies must implement the paper-version containing the updated info in the packages of the drug.

There are many ways to further improve the situation: switch to an electronic patient leaflet (ePI), that can be updated in real-time and, easily accessible to patients, physicians, and caregivers.

However, to implement this change must be updated the entire pharma-legislation, because the availability of the paper version of patient leaflet is mandatory by law. Indeed, the European Medicines Agency, in collaboration with Heads of Medicines Agencies and the European Commission, has developed key principles through stakeholder consultations to guide the development and use of ePI in the EU.

While we are looking to see the implementation of the ePI, pharmaceutical companies can take steps to reduce waste, such as implementing take-back programs for unused medications and developing more environmentally friendly packaging.

In different countries, mainly in the US, there are several initiatives aimed at reducing the waste of good drugs and promoting the appropriate prescription of medicine. Some of these initiatives include:

- Patient Education: Providing patients with information about their medications, including the appropriate dosage and how to dispose of unused medications, can help reduce waste and promote responsible use of medications;
- Medication Therapy Management (MTM): This is a service provided by pharmacists that involves a review of a patient's medications to ensure they are appropriate, effective, and being used safely. This can help reduce waste by ensuring that patients are not taking medications they don't need, and that they are taking the correct dose;

- Prescription Drug Monitoring Programs (PDMPs): These are state-run databases that track the prescribing and dispensing of controlled substances. PDMPs help identify patients who may be at risk for overuse, misuse, or abuse of prescription drugs, and can help prevent overprescribing and reduce waste;
- Drug Take-Back Programs: These are programs that allow patients to dispose of unused or expired medications safely and easily. This helps prevent the environmental damage caused by improper disposal of medications and reduces the risk of accidental ingestion or misuse of medications;
- Electronic Prescribing: Electronic prescribing (e-prescribing) allows healthcare providers to send prescriptions directly to a pharmacy, reducing the chance of errors and ensuring that patients receive the correct medication and dosage.

These initiatives not only promote responsible use of medication and reduce waste, but they also help protect the environment and promote sustainability. In Europe some of them are not allowed due to legislation system but benchmarks from other Countries should be taken into consideration, especially if those could improve the correct use of drugs, reduce costs and waste.

Regarding the shortage of the drug, the covid-19 pandemic caused disruption of global supply chain and companies learnt a lot from this unexpectable situations. In Europe, the situation led to shortages of essential medications such as sedatives and painkillers. The EMA and FDA worked with pharmaceutical companies to address these shortages and ensure the continued availability of medicines for patients.

In the United States, drug shortages have been an ongoing problem for several years, with factors such as manufacturing issues, quality control problems, and supply chain disruptions contributing to the problem. The COVID-19 pandemic further exacerbated drug shortages in the U.S. as demand for certain drugs increased and supply chain disruptions continued.

To address these shortages, the U.S. government passed legislation in 2020 that requires drug manufacturers to provide early notification of any anticipated shortages, as well as contingency plans to address those shortages. The U.S. Food and Drug Administration (FDA) also works with manufacturers to identify and address potential shortages and mitigate their impact on patients.

18.6 Conclusion

Pharmaceutical companies should take care more than in the past of the need of persons and listen their voice (patients and, general speaking, citizen). This chapter shown some of the topics that raise from social-cultural environment such as gender medicine, orphan drug and avoid waste of good product, describing some actions done in the past to address those issues.

However, pharma companies alone not always can implement solution to support the needs of the patients and community. Sometimes there are legislations, rules and guidelines that not allowed to "take actions". Therefore, companies should interact with Health Authorities to find a common solution for a common goal: the health of everyone. Companies can interact with Health/Regulatory Authorities in a variety of ways to effectively communicate the real-world needs of patients, caregivers, and healthcare providers.

Here below some of Author's suggestions:

- attend meetings and conferences organized by regulatory authorities/ministry of health where they discuss current issues and future plans related to healthcare. Pharmaceutical experts can attend these events to learn more about the needs of the community and network with key stakeholders;
- submit data and evidence: pharmaceutical companies could submit data and evidence from clinical trials or real-world studies to health authorities not only to support the development and approval of new treatments (since it is mandatory for those) but to engage them in a data-driven discussion to find new solutions to study drugs (especially through the use of real-world-evidences). This could help to provide insight into the needs of patients and healthcare providers but also caregivers;
- participate in advisory committees: regulatory authorities often have advisory committees that provide recommendations and guidance on drug development, regulatory processes and other healthcare-related issues. Pharmaceutical companies should participate in these committees to provide input and share their expertise, despite the huge preparation requested for this kind of meeting and the costs-related;
- collaborate on research projects: pharmaceutical companies can collaborate with regulatory authorities on research projects that address important healthcare issues. This can help to identify unmet needs and develop new treatments that meet the needs of patients and healthcare providers;
- engage in public-private partnerships: regulatory authorities often partner with private companies to address public health challenges (covid-19 has been a great example). Pharmaceutical companies can participate in these partnerships to leverage their expertise and resources to improve healthcare outcomes;
- collect patients voice, elaborate the unarticulated need of patients in a technical way and then engage a discussion with regulatory authorities.

Overall, effective communication, transparent mutual-relationship and, collaboration between pharmaceutical companies and regulatory authorities can help to identify and address the real-world needs of patients and healthcare providers, and ultimately lead to improved healthcare outcomes.

References

AIFA (14 aprile 2014) Determina n. 371. Criteri per l'applicazione delle disposizioni relative allo smaltimento delle scorte dei medicinali. GU Serie Generale n.101 del 03-05-2014. Retrieved from https://www.gazzettaufficiale.it/atto/serie_generale/caricaDettaglioAtto/originario?atto.

dataPubblicazioneGazzetta=2014-05-03&atto.codiceRedazionale=14A03351&elenco30giorni=true

Douw K, Vondeling H, Eskildsen D, Simpson S (2003) Use of the Internet in scanning the horizon for new and emerging health technologies: a survey of agencies involved in horizon scanning. J Med Internet Res 5(1) Retrieved from https://www.ncbi.nlm.nih.gov/pmc/articles/PMC1550552/

EIGE (2021) Gender Equality Index 2021: Health. Retrieved from: https://eige.europa.eu/publications-resources/publications/gender-equality-index-2021-health?language_content_entity=en

Elizabeth Blackwell. Retrieved from https://www.hws.edu/about/history/elizabeth-blackwell/150-years.aspx

EMA website. Getting involved. Patients, consumers and carers are involved in a wide range of European Medicines Agency (EMA) activities. Retrieved from https://www.ema.europa.eu/en/partners-networks/patients-consumers/getting-involved

EUPATI (2015) Discovery and development of medicines. Retrieved from https://toolbox.eupati.eu/resources/discovery-and-development-of-medicines/

European Institute of Women's Health Policy Brief (2017) Sex and gender in medicine regulation. Retrieved from https://eurohealth.ie/policy-brief-sex-and-gender-in-medicines-regulation-2017/

European Medicine Agency (EMA). Orphan medicine. Retrieved from https://www.ema.europa.eu/en/glossary/orphan-medicine

Food and Drug Administration (FDA). Orphan drugs. Retrieved from https://www.fda.gov/media/83372/download

Horgan RP, Kenny LC (2011) 'Omic' technologies: genomics, transcriptomics, proteomics and metabolomics. Obstet Gynaecol 13:189–195

Keteepe-Arachi T, Sharma S (2017) Cardiovascular disease in women: understanding symptoms and risk factors. Euro Cardiol Rev 12(1):10–13

Long T et al (2008) "The heart truth:" using the power of branding and social marketing to increase awareness of heart disease in women. Soc Mark Q 14(3):3–29. https://doi.org/10.1080/15245000802279334

National Cancer Institute. https://www.cancer.gov

NIH. Guideline NIH policy and guidelines on the inclusion of women and minorities as subjects in clinical research. https://grants.nih.gov/policy/inclusion/women-and-minorities/guidelines.htm#:~:text=It%20is%20the%20policy%20of,that%20inclusion%20is%20inappropriate%20with

OECD (1998) 21st century technologies. Promises and perils of a dynamic future. Retrieved from https://www.oecd.org/futures/35391210.pdf

Orlando V, Mucherino S, Guarino I, Guerriero F, Trama U, Menditto E (2020) Gender differences in medication use: a drug utilization study based on real world data. Int J Environ Res Public Health 17(11):3926. https://doi.org/10.3390/ijerph17113926. PMID: 32492925; PMCID: PMC7312791

U.S. Department of Health and Human Services, Food and Drug Administration, Oncology Center of Excellence (OCE), Center for Drug Evaluation and Research (CDER), & Center for Biologics Evaluation and Research (CBER) (2020) Male breast cancer: developing drugs for treatment. Guidance for industry. Retrieved from https://www.fda.gov/media/130061/download

Verdonk P, Benschop YWM, de Haes HCJM, Lagro-Janssen TLM (2009) From gender bias to gender awareness in medical education. Adv Health Sci Educ 14:135–152

WHO (2019) Breaking barriers: towards more gender-responsive and equitable health systems. Retrieved from https://www.who.int/healthinfo/universal_health_coverage/report/gender_gmr_2019.pdf?ua=1

WHO (2021) Gender medicine definition—Istituto Superiore della Sanità. Retrieved from https://www.epicentro.iss.it/en/gender-medicine/#:~:text=The%20World%20Health%20Organization%20(WHO,cultural%20differences%20influence%20people%27s%20health

Winkelstein W Jr (2009) Founder of modern nursing and hospital epidemiology. Epidemiology 20(2):311. Retrieved from https://pubmed.ncbi.nlm.nih.gov/19234417/

Zucker I, Prendergast BJ (2020) Sex differences in pharmacokinetics predict adverse drug reactions in women. Biol Sex Diff 11(32). Retrieved fromhttps://doi.org/10.1186/s13293-020-00308-5

Open Access This chapter is licensed under the terms of the Creative Commons Attribution 4.0 International License (http://creativecommons.org/licenses/by/4.0/), which permits use, sharing, adaptation, distribution and reproduction in any medium or format, as long as you give appropriate credit to the original author(s) and the source, provide a link to the Creative Commons license and indicate if changes were made.

The images or other third party material in this chapter are included in the chapter's Creative Commons license, unless indicated otherwise in a credit line to the material. If material is not included in the chapter's Creative Commons license and your intended use is not permitted by statutory regulation or exceeds the permitted use, you will need to obtain permission directly from the copyright holder.

Chapter 19
Medicinal Products: When Innovation Meets the Patient

Lamberto Dionigi

Abstract Therapeutic adherence is an essential element to guarantee the best benefit/risk ratio of a drug for the patient. It refers to the degree to which the patient correctly follows the recommendations on the use of the drug at the due dosage, time, and regimen, throughout the prescribed duration. A low adherence can therefore be the consequence of an incorrect, incomplete, or irregular intake of the medicine. A high adherence, on the other hand, reduces the patient's health risks, increases the likelihood of treatment effectiveness and safety, and contributes to controlling therapy costs. For this reason, both pharmaceutical companies and regulatory agencies have worked over the years to ensure that the patient is provided with adequate tools to minimize the likelihood and impact of low adherence to therapy. This chapter focuses on those medicines' elements that can influence therapeutic adherence and highlights some innovations, already in place or in development, aimed to improve it. The author will privilege the example of oral drugs, which are generally self-administered by the patient at home, an environment less controlled than a clinic or hospital.

19.1 Therapeutic Adherence: The Role of Secondary Packaging

The pharmaceutical industry is governed by several rules and requirements defined by Health Authorities across the world, with the goal of developing efficacious and safe medicines to treat and protect patients.

The box containing the drug is the first element of the packaging the patient sees and is the first tool he has available to ensure taking the right medicine at the correct dosage.

L. Dionigi (✉)
Zambon S.p.A., Bresso, Italy
e-mail: lamberto.dionigi@zambongroup.com

International standards (Directive 2001/83/EC 2001) specify the minimum information to be displayed on the box, along with where and how the essential text should be presented, to make it immediately recognizable to the patient. Some of this information is also in Braille (embossed on the outer cardboard) for tactile reading by visually impaired patients.

Several companies have adopted communication patterns and color codes that make the main information readable regardless of the orientation of the box in the shelf, in order to minimize the risk of patients picking the wrong dosage or the wrong active ingredient.

Some strategies include:

- Using clear and prominent text for the medicine name, selecting suitable and legible font and size;
- Repeating the dosage in a specific area on the packaging's front face, far from other data, to improve its visibility;
- Applying colour codes to help preventing mix-ups between LASA (Look-Alike, Sound-Alike) medicines;
- Highlighting the number of doses contained in the package by framing this information within attention-grabbing colour areas;
- Arranging primary data systematically to create a "medicine identity card", helping to reduce errors at the dispensing stage on multiple sides of the pack.

In Chap. 22 we will present examples of outer packaging, along with methodological insights, building on these redesign experiences.

When the package contains more than a single dose of the medicine, the secondary packaging should always include a writable space, in which the patient can write down the date and time of the first administration. This way, he will be able to verify adherence to the prescribed dosage over time by matching the doses taken (e.g., by counting the missing pills from a blister) with the elapsed therapy period.

Being the first interface with the user, the box must also meet the aesthetic and communications needs of marketing, especially for over-the-counter drugs. However, this should not compromise the packaging's recognisability and informativeness for the patient.

Smartphone technologies already enable an "augmented" reading of the secondary packaging and can facilitate therapeutic adherence. By scanning the box, ones could, in theory, already highlight, translate or read text, access an information link, run a video, and more; however, such of technological tools must strictly comply with regulatory guidelines and have as main objective providing support to the patient.

The package leaflet deserves a separate mention. It is certainly the primary source of detailed information for the patient and should always be read alongside the doctor's prescription (if applicable) and kept available throughout the whole therapy.

The structure of the leaflet in the European Union is defined by the QRD Template (QRD templates 2022), begins with initial recommendations, including the one of reading and storing the leaflet itself, and describes: what the drug is and what it is

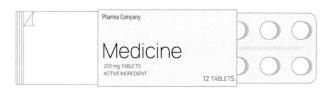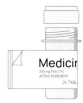

Fig. 19.1 A blister that slides, presenting a "book leaflet" from the opposite side (on the left side) and bottle with unrollable leaflet (on the right). With these types of packaging, the patient has the whole package leaflet available at every medicine intake

used for; what ones need to know before taking it; how to take it; possible side effects; how to store it; the content of the pack and other relevant information. By structuring the leaflet in this way the product designer can ensure that the patient is given the best possible conditions for using the medicine correctly.

European guidelines mandate the so-called "Readability Testing", which ensures, using a group representative of the medicine's target population, that the text in the leaflet is clear and written in a way that is understandable to users (thus avoiding overly technical medical terms) (European Commission 2009).

But despite all the precautions, the package leaflet often presents challenges: it contains a large amount of text, is bulky, difficult to refold and store, and may still not be clear or readable in all its parts. In a nutshell, it is not always "user-friendly" and this becomes a problem especially when the patient is old, visually impaired, poorly educated, taking many different medicines every day (each with his own leaflet), visiting from another country, etc. It is therefore useful to understand not only how to ensure that the patient follows what is written in the leaflet, but also how to reduce any risks related to the fact that the patient may not have read, may not have understood, or may have forgotten important information contained in that leaflet.

Some companies have sought to attach the package leaflet to the primary packaging, so that it is always available when the patient takes the medicine. For example, the picture on the left of Fig. 19.1 shows a "book" leaflet that does not need to be refolded and is exposed every time the patient takes the blister out of the secondary package. Conversely, the picture on the right shows a leaflet that unrolls or peels off from the label on the primary container, allowing the patient to carry it with him without the bulk of the outer box.

19.2 The "Augmented" Secondary Packaging

Another way to ensure that the patient never separates from the leaflet would be... having it digitally rather than physically. Some products already include on their label and carton codes readable by a smartphone, which allows one to download the package leaflet. The availability of the electronic document offers numerous advantages: the text can be enlarged or read aloud by a software, targeted searches are possible, updated information can always be available even when implemented after the drug has been released and distributed, the text can be available in other languages, videos or animations can accompany the text, the text can contain active links, and so on. However, it is important that these digital tools meet all the following three conditions:

- they must be validated by regulatory bodies to ensure that the information remains the one authorized.
- they must be extremely intuitive, safe, and easy to use.
- they must be available to those patients who are familiar with the technology (but fortunately more and more people are now daily users of smartphones and tablets).

Concerning the first requirement, regulatory agencies have already issued guidelines (e.g., European Medicines Agency 2018) to regulate the use of barcodes, Quick Response (QR) codes, or Near-Field Communication (NFC) tools.

On the market, there are several examples of the use of QR codes in medicines that have made it possible to augment the information contained in the printed package leaflet.

19.3 Therapeutic Adherence: The Role of Primary Packaging

The primary packaging is the one in direct contact with the medicine (e.g., a bottle, a blister, a sachet, etc.). As discussed, it is not excluded that the patient can dispose of the outer box, and sometimes the package leaflet, before having finished using the medicine. Again, international guidelines require you to include some essential information, such as product name, batch, expiry, etc.

Bottles for oral products generally offer ample space for the label, so it is assumed that they can also contain a suitable space to note the first opening which, as mentioned above, can favor therapeutic adherence. Conversely, blisters and sachets do not allow you to write on them. However, over the years several projects have been developed to help patients in an adherent use of drugs, for example by working on the shape of blisters, printing the days of the week (Fig. 19.2), using symbols and colors, etc.

19.3.1 Smart Containers

In other cases, more sophisticated solutions have been introduced, such as bottle lids that record openings (Fig. 19.3, on the left side), or packaging with integrated audible or visual alarms that remind the user to take the drug and warn when the

Fig. 19.2 An example of a blister combining texts, signs, and colours to support adherence to posology

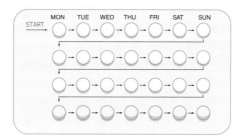

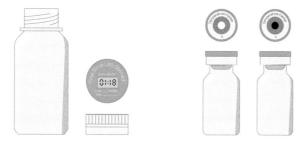

Fig. 19.3 Example of bottle lid indicating the time elapsed since the last opening (on the left); Bottle with marker that changes its color if the product has been exposed to a temperature outside the range of acceptability (on the right)

storage temperature is inadequate (Fig. 19.3, on the right side) or the product is expiring.

Electronic systems for tracking drug intake can also be applied to blisters for pills (Fig. 19.4).

This type of technologically advanced container still has costs that may not make it suitable for large productions, but it is often used for the packaging of experimental products in clinical trials, where the control and tracking of how and when the drug is used is an element that can ensure quality and integrity of the data collected.

19.3.2 Portability

Other than performing the main function of protecting the drug and informing the user, the primary packaging must be designed to make it simple and convenient to use the product in line with the prescribed dosage. It should therefore not only make available the essential information, but also have characteristics that make it suitable for the type of use done by the patient. For example, a drug or a food

Fig. 19.4 Example of a blister packaging that records the date and time when the package is opened and closed

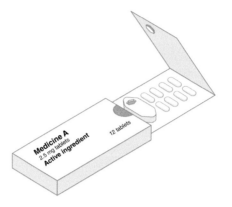

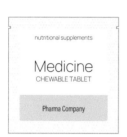 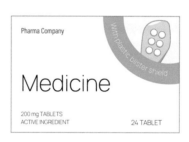 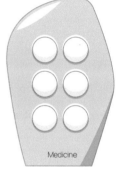

Fig. 19.5 On the left, an example of a pocket sachet containing a chewable tablet; on the right, a shaped plastic blister shield

supplement that could also be administered away from home should be easily portable and the user may find uncomfortable to keep a bottle or blister in his pocket, rather preferring a sachet instead (Fig. 19.5—on the left side).

Portability is an important aspect where the drug requires more than two administrations in 24 h or should be taken on an "as needed" basis, considering that users are often active and moving people. A packaging with good portability characteristics must withstand mechanical stress well and this excludes the classic blister among the ideal solutions, although there are innovative blisters protected by a cardboard or a plastic shield (Fig. 19.5—on the right side).

19.4 Therapeutic Adherence: Role of the Pharmaceutical Form

The pharmaceutical form can play an important role in ensuring therapeutic adherence. In the following paragraph, some examples that testimony the role of the pharmaceutical form.

19.4.1 Physical Forms and Routes of Administration

The main pharmaceutical forms can be solid (e.g., tablets, capsules, powders, granules, suppositories, etc.), semi-solid (e.g., creams, gels, ointments, etc.), liquid (e.g., syrups, oral drops, eye drops, etc.) or gaseous (e.g., aerosols, etc.) (Fig. 19.6). Depending on the route of administration, the forms will be oral, topical, parentcral, ophthalmic, nasal, vaginal, etc.

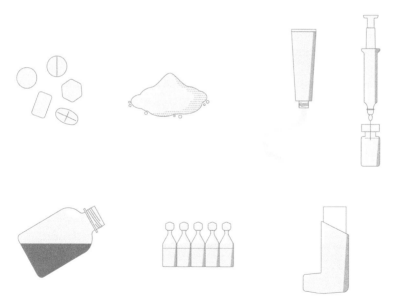

Fig. 19.6 Some examples of solid, semi-solid, liquid and gaseous pharmaceutical forms

Some pharmaceutical forms offer practical advantages over others. For example, unlike an injection, taking a tablet requires no training or searching for an isolated environment. But in its small way, even the aesthetics of a tablet offers functional spaces to improve therapeutic adherence: the unique combination of shape, colour, size, and text are all characteristics that can help the patient not to get confused. For this reason, careful research should always accompany the design of a medicine to make it as distinguishable as possible from the other drugs with which it is commonly taken in combination.

19.4.2 The Release Mode of the Active Ingredient

In addition to looking for optimal physical forms and routes of administration, scientific research and technology have made it possible to further reduce human error by acting on the release of the active ingredient into the body over time. The so-called modified release forms, compared to those at immediate release, can reduce not only the number of daily administrations but also the absorption peaks of the drug, producing a better ratio between pharmacological coverage and safety profile. The modified release finds its best application in long-term treatments and, in some cases, allows accurate matching of the desired pharmacokinetic curve (Fig. 19.7).

The release of the active ingredient can be controlled not only over time, but also in the place of the body where it can exert maximum efficacy, reducing the so-called off-target effects to the detriment of other organs. This is the case of gastro-resistant capsules and tablets, equipped with a special coating that allows them to pass through the stomach without being dissolved by gastric juices, and then release the active ingredient into the intestine.

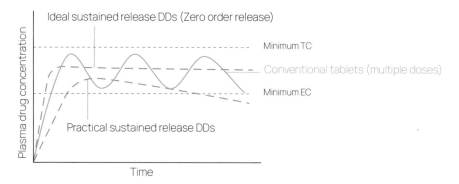

Fig. 19.7 Examples of theoretical pharmacokinetic curves, in which the levels of active substance in plasma following multiple doses of immediate-release tablets (blue line) are compared with those of a modified-release tablet (dotted lines) (Khan et al. 2022)

19 Medicinal Products: When Innovation Meets the Patient

What has been described so far can only give a raw idea of the technologies for controlled and guided drug delivery, but the field of study is vast (Vargason et al. 2021).

The design, both the drug product and the packaging, must help correctly use the pharmaceutical form. For example, a fracture line printed on a gastro-resistant tablet could lead the patient to believe the tablet can be divided mistakenly and should therefore be avoided. Similarly, the secondary packaging should communicate the nature of drug release as intuitively and clearly as possible to prevent, for example, that the patient can take it more frequently than required, exposing himself to overdose risks.

19.5 Therapeutic Adherence: Partible Units and Dispensers

19.5.1 Partible Units

Solid units, such as capsules and tablets, ensure dose accuracy with each administration. While some units can only be taken entirely (such as gastro-resistant tablets and capsules), most pharmaceutical forms must in fact be dosed at the time of intake. This applies not only to multi-dose products but also to some single-dose forms in tablets and sachets. In fact, some tablets can be divided along one or more score lines (Fig. 19.8, on the left), some sachets are bipartite to allow the intake of either the whole content or a fraction of it (Fig. 19.8, on the right), and even eye drops in single-dose containers can in fact be used partially.

In these cases, the risk of error increases compared to indivisible units, and the user should also know how to manage the part of the unused portion of the drug unit (i.e., whether it should be thrown away or it could be later safely used).

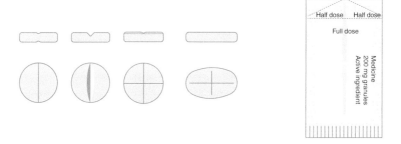

Fig. 19.8 On the left, examples of tablets with score lines; on the right, a bipartite sachet that, depending on how is opened, can release either a whole dose or a half dose

19.5.2 Multidose Containers

The previous topic is only apparently trivial, as when we break the integrity of the primary packaging by opening a blister unit, unscrewing the cap of an eye drop, or reconstituting a powder for oral solution, we enter the so-called "in-use" stability phase which is different from the "long-term" stability in the intact primary packaging. When partial use exposes the rest of the drug content to the external environment, the patient should always know whether the remaining product can be reused and, if so, under what conditions and within how long after first opening. But this implies that the patient must be able to write down the date and time of the first opening, preferably on the container itself.

When the multidose primary packaging also plays the function of a dispenser, as in the case of sprays, squeeze containers for eye drops, etc., to ensure therapeutic adherence, it will be important that the dispenser is easy to use and that it leaves as little room as possible for human errors. In those cases, it may be challenging to track doses (such as understanding whether we took our drops in the morning by checking the volume of liquid left in the bottle), so other solutions should be considered to monitor adherence through smart packaging or external tools. A new dispenser must undergo tests to evaluate its usability and complete its risk analysis (ISO 2019).

19.5.3 Dispensers Not Belonging to the Primary Packaging

If the drug cannot be dosed by the primary container, it is almost always necessary to use an external dispenser, namely a medical device that helps the user to extract and/or administer only the needed aliquot. The devices on the market are many and range from graduated syringes to cups or measuring spoons (Fig. 19.9).

Although the most widely used external dispensers are those for pharmaceutical forms that are liquid at the time of administration, there are also devices to help dosing solid forms, such as tablet cutters and tablet crushers, or more sophisticated systems capable of accurately dosing powders and granules (Fig. 19.10) (UNITAID,

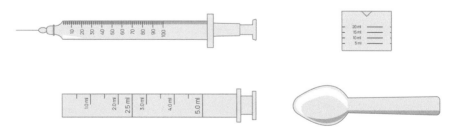

Fig. 19.9 Graduated dosing devices for liquid pharmaceutical forms (syrups, suspensions, solutions)

Fig. 19.10 System for dosing and dispensing solid pharmaceutical forms as powder, granules, or microspheres

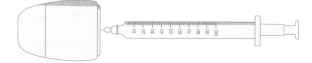

WHO 2020), avoiding that the entire bottle containing them is diluted before aliquoting (and thus preserving both stability and portability of the medicine).

19.5.4 Risk Assessment of Dosing Errors

The evolution of technology and the high standards requirements for drugs help reducing dosing and administration errors, but, as a matter of facts, any extra operation required from the user can increase the risk of non-adherence to therapy. A patient might reuse the half a tablet left that should have been thrown away, might not properly close a bottle of pills after taking one, might incorrectly dilute a powder, might be confused with the notches of an external dispenser, etc. For this reason, for example, the choice of the graduated dispenser must be compatible with the range of doses to be administered, avoiding, when possible, a dispenser having a graduation that goes beyond the maximum dosage allowed for the drug.

It should be noted that some mistakes are more dangerous than others and deserve special attention. For example, an incorrect dilution of a powder or an incorrect calculation of the dose/kg are theoretically more insidious than a missed dose, as they introduce a systematic error that will be repeated throughout the whole therapy. Therefore, the advantage of having a single presentation adaptable to many dosages should always be assessed versus multiple presentations specific to the patient groups, which reduce manipulation by the patient and allow a more targeted approach.

Last, dosing accuracy of a multidose dispenser is of varying importance depending on the route of administration. For example, the volume of a single "drop" depends on several factors (Van Santvliet and Ludwig 2004), related to both the liquid (such as viscosity) and the dispenser (such as lumen diameter), and might vary significantly between one product and another, or even for the same product, if the dispensing is made at different temperatures or the container is kept tilted differently (Fig. 19.11).

If the variability in the volume of a drop can be a problem for an oral solution, it could be to a lesser extent for an ophthalmic solution since the eye of an adult has characteristics such as to self-limit the absorption of topical solutions to a volume below 30 µL (Shell 1982), so the exceeding liquid would leak out of the treated area. A similar assessment should also be done for other products whose topical use is trivial, such as the creams, in which the variables involved do not depend only on the characteristics of the cream but also on the volume taken, the surface of application, the time taken to spread it, the integrity of the treated skin, the exposure to the environment after application, etc. Where improper use of the medicine might lead

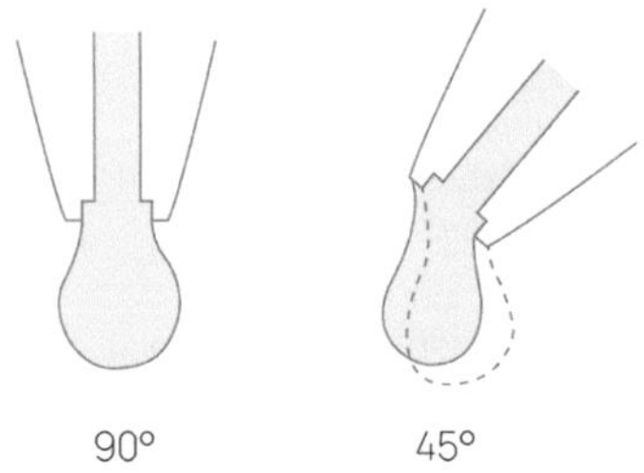

Fig. 19.11 The volume of a dispensed drop can change significantly, even when released by the same dispenser

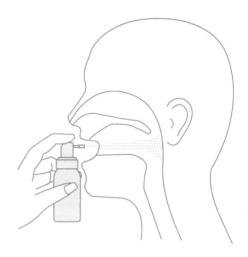

Fig. 19.12 Image taken from the package leaflet of an oro-mucosal spray. The shape of the dispenser protruding from the container and the dispensing button naturally predispose the patient to administer the product correctly

to severe complications for the patient, it will be more important to give precise instructions for use, such as recommending not to treat a damaged skin or not to bandage the treated part to avoid inappropriate systemic absorption of the active ingredient (Fig. 19.12).

19.5.5 Passive Medicine Delivery Systems

In this paragraph, it is worth mentioning passive delivery systems, such as infusion pumps (e.g., insulin) that, analogously to controlled-release active ingredients, reduce human intervention in medicine administration (and subsequently, the risk of human error), thus improving treatment adherence. It is foreseeable that an increasingly integrated and effective system of sensors that passively monitor the biomedical parameters of the patient, interfaced with drug delivery systems, and controlled by adaptive algorithms, can provide the individual with a personalized therapy capable of maximizing for him the benefit/risk ratio and could therefore go beyond the pure concept of therapeutic adherence.

19.6 Therapeutic Adherence: The Number of Units per Box

The number of units of medication included in a single pack can predispose to correct therapeutic adherence. For this reason, although certain flexibility is allowed, this number is regulated for most prescription and self-medication drugs.

For example, a pack of antibiotic tablets must be relevant to the authorized course of treatment (i.e., dosage and duration), and therefore adding extra tablets would be unnecessary or harmful to both the patient and the environment, as the excess drug could be taken by mistake, could predispose the patient to use it later even without a prescription, or (if remained unused) be disposed.

Similarly, an excessive number of units inside the pack of an over-the-counter painkiller could increase the risk of the patient abusing it since this type of medication, without strict medical supervision, is generally indicated only for short-term treatments.

19.7 Therapeutic Adherence: The Use of Organizers

For some patients with special needs and in poly-pharmacological therapy (i.e., taking several drugs during the same period), there is a need for a high level of organization for the safe administration of the products.

Patients with low vision or memory impairment (including some elderly patients) may need someone to put the units to be taken during the day in special organizers, usually consisting of multi-compartment pillboxes with text or tactile labels that indicate when to take each medication (Fig. 19.13).

These external organizers can be very useful to ensure therapeutic adherence. Although they involve an initial preparatory phase (by the patient or caregiver), they can integrate electronic components, alarms, and sensors, actively communicating with the patient.

But a much more powerful aid in the execution of the treatment plan is represented by the digital organizers. In fact, the spread of smartphones and smartwatches

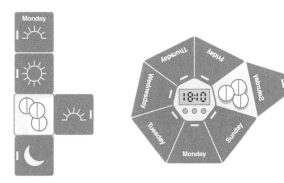

Fig. 19.13 Examples of weekly multi-compartment pillboxes with information on when to take the medication during the day (on the left) and equipped with a timer and an alarm (on the right)

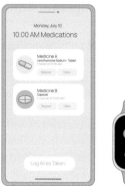

Fig. 19.14 Apps that help patients manage and track medication intake are becoming numerous. The patient receives reminders to take the medicines at the right time and in the right way, can monitor therapeutic adherence and the list of drugs to be taken

provides the patient with precise and technologically advanced tools to remember how and when to take medication. The use of specifically developed Apps (Fig. 19.14) requires at the moment an initial setting but allows the patient an advanced management of alarms to remember when to take the medicines, integrated by tools to collect and organize all the information useful for therapy.

The use of tags (e.g., Radio Frequency Identificators—RFId) integrated into the secondary packaging or in the label allows immediate interaction with a reader such as a smartphone, allowing the latter to acquire information about the medicine. It is expected that the integrated and effective use of these tools will also minimize initial preparation interventions, relieving the patient of this burden.

19.8 Looking into the Future

In this chapter, we have seen how therapeutic adherence can depend on multiple characteristics of the medicine and the packaging and how new digital technologies integrated to minimize human error, namely the risk of taking the wrong drug, the wrong dose or posology, the wrong combination, etc. Several studies evaluated these new tools' efficacy (El Alili et al. 2016).

Technologies with sensors and edible chips are a rapidly evolving reality (Litvinova et al. 2022) both in the field of "smart release" of drugs and in endoscopic diagnostics. The therapeutic areas covered by these innovations range from mental health to pain control, from cardiovascular diseases to diabetes, and from gastroenterology to oncology. The benefits that will derive from using these technologies will not only be limited to greater adherence and a better outcome of treatments but will also lead to shorter hospital stays, contributing, thanks to mobile clinical monitoring, to move patient management from the hospital to home.

An example is the capsule shown in Fig. 19.15, which contains a sensor fed by the patient's gastric fluids and emits a signal to a receiver which confirms ingestion (Flores et al. 2016).

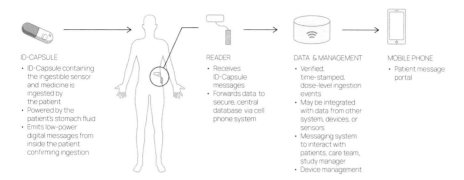

Fig. 19.15 Example of a capsule containing both an active ingredient and an edible sensor. When the capsule reaches the stomach, it sends a signal to confirm ingestion. (Source: Flores et al. 2016)

Wearable sensors, wireless technology and machine learning are already revolutionizing medicine. It is foreseeable that soon these systems will allow an increasingly automatic and smart personalization, accessing and crossing the patient's anamnestic data, the doctor's prescriptions, and the package leaflets of the drugs, so that the system can propose to the patient a therapeutic plan adhering to what is prescribed but also able to highlight warnings or detect any incompatibilities between concomitant drugs. In all this, advances in artificial intelligence and virtual assistance algorithms that adapt with use to user commands will play an increasingly important role, helping physicians and patients to interpret, filter and combine helpful information for therapy in typically faster times or in a more accurate way than the man can do. The patient will have a multi-integrated and reactive system, which will adapt in real time to his vital parameters, diet, circadian rhythms, etc. We will have a sort of virtual nurse 24 h a day who, based on the therapy described, will remind and/or suggest us to do the thing in our best interest all the time.

Through wireless technologies, helpful information will be processed and shared automatically with the doctor without depriving him of the role of decision-maker and supervisor of the therapeutic path.

And all the above opens up new perspectives that go beyond the good of the individual. The incredible amount of these "Real Word Data" collected in an increasingly passive and efficient way, once sorted, will become a valuable source of information that will increase knowledge about medicines, their efficacy and safety based on the characteristics of patients, their age, their ethnicity, etc., going to integrate and overcome the limits of what today is the primary source of this knowledge: the controlled clinical trials.

In other words, the same technology that will help a single patient to follow a therapy "better" to derive the best possible individual benefit/risk ratio will also produce helpful information for other patients, thus creating a virtuous cycle that feeds itself and allows to select those patients who will respond best to a given therapy. While waiting to find the solution to all diseases, technology will work to allow us to make the best use of the available solutions and to make them express their full potential.

References

Directive 2001/83/EC (2001) Directive 2001/83/EC of the European Parliament and of the Council of 6 November 2001 on the Community code relating to medicinal products for human use

El Alili M, Vrijens B, Demonceau J, Evers SM, Hiligsmann M (2016) A scoping review of studies comparing the medication event monitoring system (MEMS) with alternative methods for measuring medication adherence. Br J Clin Pharmacol 82(1):268–279

European Commission (2009) Guideline on the readability of the labelling and package leaflet of medicinal products for human use. ENTR/F/2/SF/jr (2009)D/869. Revision 1, 12 Jan 2009

European Medicines Agency (2018) EMA/493897/2015 Rev. 1. Mobile scanning and other technologies in the labelling and package leaflet of centrally authorised medicinal products. 26 Nov 2018

FDA (2019). www.accessdata.fda.gov/cdrh_docs/pdf18/K183052.pdf

Flores GP, Peace B, Carnes TC et al (2016) Performance, reliability, usability, and safety of the ID-cap system for ingestion event monitoring in healthy volunteers: a pilot study. Innov Clin Neurosci 13(9–10):12–19

ISO (2019) 14971:2019. Medical devices: Application of risk management to medical devices

Khan SA, Roohullah, Zeb A (2022) Modified-release drug delivery systems. In: Khan SA (ed) Essentials of industrial pharmacy, AAPS advances in the pharmaceutical sciences series, vol 46. Springer, Cham

Litvinova O, Klager E, Tzvetkov NT, Kimberger O, Kletecka-Pulker M, Willschke H, Atanasov AG (2022) Digital pills with ingestible sensors: patent landscape analysis. Pharmaceuticals 15(8):1025. https://doi.org/10.3390/ph15081025

QRD templates (2022) Centralised procedures—Quality Review of Documents (QRD) templates. Version 10.3, 09/2022

Shell JW (1982) Pharmacokinetics of topically applied ophthalmic drugs. Surv Ophthalmol 26:207–218

UNITAID, WHO (2020) Paediatrics medicines. Retrieved from https://www.who.int/publications/i/item/9789240008182

Van Santvliet L, Ludwig A (2004) Determinants of eye drop size. Surv Ophthalmol 49(2):197–213

Vargason AM, Anselmo AC, Mitragotri S (2021) The evolution of commercial drug delivery technologies. Nat Biomed Eng 5:951–967

Open Access This chapter is licensed under the terms of the Creative Commons Attribution 4.0 International License (http://creativecommons.org/licenses/by/4.0/), which permits use, sharing, adaptation, distribution and reproduction in any medium or format, as long as you give appropriate credit to the original author(s) and the source, provide a link to the Creative Commons license and indicate if changes were made.

The images or other third party material in this chapter are included in the chapter's Creative Commons license, unless indicated otherwise in a credit line to the material. If material is not included in the chapter's Creative Commons license and your intended use is not permitted by statutory regulation or exceeds the permitted use, you will need to obtain permission directly from the copyright holder.

Chapter 20
Pharmaceutical Packaging According to the "Packaging Ethics Charter"

Valeria Bucchetti

Abstract The chapter analyses the role that packaging plays in pharmacological products, starting with the communicative and instrumental aspects. Like and arguably more than other products, the medicine needs the prosthetic, synthetic and directing mediation aspect of packaging; the medicine is one of those types of things which, through packaging, take on a form, become products and usable content. The observations developed in the chapter take their cue from those in the Ethical Packaging Charter, a document for the study and analysis of packaging concerning the needs of the consumer, the user, the environment, and society.

20.1 The Project Intended as a Synthesis

The topic of packaging design is addressed here in its most profound sense, as a design act aimed at producing a synthesis whereby the different aspects involving the prosthetic—communicative and instrumental—dimensions of the packaging artefact are harmonised, according to the most evolved interpretation of this specific field of the project.[1] As is well known, a multitude of interventions can be ascribed to packaging design concerning specialised sectors, from those related to materials technology and its applications, to those referring to the use of more or less intelligent supports, to others that affect the structural and functional dimension, as well as those connected to dispensing devices in their various forms.[2] However, the

---

[1] Reference is made to packaging design as a design discipline that determines the balance between structural and communicative components and that places the semantic dimension of all the elements that make up the artefact in the foreground when carrying out the design synthesis.

[2] In this sense, to get a picture of the state of the art and its breadth, it can be useful to examine the packaging that is nominated for the competitions; the case of the *Oscar dell'Imballaggio*, organised by the Istituto Italiano Imballaggio, represents a nationwide showcase in which innovations of

V. Bucchetti (✉)
Department of Design, Politecnico di Milano, Milan, Italy
e-mail: valeria.bucchetti@polimi.it

design act and its role of synthesis are capable of virtuously bringing together in a single object choice that may be asynchronous—taken over time and not always orchestrated—or ascribable to constraints or unforeseeable needs. With its directorial intervention, a design act that has the responsibility to govern a balance, to determine it even where it is absent, to compensate for gaps, and to emphasise and exalt qualities and attributes so that users can immediately interpret them. And suppose these considerations are valid for packaging. In that case, they are even more incisive for the pharmaceuticals sector because they belong to a category of indispensable products on which the person's life may depend, and because they belong to that type of objects that, through packaging, become usable products and contents (Bucchetti 1999, 2005; Volli 2001); indeed, the medicine falls into that category which requires a prosthetic mediation.

We can thus argue that the medicine shapes itself through packaging. Sometimes it assumes its own shape, when the package is what allows granules, liquids, creams, ointments, etc., to take on an identity, in others to guarantee the manageability that enables its use (Anceschi and Bucchetti 1998), to the point of becoming, more generally, a unit of measurement of its contents (a vial of…, a sachet of…). And if these considerations refer to its function as an instrumental prosthesis, transversal to the medicine category, it is different as regards the role of communicative prosthesis performed by it. Indeed, we know the approaching extent, with specific perspectives depending on the type of medicine: hospital, ethical, or over-the-counter medicines. These product categories present three levels of communicative needs, determined first and foremost by distribution logic and channels. Where distribution and regulatory criteria refer to sales, and the processes of liberalisation place the user-consumer behind the so-called free service, and a shelf offer based on communication strategies typical of mass consumption products, which transfer onto pharmaceutical packaging, the design knowledge and appellative techniques deriving from the market experience sedimented over a century of history of commercial communication.

However, as is well known, the communicative function also performs other tasks by reversing priorities. It occurs when it supports and facilitates the product-recipient relationship during the informative and preventive phases of orientation, access to administration, and, more generally, in-depth knowledge. In developing these observations, a contribution to the theme can be fostered by a re-reading of the Packaging Ethics Chart.[3] This document was drawn up to open a shared path of reflection, helpful to promote evolution of the sector, a record that through its principles, allows us to re-examine the field under study in respect of the needs of the consumer, the user, the environment, and society.

The Charter declares itself to be:

---

a specific type emerge, which frequently concern the functionality of the artefact, and detailed technical aspects, which define the performance increase.

[3] *The Packaging Ethics Chart* has been drafted by Giovanni Baule and Valeria Bucchetti; it is a project by Baule and Bucchetti, Department of Design, Politecnico di Milano with Guidotti and Lavorini, Edizioni Dativo; promoted by Edizioni Dativo; sponsored by Istituto Italiano Imballaggio.

A document of principles to be shared to accompany packaging towards a more conscious future. The Packaging Ethics Chart stands as a tool for a "system culture": it aims to bind obligations and rights that can join production with use and consumption, individuals who are bearers of obligations and individuals who benefit from rights and expectations. The Packaging Ethics Chart connects rights, principles, and values to secure an ideal agreement between the system players so that they undertake to share principles to aim at without overlapping themselves with the regulations while making this choice public.

Therefore, the ten principles set out in the charter become keys to a review. Each principle recalls a function: it is a matter of considering each individual item as part of a whole, of a bundle of processes that act intersecting and that, depending on the primary design objective and the peculiarities of the product-content, are reconfigured from a systemic dimension.

20.2 Responsible

This is the first key term proposed by the document, intended to recall a primary principle, transversal to project action and the need to consider for each project move, beyond the fulfilment of a necessity, the effects it may have. We wish to emphasise an extended responsibility that all the actors must share in the system. A responsibility that must invest the entire community and which allows us to speak of the social responsibility of packaging.

On the design side, "designing packaging involves the analysis of its instrumental functions closely linked to the communicative functions of medium and interface with the user".[4] When we consider the pharmaceutical sector, we find ourselves in a field in which design competencies often belong to distinct groups; in which the design of the various functions (instrumental and communicative) is separate, in which the role of protecting the content and its forms of delivery requires a high technological component, therefore elaborated in technical-engineering research and development contexts, within an overall design process that separates phases and competences. Thus, the notion underlying this first principle emphasises the need to merge what the design process divides by entrusting it to the figure of a designer, who takes full responsibility for the directing role at the centre of which is the user.

20.3 Balanced

This is a principle related to the value of the *right balance*.

Packaging for pharmaceuticals is inalienable, so its presence and function is certainly not in question, as is the case for other sectors. Still, it should also deal with

---

[4] Direct reference is made to the principle of the Packaging Ethics Chart defined as responsible.

this principle, responding to the "just enough and just what is needed" paradigm. As the Charter states: "Balanced is the packaging when it is conceived and designed with a right relationship with the content and is the result of what is necessary for its correct diffusion". Hence, the packaging must be calibrated depending on the type of medicine, whether or not it is a so-called "life-saving" medicine or the organoleptic qualities and preservation of the composition.

According to this principle, technologies that load packaging with 'intelligence', for example, can be re-examined based on a balanced choice between the service offered and its necessity, but also issues more commonly labelled *overpackaging*.[5]

And if some solutions attributable to overpackaging, at first glance, should be viewed favourably as playing the role of instrumental prostheses, in which an essential service function prevails (e.g. in the forms of dispensing that allow therapy to be managed and normalized in the conduct of daily life thanks to the device), it is instead helpful to point out how often overpackaging manifests itself due to a general principle of standardisation in packaging and optimisation of dedicated machines, leading to an imbalance between content and container. Among the most apparent examples are cases where blisters are only partially filled (they contain six capsules while providing space for up to eight alveoli, etc.) to maintain format modularity for sale without modifying the packaging line. This choice optimises processes and formats (from the size of the carton to that of the shipping packaging). Still, it has an inconsistent and unbalanced impact on volumes and quantity compared to the actual content. Conversely, as a case study, it is worth mentioning the packaging solutions that leave their parallelepiped shape (cardboard box packaging) to reduce their volume in the upper part of the pack by the medicine's behaviour, meaning that the granular product contained in the vertically arranged single-dose flow packs is deposited at the base, thus leaving a significant void in the upper part of the packaging.

20.4 Safe

Safety is a crucial principle for pharmaceutical packaging. This principle interprets at the highest level that a trust contract is implicitly established, on the level of the relationship, whenever a product is trusted.

> Safe is the packaging that gives an account of its traceability, of the processes of its production chain; it is safe as regards the protection of its contents and its hygiene, safe during transport and use. And this for the entire life span of the packaging.[6]

Thus, packaging proposes itself as a device capable of transferring through its presence the necessary guarantees that the user demands or simply expects, precisely because it recognises its role, regarding conformity, adequacy, and compliance with

---

[5] On this topic, see: Bucchetti (2005), Badalucco (2011).
[6] Direct reference is made to the principle of the Packaging Ethics Chart defined as Safe.

regulations. In the case of European regulations,[7] all pharmaceutical products sold in Europe must be contained in packaging with safety features that allow their integrity to be verified. In this sense, we can refer to the various anti-tampering systems to make possible forms of tampering evident. Tamper Evident solutions whose closure is armed when the product is packaged and when the seal is broken the first time it is opened, a significant part of the carton changes shape and colour, giving irreversible evidence that it has been opened. In this case, we are talking about solutions that can be perceived by touch and whose usability is guaranteed even by visually impaired or blind users. Devices for intelligent packaging, such as Time Temperature Indicators, control these parameters through integrated sensors when the contents require compliance with the cold chain.

The safety issue cannot fail to consider the different profiles of users, particularly their temporary or permanent frailties, whether they are 'passive' users, meaning coerced or obliged to take. But also, of the seriousness and repercussions that, in many cases, the error brings with it, making the term 'safe' take on an absolute centrality for the packaging of the medicine, also because of the harmfulness that erroneous actions can produce on the subject.

It is also essential to relate another aspect to this principle, namely that about perceived safety, which involves the emotional dimension of the recipients and passes through plastic and symbolic attributes of the device, which can contribute to reinforcing or undermining the user's serenity.

Psychology of colour and shape play, in this sense, their role in constructing reassurance. For example, the case of a pre-filled device for injecting the medicine whose dark red plunger, as the colourless liquid is injected, flows taking its place and, precisely because of its red colour, triggers an association, albeit irrational, with blood, developing a consequent sensation of discomfort that is repeated with each administration. Indeed, the device does not technically compromise the administration. Still, its design seems not to have considered the emotional aspects of the human beings involved and the emotional activating role played by the instrument.

20.5 Accessible

Packaging is accessible when it is easy and intuitive to use and thus takes into account every consumer's right to approach, understand and use a product.

The notion of accessibility has multiple implications as it can relate to different dimensions of the artefact. It has to do with the idea of a threshold, understood as the space of passage that leads to the objective, which makes concrete the possibility and the right to access the medicine and to carry out the administration, with the course that decrees the outcome, the quality of which can change the sign of the

---

[7] See regulation 2011/62/EU, which stipulates that, as of 2019, all pharmaceutical products sold in Europe must be contained in cartons equipped with security features to verify their integrity.

entire act: connoting it positively or nullifying its effects. Designing accessibility means adhering to functional ethics (Fabris 2021), linked to the model of use and ease of use, guaranteeing efficiency and effectiveness to the packaging artefact. But accessibility also implies the hostile element, the barrier; it is paradoxically affirmed where it is lacking. In its resolved form, it does not manifest itself; it only becomes evident when faced with an absence or a lack. When the interaction occurs correctly and without obstacles, the device presents itself as an interface that measures the users who do not perceive its mediation, which feels as soon as they perceive a difficulty. For example, when it fails to act on a so-called child-proof closure, or as in the case of syrup packaged in "spoon" mono-doses whose shape and size are not consistent with the force that must be exerted to remove the film that seals it, producing a consequent leakage and dispersion of the medicine, or when it must load an inhaler whose instructions declare an unforeseen complexity, but also when the traceability, perceptibility or comprehensibility of the information is lacking (Ciravegna 2010; Bucchetti and Ciravegna 2014; Steffan 2014). In its more inclusive meaning of "for all", accessibility is also guaranteed by the sensory modalities of sight and touch and involves haptic perception (Riccò 2008). The packaging can be perceived as a three-dimensional object: grasped, lifted, and handled, including tactile perception (the object is touched) and kinaesthetic perception (muscular sensitivity, perception of the position of one's limbs and movement concerning the object, for example, the weight/transport ratio).[8] Modalities that guide the recipient's actions in accessing the product and that, together with the morphological properties of the structure, graphic solutions and surface finishes, favour the identification on the packaging of the different functions (opening, dispensing, etc.). A system of access to medicine that must take into account conventions, experiences, and customs; of an introjected know-how that must be able to be evaluated each time a new form of interface is introduced, to a perspective of the economy of access, to the cognitive effort required, easy to understand regardless of the experiences, knowledge or skills of the users or their level of attention, and regardless of the conditions of the context.

20.6 Transparent

The value of transparency is metaphorical. Transparent is a postural attribute, metaphorically speaking, which concerns the chosen communicative register, through which the packaging declares that it wants to address the user directly, without

---

[8] See, in this regard, Bucchetti (2007) (ed.), *Packaging tra vista e tatto* [*Packaging between sight and touch*]. See also, in the same vol., Riccò, Congruenze sinestesiche [Synesthetic congruences] (pp. 15–17). See also Calabi (2007). Percezioni aptiche e cromatiche [Haptic and chromatic perceptions], (pp. 97–147) in Bucchetti (ed.). (2007). *Culture visive. Contributi per il design della comunicazione.* [*Visual Cultures Contributions for communication design*].

mystery. This means designing to develop a relationship of trust with the recipient, a primary condition, as is well-known in the pharmaceuticals sector.

Therefore, transparent packaging tends to have a low error risk and induces virtuous behaviour. As an example, the solutions frequently adopted for medicines intended for asthma treatment are inhalers that display how many doses of medicine are left. Each time the lid is opened, the dose counter counts down, and when less than ten doses remain, the area turns partially red as an alert. It turns completely red after the last dose has been used.

A further form of transparency can be recognised when the packaging directly expresses some of its properties through certain communicative moves; for example, through the rationalisation of information on the primary area of the pack. In this case, the intention is to make communication immediate through the organisation of the graphic elements according to a signposting-type perspective[9] using images that can be immediately traced back to the disease or disorder, to the anatomical elements or organs involved, which play the role of writing in pictures. An example of this is the search for standardisation of pictogrammatic systems to make the pharmaceutical form (tablets, capsules, suppositories, etc.) immediate, and that aimed at raising the quality of typographical elements concerning the choice of font (highly readable and composed according to criteria that favour reading) and its composition (line spacing, alignments, etc.) guarantee immediate communication.[10]

20.7 Informative

"It is the packaging that ensures the best information, both useful and necessary". Packaging is a pivotal information interface connecting us with the product. In the case of pharmaceuticals, this information function is performed not only by the

---

[9] One example among many is the project realised by settepuntoquattro: the Joint Pain, Sore Muscles, Migraine product line presents a graphic layout in which illustrations, pictograms of the pharmaceutical form, typographic elements and colour codes are designed to provide information directly on the primary area with signposting functions, useful for an initial orientation. (https://www.settepuntoquattro.it/boxes/).

Also, because of both the package leaflet and the outer packaging—according to legislative decree 219/2006—may contain graphic elements aimed at making certain information useful to the patient more explicit and comprehensible, to the exclusion of any element of a promotional nature (Art. 79). The use of pictures, pictograms and other symbols must serve to clarify or highlight certain aspects of the text and not to replace the text, as indicated by AIFA provided that the signs used are widely understood and are not misleading.

[10] In the field of Pharmaceutical Packaging Design, see the research subject of Master's degree theses, in particular: "The visual communication of the medicine in the critical area", thesis by Gloria Angelini, supervisor Gianluigi Pescolderung, co-rapporteur Elisa Pasqual, IUAV, academic year 2012–2013; and "Undesirable effects. On the communicative accessibility of pharmaceutical packaging, research and design', by Agnese Rodriquez, supervisor Valeria Bucchetti, Master's Degree Course in Communication Design, Politecnico di Milano, academic year 2010–2011.

packaging but also by complementary devices, such as the leaflets, integrated with it. Information that develops today in a communicative context reshaped starting from the technological-digital transformation, characterised by an overall process of democratisation of information and determined by the apparent ease in the availability of data and news[11] and by the diffusion of tools for accessing the web, and consequently information. Changes modify the relationship between those who hold the knowledge and those who use it. But, when we refer to the information functions of packaging, we touch, in the case of pharmaceuticals, on a further issue since we face products with a high density of information content that cannot be unequivocally hierarchised. On the one hand, a large amount of information is available and, on the other, the criteria by which it is organised. This is an imposing design task for which the medical, pharmacological and regulatory reasons, with their associated need for precise expressions conveyed through technical-scientific language, are flanked by the need for comprehension on the part of a heterogeneous user base in terms of literacy, but also driven by a wide range of motivations and multiple emotional profiles that, as we know, characterise patients. Indeed, information may be sought to obtain reassurance or for reasons attributable to mistrust, to check or compare, to inform oneself and act consciously in the case of self-administration, for prudence and to protect oneself from possible incompatibilities; but also based on other motivations that have repercussions on criteria of interpretation of the corpus of information, which are highly subjective.

Today, the informational capacity of pharmaceutical packaging expands through the implementation of an *active interaction surface*[12] that transforms labels into interfaces that provide alerts and transfer information,[13] but also through the enhancement of the dialogue between communicative devices, interconnecting with other devices, delegating to them what in the past was the prerogative of the package leaflets, according to a cross-media logic that goes beyond the written surface of the packaging. Today's information dimension is made possible by smart packaging solutions capable of communicating with smartphones, tablets, PCs, etc., thanks to the evolution of digital channels, from smart labelling technologies such as Rfid tags, Nfc or QR codes that can be linked to websites and web pages, to minisites, to PDF documents, as well as to stand-alone videos, or connect to apps, thus extending the communication capabilities of the leaflet (for example by making information in different languages immediately available) and the fruition times that follow the

---

[11] A transformation that brings with it contradictory aspects since the availability of an extremely large amount of information is not matched by useful cultural tools to make a selection from the sources and disciplinary knowledge to understand them.

[12] It is interesting to recall some exploratory projects carried out in the early 2000s, in which packaging was proposed as an active interaction surface on which information could be displayed, contextualised in real time according to user input. This hypothesis was based on the use of polymer semiconductors that made it possible to transform the casing into a matrix of pixels that could be illuminated when needed. See, in this regard, Capitini (2004), pp. 143–151.

[13] Reference is made, for example, to the experiments of the start-up Inuru and the ELFI labels tested to help patients avoid mistakes when taking medication through visible light warnings on the label itself. See https://www.inuru.com/solutions/medical (accessed 17 January 2023).

parameters and dictates of digital communication. This extension of the information function is also achieved using intelligent packaging systems involving, for example, cartons made by printing conductive inks using flexographic technologies, which make it possible to connect with smartphones, as well as cartons equipped with a screen and sensors designed to support patients in monitoring and adhering to therapy.[14]

20.8 Up-to-Date

The ability to constantly relate to the society whose values it represents is a principle that distinguishes packaging and its qualities. Like any designed artefact, it also reflects the culture that determines it and, in turn, contributes to creating it. This happens regardless of the degree of awareness of the designer and the user who interprets or assimilates its values, even when these go unnoticed. The quest to be contemporary has, over time, led to a continuous evolution of pharmaceutical packaging and has determined its transformations.

From the changes that have involved formats, now articulated in a range of declinations (from the reduced ones, for example, with the revival of the *sachet of Minerva* model), to the innovation of devices according to a perspective of improved interaction and greater ease of use, from those intended for the safety of the packaging and its opening systems to the design of diversified devices concerning the functional requirements of administration, suffice it to think of the diversity of devices that contemplate the packaging in its role as an instrumental prosthesis, as a medium for dispensing; think, for example, of the variety of injectors or packaging-tools designed to allow delocalised medicine intake (and hence without the need for additional instruments such as spoons, syringes, etc.): single-dose packaging, flasks, etc.): single-dose packaging, bottles with applicators, single-dose applicators, pre-filled pens, etc. But let us also think of the set of collateral devices, often complementary, as in the case of the blister-holders designed to facilitate the storage, during everyday life, of tablets or tablets and to prevent the blister from deteriorating if transported over a long period, for example in a bag, with a consequent waste of the medicine it contains. These examples restore the adherence, though certainly still perfectible, of packaging to the *esprit du temps*.

---

[14] See what was developed with the PhutureMed project https://www.packagingstrategies.com/articles/88367-palladio-group-and-e-ink-introduce-phuturemed-advanced-packaging-solution--for-pharmaceutical-products (accessed 22 December 2022).

20.9 Forward-Looking

While packaging must fully respond to the *here and now*, it must also be able to place itself *in a correct relationship with its future*. It must respect the prefigurative principle of design, the ability to give shape to solutions not only based on an immediate advantage or adhering to an existing model, but it must be able to develop new scenarios and foresee spin-offs and consequences.

The Charter recalls that:

> Forward-looking packaging is capable of grasping changes in advance, fostering new consumption models, and evolving behaviours over time. It knows, therefore, that it must modify itself over time: it must experiment on itself to favour its future transformations. Packaging must be able to embrace all necessary changes: it must be the subject of research and forms of experimentation that make it evolve; it must have tools that enable it to foresee its transformations. Packaging must involve a constant commitment to research and innovation. As consumers, we thus know that we face an object that knows how to rethink itself for tomorrow's users.

Packaging, in its evolutionary process, reacts by facing new challenges and responds to changing habits and lifestyles, just as it cannot fail to take into account, with due anticipation, for example, the demographic transformations of the population, falling into scenarios in which the repercussions on the service functions of packaging are correlated to the increase in chronic pathologies and, consequently, to the rise in regular consumption of medicines.

But this forward-looking principle must also involve communication functions and their change, in line with the evolution of communication formats and society's digitalisation level. There are many studies, experiments, and examples. Regarding the enhancement of packaging functions to support adherence to the therapeutic plan, pharmaceutical packaging expands its information functions through a directorial orchestration of several mediums, according to a cross-media perspective.[15]

Once again, the most relevant examples concern the interaction of packaging (in many cases the case) with devices such as smartphones to monitor the correct intake of the medicine[16] to remind patients of their intake, record the date and time each tablet was taken from the packet and the position of each tablet or pill when removed from the wrapper.[17] Even extending its action by activating a dialogue, for example, with the "electronic diary" of medicines, designing an increasingly targeted

---

[15] Concerning the relationship between demographic and digital transformation, see what emerges from the research work carried out by the Università Cattolica del Sacro Cuore in Milan, a member of the 'Harvest European Project', among the winners of the European call for proposals 'Ageing and Place in a digitising world', launched by the More Years Better Lives joint programming initiative. https://www.repubblica.it/tecnologia/2018/01/30/news/italia_solo_1_anziano_su_4_usa_smart phone_e_pc-187659487/

[16] One example is Phill Solution by the Palladio Group.

[17] See: https://www.worldofprint.com/2011/02/16/stora-enso-pharma-ddsi-wireless-a-new-medical-package-offering-improved-opportunities-for-real-time-adherence-control/ (accessed 27 August 2022). See also the Cerepack project, resulting from a partnership between MWV and Cypack.

interaction in which acoustic signals, or reminders through text messages, constitute additional functionalities underpinning clinical trials aimed at integrating and increasing the service.[18]

20.10 Educative

The educative function can be traced back to an ontological principle of pharmaceutical packaging.

If every prosthetic object, and packaging among them, has in itself an educative component that has to do with how the object transfers indications through the programme of actions it contains, that is, it has inscribed in itself—in its form, in its components, in its very structural orientation—, the actions that the user is going to perform, the packaging of the medicine must interpret this component most profoundly.

Its educative function must be exercised to direct behaviour towards correct administration (respect for the therapeutic plan remains one of the nodal issues), which frequently passes through adequate interaction with the artefact, where this involves loading, assembling or, more simply, referring to the opening/closing of the package. In particular, the educative function, in the sense of a function designed to develop and refine practice through exercise, assumes a real centrality in terms of interaction whenever a new solution is introduced with which the user is unfamiliar, namely when it must accompany the user in a training path enabling use. A small example of this is the single-dose drops which, after separating the single unit from the stick that welds them together in series, require the user to act on the seal of the single opening and turn it upside down to allow it to take on the function of a resealable 'cap': an elementary but not immediately intuitive gesture.

More generally, the educative function must be extended up to the moment of disposal and, therefore, as is the case for the entire packaging sector, the packaging itself must provide the necessary indications in compliance with regulations, but also promote, through an appropriate design of the communicative elements, attentive and responsible behaviour. One thinks of the disposal of the packaging and, in some cases, of the packaged medicine, and of the need to promote and improve, through design action, the instructions of a prescriptive nature, the behaviour relating to the correct disposal of the product during the separate collection at home (what do I separate? where can I throw it?) or at the collection points in pharmacies (do I only dispose of the tablets or do I throw them without taking them out of the blister pack?).

---

[18] These are experiments that draw scenarios and models according to new paradigms. The data can be quickly downloaded into a computer for analysis by the patient or healthcare professional.

20.11 Sustainable

As is known, the sustainability of packaging concerns the materials used, the resources, and the forms of optimisation of processes and transport, according to the guidelines referring to the environmental sustainability criteria indicated by the PEF[19]—The Product Environmental Footprint—, includes multi-criteria measures of environmental performance throughout the life cycle of the packaging produced with the general aim of reducing environmental impacts taking into account the supply chain.[20] In this perspective, one essential reading focuses on a specific issue, namely the various forms of waste involving pharmaceuticals and, together with them, the packaging that carries them.

On the one hand, it refers to the shortcomings of the packaging or its weaknesses. For example, one thinks of what happens with bottles equipped with a dropper pipette when the inadequate length of the cannula prevents the entire quantity of medicine contained in the bottle from being used, not allowing the residual medication deposited at the bottom to be taken up. A waste of seemingly insignificant proportions that is only fully perceived when referring to constant administration over time. On the other hand, examples of the opposite sign: this is the case of those packages that, through the introduction of technologically advanced devices, allow the dispensing of calibrated and sterile drops, thanks to the presence of a filtering membrane that prevents bacterial contamination. A solution that, thanks to a guarantee of sterility, extends the duration of use after opening, thus allowing the entire content to be used, and thus representing a sustainable alternative to single-dose dispensers.

Regarding this issue, it is worth recalling a further question that concerns the function and role that packaging has, and can have, in combating medicine wastage, namely the forms of wastage that are most closely related to personal behaviour for which it would be interesting to address the political and financial reasons and interests that have so far prevented corrective action. This is a mighty phenomenon: eight billion tablets go unused every year in our country, or 30% of the 24 billion doses of medicine that Italian hospitals or citizens buy yearly: an enormous waste because of the expiry date.[21]

On the one hand, this phenomenon concerns the overall system and its digitalisation, the hospital's digitalised and customised distribution of medicines, and the way they are administered. On the other hand, it opens up spaces for design research

---

[19] See: https://ec.europa.eu/environment/eussd/pdf/footprint/PEF%20methodology%20final%20draft.pdf

[20] See what has been published, albeit referring to the food sector, by De Giorgi in Sustainable Packaging? A multi-criteria method for evaluating food packaging.

[21] See the statement by Carlo Gaudio, Aifa board member and director of the Department of Cardiovascular and Respiratory Sciences at Sapienza University in Rome. https://www.ordine-farmacistiroma.it/gaudio-aifa-medicinali-scaduti-spreco-da-8-miliardi/ (accessed 27 August 2022).

into the flexibility of formats, directing the study towards customised packages, since an incorrectly 'sized' package leads, as is well known, to waste.[22]

The path of a double expiry date on medicine boxes proposed by Carlo Gaudio[23] should also be read in this direction. In addition to the classic expiry date (shown in black), a second expiry date in red is hypothesised that could highlight the last months of validity.[24] A sort of *last months notice* that would help people realise that they have products that are about to expire and that, if they are no longer needed because the therapy has ended, they could be returned to municipal pharmacies or handed over to non-profit organisations that distribute medicines free of charge to people in difficulty. Medicines that are unused in their last months of validity could, in this way, be made available—ensuring the transparency of their pathway—to guarantee those 'free treatments to the indigent' envisaged by the constitutional dictate.

20.12 Principles of Design for Accessibility

What has just been outlined, with the help of the principles of the Packaging Ethics Chart, is a framework that can play an instructive role in packaging design processes for pharmaceutical products from a perspective that places at the centre, in addition to its role as an instrumental prosthesis, that of the interface, mediating device, and communicative artefact that directs behaviour, translates, and provides information. Today, packaging cannot fail to be conceived in a systemic key and, therefore, starting from the artefactual system (Bucchetti 1999; Badalucco 2011), requiring a direction capable of harmonising processes, considering instances that move from needs that are sometimes opposite, reconfiguring, if necessary, technical and technological innovations so that users remain at the centre. Thus, an area is emerging that continues to offer a field of research of particular interest (Pareek et al. 2014) and which brings to the forefront nodal themes for design, and for communication design in particular, which have their focus in the *design of accessibility* (Baule 2011; Bucchetti and Ciravegna 2014), since it is only with this form of designed mediation, of the interface in the extended sense, that the user enters into a relationship. It is on the quality of this interaction that the success of the internal process and the chain of choices that nourished it depends, or, on the contrary, its frustration. It is an area of design that requires a specific competence, a highly specialised *packaging designer* figure capable of orchestrating all the points dealt with by the Packaging Ethics Chart and knowing how to govern them in design through coherent declinations.

---

[22] On these issues see: Manifesto per la Sostenibilità Consumeristica, promoted by Federfarma.

[23] See Carlo Gaudio.

[24] Regarding expiry dates, the research work carried out within the food sector for the Ministry of Economic Development to provide improved tools for the design and use of expiry dates remains of interest. Research published in: Bucchetti and Ciravegna (2007).

References

Anceschi G, Bucchetti V (1998) Il «packaging» alimentare [The «food» packaging]. In: Capatti A, De Bernardi A, Varni A (eds) Storia d'Italia. Annali 13. L'alimentazione [History of Italy. Annals 13. Nutrition]. Einaudi, Torino, pp 947–886

Angelini G (academic year 2012–2013) The visual communication of the medicine in the critical area. Thesis, Supervisor G. Pescolderung, co-rapporteur E. Pasqual. IUAV, Venice

Badalucco L (2011) Il buon packaging [The good packaging]. Edizioni Dativo, Milano

Baule G (2011) Figure di perigrafia. Sui designer di cornici, autori di forme dell'accesso [Figures of perigraphy. On frame designers, authors of forms of access]. In: Bucchetti V (ed) Altre figure [Other figures]. FrancoAngeli, Milano, pp 63–91

Bucchetti V (1999) La messa in scena del prodotto. Packaging identità e consumo [Product placement. Packaging identity and consumption]. FrancoAngeli, Milano

Bucchetti V (2005) Packaging design. Storia, linguaggi, progetto [Packaging design. History, languages, design]. Poli.Design-FrancoAngeli, Milano

Bucchetti V (ed) (2007) Packaging tra vista e tatto [Packaging between sight and touch]. Edizioni POLI.design, Milano

Bucchetti V, Ciravegna E (2007) Durabilità e scadenza nella comunicazione di prodotto [Durability and expiry in product communication]. Edizioni Dativo, Milano

Bucchetti V, Ciravegna E (2014) Design of access. Methods and tools for packaging design. In: Steffan TI (ed) Design for All-The project for everyone. Methods, tools, applications (first part). Maggioli, Milano, pp 101–116

Calabi D (2007) Percezioni aptiche e cromatiche [Haptic and chromatic perceptions]. In: Bucchetti V (ed) Culture visive. Contributi per il design della comunicazione [Visual cultures. Contributions for communication design]. Edizioni POLI.design, Milano, pp 97–147

Capitini M (2004) Imballaggi intelligenti [Smart packaging]. In: Bucchetti V (ed) Design della comunicazione ed esperienze di acquisto [Communication design and shopping experiences]. FrancoAngeli, Milano, pp 143–151

Ciravegna E (2010) La qualità del packaging. Sistemi per l'accesso comunicativo-informativo dell'imballaggio [The quality of packaging. Systems for communicative-informative access to packaging]. FrancoAngeli, Milano

De Giorgi C (ed) (2013) Sustainable packaging? Metodo multicriteria di valutazione del packaging alimentare [Sustainable packaging? Multi-criteria method for evaluating food packaging]. Umberto Allemandi & C, Torino

Fabris A (ed) (2021) Guida alle etiche della comunicazione [A guide to communication ethics]. Edizioni ETS, Pisa

Pareek V et al (2014) Pharmaceutical packaging: current trends and future. Int J Pharm Pharm Sci 6(6):480–485

Riccò D (2007) Congruenze sinestetiche [Synesthetic congruences]. In: Bucchetti V (ed) Packaging tra vista e tatto. Edizioni POLI.design, Milano, pp 15–17

Riccò D (2008) Sentire il design. In: Sinestesie nel progetto di comunicazione [Feeling design. Synaesthesia in communication design]. Carocci, Roma

Rodriguez A (academic year 2010–2011) Undesirable effects. On the communicative accessibility of pharmaceutical packaging, research and design. Thesis, supervisor V. Bucchetti. Politecnico di Milano, Milano

Steffan TI (ed) (2014) Design for All-The project for everyone. Methods, tools, applications (first part). Maggioli, Milano

Volli U (2001) La grammatica dell'imballaggio [The grammar of packaging]. In: AA.VV. PackAge. Storia, costume, industria, funzioni e futuro dell'imballaggio [and future of packaging]. Lupetti, Milano, pp 12–35

Open Access This chapter is licensed under the terms of the Creative Commons Attribution 4.0 International License (http://creativecommons.org/licenses/by/4.0/), which permits use, sharing, adaptation, distribution and reproduction in any medium or format, as long as you give appropriate credit to the original author(s) and the source, provide a link to the Creative Commons license and indicate if changes were made.

The images or other third party material in this chapter are included in the chapter's Creative Commons license, unless indicated otherwise in a credit line to the material. If material is not included in the chapter's Creative Commons license and your intended use is not permitted by statutory regulation or exceeds the permitted use, you will need to obtain permission directly from the copyright holder.

Chapter 21
Sensory Qualities of the Medicines: From Problems to Proposals

Dina Riccò

Abstract The text reviews the studies conducted on the sensory qualities of the medicines. It considers the medicine as a product, therefore as a project object of which to examine its tertiary qualities—the experienced object and therefore evaluates its visual (e.g., colour, shape, etc.), gustatory (e.g., bitter, sweet, pleasant, unpleasant, etc.), the qualities of the surface (e.g., smooth, rough, etc.), its consistency, etc., together with the connotations that these induce, noting the problems, the recognition in visual impairment and the incidence that these have on adherence to treatment and correct intake. Compare the sensory characteristics of the medicine with the formal/chromatic characteristics of the tablets in pharmaceutical production. It concludes by noting how the research carried out on the sensory characteristics the medicines is limited to studying these characteristics separately, not considering the interaction between them and the perceptual hierarchies, the prevalence that one can hold over the others. Very few studies address the issue of accessibility for people with sensory disabilities, the latter are addressed in the medicine packages by providing Braille text, but no indication allows communication and discrimination of the tablet for people with visual impairments.

21.1 Sensory Properties of Artifacts: Affordances and Proximity of Use

The concept of *affordance*, which Gibson introduced by referring to the studies of Gestalt psychologists, Koffka and Lewin in particular,[1] assumes that given properties of an object (such as shape, size, weight, texture, etc.) or an environment (sound

---

[1] Gibson (1999, pp. 221–222) coined the term affordance referring to the term *Aufforderungschrakter*, coined by Kurt Lewin, understood, and translated by some scholars as "character of invitation" (by

---

D. Riccò (✉)
Department of Design, Politecnico di Milano, Milan, Italy
e-mail: dina.ricco@polimi.it

fields, smell fields, etc.) become such only when they are perceived by a subject. An *affordance*, writes Gibson, is "at the same time an environmental fact and a behavioral fact. It is both physical and psychic" (Gibson 1986). Therefore, the *affordances*, and with them we could say more generically the sensory characteristics of the artefacts, since they are not proper to either the object or the individual, take place only in the interaction, in the relationship that is established between the individual and his environment. It is not so much the individual sensory characteristics, their recognizability and identification, that define these relationships and suggest their possible interactions, but rather a specific combination of them, as Gibson says, an affordance "is an invariant combination of variables" (Gibson 1986).

The sensory relationships that can be defined with the artefacts are first and foremost linked to the physiological limits of each perceptive system. A limited distance of use allows an artifact to solicit a sensory quantity/quality which, for obvious reasons related to the range of receptive capacities of our senses, are not possible for large distances. Therefore, already the mere definition of the *degree of proximity* of use necessary for an artifact, allows the designer to determine specific levels of involvement of the senses and which of these to privilege.[2]

Already in the sixteenth century, the physician and mathematician Gerolamo Cardano had formulated a classification of the senses which, precisely starting from the distance of objects from a perceiving subject, specifies three categories of objects: *distant objects*, *external close objects* and *internal close objects* to the body (Riccò 1999, pp. 32 et seq.).

In this context, drugs—like foods, with which we find great affinities in terms of possible sensory involvement and even with a different hedonistic purpose—can be classified as *close internal objects* that enter the body and which, considering the classification of artifacts in relation to the degree of proximity and the level of sensory involvement, we can include *pseudoscopic artifacts*, i.e. artifacts in which the visual component is active before use, while during use other sensations, such as tactile, proprioceptive, gustatory, become prevalent (Riccò 1999). In the following we will dwell on this passage in which the visual observation with its characteristics acts—taking an expression from Ulric Neisser—as a *perceptive anticipation* for other modalities, that is, it activates the formation of mental images that precede the perception of the object in all its characters.[3] This is what happens when we are in

---

Brown, in 1929) and by others as "valence" (by Adams, in 1931). It is the latter term that entered general use to mean a phenomenal fact conferred on the object by experience (Riccò 2004).

[2] The reference is to the studies on proxemics by the American anthropologist E. T. Hall (1966).

[3] Thus Neisser writes: "Imagining is not perceiving, but images are essentially derivatives of perceptive activity, in particular, they are *anticipatory phases* of this activity, schemes that the perceiver has detached from the perceptive cycle for other purposes". And again: "Our perceptual anticipations are so fully integrated that things can feel hard or rough or heavy (even if the definitive information about these properties comes from touch) and their greatness can be grasped (even if experiments have proved that in case of conflict the decisive information about size and position is usually of a visual nature). The perception of objects and events is the fundamental process, and it employs whatever information is available" (Neisser 1976, pp. 137 and 150, It. Ed.).

front of a food and we are preparing to taste it, to anticipate it, with the eyes even before the mouth, as chefs well know.

21.2 Sensory Aspects of Drugs and Adherence to Treatments

Colour and shape of medicines have clinically relevant effects, i.e. they can condition adherence to treatment (the *compliance*) (More and Srivastava 2009). A study performed by Kesselheim et al. (2014) at Harvard Medical School to detect tablet drug taking habits—conducted in the United States on more than 10,000 patients hospitalized between 2006 and 2011 following a heart attack—found that when refilling a prescription for drugs, in that case statins and beta-blockers, the pills of the generic equivalent drug change shape or colour, the probability that you stop taking it increases significantly: 34% when it is the colour that has changed and even 66% when it changes it is pill shape. This does not explain all the reasons for non-adherence to treatment—the researchers argue—but certainly these data are statistically and clinically significant.

The study concludes by inviting the FDA (Food and Drug Administration) to request the production of generic drugs that are also perceptually similar to the original brand drugs, inviting doctors to inform patients about the potential changes in shape and colour of the pills, reassuring them that that even if they are different in colour and shape, the drugs work in the same way.

21.2.1 Influence of Colour

There are numerous studies conducted on the effects produced by the colours of drugs (see the extensive review by Tao 2018) and testify how these can influence correct identification and adherence to treatments. Colour assumes particular importance for the correct discrimination of the drug when the drugs are small, therefore difficult to discriminate due to their shape, and for patients with impaired cognitive and memory functions.

We also consider that colour is processed in a pre-attentive perceptual phase, leading to automatic executions, therefore correct design assumes great importance.

However, in the large number of research, data and studies are not available, as far as we know, which quantify and justify the percentages of tablets that pharmaceutical companies produce in different colours. What are the most and least produced colours in the tablets? What colours do patients prefer? Are there differences between adults and children? An attempt has therefore been made here to collect and compare these data. By searching Drugs.com's *Pill Identifier*—a database that queries over 24,000 drug pills—we can detect the colour and shape prevalence of pills manufactured by the US pharmaceutical industry (we have not found an equivalent system relating to the distribution of European medicines).

Below we indicate the absolute numbers (of which we have calculated the percentages) of the data collected (Table 21.1).

The "Pill identifier" tool does not specify the range of colours included for each colour name—namely, we know that the name "red colour" includes different gradations of colour—moreover it does not specify the method used for the classification, namely whether the operators of the classification are being trained.

Added to this is a technical difficulty due to the display devices: on the screen, in print or live in a different environmental context we will have a different colour rendition. However, consulting the tool it is evident that a wide range of gradations have been inserted in the same colour name (Figs. 21.1 and 21.2) intends to exemplify the extremes of colour for each category.

Despite all the limits that this comparison can give us, the data still appear to be extremely interesting. Beyond the clear dominance of white pills (41.63%, which together with Beige and Yellow pills exceed 50%), one wonders: is there a reason that justifies the extremely low number of dark pills?

Adding up the Black (33) and Maroon (75) pills, we arrive at only 0.4% of the total pills. This data appears to contradict some studies in which users perceive black coloured pills as highly effective drugs. According to a study by Tao et al. (2018)—on a sample of 224 Chinese participants who were asked about the expected

Table 21.1 The table indicates the distribution of pills in relation to the colour in distribution in the pharmaceutical market in the United States

Pill color	Absolute number	% number
White	11,078	41.63%
Yellow	3348	12.58%
Blue (include turquoise)	2360	8.86%
Pink	2252	8.46%
Orange	1906	7.16%
Green	1536	5.77%
Brown	876	3.29%
Red	847	3.18%
Purple	648	2.43%
Peach	561	2.10%
Beige	413	1.55%
Gray	327	1.22%
Tan	169	0.63%
Clear (capsules with transparency)	145	0.54%
Maroon	75	0.28%
Gold	34	0.12%
Black	33	0.12%
Total	26,608	

The data was obtained by querying the "Pill identifier" of Drugs.com (data updated to March 5, 2023). The website claims to use a database with over 24,000 pills, without stating the exact absolute number. It should be considered that the absolute numbers relating to each colour include both single-coloured pills and two-coloured pills

White and neutral color

Pill color	Images	Absolute number
White	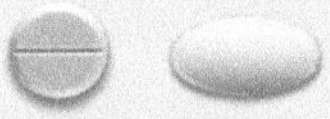	11078
Gray	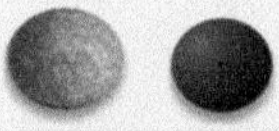	327
Clear (capsules with transparency)	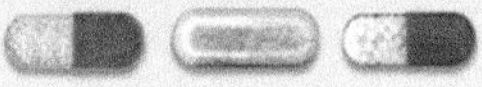	145
Total		11550

Yellow and gold

Pill color	Images	Absolute number
Yellow	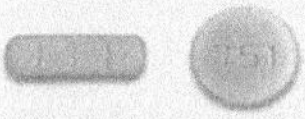	3348
Gold	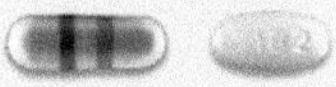	34
Total		3382

Light pastel colors

Pill color	Images	Absolute number
Beige	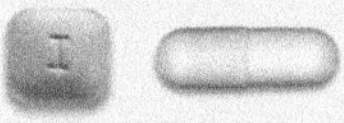	413
Orange	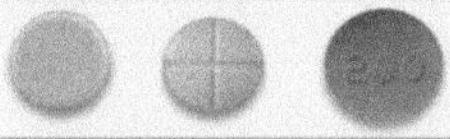	1906
Peach	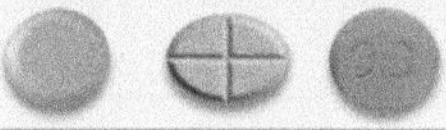	561
Tan	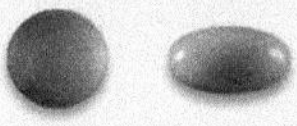	169
Total		3049

Fig. 21.1 The figure exemplifies the pill colour categories listed in Table 21.1. The colour categories are grouped by similarity, thus defining six combinations of colours, ordered from lightest to darkest: White and neutral colours, Yellow and Gold, Light pastel colours, Saturated and cold colours, Saturated and warm colours, Black and Maroon

Saturated and cold colors

Pill color	Images	Absolute number
Blue (includes turquoise)	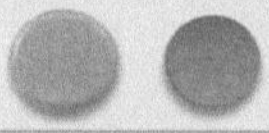	2360
Green	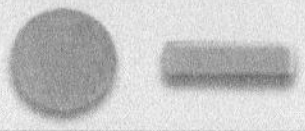	1536
Total		3896

Saturated and warm colors

Pill color	Images	Absolute number
Pink	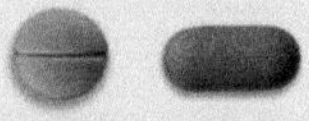	2252
Purple	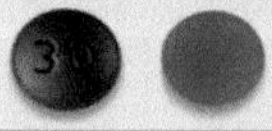	648
Red	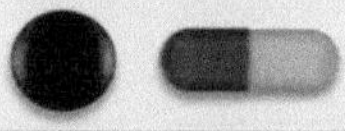	847
Brown	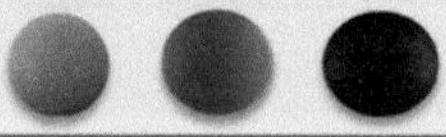	876
Total		4623

Black and maroon

Pill color	Images	Absolute number
Black (also bicolor with black)	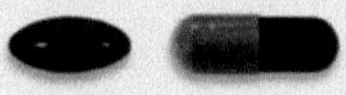	33
Maroon	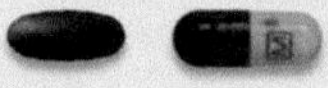	75
Total		108

Fig. 21.1 (continued)

efficacy of pills of different colours—red and black were the first colours (Fig. 21.2). Similar results had previously been reported by Sallis and Buckalew (1984).

This apparent contradiction—between the small number of black medicines and the high efficacy perceived by users—could be explained by considering the underestimation of the influence of colour by pharmaceutical companies.

In fact, the reasons that lead to the attribution of a given colour to the pills are of a different nature, among which we indicate the following:[4]

---

[4] See: "The colouration of tablets and capsules", by Paul Smith (2004) from Sensient Pharmaceutical Technologies, a leading global manufacturer and marketer of colours, flavors, and other specialty ingredients, which develops specialized solutions also for pharmaceutical industries (https://www.manufacturingchemist.com/news/article_page/The_colouration_of_tablets_and_capsules/34905; https://www.sensient.com/). This diversification of functions only considers the colour component.

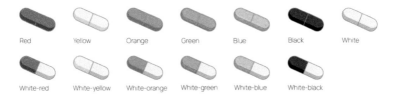

Fig. 21.2 The figure represents the 13 coloured capsules examined by Tao et al. (2018)

Table 21.2 Comparison of perceived therapeutic effects of coloured drugs for five population groups by Tao et al. (2016)

	Population Group				
Color	Chinese	Italian	White American	Black American	General American
Red	Stimulant	Stimulant	NA	NA	Stimulant
Yellow	Hallucinogenic	Stimulant	Stimulant	Hallucinogenic	Stimulant
Orange	Analgesic	Stimulant	Stimulant	Stimulant	NA
Green	Depressant	Depressant	Analgesic	Depressant	/
Blue	Depressant	Depressant	Depressant	/	Depressant
White	Depressant	Depressant	Analgesic	Stimulant	/
Black	Hallucinogenic	NA	Stimulant	Analgesic	/

Data for Italian from Sebellico (1989)
NA: data were not available

- Identification. Colour can help patients and pharmacists recognize different dosages of a drug;
- Flavour perception. The expectation in the perception of the taste of a tablet can be modified with the colour (for example from a red tablet I expect a cherry taste, and vice versa);
- Brand identification. It allows the manufacturer to stand out and be characterized in a highly competitive market;
- Quality perception. Colour can be used to add aesthetic value and with it characterize the perception of quality;
- Counterfeit prevention. Unique colour development, coupled with full colour printing, helps reduce the risk of drug counterfeiting.

The chromatic choices of pharmaceutical companies evidently consider other factors as priorities, underestimating the importance that these cover in the perception of use by patients (Table 21.2).

As Spence (2021) points out, sometimes it becomes a priority for the pharmaceutical company to define colour to support the personality of the brand or avoid counterfeiting, and not to encourage correct identification or adherence to treatment on the part of the patient.

Other aspects of interest to consider in the applications of colour—but which we have not found to be applied in pill drugs—are the *colour codes* which allow to facilitate discrimination and avoid errors. They are applied for example in the drugs used during anaesthesia,[5] and in the topical ophthalmic medications.[6]

21.2.2 Influence of Shape and Size

The same "Pill identifier" tool indicated above allows us to query the database, also in relation to the shape of the pill. There are 18 categories of shapes, as shown in the Table 21.3. As could be expected, the Capsule/Oval and Round category are largely dominant, while the other shapes are secondary and, together, represent only 4.2% of the total. However, it is interesting to note the variety of pills: polygons with different number of sides, characterized by angularity or roundness, with symbolic shapes, and also the attempt to design affordances that suggest and favor divisibility, as is the case with the shape Fig. 21.3—"8 shaped".

Shape and size of pills are less studied than colour, we have a limited number of studies in this regard, Spence (2021) summarizes the current state of knowledge well. Different product forms and methods of administration constitute different degrees of desirability and efficacy for patients. Not only if we compare methods of different invasiveness—injections versus oral administration—but also within the same mode of administration: pills of different shapes are evaluated differently by patients.

Shape A study conducted by Hussain (1972, in Spence 2021) found that the shape in which a drug is presented can influence the outcome of the treatment. The study conducted with 44 outpatients treated for anxiety found better efficacy of the drug when presented in capsule form, instead of tablets. Other studies confirm that patients find capsules stronger than tablets (Buckalew and Coffield 1982, in Spence 2021).

---

[5] See: BS EN ISO 26825 (2022): "Tracked Changes. Anaesthetic and respiratory equipment. User-applied labels for syringes containing drugs used during anaesthesia. Colours, design and performance".

[6] See: *Guidance for Industry. Container Closure Systems for Packaging Human Drugs and Biologics* (1999, p. 27).

Regarding topical ophthalmic medications, the colour coding of the pharmaceutical classes recommended by the AAO (American Academy of Ophthalmology) are presented using the pharmaceutical class, the colour name, and the Pantone Code Number, as follows:

- Anti-Infectives/Tan (467);
- Anti-Inflammatories-Steroids/Pink (197, 212);
- Mydriatics and Cycloplegics/Red (485C);
- Nonsteroidal Anti-Inflammatories/Gray (4C);
- Miotics/Green (374, 362, 348);
- Beta-Blockers/Yellow or Blue, Yellow C (290, 281a);
- Adrenergic Agonists (e.g., Propine)/Purple (2583);
- Carbonic Anhydrase Inhibitors/Orange (1585);
- Prostaglandin Analogues/Turquoise (326C).

21 Sensory Qualities of the Medicines: From Problems to Proposals

Table 21.3 The table indicates the distribution of the pills—in distribution in the pharmaceutical market of the United States—in relation to their shape

Shape		Absolute number	% number
	Capsule	14,586	52.51%
	Oval		
	Round	12,007	43.22%
	4 sided	265	0.95%
	Rectangle	234	0.84%
	3 sided	186	0.66%
	5 sided	120	0.43%
	6 sided	103	0.37%
	Egg	82	0.29%
	8 sided	59	0.21%
	U shaped	57	0.20%

(continued)

Table 21.3 (continued)

Shape		Absolute number	% number
	8 shaped	31	0.11%
	Barrel	25	0.09%
	Character	6	0.02%
	Heart	6	0.02%
	7 sided	4	0.01%
	Kidney	3	0.01%
	Gear	2	0.007%
	Total	27,776	

The data was obtained by querying the "Pill identifier" of Drugs.com (data updated to March 5, 2023).[a] The website claims to use a database with over 24,000 pills, without stating the exact absolute number. It should be considered that the search for Capsule and Oval, while representing two different categories, return the same number of drugs

[a]The Drugs.com Drug Database contains over 24,000 drugs, including both prescription and non-prescription drugs. The sources of information, as stated on the site, are supplied by various independent suppliers such as: *American Society of Health-System Pharmacists, Cerner Multum* and *IBM Watson Micromedex*. Individual drug (or drug-class) content compiled by these sources is peer reviewed and delivered by Drugs.com. See: https://www.drugs.com/pill_identification.html

Angular vs. Curvy Diamond-shaped pills are perceived to be more difficult to swallow than round or oval pills (Wan et al. 2015). Three studies conducted by Blazhenkova and Dogerlioglu-Demir (2020) using three different types of stimuli—abstract drawn shapes (Fig. 21.3), 3D-printed mockup pills and photographs of the existing pills—reveal that angularity is associated with an energizing effect, while the roundness to a calming effect (Fig. 21.3). Furthermore, the congruence between the design of the pill and the expected benefit of taking the drug increases the perception of efficacy.

Size The size of the pills is obviously very important to facilitate swallowing. The active ingredient in a pill constitutes only a small percentage of its total, this allows pharmaceutical industries to define the size in relation to other factors (e.g., brand or acceptability), but the choice is strongly influenced by the ease of swallowing perceived by patients. In fact, many attempts to scale up generics have been rejected for that very reason (Spence 2021).

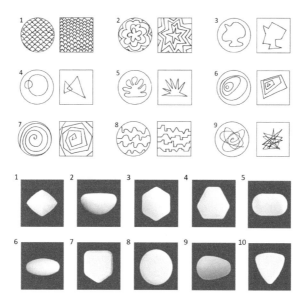

Fig. 21.3 Above: Angular vs. curved drawn pill stimuli; below angular vs. curved photograph pill stimuli used in study 1 and 3 of Blazhenkova and Dogerlioglu-Demir (2020)

In all of the correspondences reported above between the characteristics of the shape and the expected efficacy, two factors must be considered: on the one hand, the studies were carried out over a very long period of time, from 1970 to today, which means that the same experiment proposed 50 years later it could give different results because the consumer experience is different; and at the same time the perceived character/effect association can be the result of learning, of the experience acquired through use (Spence 2021).

The pills are distributed in a container and this also affects the use. Changes in the format of the packaging, or making it more difficult to open the package, have been shown to affect the amount of pills ingested, in particular it has been shown that just changing the format of the container –from the bottle to the single blister— have reduced the incidence of people who attempt suicide with analgesic overdose (Chan 2000). For this reason, legislation was introduced in the UK (in 1998) to limit the size of packs of over-the-counter analgesics (Hawton et al. 2004).

Overall, the associative factors specific to the shape and distribution formats of the drug appear to be perceived as more constant and universal than those of colour.

21.2.3 Influence of Flavour

Drugs with a more pleasant taste can improve adherence, especially in children, to drug therapy. More than 90% of pediatricians report that the greatest barriers to completing treatment are their own taste and palatability (Milne and Bruss 2008, in Mennella et al. 2013). Many active ingredients of drugs have a bitter taste, which is why they are unwelcome to adults and to children who are more sensitive to the bitter taste, this creates compliance problems for both. An effective method to avoid the unpleasant taste is encapsulation, which however cannot be applied for children before the age of 6–8, when liquid formulations are needed. Another possibility is the application of flavor masking techniques: sugars, acids, salt, and other substances reduce the perception of bitterness (Mennella et al. 2013). The addition of sucrose, sweeteners, flavourings, acids to medicines reduce, but do not eliminate the bitterness of medicines, furthermore sweeteners create other problems (e.g., dental caries).

In addition to taste, other sensory attributes contribute to compliance, such as consistency, acidity, or bad smell. People speak of taste actually meaning the *flavor* which is instead composed of a perceptive integration, therefore of a set of gustatory, olfactory and trigeminal sensory characteristics (Mennella et al. 2013). The visceral system is also involved if we consider that the ingestion of bitter compounds can act in the intestine and cause nausea, or salivation triggered by some acids (e.g., lemon).

As is the case with food, pharmaceutical companies also apply sensory analysis methods to evaluate and improve the aromatic-gustatory profile of their products, above all to limit the bitter taste, particularly when the drugs are aimed at children.

Compared to studies of sensory analysis of food, the sensory analysis of drugs collides with the difficulty of recruiting panelists, with the risks of drug toxicity, with the difficulty of quantitative measurement.[7] The detection of the subject's behavior and the subject's facial expression are among the most used methods. We point out the interesting study conducted by Hofmanová et al. (2020), in which researchers recorded negative facial expressions (e.g., pursed lips, wrinkled nose, disgusted voice, lowered eyebrows and head snake) to gauge aversion to a pill. The study evaluated the acceptability of 7.5 mm round tablets with five different coatings in both children and adults. However, the ability to swallow tablets was independent of the coating applied. Instead, other correlations were observed, in particular:

- the more bitter the tablet, the less liked;
- the more unpleasant the aftertaste, the less liked;
- the smoother the tablet, the more slippery;
- the more bitter the tablet, the more unpleasant the aftertaste.

In summary, women are more sensitive to taste, and rated the tablets more bitter than men. Furthermore, although the palatability between adults and children was similar, children perceived the tablets as more bitter, smoother, less sticky, and less palatable than adults. In particular, the researchers note that there is a direct correlation between the palatability and aftertaste, smoothness, and slipperiness of the tablets. It is therefore necessary to analyse the palatability of the medicinal product as a multifactorial attribute, and not a simple hedonic factor (Hofmanová et al. 2020).

21.3 Medication Error Risk for Visually Impaired Population

Evaluation of the sensory qualities of drugs cannot exclude the necessary requirements for drugs for use by people with sensory impairments. Visually Impaired Population are particularly at higher risk for experiencing a medication error (Zhi-Han et al. 2017; Alhusein et al. 2018).

A study conducted by Ling Zhi-Han et al. (2017) identifies which are the main difficulties encountered in the self-administration of drugs concerning both the discrimination of the packaging and of the drug itself. The study was conducted on 100 subjects, including 62 blind and 38 visually impaired (with visual acuity <6/60; ≥3/60). According to the study, the greatest difficulties lie in the impossibility of differentiating the various types of pharmaceutical forms (tablets/capsules) and in forgetting to take them within the prescribed times.

A study by Alhusein et al. (2018)—which it believes to be the first to address the pharmaceutical care needs of older people with sensory impairment—reports that

---

[7] Mennella et al. (2013) indicate among the types of psychophysical tools used to assess bitter taste and medication palatability in pediatric populations: Facial reactivity, Brief-access tests, Suckling response, Suprathreshold taste thresholds, Scaling methods.

medicines are difficult to identify, particularly when they change their name, shape or colour.

McCann et al. (2012) reports that almost 30% of the visual impairment subjects interviewed (BCVA 6/18 to 3/60) needed daily help to take the prescribed drugs, even using optical aids, with difficulty distinguishing the drugs and difficulty in opening packages. The knowledge we have on medication self-management in people with visual impairment, compared with sighted peers (BCVA 6/9 or better), is limited.

The conclusions are evident: greater attention is needed by researchers to detect the specific needs of people with sensory disabilities, and at the same time greater attention also by pharmaceutical companies to the requirements necessary for drugs to avoid errors in taking them by of visually impaired people. The characteristics that we have indicated above are mainly visual, they concern the colour, the shape intervenes as a discriminant only to a limited extent, 52.51% of the pills are capsules or oval-shaped tablets, the incisions and signs of tactile discrimination are equally limited. For blind people, self-administration of medication carries a high risk of errors.

21.4 Conclusion

Despite the difficulty of defining generalizations, both for technical reasons and for gender and cultural differences (Tao et al. 2018), many studies demonstrate the influence that colour exerts on the expectation of efficacy of a drug, with important implications for adherence to treatment. We know that the study of colour—not only when applied to drugs—presents difficulties related to constancy, the phenomenological yield in relation to the devices, the print and screen in which it is represented, the names of the colours, the culture. In addition, many of the studies on the colour applied to drugs detect only the "name of the colour", therefore the tint, without specifying the colour composition.[8]

To the colour are added other perceptual characteristics that influence adherence to the treatment such as shape, size, texture, aroma (Tao et al. 2018) or that favor the error due to phonosymbolic factors of the name not congruent with the properties of the drug (Spence 2021), the so-called "Look-Alike/Sound-Alike" (LASA) drugs.[9]

Despite the multifactorial nature, most of the research carried out on the sensory characteristics of drugs is limited to studying these characteristics separately, not considering the interaction between them and the perceptual hierarchies, the prevalence that one can hold over the others. That is, as Spence (2021) points out, it is not

---

[8] An exception is the study by Tao (2016) which specifies the CMYK composition of the colours being tested.

[9] They are the drugs that can mislead and mistaken for phonetic, graphic or packaging similarity (https://www.salute.gov.it/portale/sicurezzaCure/dettaglioContenutiSicurezzaCure.jsp?lingua=italiano&id=2459&area=qualita&menu=sicurezzasicurezzaterapie).

currently clear which of the attributes of the product (colour, shape, sound symbolism, etc.) dominates in the coexistence of factors.

Charles Spence (2021)—head of the Crossmodal Research Laboratory at the University of Oxford—presented an extensive and up-to-date review of the literature related to the sensory qualities of drugs that we can only join in his call for a multifactorial approach that consider the perceptual complexity to reduce the cognitive dissonance between the patient's expectations and the properties of the drug, to reduce errors and illogical behaviors.

As Hofmanová et al. (2020) argues, there is also a need to analyze desirability as a multifactorial attribute rather than a simple hedonic parameter.

In summary, we must therefore consider that the information offered synchronously on different sensory registers interact, and not always in the expected or desired direction. In the presence of a perceptual "disagreement" the overall character of a piece of information is transformed and, at the same time, leads to the formation of hierarchies among the pieces of information, namely imposes the need to choose which of these to give priority to. In some conditions the visual, the colour or the shape may be prevalent, but the opposite can also happen. As Shams, Kamitani and Shimojo (2000, p. 788) write and demonstrate, it can happen that "you see is what you hear",[10] namely the visual perception of an event is influenced and marked by the characters of an audio event concomitant. An artifact can therefore change the characters and intentions that led to its *visual project*—amplifying or reducing the communicative effectiveness—also because of *non-visual* perceptive factors.

Finally, we note the insufficient attention to communicative accessibility, to allow the recognition of the drug to people with visual impairments. Very few studies address these aspects, if not applied to drug packages, by law in Italy provided with Braille text, but no indication allows communication and discrimination of the tablet for people with visual impairment.

The design of the totality of sensory qualities and their congruent relationships would allow addressing these aspects as well.

References

Alhusein N, Macaden L, Smith A, Stoddart KM, Taylor AJ, Killick K, Kroll T, Watson MC (2018) Has she seen me?: A multiple methods study of the pharmaceutical care needs of older people with sensory impairment in Scotland. Br Med J Open 8:1–8

Blazhenkova O, Dogerlioglu-Demir K (2020) The shape of the pill: perceived effects, evoked bodily sensations and emotions. PLoS One 15(9):1–23

Buckalew LW, Coffield KE (1982) An investigation of drug expectancy as function of capsule colour and size and preparation form. J Clin Psychopharmacol 2(4):245–248

---

[10] Shams; Kamitani; Shimojo (2000), describe a case, which they discovered, of sound-induced visual illusion: when a single visual flash is accompanied by multiple auditory beeps, the visual flash is not perceived correctly, but as a function of the number of acoustic beeps.

Chan TY (2000) Improvements in the packaging of drugs and chemicals may reduce the likelihood of severe intentional poisonings in adults. Hum Exp Toxicol 19(7):387–391

Gibson JJ (1986) The ecological approach to visual perception. Erlbaum, Hillsdale/London

Hall ET (1966) The hidden dimension. Doubleday & Co. Inc., New York. (Tr. It. Bompiani, 1968)

Hawton K, Simkin S, Deeks J, Cooper J, Johnston A, Waters K, Arundel M, Berna W, Simpson K (2004) UK legislation on analgesic packs: before and after study of long-term effect on poisonings. Br Med J 329(7474):1076

Hofmanová JK, Mason J, Batchelor HK (2020) Sensory aspects of acceptability of bitter-flavoured 7.5 mm film-coated tablets in adults, preschool and school children. International Journal of Pharmaceutics 585:119511.

Hussain MZ (1972) Effect of shape of medication in treatment of anxiety states. Br J Psychiatry 120(558):507–509

Kesselheim AS, Choudhry NK, Avorn J (2014) Burden of changes in generic pill appearance. Ann Intern Med 161(2):96–103

McCann RM, Jackson AJ, Stevenson M, Dempster M, McElnay JC, Cupples ME (2012) Help needed in medication self-management for people with visual impairment: case-control study. Br J Gen Pract 62(601):e530–e537

Mennella JA, Spector AC, Reed DR, Coldwell SE (2013) The bad taste of medicines: overview of basic research on bitter taste. Clin Ther 35(8):1225–1246

Milne CP, Bruss JB (2008). The economics of pediatric formulation development for off-patent drugs. Clinical therapeutics 30(11):2133–2145

More AT, Srivastava RK (2009) "Aesthetic considerations for pharmaceutical OTC (over the counter) products", in Oxford Business & Economics Conference Program, June 24–26.

Neisser U (1976). Cognition and Reality: Principles and Implications of Cognitive Psychology. W H Freeman and Company.

Riccò D (1999) Sinestesie per il design. Le interazioni sensoriali nell'epoca dei multimedia. Etas, Milano

Riccò D (2004) Design e sensorialità. In: Bertola P, Manzini E (a cura di) (eds) Design Multiverso. Appunti di fenomenologia del design. Polidesign Editore, Milano, pp 101–115

Sailis RE, Buckalew LW (1984) Relation of capsule color and perceived potency. Perceptual and Motor Skills 58(3):897–898

Sebellico A (1989) Il coloure del farmaco: Inchiesta preliminare. Boll Soc Ital Biol Sper 65(7):685–687

Shams L, Kamitani Y, Shimojo S (2000) What you see is what you hear. Nature, 408(6814):788

Smith P (2004) The colouration of tablets and capsules. Retrieved from: https://manufacturingchemist.com/the-colouration-of-tablets-and-capsules-34905

Spence C (2021) The multisensory design of pharmaceuticals and their packaging. Food Qual Prefer 91:1–17

Tao D, Wang T, Wang T (2016) Effects of colour on expectations of drug effects: a cross-gender cross-cultural study. Col Res Appl 42(1):124–130

Tao D, Tieyan W, Tieshan W, Qu X (2018) Influence of drug colour on perceived drug effects and efficacy. Ergonomics 61(2):284–294

Wan X, Woods AT, Velasco C, Salgado-Montejo A, Spence C (2015) Assessing the expectations associated with pharmaceutical pill colour and shape. Food Qual Prefer 45:171–182

Zhi-Han L, Hui-Yin Y, Makmor-Bakry M (2017) Medication-handling challenges among visually impaired population. Arch Pharm Pract 8:8–14

Open Access This chapter is licensed under the terms of the Creative Commons Attribution 4.0 International License (http://creativecommons.org/licenses/by/4.0/), which permits use, sharing, adaptation, distribution and reproduction in any medium or format, as long as you give appropriate credit to the original author(s) and the source, provide a link to the Creative Commons license and indicate if changes were made.

The images or other third party material in this chapter are included in the chapter's Creative Commons license, unless indicated otherwise in a credit line to the material. If material is not included in the chapter's Creative Commons license and your intended use is not permitted by statutory regulation or exceeds the permitted use, you will need to obtain permission directly from the copyright holder.

Chapter 22
Compendium: Step Toward Design-Oriented Practices in the Pharma Industry in a Multidisciplinary Perspective

Antonella Valeria Penati

22.1 Introduction

In the first chapter of this volume, we began our exploration by stating that "from a regulatory point of view, the pharmaceuticals sector—given the peculiarities of the product and its impact on consumer health—has always been hyper-regulated" (see Chap. 2 and Addendum 1). The power of this regulation stems not only from legislative documents at the EU and international levels but also from national regulations. The regulatory landscape is further complicated by the addition of documents such as Guidelines, Product and Process Regulations, and Recommendations from individual states over time, creating a highly stratified and complex legislative framework in the pharmaceutical field. Throughout the various chapters, regulatory milestones have been revisited, aligning with the topics addressed by different authors (refer to Addendum 1 for the regulations or sections of regulations framing the design of primary and secondary packaging, as well as the package leaflet). Our specific focus is on the role of current legislation in guiding the design of the 'medicine system' toward the patients and their needs. As elucidated in the text, the 'medicine system' encompasses the ensemble of physical artifacts and information apparatus—primary packaging, secondary packaging, package leaflet—that, alongside the medicine, undergo evaluation by regulatory bodies for its 'marketing'(Fig. 22.1).

Among the several classifications in literature, delving into indispensable aspects for the correct knowledge and management of pharmaceutical forms, here we choose to deepen the one referring to the route of administration. We believe this is the description closest to the end user's experience. Since the topic is the result of consolidated manuals to which all pharmaceutical companies refer, we will include extensive excerpts from scientific references describing the various pharmaceutical

---

A. V. Penati (✉)
Department of Design, Politecnico di Milano, Milan, Italy
e-mail: antonella.penati@polimi.it

© The Author(s) 2025
A. V. Penati (ed.), *In-Home Medication*, Research for Development,
https://doi.org/10.1007/978-3-031-53294-8_22

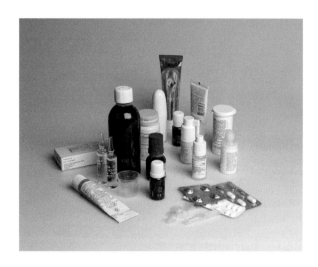

Fig. 22.1 The term medicinal shapes, in this context, can be understood to mean the set of formal properties of the medicines and their containers, including packaging, blisters, and any auxiliary devices such as dispensers, measuring, regulating and storage instruments. Medicine delivery devices may facilitate, or not, the ability to dose and control the dispersion of content

forms. All the following pharmaceutical forms and their description follow the guidance provided by the Council of Europe (2019).

In this context, we will set aside the expansive role of regulatory impetus for innovation, acknowledging its broad scope, particularly concerning environmental and counterfeiting issues. Similarly, we will not accord predominant attention to technological innovations, despite their potential to ameliorate issues encountered in various phases of the treatment process, such as prescription, dispensing, and the patient's medicine management in the home.

Instead, in this concluding section, we will delve into many of the challenges highlighted by the various authors in the book. We will draw upon research findings from the international literature, insights gained from observing the daily behaviour of patients, and understanding how 'domesticity' significantly influences the gestures of care. Additionally, we will analyse specific types of products that exhibit functional and communicative shortcomings. Some authors have captured, through their contributions, the endeavours of companies to move in the direction of the user, presenting them as 'examples to follow'. They have identified, within existing innovative products, procedures, and services, the principles that can guide design in this sector. From the multitude of innovations available, we have chosen to highlight those most relevant to the objectives of this text—innovations oriented towards the user and aimed at simplifying the gestures of care.

N.B. In the introductory chapter, it has been previously highlighted that the editorial approach employed in this text to delineate specific issues encountered in existing products, along with instances of innovative proposals in product usability, deliberately avoids making direct references to the medicines used as examples. This approach is adopted to prevent the potential discrediting of these medicines or, conversely, to steer clear of improper advertising. Instead, the chosen strategy involves utilizing the Active Ingredient as the primary reference element in textual segments. In illustrated sections, a fictitious packaging has been employed, presenting the information, graphic elements, and formal attributes that are the focal points of attention. Each reference to the encountered problems is intended to contribute to the broader discourse on potential enhancements to medicines, which represent intricate products with established standards in design and production quality. It is essential to note that, due to the expertise of the writer and the research's specific objectives, each medicine used as an example has never been scrutinized from a medical-pharmaceutical standpoint concerning the benefits and effects produced by its active ingredient. The examination is limited to the 'medicine-system,' encompassing the medicine along with the ensemble of physical and informational artifacts that render it usable. From this perspective, 'usability' refers to the amalgamation of formal, textual, and visual qualities and characteristics that facilitate intuitive and straightforward access to information and products related to the treatment.

N.B. Simplifying as it may be, we shall use the term 'form' in this chapter to refer to the typological characters of medicines as used in the pharmaceutical industry—e.g. pharmaceutical forms, oral solid forms, etc. To refer to the sensible characters of the medicine—dimensional, geometric, chromatic, surface, etc., we will use the term shape.

This concluding chapter is designed as a 'virtual round table' featuring the book's authors. Each contributor, with their specific expertise and professional roles in either corporate or academic settings, has provided valuable insights. The legal expert, regulatory affairs specialist, biotechnologist, packaging manufacturer, bioengineer, doctor, nurse, industrial products expert, and experts in communication and information processes, user behaviour, and use practices have all played essential roles.[1]

The conclusions draw upon the problematic and propositional elements, along with 'good practices' and virtuous examples presented by the authors throughout their respective chapters. These elements serve as the foundation for the reflections and recommendations put forth in this section. The recommendations are rooted in adherence to the existing regulatory framework, sometimes specifying its

---

[1] The contributors to the chapters of this book participated in the revision process of the concluding chapter. Specifically, Annabella Amatulli and Lamberto Dionigi, leveraging their expertise in regulatory affairs, not only engaged in the revision work but also made substantial contributions to the integration of paragraphs across the entire concluding chapter. Their input was comprehensive and touched upon various aspects of the text. Elena Piovosi focused on the revision and integration of paragraphs related to the *Primary Pack*, *Primary Pack: Recommendations concerning blister packs*, and *Premises towards a system of recommendations to improve primary packaging*, particularly blister packs for oral solid forms. Giuseppe Andreoni dedicated his efforts to the revision and integration of paragraphs addressing *Prescription—prescription and Premises towards a system of recommendations to improve the prescribing process*. Dina Riccò took charge of revising and integrating paragraphs related to *the form of medicine, Focus: Solid forms for oral use, Solid forms for oral use: types and morphologies*, and *Premises towards a system of recommendations for better use of medicines*; *Secondary packaging: labelling; Summary notes: premise to recommendations; Secondary packaging: Reccomandation*. Her contributions spanned a range of critical topics. Elena Caratti, in her role, meticulously revised and integrated paragraphs pertaining to the *Package leaflet* and *Premises towards a system of recommendations to improve the packaging leaflet*. Her expertise significantly enhanced the overall quality of the text in these areas.

indications, at other times advocating for more careful application, and in some instances proposing indications with partial dissimilarity, accompanied by reasons supporting such choices. Concrete examples of existing solutions are often provided as paradigmatic illustrations. The path of best practices, acting as a reference, appears to be the most promising route for initiating virtuous processes of innovation.

It is important to clarify that in this context, the term "best practices" is not used as conventionally in literature. Rather than engaging in a comprehensive analysis of objectives, contextual elements, organizational culture, and evaluation systems (Kahan and Goodstadt 2001), our focus centres on the everyday use and domestic sphere, primarily observing the attitudes and conduct of patients in acts of care. Here, we identify "good practices" in the behaviours of patients—sometimes spontaneous, not entirely conscious or planned, yet effective in achieving specific results. This term is also extended to encompass artifacts such as medicines, packaging, and accompanying informational elements that exhibit elements of innovation. While the impact may be modest and not necessarily affect company economies, these innovations hold significance when considered in the context of improving the user experience. Throughout the chapter, positive examples are juxtaposed with problematic cases to highlight critical issues and propose virtuous solutions. The primary observation of medicines as objects of care emphasizes inappropriate patient behaviour, often influenced by product characteristics and communication methods.

The outcome of this exploration is not a complete or systematized platform but rather a set of premises for Design, an initial collection of examples, principles, suggestions, criteria, and reflections. This compilation does not claim to constitute a definitive reference manual but aligns with the design culture's metaprojectual activity (Deserti 2003; Collina 2005). This activity evaluates individual and social instances, value systems, lifestyles, behaviours, and technological trends to build an open platform of instances that can inspire diverse projects.

The purpose of this activity is not to define the premises for the design of a product, but to build an open platform of instances that can feed different projects. The meta-design activity serves as a guideline, orienting and not excluding *a priori* design paths, offering principles and starting hypotheses that can be adapted and interpreted in design without imposing standardized outcomes, encouraging contextualized solutions.

When examining the medicine-system from the perspective of use, attention is directed towards analysing existing products and their propensity in incorporating rules and prohibitions in the product's shape (persuaders, dissuaders). This includes directing user actions through formal characteristics like affordance, mapping, and usability, and supporting correct usage sequences.

The use-related perspective of analysis also allows us to observe the impact of organisational techniques in the daily management of therapy and the techniques of the body for the correct use of the medicines.

Observing the medicine-system from the point of view of its impressive array of information, we find all the prerogatives of communicative artefacts: describing, prescribing, explaining, and informing The forms of verbal and visual communication in pharmaceuticals reveal communicative artifacts with varying degrees of criticality, including absence or inadequate use of information hierarchies; absence of a defined and/or adequate collocation of information with consequent difficulty in tracing specific contents; inadequate treatment of individual warnings often handled as if they were a single text; use of a polished and technical language, aimed more at the world of doctors and pharmacists than at that of the patient.

Consequently, these information texts are often unread and misunderstood by users The viewpoint adopted in this text prioritizes the user-patient and their experience of use throughout the observation, reflection, and recommendation phases.

22.2 General Comments on the Regulatory Framework

The existing regulations, along with the Guidelines and Formats required from companies for new products and/or new packaging and/or a new package leaflet (see Chap. 2 and Addendum 1), provide adequate tools to ensure the legibility of information on medicinal product packaging. These regulations cover various aspects, including font size, the use of italics, bold type, and capital letters for creating information hierarchies.

The Guidelines also define spacing, colour contrast between text and background, coordination of the graphic image between primary and secondary packaging to ensure the medicine's recognizability once taken out of the carton, and recommendations for inserting Braille characters on the free part of the packaging to avoid interference with written parts. Additionally, the 2004 revision of Directive 2001/83/EC introduced an obligation to provide competent authorities with the results of the assessment of the package leaflet by targeted groups of patients and the labelling carried out by the relevant EMA committee (European Parliament and of the Council 2004). This obligation applies to all marketing authorizations granted after October 30, 2005, as well as to amendments to previously granted authorizations resulting in significant changes to the package leaflet.

We would like to point out a few general considerations on the regulatory text.

A first consideration pertains to the criteria established for composing text to ensure easy readability. These criteria are initially defined for the package leaflet and then extended to the information displayed on secondary and primary packaging. However, these general rules, designed for a lengthy text with connected propositions (typical of the package leaflet), may not be as effective when applied to short texts, such as those found on secondary packaging. Unlike the cohesive text of a package leaflet, the information on secondary packaging resembles a "data record" or "labelling", consisting of short, autonomous propositions that do not form a unified text. Each notice on the packaging functions as a complete text, requiring user understanding of its autonomy and independence from other information.

A second consideration pertains to the Guidelines, particularly the points addressing the normative dictate and the indications regarding the recruitment of patients and the modalities for submitting products to end users for testing regarding readability and comprehension.

First, it is observed that the readability test by users is exclusively designated for the Package Leaflet and is not extended to the secondary and primary packs. Additionally, user involvement is limited to assessing readability, with no tests focusing on the usability of the product, including the ease of understanding and use of the medicine packaging throughout all necessary steps. There are no tests concerning the usability of the product (the ease of understanding and use of the packaging of the medicine in all the steps necessary to get to it). It is crucial to highlight that readability cannot be adequately evaluated without considering usability.

As discussed in Chap. 17 and revisited below, various critical points (resembling "impediments") are encountered by patients attempting to read the Patient Information Leaflet. These impediments are associated with different phases characterizing the patient's interaction with the secondary, primary, and package leaflet, starting from the initial stages of opening the pack.

Moreover, many of the patient's challenges (e.g., cognitive, organisational, memory etc.) arise not solely from the use of a single medicine but from the complexity inherent in polypharmacy, especially when managing multiple medicines at various times of the day. In this intricate context, readability, comprehension, and the ability to distinguish and recognize play a crucial role in demonstrating how the instructions in a package leaflet "enable the user to act appropriately" (point 3.1, *User testing, Guideline on the Readability of the Labelling and Package Leaflet of Medicinal Products for Human Use,* European Commission 2009).

The context within which the leaflet is read further influences the results obtained. The daily domestic life characterized by the multiple actions and their promiscuity introduces various elements affecting both the reading activities and medicine intake, such as situations, people, needs, noise, light, and environmental conditions, that may significantly diminish the comprehension of the information read.

Continuing with general considerations on the regulatory framework, it is imperative to acknowledge that the recommendations, including Recommendation No. 19 on the *Handling of Solid Oral Forms*, primarily target hospitals and caregivers.

Unfortunately, patients and caregivers managing medicine therapy in a home setting do not receive sufficient guidance on behaviours to mitigate medication errors. In the home environment, even before addressing concerns related to inappropriate medicine handling, one must consider the early removal of the medicine from its packaging, a practice that frequently occurs well before the medicine is taken. Specifically, in the case of blister tablets, a prevalent and initial form of handling involves 'unblistering' the medicines and storing them unprotected in contact with one another. Additionally, common practices, such as the storage and reuse of portions of residual medicines, and the handling of medicines without taking precautions regarding contact, inhalation, and hygiene of the instruments used, are well-known. While these situations are closely monitored in hospitals where care professionals work, they often take a back seat when performed at home by the patient or caregiver.

Both the doctor and pharmacist play pivotal roles in ensuring patient safety. The doctor should consistently inform the patient of the precautions that must be observed when altering the pharmaceutical form, and similarly, the pharmacist should ascertain whether the patient has swallowing problems. If swallowing difficulties are identified, the pharmacist should always check the availability of alternative and easier-to-take pharmaceutical forms, such as drops, syrups, powders, etc.

Pharmaceutical formularies should always present the shape and size of the medicines, especially when they are solid oral forms, so that they are not prescribed to patients with swallowing problems.

It is essential to underscore the significance of this recommendation due to the lack of care education that provides precise guidance on the behaviours exhibited by patients in their homes.

Patients may inadvertently engage in improper actions with medicines, actions that have the potential to compromise the efficacy of the active ingredient or even lead to adverse reactions, precisely due to alterations in the pharmaceutical form.

22.3 Prescription—Recipe

Throughout the regulatory passages encompassing Regulations, Implementing Decrees, and Guidelines related to medicines, there is a notable absence of consideration for the roles of prescribing physicians and dispensing pharmacists. The limited reference to these crucial actors is encapsulated in the brief passage from the *Guideline on the Readability of the Labelling and Package Leaflet of Medicinal Products for Human Use* (European Commission 2009), which emphasizes the package leaflet's clarity for users, suggesting their potential need for assistance from health professionals.

This text recognizes that users, when not autonomous or facing difficulties, may seek help from health professionals to understand the information on the medication. As highlighted elsewhere (refer to Chap. 8), during the lifecycle of medicine therapy, the user, whether a patient or caregiver, relies on three primary sources of information: the prescribing doctor, the dispensing pharmacist, and the package leaflet. A closer examination of this information cycle reveals the involvement of at least four actors, acknowledging the distinct roles of general practitioners and specialists or hospital doctors. However, these sources are not always aligned in their information functions toward the patient. The boundaries of information prerogatives for each actor are often blurred, leading to potential overlaps and the provision of divergent information to the patient. Some content areas may be addressed by one or more sources, while others risk being neglected, creating gaps in the interface between patient and therapy.

Several noteworthy observations supplement these reflections:

- it is well documented that the moments in which the patient has the most difficulty—and these are the moments in which errors and discomfort in taking the medication are most likely to occur—are those of so-called 'transition of care' (Ministero della Salute 2014). They are represented by the moments of transition: from home to hospital regimen and vice versa or the change of therapy after

a specialist visit. In general, these moments occur whenever treatment is interrupted by the doctor's instructions and, even more so, whenever a new medicine or several newly prescribed medicines are introduced into the usual therapy. In these moments of transition, communication between patient and doctor is crucial because it is precisely here that "intentional omissions" and "unintentional omissions" can occur in the information that the patient transfers to the doctor and vice versa (Ministero della Salute 2014);
- the role of the pharmacist and the family doctor has remained substantially unchanged in the face of profound changes which have affected the system of relations between the various parties involved in care. For example, the direct relationship between the family doctor and the pharmacist, fostered by proximity, is no longer an element that can be relied on; the increasingly frequent referral of patients to the specialist profoundly alters the role of the family doctor and the direct knowledge he had of the patient; the weakening of the relationship of loyalty between patient and pharmacist—which is still typical of small realities—is less and less so in large cities; the use of increasingly shorter hospital stays, with parts of the treatment process that used to take place in the hospital system now tending to be transferred to the patient's home, investing him with complex care tasks. These factors undermine the virtuous triangulation between patient, family doctor and pharmacist that, in the past, allowed a more complete knowledge of the patient and his health problems. The Covid19 pandemic has helped to highlight the transformation of the historical roles of family doctors and pharmacists, attributing to the latter several tasks and functions that were not previously his responsibility. Let us close this aside with a datum taken from the literature: in hospitals, where there is proximity and dialogue between doctors and pharmacists and where the pharmacist becomes a critical contact person with whom it is possible to collaborate in setting up the patient's therapy, fewer prescription/dispensing errors are detected than in territorial pharmacies (Hoxsie et al. 2006);
- the lack of a unified design of the documentation accompanying medicine therapy. Documentation makes it possible to connect the information on the pathology from which the patient suffers with the information on the medicines prescribed. The recommendations of the Italian Ministry of Health expressly provide that 'To facilitate the reconnaissance [i.e., the activity of collecting complete and accurate information by the hospital doctor or specialist about the patient and the medicines intake], it is important to compare it with the list of medicines, if any, drawn up by the family doctor, which should always be shown every time the patient makes a visit or enters a health facility for treatment' (Ministero della Salute 2014, p.9). We know very well that the family doctor does not draw up this document, and the patient often finds it difficult to account fully for the treatment he is receiving. Again, based on literature data (see Chap. 8), it also seems appropriate to note the information asymmetry between doctors and pharmacists. While the doctor owns the information on the pathology and the medicines to be taken by the patient, the dispenser only sees part of this information (that relating to the

medicine prescription). The much-desired counselling activity requested by the pharmacist to support the patient in the proper therapy intake, is carried out without all the information necessary to carry out this task effectively. Recommendation no. 17 (Ministero della Salute 2014) entrusts the pharmacist with an essential role in assisting the physician in the Recognition and Reconciliation therapeutic phase. However, if this collaboration is possible within hospital facilities, it is not so in the case of specialist visits. Hence, the importance of a shared document makes the information needed to set up a therapeutic plan adapted to each patient's condition available to all those involved in treatment.

These reflections underscore the complexity of the healthcare system and highlight the necessity for coordinated efforts among healthcare professionals to ensure comprehensive and coherent information delivery to patients.

22.3.1 Premises for a System of Recommendations for Improving the Prescribing Process

[Prescription 1] In prescriptions, encourage the simplification of daily therapy and the organisation of care activities:

- whenever possible and wherever the characteristics of the medicine allow it, group the intake of medicines (e.g. once or twice a day, in conjunction with meals). The meal ritual continues to constitute one of the activities that can mark the day, characterising it with elements of diversity (e.g., the food taken, the place, the diners) that constitute effective anchors for memory activities. Medicines, especially for oral use, find a natural insertion in meal rituals (e.g., food and table preparation activities);
- inviting the patient to put the medicines at the table when preparing breakfast, lunch or dinner so that the therapeutic container becomes a habitual presence on par with plates, cutlery and glasses;
- in the case of weekly or monthly therapies, suggest to the patient to place the intake on a day of the week characterised by peculiar elements that facilitate memorisation processes (e.g. Sundays after lunch with family, market day if one is used to going there). For monthly therapies, favour the beginning of the month, a date that is easy for everyone to remember;
- if the therapy is not urgent, suggest that the patient start taking the newly prescribed medication on Monday. Especially in the case of treatments that involve taking only one tablet per day, this may make it easier to keep track of the medicines taken and any omissions;
- invite the patient to organise medicines by dividing and grouping those with the same intake time. If one or more of the medicines that are part of the patient's therapy have to be taken several times during the day, suggest to the patient put in a sachet for each 'group' of medicines that have to be taken at a specific time;

- if some medicines cannot be kept together with the others (e.g. medicine stored in the fridge), suggest that the patient insert the packaging tag of the missing ones into the group of medicines, to be used as a 'reminder'.

[Prescription 2] In prescriptions that introduce significant changes in the current therapy, as may occur after hospitalisation or after a specialist visit, it is recommended that the new daily treatment be fully rewritten, favouring, if possible, its display in the form of a 'daily schedule' rather than a simple list. This is in addition to *Recommendation No. 17—Recommendation for medication therapy reconciliation*, which sets out several measures to promote the rationalisation of therapy and prescribing processes.

[Prescription 3] Due to the technological transition to digital document formats, it is recommended to move to the formalisation of a Therapy Record, drawn up by the family doctor together with the patient and validated by the family doctor. This record should contain all the medicines that are part of the patient's daily therapy, medicines of occasional use, and medicines to which the patient is allergic or intolerant. It should also contain the patient's habits and lifestyle (e.g. food intolerances, alcohol use, smoking). The patient can complete a section of the card to supplement the list of prescribed medicines, with a list of substances such as supplements, phytotherapy, homeopathics, etc. The therapy card is helpful both in the case of admissions with an uncooperative patient, and in the case of specialist visits where there is a risk of not remembering some of the medicines being treated (e.g. eye drops and ointments, which are rarely declared by the patient to the doctor); the card is also helpful for the pharmacist, who can thus advise the patient more appropriately.

[Prescription 4] The therapeutic record must contain information on the active ingredient, the pharmaceutical form, the dosage, and the daily intake time. It should also include information on who prescribed the medicine, the prescription date, the expected duration of therapy, any examinations required when taking certain medicines, and the deadlines to continue therapy (e.g. liver function, kidney function, etc.). Finally, it helps provide information on the patient's particular difficulties (e.g., swallowing difficulties, needle phobia, low vision, etc.), which may guide the doctor towards pharmaceutical forms that are better tolerated and easier for intake.

[Prescription 5] In case of hospitalisation or medical examination, in the absence of a certified medical record from the general practitioner on the medicine therapy used by the patient, the hospital doctor must ask the patients to bring with them the packages of the medicines in use, so that they can rely on the information on the therapy taken.

[Prescription 6] It is wise to ask patients to return the medicine packaging to the prescribing doctor. It is helpful to write the therapy's beginning and opening dates on these packaging so the doctor can check therapy adherence. In fact, in some studies conducted on therapeutic compliance, the prescribing doctor's request to be able to check the packages used proved to be a helpful incentive to follow the therapy correctly. This allows the doctor to check whether the patient has failed to take the prescribed medicine.

[Prescription 7] It is recommended that the family doctor ask the patients to note on the outer packaging of the medicine for which condition they are taking it, by which doctor it was prescribed and the opening date.

[Prescription 8] For proper prescribing, it is recommended that pharmaceutical formularies available to doctors include information on the shape and size of the medicine, any unpleasant tastes, and effects that may occur immediately after intake (e.g. burning, pain, bitterness in the mouth, etc.). Thus, the doctor will be able to assess with the patients which pharmaceutical form is most acceptable to them, and the latter will be alerted to any minor manifestations closely related to the intake time.

[Prescription 9] Since several research shows that patients are reticent about taking medicines that, despite having the same active ingredient, present themselves with different colour and formal characteristics, it is recommended that the doctor, when prescribing, and the pharmacist, when dispensing, inform the patient about the efficacy of medicines that are identical in formulation even though they have different perceptual characteristics.

[Prescription 10] As required by current legislation, the prescription must be filled in its entirety, including the date and the doctor's signature, legibly, without using acronyms and abbreviations.

[Prescription 11] In prescriptions for 'non-standard' medicines (i.e., combinations or dosages for unconventional medicines, due to possible interactions between active ingredients in use in the patient's therapy, or due to the presence of pathologies that advise against the use of the medicine indicated by the doctor), it is recommended that the prescriber add an explanatory note informing the family doctor (involved in the prescription transcription operations) and the pharmacist (engaged in the dispensing operations) of the appropriateness of the prescription based on the clinical evaluation carried out by the doctor. This is to avoid requests for clarification to the prescribing physician and/or delays/suspensions in dispensing the prescribed medicine (Chen et al. 2005).

[Prescription 12] In the 'first prescriptions' of new medicines, it is a good idea for the prescriber to include the wording 'new medicine prescribed' in the prescription (similarly to the language already present in prescriptions for specialist visits in which it is possible to distinguish 'first visit' from 'follow-up visit') to make the patient aware of the different stages of medicine integration in the treatment. In the transcription phase, the general practitioner will pay more attention to possible interactions between the prescribed medicine and the patient's overall therapy, to possible contraindications concerning the pathologies from which the patient suffers, to the concomitant prescription/scheduling of laboratory tests or other diagnostic practices required by the use of the medicine, to verify that the patient has understood the indications relating to the daily dosage to provide the patient with information for a possible customisation of the dosage concerning the dosages available on the market, to schedule intake before or after meals, to make the patient aware of any foods or drinks that may render ineffective or potentiate the effect of the medicine, to advise or prohibit the handling of the pharmaceutical form, to direct the patient towards alternative pharmaceutical forms that are easier to manage. In the dispensing phase, the pharmacist will need to devote more attention to the counselling phase, to guide any procedures/methods of use to be observed when taking the medicine, advice and information on any side effects and ways to reduce them (Al-Khani et al. 2014), and in instructing the patient on the first use of the devices.

[**Prescription 13**] In 'first prescriptions', it is recommended that the prescriber include the reasons for prescribing the new medicine to inform the general practitioner (involved in the prescription transcription process) and the pharmacist (involved in the dispensing process). Regarding this recommendation, we refer to the publication by Al-Khani et al. (2014), concluding that: "the inclusion of the prescription statement in every prescription could help the pharmacist to detect medication errors […]"; "the statement could help the pharmacist to detect medication errors […]"; "the statement would improve the pharmacist's communication with the patient and, consequently, the patient's adherence to the prescribed therapy […]"; "some modifications to the current medicine prescription form that include additional fields, such as a special field for the physician to write the medicine indication at the time of prescription, helps to reduce medication errors (Kennedey et al. 2011) […]". The same document also states that "the American Society of Health-System Pharmacists (ASHP) has recommended that, to prevent medication errors, the desired therapeutic outcome for each medicine should be expressed at the time of prescription (Best Practices, ASHP) […]". In addition, the Institute for Safe Medication Practices (ISMP) recommended that prescription orders include a brief notation about the purpose or indication for the use of the medicine unless it is considered inappropriate by the prescriber; "an indication about the use of the medicine can help to ensure that the correct medicine is prescribed, and this is considered an additional safety checkpoint in the medication use process (ISMP) […]". And again, for the authors, the indication on the prescription of the reasons for prescribing allowed pharmacists to check the indication for prescribing a medicine and to check the correspondence with the medicine dispensed; that "review of the patient's history before dispensing were the main factors (60%) that helped pharmacists detect and thus prevent medication errors […]". The studies by Lizano-Díez et al. (2020) lead to the same conclusions.

[**Prescription 14**] In prescriptions for medicines, which are known to fall into the group of LASA medicines, it is recommended that the prescriber include a warning LASA medicine and, if it is a specialty, in addition to the proprietary name, the name of the active ingredient of the medicine prescribed should be written in brackets. (Lizano-Díez et al. 2020; Berman 2004).

[Prescription 15] In prescriptions, and especially in handwritten prescriptions, the use of block letters is recommended. As a result of current legislation, it is also recommended that the dosage should always be separated from the name of the medicine/active ingredient so that there is no confusion in the case of a medicine name ending in letters; in fact, these can be confused with the numbers that make up the dosage (e.g. the letter l with the number 1 or the letter O with the number 0) (Berman 2004; Ministero della Salute 2018).

[Prescription 16] To avoid patient stockpiling of medication, in the hypothesis of a fully digital transformation of the prescribing system, the inclusion of a refill interval is recommended, meaning a time interval since the last prescription made, within which the medication cannot be re-prescribed unless the physician removes the time restriction.

[Prescription 17] In a fully digital transformation of the prescribing system, introducing a refill interval is also recommended to intervene in non-adherence to therapy. If the chronically ill patient does not request a 'refill' prescription within the prescribed time interval, a warning message for the family doctor can be activated.

[Recipe 1] The white sheet of prescriptions is challenging to recognise and may not be easily identifiable among other sheets and documents. It is recommended that the 'prescription leaflet system' be redesigned (in the Italian context, these are red, white, psychotropic medicines, hospital medicines, medicines with a therapeutic plan, etc.) following a basic format 'adapted' to the different types of prescription, but which guarantees easy recognisability and uniform graphic language.

[Recipe 2] The white prescription for non-medicinal medicines must always bear the patient's name, date, and doctor's signature. It should be labelled with a graphic element (e.g. the green pharmacy cross) to make it recognisable from other documents.

[Recipe 3] It is recommended to redesign the information content of the prescription. This should contain a detachable part that remains with the patient, indicating the prescribed medicine, dosage, and directions for the use of the medicine.

[Recipe 4] In the hypothesis of a fully digital transformation of the prescribing system, it is recommended that the prescription contain a link to a multimedia document (e.g. hypertext, video, animation, etc.) illustrating the correct way to take and/or interact with other substances. In the case of a diagnostic examination, the link is helpful to show its stages.

[**Recipe 5**] In the hypothesis of a digital transformation of the prescribing system, it is recommended that the prescription contain a link (e.g. web address or QR code) to the website of the National Medicine Agency (for Italy) and in particular to the web page that allows retrieving information on the prescribed medicine (e.g., active ingredient, excipients, etc.), on possible interactions with other medicines, on its manipulability, on the different dosages available and on the recommendations necessary to maximise adherence and therapeutic efficacy. A link to the scientific literature supporting its use (e.g. clinical trial outcomes, recorded adverse events, etc.) is also conceivable.

[**Recipe 6**] In the hypothesis of a fully digital transformation of the prescribing system, it is recommended that the prescription contain a link to the therapeutic plan established by the prescribing physician to generate an e-calendar file to be downloaded on one's smartphone or mobile device to support patient adherence to therapy.

[**Recipe 7**] In the hypothesis of a fully digital transformation of the prescribing system, it is recommended that the prescription for an examination and/or instrumental examination contain a link to the prescribing doctor's treatment plan for the generation of an e-calendar format file to be downloaded to one's smartphone or mobile device to help the patient remember the date of execution, as well as any instructions for online payment.

22.4 Premises Towards a System of Recommendations to Improve the Dispensing Process

In the literature, beyond an abundance of research focused on analysing errors in the dispensing process, a wealth of propositional studies exists. These studies, characterized by their emphasis on suggesting improvements, revising current procedures, or experimenting with novel practices, present a range of strategies aimed at intervening in various problematic aspects of the dispensing process. The overarching objective of these endeavours is to mitigate the risk of errors (Campmans et al. 2018).

Numerous suggested interventions address various phases and activities within the dispensing process. These encompass:

- the definition of new prescription formats: as previously mentioned, exploring innovative prescription formats is proposed to enhance clarity and accuracy;
- the definition of management protocol for the dispensing process;
- the definition of control strategies for the dispensing process, such as the introduction of "double-checking" and the incorporation of a "secret shopper", suggested to monitor operator compliance with internal rules and guidelines of dispensing bodies (Hoxsie et al. 2006);

- the re-engineering of procurement and distribution process for medicine stocks within the pharmacy;
- the re-engineering of the dispensary, studying the arrangement of Look-Alike Sound-Alike (LASA) products, avoiding alphabetical order, and maintaining a physical distance between them. This aims to reduce distractions during the selection phase and minimize the occurrence of medicines with similar names (distractors) in the health worker's field of vision (Lizano-Díez et al. 2020; Weir et al. 2020);
- the redesigning of medicine arrangement, in the pharmacy and in its warehouse;
- the reformulation of error sharing and reporting procedures;
- the design of patient education tools dealing with medicine safety;
- the design of patient education services;
- a staff training on operational procedures, and protocols, and cultivating a culture of error prevention.

In a research study conducted in Alberta, Canada, focusing on the advisory role of pharmacists during dispensing, the proposed Chat Check Chart (CCC) protocol was introduced and tested. This protocol aimed to assess the extent to which pharmacists, in their daily practice, gather information about the patient and their health status. Additionally, it sought to evaluate the pharmacist's preparation of therapy by assessing the prescription's efficacy, safety, and manageability to enhance patient therapeutic adherence. The CCC protocol also emphasized documenting activities to maintain a comprehensive record (Nusair and Guirguis 2017).

The protocol proposed by Dyck et al. (2005) and Nusair and Guirguis (2017) aimed to manage the interaction between pharmacists and patients, ensuring a safer dispensing process. This protocol involved a series of verifications, including confirmation of patient identity; checking for medicine allergies; verifying the correctness and completeness of prescription data; assessing the patient's understanding of medication use modalities; providing information on expected therapeutic responses and timeframes; explaining common or important side effects and their management; and specifying storage requirements for the prescribed medicine. Despite these proposed measures, numerous studies in the literature highlight the frequent non-observance of these procedural steps.

Hoxsie et al. (2006), in their study based on observations at medicine dispensing stations, identified frequent non-compliance with the provided protocol among operators. The protocol included checks such as confirming patient's name and date of birth; determining the number of prescriptions to be picked up; assigning only one task to the operator; prohibiting interruptions during dispensing procedures; using trays for prescribed medicines alongside prescriptions; showing patients the items to be dispensed; restricting patient consultations to pharmacists rather than technical staff; providing advice to patients with new prescriptions; differentiating dispensing procedures for high-risk patients; and utilizing receipts to verify the correspondence between individual prices and dispensed medicines.

It is important to tell patients about the protocols they should follow to actively participate in dispensing activities, encompassing verification, control, and adherence to the pharmacist's instructions. Hoxsie et al. (2006) emphasized the detrimental impact of interruptions on dispensing errors, proposing measures such as displaying a "do not disturb" sign to mitigate interruptions during dispensing.

Lizano-Díez et al. (2020) echoed the importance of minimizing distractions during prescribing, dispensing, and administration, suggesting the use of "Do not disturb" tags in hospital settings. Dispensing errors are often attributed to poor communication between prescribing doctors and pharmacists (Chen et al. 2005). To address this, recommendations include including additional information in prescriptions to enhance understanding, as verbal instructions from patients may be confusing or inconsistent.

Among the factors contributing to a high incidence of dispensing errors, pharmacists often identify poor communication between prescribing doctors and dispensing pharmacists (Chen et al. 2005). The recurring recommendation is to augment the prescription with additional information regarding the reasons for the prescription. The authors of the study highlight several challenges, including the difficulty pharmacists face in providing adequate instructions and directions in the absence of written information from the doctor. Oral information provided by the patient regarding the reasons for using the medicine can be confusing or contradictory to the prescription. Inconsistencies between the oral instructions of general practitioners (as interpreted and relayed by patients to the pharmacist) and the written instructions on the prescription are also noted. Additionally, the lack of awareness among general practitioners about the challenges patients encounter in using medicines, coupled with the difficulty in assessing the safety of medicines without essential information such as blood test results or patients' medical history, further emphasize the need for improved information sharing between doctors and pharmacists.

These issues underscore the importance of enhancing information sharing between doctors and pharmacists. The recommendation emerges that prescribing recipes should include more comprehensive information, encompassing a range of clinical data related to the patient's health, thereby aiding pharmacists in ensuring safe and accurate dispensing. Several recommendations advocate the use of digital technologies to address information-sharing problems and reduce prescription/dispensing errors. These include:

- shared electronic medical records;
- prescription tracking technology;
- barcode scanning technology to verify the correspondence between the medicine prescribed and the medicine dispensed by exploiting the unique serialisation codes of each pack. In other words, serialisation, implemented by the pharmaceutical industry to track medicine and hinder counterfeiting, can also become a tool for error detection between prescription and dispensing (Aldughayfiq and Sampalli 2021);
- automated dispensing technologies;
- computer applications to detect an interaction between medicines, identifying potentially dangerous combinations (Chen et al. 2005);

- inclusion of warning messages in digital prescription programmes to alert potential LASA medicine pairs. Warnings can indicate the pathology of a prescribed medicine to provide feedback on the correctness of the prescription. For example: "This medicine is typically used for hypothyroidism. There is no such problem listed for this patient. [Cancel/Ignore/Add diagnosis]", (Lizano-Díez et al. 2020). Such applications can be used to digitise the prescription/dispensing system.

While many recommendations go in the direction of supporting the use of digitisation to overcome the many error problems between prescription and dispensing and to share information between the different actors in the process, other works warn against the hypothesis that technologies alone can be decisive, pointing out new error cases dependent on their use. In the face of advantages such as speed, better readability, and the obligation to complete the prescription format, several potential fallacies of computerised prescriptions are highlighted. These include: the use of 'drop-down menus' that can easily lead to selecting the wrong medicine from a list of medicines arranged in alphabetical order or selecting the wrong patient from a list of names in alphabetical order with the possibility of repeating the error in subsequent prescriptions. The most significant chance of error occurs in therapies that need to change medicines and dosages since, in computerised systems, the prescription filled frequently remains in memory, and its data are recalled (Chen et al. 2005).

The authors caution against the excessive use of warnings: the continual drawing of attention to reduce issues may produce, as a consequent effect, inattention to all reports, including those referring to more serious risks.

In addition to digital technologies, automating processes is a further avenue that the dispensing system is taking to remedy dispensing errors. These systems have spread, first and foremost, in hospital pharmacies in both the US and Europe and are beginning to be used equally in community pharmacies. In some cases, they are combined with repackaging technologies aimed at facilitating the taking of the medicine at home, facilitating adherence in the case of complex therapies to be managed by the patient. The technologies in question, starting with the patient's treatment plan, can remove the medicines from the original manufacturer's packaging and repackage them into sealed sachets containing the medicine doses to be administered at a given time of day. The system also automatically prints the label on each sachet with the patient's data, the names of the medicines with their dosage, and the day and time of intake (James et al. 2009; Comelli 2021).

The dispensing of medicines unpacked from the original packaging and repackaged according to the patient's therapeutic needs is an example of a service provided by the pharmacy to meet the needs of patients, which is recommended in the case of people with little autonomy in therapy management.

A further example of a change in the prescription/dispensing system, which goes in the direction of offering the patient a more efficient and effective treatment service, is represented by those Centres or Outpatient Clinics that, in the case of pathologies requiring complex therapy (such are, for example, therapies with antiretroviral medicines; chemotherapeutic medicines; psychopharmaceuticals, etc.)

have activated experiences of unification of prescription and dispensing activities. When taking these medicines, it is essential to check the correct intake; to change dosages during therapy; to check the interaction of therapies, such as the current one or to temporarily suspend the consumption of certain medicines; and to monitor the functionality of specific organs before starting, during and after treatment. The unification of prescribing and dispensing activities enables the physician to monitor the benefits or side effects of medicines as they occur and to modify the overall therapy under close supervision.

Although recommendations on the numerous procedural aspects accompanying the act of dispensing are very frequent in the literature—a sign of the multiple critical elements found in practice, even in the face of highly regulated activities—, we have confined our attention to the problems and possible recommendations relating to the secondary packaging of the medicine and the prescriptive prescription.

These are two elements to which, in the text, we have given prominence as artefacts invested with the 'responsibility' of facilitating or hindering—by making them more complex—the actions that take place in the decision-making chain that, from clinical diagnosis led to the prescription of the medicine and its dispensation. In Chaps. 9 and 22, we have dwelt on the hypotheses of their redesign and concerning a digital format transformation.

22.5 The Form of the Medicine

In Chap. 4, we explored the relationship between the "pharmaceutical form", namely the form taken by the active ingredient along with excipients after the pharmaceutical manufacturing process, and the route of administration. In fact, medicines can:

- be taken by mouth—these are the so-called 'oral pharmaceutical forms'. They can be liquid, powder, solid, etc. Oral intake presupposes that the medicine is ingested, thus following the digestive processes typical of food, which, passing through the stomach, enters the intestine and is metabolised by the liver and kidneys. Among the oral forms, some medicines enter the body by the sublingual or buccal route (i.e., tablet held under the tongue or between cheek and tongue). In this case, the medicine enters the bloodstream directly without passing through the digestive process;
- be administered by injection, intravenously; intramuscularly; subcutaneously, etc.;
- be taken rectally or vaginally;
- be taken via the ocular or auricular route;
- be taken nasally;
- be inhaled into the lungs by mouth or nebulised by nose and mouth;
- be applied to the skin via the skin;
- be absorbed transdermally.

The choice of the pharmaceutical form depends on factors such as physico-chemical properties, bio-availability considerations, storage characteristics, absorption speed, age of the user, and the target area of the body. Certain routes of administration imply a local action of the medicine (e.g., eye, ear, vagina, skin), while others are associated with systemic effects (e.g., tablets, injections, drips, suppositories). Some pharmaceutical forms, such as patches, powder preparations, and drops, can ambiguously exert both local and systemic actions.

In Chap. 16, we observed the ambiguity in the relationship between pharmaceutical form, route of administration, and local/systemic action can lead to user errors. For instance, a powdered preparation intended for local use may be mistakenly dissolved in water and ingested if the route of administration is not clearly communicated on the packaging. Changes in the relationship between pharmaceutical forms traditionally linked to a route of intake (e.g., capsules: oral route; ovules: vaginal route; suppositories: rectal route) and changes route of intake (e.g., substitution of vaginal ovules with vaginal capsules or vaginal suppositories) may pose comprehension challenges for users.

Beyond functional characteristics (e.g., the rounded ogive shape, typical of an ovum, is more functional for introduction into the vagina than the tapered ogive shape of a suppository and is even more so than a capsule-shaped medicine), there's an issue of the user's established relationship over time between the shape of the medicine and the route of administration.

In the world of objects, Chap. 16 pointed out that typologies represent the shape established over time of class objects (e.g., the bottle, the table, the scissors and, in the world of the medicines, the tablet, the suppository, the ampoule). The function of typological archetypes is precisely that of referring—even in the presence of multiple morphological variants of the same object—to the immediate recognizability, function, context of use, and mode of use.

Typologies generate expectations in the user concerning the way objects are used. Typologies are effective because they allow the user to save cognitive energy and establish a habit of use with the object, which is part of the automatism of the user/object relationship. Changing the function of a typology and modifying its usage, can generate a disorientating effect in the user that can lead him to error. In the case of pharmaceuticals, in addition to the well-established habits of use, capsules and suppositories (two archetypal types) are known for their systemic action, contributing to the possibility of error. For the user, drinking a tablet (vaginal) or inserting rectally a suppository (vaginal) does not constitute an immediately noticeable anomaly. The user is aware that both pharmaceutical forms (capsule and suppository) can generate curative effects even in districts distant from the route of intake.

Interviewing some users about their habits, we also found that keeping vaginal suppositories in the refrigerator, whose use generally takes place in the bathroom, generates actions (e.g., opening the fridge, taking the packet, taking the suppository out of the pack, putting it back in the fridge, reaching the bathroom with the 'dose' separated from the pack, etc.) that choose how to use the medicine even more ambiguous. The separation between the place of storage and of use can lead the medicine, at the time of its use, to be 'far' from its packaging and thus from the information needed to support its correct use. Even in the presence of the packaging, however, the interpretation to be given to the adjective 'vaginal' in the context of the use of the medicine remains ambiguous. It may characterise the nouns 'capsule' and 'suppository' by indicating the route of ingestion. Still, it may also be interpreted as an adjective, meaning the part of the body on which the curative effect may be felt. Especially in the case of the vaginal suppository, this interpretation is credible.

We have chosen to focus our attention on the dynamics surrounding solid oral forms. Specifically, we are placing particular emphasis on the theme of morphological variants in medicine recognition activities, exploring how different shapes, sizes, colours, and markings of solid oral forms can impact the ability of users to identify and distinguish between medications. Additionally, we are examining the relationship between the form and function of the medicine-object, studying how the physical characteristics of solid oral forms can affect their usability and administration.

Furthermore, we are exploring how the shape of solid oral forms can effectively communicate the correct mode of use to users, considering the importance of clear instructions, labelling, and packaging design in ensuring proper medication usage.

22.5.1 Focus: Solid Forms for Oral Use

We have chosen to focus our attention on oral solid forms due to their widespread use among adults in clinical practice and home care. The reason for this primacy relies on the simplicity of the production methods compared to other pharmaceutical forms, the high stability of the finished product, the availability of this form for different pathological conditions, the safety of storage—especially when packaged in blister packs—, the precision of dosage—when taken in their intact form—, the ease of use both indoor and outdoor (Abrate et al. 2016). Even at the level of distribution and storage, both in the warehouses of pharmaceutical companies and the pharmacies' warehouses, they are among the forms that best allow a rational use of space. Despite these advantages, challenges arise in special cases, such as:

- patients with difficulties in swallowing tablets, as in the case of dysphagic patients or patients with a nasogastric tube;
- paediatric patients, frail patients, elderly, and patients undergoing polypharmacy;
- patients needing to 'tailor' the dosage according to weight, age, or other factors;
- patients requiring initiation of therapy and/or termination of treatment at graduated dosages, as is typical of some medicine classes.

In these conditions, the oral solid form becomes problematic because it must be broken, crushed, and sometimes reduced to powder for intake. The alteration of the oral solid form takes tablets and capsules from being a safe, easy, precisely dosed solution with long stability of the active ingredient, to being an unsafe medicine;

with dosage that is difficult to control; with difficult preservation of the pharmaceutical characteristics. Its administration, in these cases, can lead the user to make mistakes that can compromise the treatment process to the point of becoming hazardous to health. Incorrect handling of a solid oral pharmaceutical form poses risks to both patients and caregivers. Alteration of the coating, for example, can bring carcinogenic, teratogenic, or hormone-based substances into contact with the skin. During rupture of the medicine, the dusts produced can also be inhaled. Some of these may be irritating in contact with the eyes or external mucous membranes or even internally. Sometimes the fractionation of the medicine can alter the stability of the active ingredient. This may also degrade through exposure to light. Sometimes, on the other hand, disruption of the coating can alter the bioavailability of the medicine. Alteration of the coating may cause the patient to experience an unpleasant taste, and unpleasantness is one of the elements that prompts the patient to discontinue therapy.

The widespread issues arising from improper handling prompted the Italian Ministry of Health to issue Recommendation No. 19, *Recommendation for the Handling of Oral Solid Pharmaceutical Forms* (Ministero della Salute 2019). Similar recommendations exist at the European and non-European levels (Royal Pharmaceutical Society 2011; Good Practice Guidance 2011; Gruppo Regionale sul rischio clinico da farmaci 2015).

It is noteworthy that these recommendations primarily target healthcare professionals, indicating a lack of communication regarding the proper handling of oral solid forms to non-expert users. We note here a significant fact for our research: the Recommendation just referred to, like all ministerial Recommendations, is addressed to healthcare professionals. Similarly, international publications have a manualistic character and are addressed to the professional world. This is an indication of the extent to which tablets, capsules, candies present a shape that is unable to communicate, even to 'expert users', its characteristics of use because, even for professional figures—as is the case with nurses, who are trained in the use of medicines—it is not easy, let alone intuitive, to establish whether a given medicine can or cannot be manipulated.

In our exploration of medicine handling in the home environment, it is readily apparent how little consideration is given to problems encountered by patients in such a context precisely because they are users without specific knowledge of the medicine object.

It seems interesting to reflect on the shape of medicines for oral use and to trace in its connotations—or absence of connotations—some reasons for the lack of compliance with rules of use which recurs in the professional context.

In the Ministerial Recommendations and the manuals, the forms of medicine handling are basically reduced to the two main ones: breaking the medicine; crushing/masticating/powdering the medicine.

Based on the observation of how users handle medicines, it is useful to integrate the two main modes of management found in the literature with these additional ones:

- unblistering the medicine at times (even days) before its intake. This does not occur in the hospital world, whereas it frequently happens in the home environment;
- storage the medicine residual doses (even days) after its division. This operation does not occur the hospital world, whereas it is typical of domestic use;
- mixing medicines (even split) due to the early preparation of the daily therapy. Our observation of the medicine preparation and storage methods has revealed a wide range of 'do-it-yourself' solutions, prepared by users (e.g., small bags, cling film, small cups, saucers, tins, favours, etc.) and used to 'store' the medicines which make up the daily therapy, subdivided by time of intake;
- ingestion of medicine, formulated to be dissolved in the mouth.

In the following discussion, coming from what emerged in Chap. 16, regarding the shape of solid oral medicines and how formal characters (e.g., geometry, colour, surface, surface markings) are capable or not of communicating the correct ways of using the medicine.

At the end of the paragraph, we define some recommendations aimed at introducing, in the form of the object, persuasive or dissuasive elements capable of orienting the user's behaviour. We suggest Recommendations of an informative nature intended expressly for the patient and aimed at inducing correct usage behaviour.

22.5.2 Solid Oral Forms: Typologies and Morphologies

In Chaps. 12 and 16, we explored, both theoretically and from the user's perspective, how the form of a medicine significantly influences its correct usage and the information it provides to the patient, either effectively or ineffectively. Here, we provide a summary of key concepts, directing readers to the mentioned chapters for more in-depth analysis.

Oral pharmaceuticals such as tablets, capsules, granules, and pearls have maintained archetypal structures over time, making them easily recognizable.

The relationship between the form and the route of intake is equally clear. However, the morphological differentiation within the same typology—the presence of formal variants—often makes these shapes indistinguishable. This issue is particularly challenging for patients undergoing polypharmacy, where distinguishing one medicine from another becomes difficult based on formal characteristics alone.

Morphological peculiarities, including base geometry, section profile, size, colour, surface marks, and treatments, may lack distinctive details for effective medicine identification. Once removed from their blisters, capsules, tablets, and pills can become indistinguishable to users due to limited geometric and chromatic variations. In cases where tablet shapes are very similar, surface imprints become crucial for distinguish two different medicines or two different dosages of the same active ingredient. Moreover, we noticed how much the colour characterisation supports the patient in recognising the medicine, with the point that, especially in the

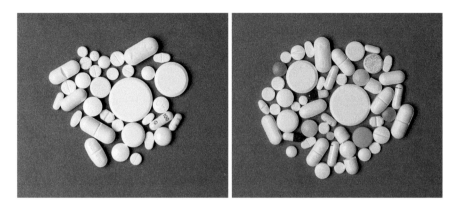

Fig. 22.2 Common formats for solid pills, dragees, tablets and capsules. A striking image of the enormous variety of shapes distinguishable by a few formal traits. The clear predominance of white colour in oral solid forms means that medicines with colour characterisation become immediately distinguishable from others

elderly, a change in the colour of a medicine (e.g. caused by the administration of the same medicine of another brand during a hospital stay) generates a lot of mistrust, if not outright rejection, in the patient (Fig. 22.2).

The colour element, although essential for patient recognition, is poorly designed when present. And, it may not be used appropriately on the medicine's surface or in the secondary pack to distinguishing, for example, between two different dosages of the same active ingredient. Patients with multiple dosages of the same medicine in their daily therapy may encounter issues with colour characterization, leading to confusion.

To sum up, morphological variants, including size, shape geometry, colour characterization, and surface signs, extensively used in the realm of objects for product distinction, brand identity, and functional indications, are often undervalued in the pharmaceutical domain. In pharmaceuticals, where the shape and its connotations should serve a purely functional purpose—helping users discriminate between medicines—morphological features are not always given due consideration.

This underscores the need for improved design considerations in pharmaceuticals to enhance user understanding and ensure correct medication usage. For a detailed exploration of these issues, see Chap. 17.

22.5.3 Manipulability of Oral Solid Forms: Informing the Patient to Overcome the Hermeticism of the Technique

The tablet coating is essentially a 'technique,' deviating from the typical appearance associated with 'devices,' 'machines,' and 'instrumental apparatuses'. Instead, it presents itself as a simple, sometimes coloured surface that lacks any apparent implications regarding its use. Like any technique, the tablet coating serves as a device with specific functions, addressing practical needs. Our technological imagination, shaped by the products of the mechanical age, often overlooks the presence of technicality in the world of surfaces, a characteristic more closely associated with electronics and chemistry.

The surfaces of medicines are never innocent. Due to their role in concealing technological aspects, they have an increased need to convey themselves, making their functions explicit. This necessity for comprehensibility is particularly crucial for a product like medicine, which, due to its societal function, cannot be considered an elitist product limited to a circle of specialists Medicine must guarantee the broadest accessibility, akin to the principles outlined in the EU Directive 2016/2102 for website accessibility, ensuring perceivability, operability, understandability, and robustness. Ease of use and comprehensibility become even more critical in the case of medicines, given their integration into our daily lives, characterized by carelessness and approximation. The world of surfaces possesses its depth, and it is only by delving into it that one can transition from a purely descriptive level (smooth, rough, shiny, matte, coloured, white, etc.) to understanding the functional significance these surfaces hold. The surface of objects serves as both a place of signs with signal value and a space of multiple functions, emphasizing the interconnectedness of signs and functions.

A brief technical premise is necessary. Tablets may or may not be coated, and coated tablets may feature different types of coatings. The most common types include sugar coating, as well as coating with polymer films or natural resins. The latter type of coating is achieved through various substances selected based on the barrier function required for the surface. These coatings serve multiple functions, including:

- masking unpleasant odours and tastes;
- promoting swallowing by smoothing the surface;
- protecting unstable or photosensitive medicines;
- improving mechanical resistance;
- making the tablet gastro-resistant;
- scheduling the release time of the active substance(s);
- preventing the patient from encountering the active substance (Lai 2023).

Certain coatings, such as sugar coating, generally do not alter the release kinetics of the medicine. Sugar coating is commonly employed in the first four functions listed.

In some cases, the coating allows for unconventional forms of active ingredient release, such as modified release, controlled release, sustained release, and delayed release. The outcome depends on the technological characteristics of the formulation. Gastro-resistant formulations, for example, are characterized by polymer coatings that remain intact in the stomach and release the active ingredient in the small intestine (Abrate et al. 2016). Excipients may enable direct absorption of the active ingredient through the mucosa, leading to a rapid increase in its concentration in the blood, bypassing first-pass metabolism in the liver. Additives in capsules and excipients also influence the speed of absorption of the active ingredient.

Consequently, the same active ingredient in different pharmaceutical formulations can result in varying effects concerning release time and site of release. The choice of excipients and surface-forming substances, along with the route of administration, plays a crucial role in defining the medicine's effect. The effect of an active ingredient, even at the same doses, can differ significantly between pharmaceutical formulations with different excipients and coatings (Lai 2023). When the coating consists of a very thin polymer layer, the tablets are termed film-coated tablets. These coated tablets have a smooth surface, often coloured and polished.

As outlined, the diverse functions a surface can assume have implications for the safety of the active ingredient once the medicine has been handled. Despite these varied functions, the medicine surface lacks formal or visual connotations that aid users in understanding the distinct pharmacological action performed by the coating in each medicine.

This information is crucial for users to avoid unintended consequences and ensure the safe and effective use of oral solid forms.

On the secondary packaging, alongside information about the pharmaceutical form, various characterizing elements are typically provided. For instance:

- Atorvastatin: film-coated tablets. The designation 'film-coated tablets' alone fails to elucidate the purpose of the surface film. Indeed, in packages labelled as 'film-coated', the package leaflet, under the 'Method of administration' section, presents diverse instructions regarding the necessary user behavior. For instance: The package leaflet specifies: "to be swallowed whole with water".

Conversely, in other medications with a film coating, the prescribed usage behavior differs. Examples include:

- Naloxegol: film-coated tablets. The package leaflet suggests: "May be crushed and reduced to powder, mixed with half a glass of water and drunk immediately";
- Ciprofloxacin: film-coated tablets. The package leaflet indicates: "divisible";
- Azathioprine: film-coated tablets. The outer packaging provides no additional information. But in the package leaflet under "Method of administration" it states: "The tablet must not be divided or broken". A concluding paragraph in the lengthy package leaflet states: "The following information is intended exclusively for medical doctors or healthcare professionals. Instructions for use, handling, and disposal: There are no risks associated with handling tablets with the coating intact. No special safety precautions are necessary in this case. But, immunosuppressive agents should be handled in strict accordance with instructions when healthcare personnel halve tablets […]. Surplus medicines and contaminated devices should be stored temporarily in clearly labelled containers. Unused product or waste materials should be disposed of in accordance with local regulations";
- Oxycodone Hydrochloride/Naloxone Hydrochloride. Despite being a film-coated medicine, the secondary pack lacks this designation, unlike the medicines. In this case, the secondary pack is labelled "extended-release tablets".

Both the secondary pack and the package leaflet include warnings: "tablets must be swallowed whole, not broken, chewed or crushed".

These examples show that simply characterizing a medicine as 'film-coated' may not sufficiently inform patients about the correct actions to take or prevent incorrect actions. Such actions could potentially alter the efficacy of the active ingredient, impede its delivery to the intended organ, or result in contamination for those handling the medicine and the surrounding environment.

Substituting the description 'film-coated tablets' with 'extended-release tablets', as seen with Oxycodone Hydrochloride/Naloxone Hydrochloride, does not uniformly aid patient understanding of appropriate actions. Both designations, crafted by pharmaceutical professionals and tailored for an expert audience, employ language that may remain unfamiliar to end consumers.

The examples highlight the sophistication of pharmaceutical technology and the multifaceted functions that a medicine's coating can achieve based on the substances used. As argued earlier, the surface of the medicine, does not convey its function. In the absence of crucial information, descriptors such as 'film-coated' or functional descriptions like 'sustained-release tablet' fall short in guiding the user toward the correct behavior.

A review of the pharmaceutical handbook (AA VV 2023), focusing on oral solid forms, heightens awareness of the operational complexity to which a medicine is subject. It presents various case, including:

- Oral solid forms: divisible and breakable;
- Oral solid forms: non-divisible and non-breakable;
- Oral solid forms: divisible but not breakable;
- Oral solid forms: non-divisible but breakable.

The listed prerogatives of a medicine encompass authorized or prohibited operations, determined by the intended function of the medicine, how the pharmaceutical action is to be executed, and the physical, chemical, and organoleptic characteristics of the medicine itself.

Examining the issue of medicine manipulation from the user's perspective reveals two primary needs:

- dosing/customizing the dose: this involves dividing the medicine into two or more parts to achieve a customized dose;
- facilitating swallowing: in this case, both dividing and crushing are operations that users may resort to make swallowing the medicine easier.

In the case of dividing the medicine to obtain a customized dose, the remaining fraction of the medicine will be used later. This practice, often employed in weekly preparations of daily therapy, raises concerns about tablets and half-tablets being stored together for days, leaving the active ingredient unprotected.

Interestingly, in the examples mentioned earlier, the instructions regarding medicine handling are never explicitly directed to the user to guide their actions. Instead, they are formulated to inform about the technological or functional characteristics of the medicine, lacking explicit guidance on user behavior. For instance:

- Naloxegol: 'the tablet can be crushed and reduced to powder, mixed with half a glass of water and drunk immediately'. In this description of the actions the user should perform, it remains implicit that crushing is only permitted to make swallowing easier. On the other hand, it is not possible to fractionate the dosage (and possibly keep the half dose for later use). This is deduced from the requirement to take the medicine 'immediately'. But this is not explicitly mentioned in the Packaging Leaflet.
- In the case of Ciprofloxacin, the label indicates: "divisible tablet". leading users to assume it is also breakable, which is not universally true for all medicines.
- In the case of the active substance Azathioprine, the package leaflet explicitly states "The tablet must not be divided or broken". The tablet, however, bears the pre-break mark on its surface and this sign, for the user (who often does not read the package leaflet) is a clear 'invitation to use' that contradicts what is written in the package leaflet. The final paragraph of the package leaflet, which provides indications for the exclusive use of doctors and healthcare professionals, effectively excludes from the information the patient, who is already reluctant to read such lengthy texts. In our observation we found two patients who had been prescribed half a tablet dose by their doctor and, in both cases, the handling (the tablet being very resistant) was done using a chopping board and knife, put away or used afterwards for normal kitchen use, without particular attention to the contamination problems inherent in this medicine.

Addressing the use of customised medicine dosages in prescriptions requires careful consideration of the implications of fractionation. When crafting package leaflets, it is crucial to define how to provide correct information to patients and the actions that information should induce.

The instruction 'do not fractionate the medicine' can be communicated in various ways, as illustrated in the following examples:

- Adenovir Dipivoxil: "*The recommended dose, in each case, is one tablet. If dosage adjustments are necessary, variation of the intake interval is recommended*";
- Alfusozine: "*The recommended dose is 2.5 mg or multiples thereof. No further dosage reductions are planned*";
- Acetylsalicylic acid: "*No dosage reductions are planned, however, the tablets are technically divisible*";
- Ambroxol: "*The dosage is 1 tablet three times a day, possibly to be reduced by reducing the number of tablets/day*";
- Acetylsalicylic acid: "*gastro-resistant tablets*";
- Biperiodene hydrochloride: "*is an extended-release formulation. Splitting the tablet alters the pharmacokinetics of the active substance. Tablets should not be cut, crushed or chewed, as this may lead to an increased risk of adverse effects including convulsions*";

- Minocycline: *"The medicine is highly irritating to the oesophagus, so capsules should not be opened. Instead, they should be swallowed with an adequate amount of water, in an upright or sitting position and at least 1 hour before going to bed"*;
- Risedronic acid: *"Tablets should be swallowed whole and not sucked or chewed. To promote tablet transit in the stomach, take risedronate with a glass of still water, maintaining an upright position (standing or sitting). Patients should not lie down for 30 minutes after swallowing the tablet"*.

The examples from the SIFO handbook, *Evaluation of the divisibility and breakability of oral solid pharmaceutical forms* (Abrate et al. 2016), concerning information for the proper medicine intake and the possible forms of manipulation, reveal a diversity of ways in which these indications are given to the patient. Sometimes, the indication *not to fragment* the medicine is accompanied by medical reasons for not taking lower dosages (e.g., no need to adjust or reduce the dosage). The medical reasons are not always supplemented by an explanation concerning the effects that the medicine may have on the patient if it is not taken correctly or the effects of reduced efficacy of the active ingredient due to handling the medicine (e.g., the meaning of the term gastro-resistant is not necessarily understood by the patient and, even if understood, it is not easy for everyone to deduce that this characteristic implies that the tablet should not be handled). In still other cases, the physical effects that the medicine may produce on the patient if it is not taken correctly are described (e.g., increased risk of adverse effects, including convulsions; medicine highly irritating to the oesophagus). In other cases, no medical or pharmaceutical explanations are given to the patient, but the actions the patient must take to take the medicine effectively are defined in detail. Finally, in other cases, the indications given to the patient are contradicted by the shape attributed to the medicine. We see this in the case of Azathioprine, which is presented as a tablet characterised by a split line, even though the package leaflet states that the medicine cannot be split.

The case of the medicine containing the active ingredient Azathioprine is an example of 'reasons of shape' which, with their plastic evidence, immediately reach the user. In this case, the shape and its signs convince the user to take an action. There are examples of tablet shapes that, in a not-so-direct way, can constitute an 'invitation to use' that makes it easy to break into action. These medicines have an oblong, ovoid shape and thin thickness. Due to their greater prehensibility (precisely because they provide the user with a larger gripping surface), they facilitate the tablet-breaking action. Powerful oxycodone hydrochloride/naloxone hydrochloride painkillers fall into this class of medicines precisely because of their elongated shape (a shape that does not constitute a clear invitation to use); they do not hinder the user from breaking the medicine. Lenticular tablets with a double convex surface would have a more significant deterrent effect. Implicitly, this shape discourages breaking the medicine by making it more difficult to grip and not providing a flat surface on which a knife blade could easily rest.

So far, we have taken the traditional tablet, designed to be swallowed, as a reference. However, there are—and recently, they have become increasingly popular—tablets whose absorption does not involve swallowing and subsequent filtering by the digestive organs. In the case of sublingual tablets, the active ingredient enters the bloodstream through absorption by the oral mucous membranes. These medicines are sometimes designed precisely to avoid what is referred to in medical terminology as the 'hepatic first-pass effect'. In these cases, swallowing would defeat this very purpose. In some medicines, even swallowing would render the active ingredient ineffective. Below are some examples from the SIFO manual, *Evaluation of divisibility and breakability of oral solid pharmaceutical forms* (Abrate et al. 2016):

- Desmopressin: sublingual administration;
- Deferasirox: dispersible tablets. They should not be chewed or swallowed whole;
- Nitroglycerin: tablets must be crushed with the teeth and allowed to dissolve under the tongue. Ingestion nullifies the therapeutic effect.

Therefore, even with this pharmaceutical form, mistakes can be made when taking the tablet. The distinction between the orally-dispersible formulation (for which the medicine, in tablet or granulate form, is dissolved in the mouth and then swallowed) and the sublingual formulation (for which the medicine is dissolved and absorbed by the mucous membranes of the mouth) is not sufficiently known. In the former case, the medicine follows the 'digestive route', but arrives in the stomach already dissolved. Therefore, it has a faster effect than the traditional formulation, although less rapid than the sublingual formulation. It also makes it easier for those with swallowing problems. In the second case, the digestive route is completely avoided. The possibility that the patient, unaware of these subtle differences, swallows the tablet instead of holding it in the mouth is high. Also contributing to this is the complete lack of formal characterisation of tablets with such different modes of intake.

A final consideration concerns oral capsule forms. The formal characteristics of the product may lead to the capsule being opened and its contents dissolved in water. In some cases, this is possible and permitted. But, as always happens in the relationship between user and object, there is a imprinting in the user's experience that may lead the user to repeat the same experience in the same way for the same type of object. Since the universe of active ingredients available in capsule form is at least as varied as that of tablets (e.g., capsules that can be opened, capsules with an active ingredient harmful to the gastric mucosa, capsules with an active ingredient with a reduced effect if not taken in its entirety; capsules containing gastro-resistant granules that can be removed from the capsule, swallowed with water but not chewed, etc.), it is essential, as with tablets, to provide the patients with indications as to what they can or cannot do to take the medicine.

Again, these are technological sophistications with no formal connotations such that they can be distinguished by the patient to direct them to the correct use. The surface of the medicine, as well as the secondary packaging and the package insert, are called upon to supplement verbal and visual information to prevent misuse of the medicine.

In the case of capsules, an example of how the shape of the medicine can direct the patient to act, without the certainty of correct usage behaviour, we have with ursodesoxycholic acid capsules (Fig. 22.3). The medicine is presented in rigid capsules 22 mm long. The capsules are transparent, and the user can see three coated tablets inside each capsule. The secondary packaging is labelled 'extended-release hard capsules'. Nothing is said, not even in the package insert, about the possibility of opening the capsule and swallowing the three tablets separately. The stated feature (i.e., 'sustained-release hard capsules' and not 'sustained-release tablets') should impede opening and swallowing the three tablets contained therein. On the other hand, the transparency of the capsule, which allows the three coated tablets inside to be clearly seen, would also invite the patient to open and swallow the three tablets separately. This is an example of how the lack of clear verbal communication in the presence of an implicit visual invitation—'the transparency' allowing a glimpse of the three tablets inside—can create problems in the patient as to how to proceed.

22.5.4 Premises Towards a System of Recommendations to a Better Use of Medicines

[**Form 1**] Pharmaceutical forms that over time have crystallised into a functional typology for use and recognised by the user, and around which gestures, practices and habits of use have been consolidated, should not be replaced by other formal typologies that have, in turn, accustomed the user to sequences of actions and modes of intake that are part of the automatisms of everyday actions. Unless patients have a particular need (e.g., tablets for eye use, mostly for hospital use), capsules and tablets should be used for oral intake, the suppository for rectal use, the ovum for vaginal use, etc.

[**Form 2**] Pharmaceutical forms that by their nature do not explicitly refer to the route of administration (e.g., powder preparations, drops, nebulised substances) should indicate the route of administration on the packaging, paying attention to the fact that the adjective 'vaginal' or 'nasal' does not always make it clear whether the adjective refers to the route of administration or to the part of the body on which the

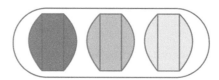

Fig. 22.3 Example of a medicine consisting of a transparent capsule containing three tablets. There is no indication in the package leaflet that the capsule can be opened to swallow the three tablets separately. The transparency, however, in allowing a glimpse of the three tablets contained (a pharmaceutical form that we are used to swallowing individually), constitutes a permission/incentive to open the capsule to take the three tablets one at a time

medicine will act (e.g., *Granules for external genital skin solution—do not ingest—* is more effective than *Granules for vaginal solution*).

[Shape 3] The good practice of placing distinctive information directly on the surface of the medicine should be extended as far as possible. Making medicines distinguishable from others helps provide information essential to the user. Therefore, wherever possible, it is recommended that the surface of tablets or capsules be marked with signs (e.g., company logo, name of the medicine or its abbreviation/symbol/acronym or pictogram of the organ) and/or information (e.g., dosage of the tablet or capsules; pre-breakage sign; pictogram prohibiting opening of the capsule, etc.). This information is already present in many medicines (Fig. 22.4).

[Shape 4] Using colour as an element of medicine identification is recommended. Where possible, the same colour could be used to indicate the surface of the medicine and the secondary packaging containing it. This is particularly useful for patients undergoing polypharmacy: the colour association allows easy tracing of the secondary packaging and accompanying information once the medicine has been unpacked for consumption (Fig. 22.5).

[Shape 5] It is recommended that the shape and size of the tablet/capsule should always be drawn on the secondary packaging, to avoid patients with swallowing difficulties purchasing medicines they cannot take.

[Form 6] At the prescribing stage, it is recommended that the physician verifies patients' ability to take solid oral medicines, to guide them towards using other bioequivalent pharmaceutical forms if necessary.

[Form 7] It is recommended to indicate in the package leaflet, next to the directions for use prohibiting tablet breakage or fragmentation, alternative pharmaceutical forms (e.g. syrup, granules, drops) commercially available for that active ingredient as a substitute for the solid form. The indication is intended to prevent patients with swallowing problems or with a need to customise the dosage of the medicine from deciding to fragment the medicine despite the prohibition and being supported by information on accessible alternatives of choice. This good practice is already in use in the package leaflets of some pharmaceutical companies.

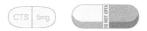

Fig. 22.4 Left, marks on the tablet indicating the active ingredient contained and the dosage. The tablet also bears a break line, indicating the possibility of breaking the medicine. The elongated shape helps in this operation. On the right, capsules with the prohibition to open the capsule clearly marked on the surface

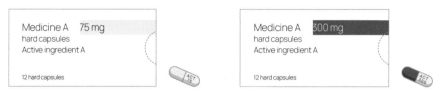

Fig. 22.5 Colour coherence between secondary packaging and medicine

[Form 8] When dispensing oral solid forms of medicines for the first time, it is recommended that the pharmacist provide the patient with information on the size of the tablet/capsule and on the possibility or impossibility of breaking/crushing the medicine. It is recommended that the pharmacist check with the patients about the prescribed dosage and the possible need for personalised dosage. In this case, the pharmacist should direct the patients towards the correct method of use.

[Form 9] If it is necessary to crush the medicine, and this is permitted, it is recommended that patients wash their hands thoroughly before and after handling. It is also recommended to wash the tools (e.g. cutting board, knife, etc.) used to split the tablet so that other people do not come across the active substance. The package leaflet should include these recommendations.

[Shape 10] In the case of a divisible tablet, the pre-break line or cross should be stamped on the tablet. Studies show that dividing tablets results in a weight loss of the medicine (e.g., active substance plus excipients) of about 15% compared to the weight of the whole weighed tablet. The change in dose is more significant in the case of tablets without a dividing line (Abrate et al. 2016, p. 21).

[Shape 11] It is recommended not to characterise the surface of tablets that cannot be split with pre-break lines or crosses. These 'marks-signs' are an explicit 'permission' to fragment the medicine and should not be used in tablets that must be swallowed.

[Shape 12] If it is necessary to break the medicine and this is permitted, it is recommended that this be done following the breaking line, if present.

[Shape 13] It is recommended to avoid the oblong shape in oral medicines for which fragmentation is highly undesirable. Indeed, due to its greater prehensibility, the elongated shape facilitates tablet breakage. In such cases, lenticular forms with a double convex surface are preferred, discouraging division because they are less manageable and challenging to fragment with cutting instruments (Fig. 22.6).

22 Compendium: Step Toward Design-Oriented Practices in the Pharma Industry...

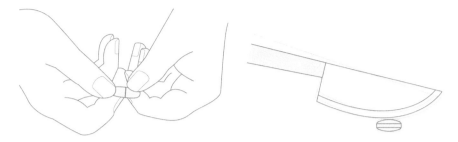

Fig. 22.6 The shapes of the tablets favour or inhibit their manipulability

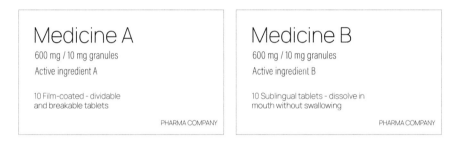

Fig. 22.7 In addition to the description of the characteristics of the medicine (film-coated or gastro-resistant), indications concerning the handling of the medicine and the correct way to take it have been added

[Form 14] Storage Instructions: Package leaflets, especially for oral solid forms, should include specific instructions on how to store the medicine once removed from its primary packaging.

[Form 15] It is recommended that instructions for use accompany devices for cutting and/or crushing tablets and contain, as a minimum, the following indications for the user: check the medicine handling conditions before using the instrument, always remove medicine residues after use, especially if more than one patient uses the tool. In the case of devices containing and storing tablets, the patient should constantly be reminded to inquire about the stability conditions of the medicine outside the packaging.

[Form 16] In secondary packaging, besides the pharmaceutical form and the description of its coating, it is recommended to explicitly indicate what the user can or cannot do regarding handling the pharmaceutical form. Thus, the suggested description is 'Film-coated tablets, dividable and crushable' or 'Film-coated tablets, dividable but not crushable' or 'Sublingual tablets, dissolve in the mouth without ingesting' etc. (Fig. 22.7).

[Form 17] In the case of sublingual tablets, it is recommended to inform the user of the correct way to take them, indicating that the tablet should not be ingested to prevent the active ingredient from losing its efficacy.

22.6 Primary Packaging

As discussed in Chap. 16, the primary packaging is significantly affected by usability issues. It serves the dual purpose of storing and dispensing medicine while playing a crucial role in enhancing recognizability between the outer packaging and the medicine itself. It is precisely because primary packaging has important functional aspects that sometimes monitoring seemingly negligible details defines its quality. In this volume, we have dealt with one type of primary packaging: the blister for tablets or capsules. During our research, we found several problems perceived by users when dealing with the primary packaging of medicines. Sometimes, the discomfort is due to formal details, upon which it is easy to intervene to improve the usability of the medicine and promote better adherence to therapy. Before delving into the specifics of the blister pack's shape, let us review the recurrent problems encountered:

- the corners of the flap of plastic packages of ointments or single-dose vials are often sharp. For this reason, companies receive reports and complaints from users. Today, many examples on the market of products have paid more attention to this detail by rounding off the sharp edges. As we will discuss later, this is also a problem in the production of blister packs (Fig. 22.8).
- the shape of eye drops vials, due to their size and the pressure required for use, are not always user-friendly. Some packages feature a container with a slightly flattened shape on two sides to ease grip and pressure actions (Fig. 22.9);
- the single dose of suppositories packaged in strips is never easy to open. It is challenging due to a lack of a clear 'invitation to use' and because, in some packages, the opening is on the nose-tip side, whereas use requires the suppository to be grasped from the flat side. A thoughtful redesign does not only place the single-dose opening on the underside of the suppository to facilitate proper grip and use. Still, it emphasises the elements that enable opening, making the scissors unnecessary and designing 'prehensile' opening flaps (Fig. 22.10);
- some devices combine two functions (e.g., the opening movement of the device also activates the dose refill function); these should be redesigned because the action of opening and closing, repeated several times by the patient, induces to a dispersion of the medicine (e.g., this happens in some powder inhalers for broncho-obstructive diseases);

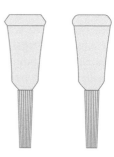

Fig. 22.8 Example of a micro-design intervention to promote user usability of the medicine

Fig. 22.9 Example of a micro-design on the shape of the eyedrops vial to favour prehensibility and make it easier to exert pressure to get the drops out. The shape of the elongated cap and its facets also better the grip

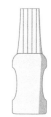

Fig. 22.10 Example of a micro-design intervention on the shape of the suppository strip to ease opening. The opening side is placed at the base of the suppository, i.e. at the point where the suppository is gripped, and the two opening tabs are not overlap-ping but separated (a project by C. Motta, A. Rocca, M. Pasquini, S. Papisca, F. Sergi, H. Zuang, School of Design, Politecnico di Milano, 2021)

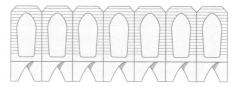

- the tab on the caps of tubular containers should extend beyond the contact surface to facilitate opening with the thumb (Fig. 22.11);
- it is helpful to draw a 'tear-off invitation' to facilitate and direct the opening tear on aluminium or multilayer pouches containing single-dose medicines (e.g. eye drops) or powdered medicines. In the absence of this invitation, the user is forced to use scissors or, in the act of tearing, may end up breaking the entire aluminium pack, which is helpful for the correct storage of the medicine (Fig. 22.12);
- the legibility of information on single-dose packs is always an issue. For example, in the case of eye drops, some shapes, as opposed to others, favour the legibility of the information through an information palette that simultaneously improves the prehensibility of the object (Fig. 22.13).

Keeping with the example of single-dose eye drops, recommendations to promote product usability should include:

- a design focus on allowing the patient, in case of infection, not to use the same vial for the right and left eye;
- a design focus on opening methods. For example, those that involve twisting the cap around and the consequent breaking of the protective material, leaving a residue of indistinguishable material on the neck part, which can injure the eye during the administration of the eyedrops;
- a design focus on the gestures performed by the user. For example, opening and using the inverted cap to close the container and protect the remaining eye drops is a simple gesture but, on the contrary, not intuitive;
- a design focus on the shape of the flap at the base of the vial, which can injure the user and must be rounded;

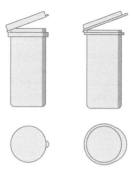

Fig. 22.11 Example of a micro-design that facilitates the thumb lever action when opening

Fig. 22.12 Example of a micro-design to indicate to the user the 'tear-off' opening point of the package. The point should be placed on the left to accommodate the gestures that are normally made by the user

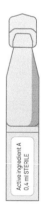

Fig. 22.13 Example of a design improvement in single-dose eye drops containers already on the market. The shape allows easier prehension of the vial and easier recognition of the medicine due to the information that can be printed on the flat surface

- a design focus on the possibility of re-closing the vial in the presence of medicine residues. Single-dose eye drops currently on sale can be resealed and re-used, and single-dose eye drops that, once opened, can no longer be resealed.

However, there is no rigorous logic linking this possibility or impossibility to the characteristics of the medicine. For example, it is recommended that single-dose antibiotic eye drops should not be resealed and, therefore, re-used. This is because, during use, any contact with the eye could contaminate the remaining contents.

Re-closing for eye drops without preservatives should not be permitted because the opening could affect the stability of the active ingredient.

These are examples, certainly not exhaustive, allowing us to focus on the many possible micro-improvements that can be obtained by redesigning several formal details of the primary packaging for better usability.

In addition to usability, the primary packaging assumes, in a privileged way, the functions of preserving and protecting the medicine. In this regard, it is helpful to recommend that:

- the packaging format of medicines (e.g. ointments, eye drops, syrups and drops) that, once opened, have a short shelf life (15 days to 1 month), should be adapted to the most common therapeutic needs, avoiding the marketing of overdosed packages that force large quantities of medicine to be thrown away;
- the expiry date is placed on the part of the primary packaging, making it visible to the user until the last dose of medicine's intake, compatible with the machinability of the product. In this respect, a problem arises with ointments in aluminium tubes: the expiry date is placed on the closure flap, and it is the user's habit to roll up the tube while consuming the ointment. The solution of printing on the tube is preferable, taking care to move the expiry date as close as possible to the neck of the tube, making this information visible until the end (Fig. 22.14);
- the primary packaging should always display the legally prescribed expiry date, but it would also be helpful to include the expiry date of the product after first opening (see next section on secondary packaging);
- if the medicine has special storage requirements, these must also be indicated on the primary packaging, even if they are already present on the secondary packaging.

Communication aspects are often neglected in the design of the primary packaging, almost entirely relying on the secondary packaging and the package leaflet.

In contrast, as we pointed out in the case of expiry date information, this is most effective if placed (even repeatedly, if necessary) as close to the 'moment of use' as possible. On secondary packaging, finding information on the expiry date and the correct medicine storage is helpful. Information should be available to the user from the moment of purchase, regardless of whether the pack is opened.

The same information, however, is also helpful on the primary packaging because:

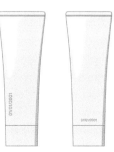

Fig. 22.14 The expiry date has been moved from the fin to the body of the tube for greater legibility

- the user does not always keep the secondary packaging after the first use of the medicine (especially in some types of packaging, such as ointments);
- storage conditions change after opening the primary pack, and it is useful to provide this information to the patient visibly and at the appropriate time.

'Mapping' (Norman 1997) represents one of the principles underpinning the ease of use of products. This term refers to the study of the spatial location of signals, command, and control devices (e.g. buttons, switches, etc.) and activators of functions, at points that have a logical (also temporal) connection with the desired effect.

If placed in proximity to the action, a use indicator enters the users' field of vision just as they are about to act and can thus direct the gesture effectively.

In the world of medicines, a positive example is the pictogram indicating the gesture of pressing and twisting, placed directly on the 'childproof' cap of a syrup. Or, in the case of smaller caps such as those of drops, where this signal may not be visible, this same indication has, in some cases, been moved from the package leaflet to the two closure flaps at the top of the secondary packaging (Fig. 22.15).

In this regard, a digression must be made concerning the still unresolved problem of 'child-proof' caps. Although these caps are difficult for children to open and sufficiently intuitive for the adult, they represent a real difficulty for the elderly patient and those with motor difficulties.

Back to the communication issues, it is useful to remember that some pharmaceutical forms (e.g., drops or powder preparations) do not have a close and intuitive relationship with the intake route.

In such cases, it is useful to include the usage instructions in a clear and comprehensible manner on the primary packaging, as well as on the secondary packaging and package leaflet (when these are required by law), accompanying the verbal instructions with illustrative forms whenever possible.

Lastly, let us consider an 'implicit' communication aspect which we have already developed in Sect. 22.4 of this chapter and to which we will return later in the section on blister packs (see Sect. 22.5.1), mentioned here in connection with the other types of packaging. It concerns the colours co-ordination between the outer and inner packaging to facilitate the recognisability of medicines. In the case of oral

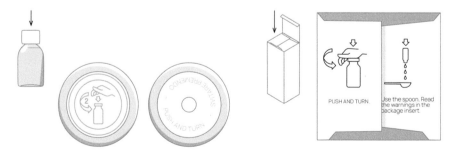

Fig. 22.15 Example of visual information displayed near the point where the user is to perform the action

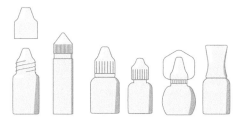

Fig. 22.16 Eye drops bottles with different shapes of container and cap can be a valuable aid in recognising medicine in the case of low vision

solid forms, such coordination should also concern the colour appearance of the surface of the medicinal product itself: once removed from the primary packaging, it no longer has any 'immediate' visual connection with it. In the case of eye drops, ointments, syrups, the recommendation is to coordinate the primary packaging with the colour of the outer packaging (e.g. line, band, coloured box, etc.). In the case of eye drops, it is recommended to co-ordinate the colour of the eye drop cap with the colours of the secondary packaging, as the possibility of these products being used by visually impaired patients is high. The shape of the eye drops bottle, as well as that of the cap, are also important elements for visually impaired users. In these products, it is useful to support the visual recognition and distinction of medicines with tactile feedback. In this case, a formal diversification of the container and closure elements is recommended (Fig. 22.16).

22.6.1 Primary Pack: Blister Pack

In Chap. 16, we examined the blister pack, a prevalent form of packaging, particularly popular in Europe where capsules, confections, and tablets are sold in packages that preserve and separate them individually. This type of primary packaging can be composed of a thermoformed sheet of thin plastic material, heat-sealed with an aluminium film, or consist of two aluminium sheets. In the first case, the medicines can be extracted by finger pressure on the part of the alveolus containing the pill; in the second case, the opening can be done by pressure or, in the case of the so-called 'peelable' forms, the pill chamber is uncovered by 'dragging' a flap of aluminium foil.

For plastic blisters, the foil may be transparent or opaque, while aluminium-aluminium blisters are always opaque. In some cases, the characteristics of the medicine guide the company to select transparent or opaque packaging or a squeezable or peelable form. In other cases, this choice aims to make the blister 'child-proof', as opacity and a 'peelable' opening are less attractive and more difficult for a child to open.

Whether a plastic/aluminium blister or an aluminium/aluminium blister, the bottom foil—made of aluminium—constitutes the sealing element of the pack and the 'page' containing all information about the medicine, the manufacturer, and the expiry date.

In the chapter on primary packaging, our focus shifted to the extent to which the patient's experience of use can be influenced by the signs and formal elements that characterise it, even though most of them are conceived as a function of the production process and not of the patient. We focused on the alveoli's shape and rhythm, the 'unit of measurement' implicit in this type of packaging, and the linear order that seems to support the temporal logic that oversees the treatment process. Moreover, we verified how observing users' behaviour contradicts the assumptions of simplicity and ease of use that this type of packaging seems to invoke.

In particular:

- The Blister pack does not appear simple, easy, and quick to open for those whose gestures of grip and pressure are missing. Difficulties in opening are influenced by the following:

  – the size of the medicine;
  – the consistency of the medicine;
  – the height of the array of alveoli;
  – the presence or absence of 'grip areas' on the blister;
  – the elasticity of the aluminium foil and the resistance to pressure of the alveolus containing the medicine;
  – the difficulty of distinguishing the two different types of opening (i.e., pressure and peelable).

There is also the difficulty of preserving residual medicine fragments when prescribed doses involve customising the quantity by breaking the original unit. Furthermore, in aluminium-aluminium blister packs, there is an overall deformation of the blister after the opening of several cells, which makes the blister pack challenging to handle and store in secondary packaging.

- The Blister pack does not prove to be simple, easy, and quick in providing all necessary information in the vicinity of the medicine, even though the clarity of legislation (European Commission—Guidelines on the legibility of labelling and package leaflets of medicinal products for human use, Art. 7.1. Presentation in blister packs). This is because:

  – information about the name of the medicine, the dosage, the proprietary pharmaceutical company, and the expiration date is often sparsely distributed on the surface of the closure. In most cases, they are not present on each dose at the same time (although the regulations indicate that the information necessary to recognise the medicine must be printed on each dose);

- the integrity of the aluminium foil is decidedly short-lived: it ends as soon as use of the medicine begins. Tearing the aluminium foil removes any information;
- the practice of portioning out the blister pack, especially for external use, using scissors or pre-cut blisters, means that the patient only has the information on the cut-out part of the pack with him;
- the aluminium surface is reflective and, in the case of visually impaired patients, it is not always easy to read the information on this surface;
- the expiry date is sometimes only printed on the edge of the blister pack. It is rarely present on the individual doses in the blister pack. For example, medicines for occasional use (e.g. painkillers) may remain in the wallet or purse for some time: it is possible that the patient no longer recognises the medicine, and the expiry date is uncertain.

- The Blister packs are not simple, easy, and quick to display and allow control of the doses taken and those still in the packaging. For example, in aluminium-aluminium blister packs and those using opaque plastic, it is not easy to identify the medicine contained, doses already taken, and those still available. The function as a unit of measurement, as a calendar, and as an indicator of whether the proper medicine intake, since:

  - the number of doses contained in the individual blister pack often bears no relation to the patient's therapy;
  - the start of therapy may occur on any day of the week, and this does not make it easy to count doses taken and doses forgotten;
  - there is no space on the secondary packaging or on the blister pack itself where the user can note the day of the start of therapy;
  - there is rarely a sequence order on the blister pack, which facilitates checking the correspondence between days and medicines taken.

22.6.2 Premises Towards a System of Recommendations to Improve Primary Packaging: Blister Packs for Oral Solid Forms

[Blister 1] The blister packs available in the market exhibit a wide range of configurations for medicine placement, and the separability of individual doses varies significantly. On the market, blisters can be found with doses without pre-cuts, with doses that can be separated by pre-cuts, with doses that can only be separated with scissors, with doses arranged in dense succession or in irregular geometries, not allowing the separation of individual doses from the blister without affecting the integrity of the cell. However, a close correlation does not always exist between the portionability permitted or prevented by the blister design and the characteristics of the medicine contained. In the case of medicines with a high risk of generating side effects, not only should the fractionability of the blister be prevented by formal precautions (e.g. by playing on the misaligned positioning of the alveoli), but the entire packaging design should be designed so as not to allow the primary, secondary and package leaflet packs to break apart (see Chap. 19). Some commercial medicines are designed precisely for this purpose. The case of over-the-counter medicines or those for occasional use is different, for which there should be the possibility of reducing the traditional blister to a pocket packaging, allowing the user to carry all the information necessary to recognise the medicine even at a distance.

[**Blister 2**] In the case of pre-cut blister packaging, particularly suitable for portioning individual doses and allowing for outdoor use, it is recommended to ensure that the information necessary for the patient to identify the medicine and its correct intake is provided. This can be achieved by marking each blister with the medicine's identification information, including the expiry date. Or by designing the distribution of information so that there is always data or parts of data on each dose that make the medicine recognisable even without secondary packaging. Or by designing an outdoor packaging that expressly covers this requirement. Besides, current legislation already provides this indication.

[**Blister 3**] It is recommended to indicate the method of storage of the medicine clearly. In the case of oral solid forms, removing the medicine from the packaging often takes place well before the intake. The user should be informed if this behaviour compromises the stability of the medicine and how long it may lie unpackaged.

[**Blister 4**] The user should be warned not to keep tablets with different active ingredients in contact with each other for long periods after unpacking.

[**Blister 5**] In pre-cut blister packs, it should be noted that the aluminium foil is prone to easy breakage, which may occur through accidental contact (e.g. with objects contained in the pouch such as pens, keys, etc.). In the case of blister packs for outdoor use, the design of a protection system that prevents accidental breakage of the aluminium foil is recommended.

[**Blister 6**] In pre-cut blister packs, it is recommended that, after portioning, no sharp sides or corners are formed for individual doses that could injure the user. It is recommended that these connection parts be redesigned so that all sides are rounded when dividing into individual doses (Fig. 22.17).

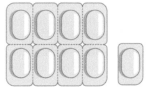

Fig. 22.17 Example of a micro design intervention aimed at reducing the sharp sides of the blister and individual portions

[Blister 7] Blister cells that are too close together can cause multiple openings even if pressure is directed on a single pocket. It is recommended to design the correct cell spacing to avoid this problem.

[Blister 8] Therapy may involve using parts of tablets, rather than the entire dose. The patients usually place the remaining portion in the empty blister pack without a secure closure method, or in other ways, such as using food film, compromising the medicine recognisability. It is advisable to encourage innovation in blister packs to allow proper storage of the medicine fragments in the case of dosage regimes involving customised use instead of full dose.

[Blister 9] It is recommended to design tabs that are easy to grasp with the fingers to facilitate blister opening actions and allow the patient to distinguish between opening modes (e.g., pressing or peeling). It is also recommended to make affordance marks clearly visible (e.g., using a glossy/opaque contrast, as is already the case in some pharmaceutical company products) (Fig. 22.18).

[Blister 10] It is recommended that a prehension area be provided in the blister pack to facilitate the opening of the alveoli. Considering the numerous cases where some cells are not filled with tablets, it is recommended to take advantage of this to design a more ergonomic blister. In any case, favouring one side with generous margins is advisable to facilitate prehension and include markings that make the actions clear to the user (Fig. 22.19).

[Blister 11] Blister packs, especially aluminium-aluminium, are soft and deform during use. It is recommended to limit their size by favouring more blisters per pack, with a reduced number of tablets per blister (Fig. 22.20).

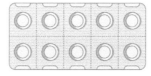

Fig. 22.18 Example of a micro-design intervention that makes it easier for the user to open the cell by signalling with glossy/opaque contrast the tabs that the user must grasp and drag

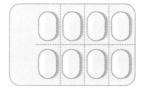

Fig. 22.19 Example of micro-design intervention to ensure an easy grip of the blister for the user to facilitate opening

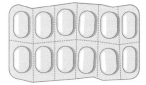 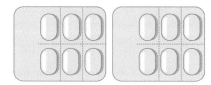

Fig. 22.20 In aluminium/aluminium blisters, it is preferable to have a small size to prevent the blister from bending and no longer being placed in its packaging

[Blister 12] The expiry date printed on one side of the blister according to the standards must be visible to the user. To this end, it is recommended to interrupt the knurling of the plastic foil in the area where the date is printed to avoid visual interference. For the same purpose, it is helpful to interrupt the lettering on the aluminium foil so that it does not overlap with the expiry date.

[Blister 13] Preferably print the expiry date on aluminum foil for better visibility. The visual quality is superior to the result of printing on plastic foil.

[Blister 14] Use matt-coated aluminium foil for the surface of the blister closure whenever possible. This treatment, already used by some pharmaceutical companies, makes it possible to print and make the data visible.

[Blister 15] Medicines whose intake follows a dosage schedule that varies radically according to the pathology and presents a severe risk of error (e.g., the medicine containing the active ingredient Methotrexate sodium salt), must be placed in separate packs, specifically dedicated to each of the two different modes of intake.

[Blister 16] The arrangement of alveoli in the blister pack—such as medicines used in weekly or monthly treatment regimens—should be spaced to suggest the intervals at which they are taken. This aligns with patient perceptions, as observed, where the density of cells in the blister pack is correlated with the frequency of intake. Some blister packs are already designed following this principle, enhancing patient understanding and adherence to the prescribed treatment schedule (Fig. 22.21).

[Blister 17] Blister packaging establishes a predetermined quantity of dispensed medicine doses. In the context of medications intended for specific and temporary use, such as antibiotics, this predetermined quantity often does not align with the doctor's prescribed doses. The packages available for purchase thus come with pre-assigned doses, introducing an inherent limitation as they are not tailored to individual requirements. To address potential surpluses, the redesign of blister packs should incorporate a foundational unit, termed a 'base pack', supplemented by modular packs. These modular packs would contain additional doses necessary to fulfil the complete treatment plan following medical guidelines. This concept aligns with existing legislation, specifically the European Medicines Agency's guideline on the packaging information of authorized medicinal products for human use

22 Compendium: Step Toward Design-Oriented Practices in the Pharma Industry… 473

Fig. 22.21 The number of tablets in a blister and their spacing become a visual indication for the user of the frequency of use of the medicine. The blister shown is of an Alendronic Acid medicine that is taken weekly. The blister has a monthly duration

(EMA 2011). In Section C, it states: *"The appropriate range of pack sizes should be chosen in accordance with the duration(s) of treatment and in accordance with the posology in the summary of product characteristics, and not in accordance with local traditions or prescription habits"*. Various pack sizes could be offered, including one for a short course of treatment and a foundational pack for initial prescribed doses, complemented by modular packs for additional doses as needed.

[Blister 18] To support the patient in verifying the correct medicine intake, it is recommended to mark the blister pack with an initial sign to be placed on the first alveolus used. In the absence of a formal solution, it is helpful to recommend that the patient mark the date of the first opening on the pack. Similar precautions already exist in several medicines, including contraceptive pills.

[Blister 19] It is always recommended to support the patient in following an orderly sequence when opening blister packs and use one blister pack all the way through before starting to open subsequent blister packs. The suggestion of the sequence of intake is already present in several medicines, including contraceptive pills, and makes it easier to check whether the therapy has been taken without interruption.

[Blister 20] Almost no blister packs are designed with the idea that the week is, in fact, the time to check our daily fulfilments/failures. The cells that make up the blister rows, or the blisters themselves, hardly ever correspond to the number seven (e.g., the number of days in the week). Particularly in therapies with a fixed dose of a single tablet per day, to facilitate the verification of the correct intake of the medicine, it is recommended to design the blister so that it corresponds to the days of the week.

[Blister 21] In the case of initiating a new non-urgent therapy, it is good practice to suggest that the patient start the first intake on Monday to facilitate the monitoring of the medicine intake.

[Blister 22] Where technically possible, it is recommended to help the user monitor the amount of medicine doses remaining using devices, including graphic ones, reminding the patients of the need to prescribe and purchase new packs (Fig. 22.22).

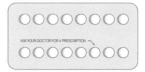

Fig. 22.22 Example of a micro design intervention to remind the patient to make the prescription

These recommendations aim to address the challenges identified in the use of blister packs and improve their functionality for both patients and healthcare providers.

The packaging of contraceptive pills serves as a noteworthy example of effective design, incorporating features such as a therapy timetable, a visual timeline guiding the patient on pill direction, and the initiation day of the therapy.

The contraceptive pill case is an example of a good packaging design which considers employing certain formal and communicative expedients, many problems of memory of use encountered by every user in the management of therapy.

These expedients could easily be applied to the packaging of all those medicines that, regardless of the physical characteristics of the patient (e.g., gender, age, body weight, etc.) and the severity of the pathology, need to be taken according to a fixed dosage (e.g., one tablet per day).

22.7 Secondary Packaging: Labelling

What users commonly refer to as "the little box" is, in fact, a complex system that serves multiple functions beyond containment. It fulfils important roles in information function, along with the package leaflet and the primary packaging.

Among the various functions associated with packaging—such as preserving and protecting during transport, storage, display, and sale; shaping the contents; allowing and managing the access to contents through openings and closures; making the product recognizable; and informing—the most crucial are undoubtedly linked to ease of recognition, identification, and distinction. These functions significantly impact the pharmacist's choice of medicine during the dispensing process, where informed choices must be made. Simultaneously, the outer packaging is of great importance to the patient during the purchase and pre-opening phases.

The external packaging must provide clear information on the contents, complying with current legislation. This legislation refers to these information elements as 'labelling,' covering all product characteristics 'placed on the market' (Directive 2001/83/EC of the European Parliament and of the Council of 6 November 2001 on the Community code relating to medicinal products for human use). The legislation designates these information elements as 'labelling' (*25. Labelling: Information on the immediate or outer packaging*). These elements describe all the characteristics of the product 'placed on the market' (this is the legal definition) and attest to the authorization process. They are:

- Name of the medicinal product: may be an invented name or a scientific name;
- Name of one or more active ingredients;
- List of excipients: Includes excipients with known action or effect; for injectable products or eye drops, all excipients must be listed (visibility is not further specified in the standard);
- Dosage: corresponds to the proportion of the active substance (or several active substances) per unit of volume or weight. Indicated by a number and a unit of measurement for each active substance;
- Pharmaceutical form: expressed according to standard European designations (e.g., 'film-coated tablets' or 'capsules');
- Method of administration: provides information on the method of use and, if necessary, the route of administration;
- Dosage form: expressed by weight (e.g., ointments), nominal volume (e.g., drops), or the number of units (e.g., capsules);
- User Indication: Information indicating whether a medicine is intended for infants, children, or adults;
- Marketing authorisation number: states and allows verification of whether a preparation has been authorized as a medicinal product by the authorities;
- Batch name or date of manufacture: allows the traceability of medicinal products placed on the market belonging to the same production batch;
- Pharmaceutical Company: expressed through name, company name, and address;
- Expiry date: provides information to consumers on the date by which the medicinal product can be safely used;
- Pharmaceutical Stamp for Medicines Dispensed by the SSN (National Health Service): Required for reimbursement by the National Health Service;
- Price.

The regulations mandate that secondary packaging carries a series of 'Warnings' and 'Precautions' essential for the correct and safe handling of the medicine:

- "Read the package leaflet before use";
- "Keep out of sight and reach of children";
- "Do not store the medicine above a certain temperature";
- "Do not dispose of the container in the environment after use";
- "The expiry date refers to the product in intact packaging, correctly stored";
- To be sold with a medical prescription" (for medicines requiring a medical prescription);
- For certain medicines, "Special Warnings" may be necessary. Examples include warnings restricting the use of the medicine in pregnant women, cautions about driving vehicles or operating machinery after taking the medicine, warnings related to dual treatment of the medicine, etc.

These various pieces of information, categorized by function, duration of use, and purpose of reading, serve different purposes for the two main users: the pharmacist and the patient, who, concerning the information on the secondary pack, exhibit selective interests.

22.7.1 Secondary Packaging: The Information Function During Dispensing

For the pharmacist during the dispensing phase, the clarity of multiple information elements, typically arranged on the main page of the packaging and, as per regulations, on at least three contiguous sides (European Medicines Agency 2011), is of paramount importance. Each of these information elements plays a fundamental role in unambiguously identifying the medicine to be dispensed and distinguishing it from others. Specifically, the Name of the medicine, Active ingredient, Dosage, Pharmaceutical form, and Number of doses/units per pack constitute a sort of 'Identity Card' for the medicine. Their purpose is to establish an unambiguous relationship between prescription and pharmaceutical dispensing. Furthermore, the design of the information component must ensure the communicative effectiveness of the secondary packaging (Fig. 22.23, 22.24, 22.25 and 22.26).

This ensures easy verification that what was ordered by the pharmacy corresponds to what was delivered by the supplier. It facilitates the rational organization of medicine stock in the warehouse, arrangement in drawers, and on sales shelves, and, most importantly, it ensures proper dispensing. To be easily readable, the

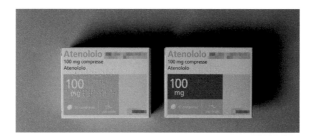

Fig. 22.23 Further example of secondary packaging that can create dispensing problems: two packs of the same medicine (active ingredient Atenolol) highly differentiated by two colour code on the dosage. The medicine, however, has the same dosage. The difference in the two packs is in the number of tablets contained. This is not sufficiently highlighted by the graphic treatment

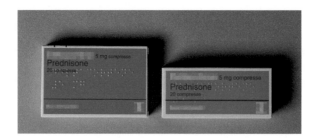

Fig. 22.24 A further element of confusion during dispensing is represented by medicines, sold by the same company, that are identical in terms of number of doses contained and active ingredient but have different packaging sizes

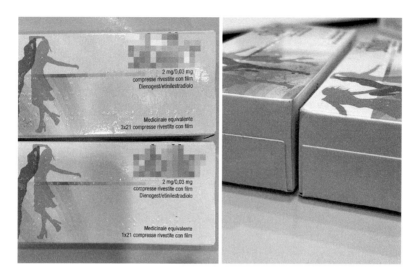

Fig. 22.25 Examples of secondary packaging that can create dispensing problems: two packs of the same medicine (active ingredient Dienogest/etinilestradiolo), with no colour difference, but only an imperceptible difference in thickness. These two packaging contains a different number of blisters of 21 pills each

labelling information must incorporate careful considerations for the choice of font(s), the font size for each piece of information, the hierarchical arrangement of elements on the page, and the logical relationship or complementarity between two or more information elements, among other factors.

The expiry date serves the pharmacist as a useful element for planning and verifying how long a medicine will remain in the pharmacy's stock. It aids in managing correct stock rotation and imposes restrictions or bans on dispensing medicine too close to its 'end of life' date.

Additional data, present in the labelling, are not used during dispensing. Instead, they serve specific circumstances, such as certifying the completion of the 'placing on the market' procedure and addressing situations like the need to withdraw a production batch by the Ministry of Health.

Certain elements, such as the sticker marking, are strictly functional for administrative procedures overseeing the economics of the medicine. They contribute to serialisation, ensuring traceability for anti-counterfeiting purposes, and they play a role in defining a future bi-univocal correspondence (according to evolving technological experiments) between the prescribed and dispensed medicine.

In accordance with current legislation, the secondary pack also carries 'Warnings and Precautions'. While not primarily intended for the pharmacist, they provide indications on correct storage temperature. Additionally, information on excipients and 'Special Warnings' may be useful for patient counselling.

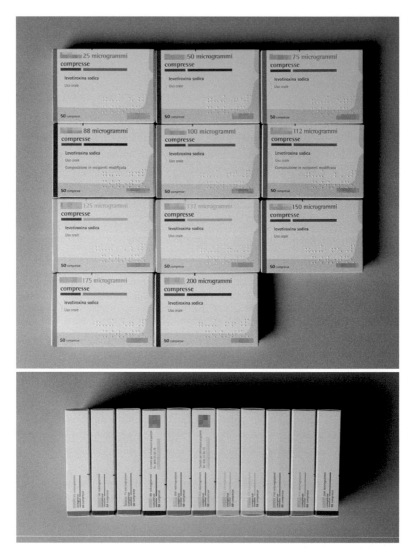

Fig. 22.26 A final example of secondary packaging that can create dispensing problems: a medicine available in multiple dosages, which is difficult to recognise with the help of the colour code. Below, the view presented to the pharmacist when choosing between different dosages, during dispensing

22.7.2 Secondary Packaging: The Information Function During Use

As seen above, in the context of the pharmacy, the communicative purpose of the packaging is paramount. Once the medicine enters the patient's sphere of use, the packaging fully and tangibly manifests all its functional prerogatives (e.g. containing, preserving, facilitating access to the contents, dosing, informing, etc.); moreover, the information apparatus itself, and even how it is "displayed on the page", assume a different utility concerning the specific needs of those who dispense the medicine. As we pointed out at the beginning of this chapter, the information necessary for the correct identification of a medicine is hyper-normed, as are certain principles of a hierarchical arrangement of the information on the different sides of the package, as well as which information must necessarily be present on the main page of the package and, according to what logic, some of it must be close together to create connections of meaning.

However, although the regulatory repertoire has been enriched with Guidelines and Recommendations, there are still many gaps in the effectiveness of the information elements that support the patient's correct use of medicine.

Several elements contribute to these considerations, which it is useful to summarise (for a detailed discussion, see Chap. 17):

- For the patient, the name of the medicine holds significance, especially on a visual level, aiding in remembering when to take it. Among the names assigned to medicines, references to the time of intake, such as 'the morning one' or 'the noon one,' are common. However, patients often struggle to recall details about the pathology, organ, or the reason for taking the medicine, particularly those on polypharmacy or using medicines temporarily or occasionally.
- For the patient, distinguishing one medicine from another is less about 'registry' elements and more about overall graphic elements perceived *at a glance*. This recognition approach becomes challenging when the patient has medicines from the same pharmaceutical company in their therapy. Graphic similarity due to the visual identity of the brand can easily lead to mistakes in exchanging medicines. Fortunately, this occurrence is not so common and depends on the quantity of medicines and the number from the same pharmaceutical company.
- For the patient, especially in polypharmacy, the organization according to a set sequence or subdivision into recipients arranged by the user or caregiver aids in recognising medicines. Once medicines are organized based on intake times, the visual identity of the medicine becomes less crucial, and routine gestures take over (see Chap. 17).
- For the patient, the information function of secondary packaging is short-lived. Reading information on the outer packaging, including warnings, recommendations, and prescriptive elements, occurs immediately before opening the package and is done almost exclusively after the first purchase. Subsequently, the package leaflet takes over, and patients are unlikely to refer to the secondary pack for specific information.

- Not only is the information short-lived, but the secondary packaging itself is often discarded by users, who retain only the primary pack, particularly with blister tablets.
- As noted in Chap. 17, many patients do not thoroughly read the 'labelling' data on the medicine's secondary packaging, except when repurchasing. Doctors need to focus on details such as the name of the medicine, pharmaceutical form, dosage, and number of doses per pack. Patients often overlook other elements of the labelling, including the active ingredient. The dosage becomes crucial only when the patient has two different dosages of the same medicine in therapy. Conversely, this information takes a back seat, especially during hospital admission or specialist visits, where patients may not have their therapy data.
- It is essential to consider that the verification of correspondence between the prescribed medication and what was dispensed by the pharmacist is challenging for patients due to the lack of a prescription record (this verification requires the comparison of all medicine data). If the prescription was made by a specialist or hospital doctor and re-transcribed by the family doctor, patients would need to reread documentation from the visit or hospitalization to verify correspondence. This rarely happens because of the high tendency to archive these documents for safekeeping. Additionally, therapy data are included in documents containing reports of hospitalization, descriptions of the pathology, examinations, etc. This information has different 'times of use' and 'occasions of use' and should be made autonomous. Finally, the failure to check that the prescription corresponds to the therapy purchased also depends on the patient's cultural attitudes, with many considering it a remote possibility for errors to occur between the prescription, re-transcription, and dispensation phases.
- The extent to which patients disregard the possibility of errors in the prescription and dispensing phases is highlighted by an exercise involving 160 students from the B.Sc. in Industrial Product Design. They were tasked with analysing the legibility of information on the secondary packaging of certain medicines, along with corresponding prescriptions provided by the teaching staff. In the exercise, despite alterations to some data in the prescriptions given by the teaching staff, only 32 out of 160 students read the prescription. Of these 32, only 1 student detected discrepancies between the data on the prescription and the dispensed medicine. This exercise reflects a behavior observed frequently—patients generally do not habitually read prescriptions. This may be because patients view prescriptions as a communication tool between the doctor and pharmacist, not directly involving them. Additionally, patients often trust the doctor's work to the extent that they do not consider errors a plausible occurrence in the prescription or dispensing phase.

The communicative and informative function of secondary packaging has gained significance due to anti-tampering legislation mandating the sale of sealed packages without inspection (European Parliament, Directive 2011/62/EU). It is required that the user has much more information than before. Some of this is necessary to anticipate the contents usually in the packaging leaflet.

In addition to the medicine's 'master data', the packaging also contains several textual propositions with prescriptive value (e.g., warnings, recommendations, etc.). The patient rarely reads this information and, even when read, its prescriptive meaning is not necessarily grasped, probably because it is written in an insufficiently persuasive or normative manner. Again, it may be misunderstood for several reasons: it is not sufficiently explicit, or misplaced concerning the action to be performed, or it presupposes knowledge the patient does not always possess, or it is expressed in a technical language inaccessible to those.

Factors contributing to the diminished effectiveness of this information, as discussed in Chap. 17, include:

- A lack in their precise positioning. Warnings are sometimes positioned on the back or minor sides of the medicine pack, contrary to guidelines recommending placement on the main sides. This discrepancy may contribute to confusion and medication errors; [2]
- Absence of grouping by 'areas of meaning' or priority 'time of use,' resulting in haphazard listing, mixing storage indications with warnings on precautions for use;
- Frequent lack of proper spacing between warnings, hindering their individual significance; in some medicines, the different warnings are even written as if they were a whole text;
- Varied use of bold type, capital letters, and colour to create information hierarchy, differing among companies. Even the 'special warnings' do not have a 'dedicated space' and a graphic mode that puts them in the foreground compared to the general warnings required by law;
- The general 'warnings' required by law are repeated on all packages and have now become part of everyday use and, precisely because of this, are taken for granted and tend not to be read by the patient;
- Among these general warnings, some (e.g., the storage temperature of the medicine) contain information specific to the individual medicine. It does not stand out because it is written together with the other information. Therefore, it does not have the force necessary to indicate to the patient the correct behaviour to adopt after purchasing the medicine. If the patient does not observe the proper storage methods, the effectiveness of the medicine may be compromised even before it is used.

---

[2] The placement of warnings varies among different companies, with some choosing to position them on the rear surface or smaller sides of the medicine packaging. Notably, this practice diverges from the guidelines, such as those outlined by the European Medicines Agency (EMA) in its 4th edition guidelines of 2022. The EMA strongly advises applicants/MAHs to optimize available space to ensure crucial information about the safe use of the medicine is not only legible but also prominently featured on the principal surfaces of both the packaging and the accompanying leaflet. This emphasis on prime spaces is intended to minimize confusion and reduce the likelihood of medication errors, as outlined in EMA guidelines from 2006. For more detailed information, refer to the source document available at https://www.ema.europa.eu/en/documents/regulatory-procedural-guideline/checking-process-mock-ups-specimens-outer/immediate-labelling-package-leaflets-human-medicinal-products-centralised-procedure_en.pdf

In summary, for the pharmacist:

- The legibility of the elements constituting the medicine registry is crucial for correct dispensing;
- Warnings and prescriptive components are generally known to the pharmacist, who may not need to read them unless there are 'special warnings';
- The overall graphic image of the medicine is significant in discriminating between two different medicines, along with the name, influencing dispensing errors.

For the patient:

- Dealing with the medicine's 'master data', visual aspects of its name as well as the overall graphic appearance, are memorized and used by the patients in daily therapy management. Dosage becomes relevant only if the patient takes different dosages of the same medicine. Analytical information defining the medicine's 'registry,' including the name, dosage, pharmaceutical form, and—if the medicine is available in different formats—doses per pack, is useful during prescription renewals;
- Warnings and prescriptive components have a brief lifespan and tend not to be read carefully by the patient due to various reasons;
- Some information should be prominently placed on the secondary pack to guide or deter the purchase of the medicine, considering not all medicines are suitable for all patients.

The complexity of the use of those several information elements, necessary as a whole and in their individuality for the correct dispensing actions, for the recognition of the medicine during home therapy, for the proper prescription request for refills and the appropriate return of the data to the specialist or hospital doctor, are indicators of how much thoughtful project design is required.

Despite legislation, certain medicines still fall short of fully complying with standards and recommendations for effective visual representation (see Chap. 17).

In 2004, Adrienne Berman's article has been a cornerstone for studies addressing the analysis of dispensing errors related to poor graphic design of medicine packaging (Berman 2004). The key issues highlighted in her work include:

- Easy confusability of the names of different medicines;
- Small size and poor legibility of information;
- Insufficient emphasis on the route of administration (e.g., intravenous or intramuscular);
- Poor differentiation between normal-release and sustained-release medicines;
- Little or no use of colours to differentiate products;
- Limited or no use of colours to differentiate different dosages of the same product;
- Prevalence of company logos over product-identifying information;
- Incorrect positioning of information on the page, hindering the creation of connections of meaning between individual elements or making individual pieces of information autonomous.

Berman's article closely aligns with the timeline of Directive 2001/83/EC on the Community code related to medicinal products for human use and predates the Guideline on the readability of the labelling and package leaflet of medicinal products for human use (European Commission 2009). It anticipated many problematic issues later addressed through specific recommendations within the complex regulatory system overseeing the 'placing on the market' of medicine.

Regrettably, some of these design-related problems persist in products currently available on the market, including those in Italy. This emphasizes the ongoing need for improvements in medicine packaging to enhance patient safety and reduce dispensing errors.

22.7.3 Secondary Packaging: The Information Function of the Colour Code

The use of colour for functional purposes in the context of medicines presents a complex design challenge, warranting a comprehensive discussion. Here, we'll provide a summary of considerations, highlighting the intricacies of the problem from a design perspective.

One critical consideration is that the colour design of medicines can lead to ineffective solutions if not approached systematically beyond individual medications. A brief case study reveals key issues:

- for the same company brand, identical colours are used to identify the same dosage in medicines with different active ingredients;
- for the same trademark, different colours are used to identify the same dosage in medicines with different active ingredients;
- for the same trademark, the same colours are used to identify different dosages in medicines with different active ingredients;
- for different company brands, different colours are used to identify the same dosage in medicines with the same active ingredient.

While this summary is indicative, it underscores the discretionary use of colour, lacking a systemic perspective, even when designing the portfolio of medicines produced by the same company. This discretion significantly impacts the user experience and recognsability of the medicine. It is crucial to emphasise that the colour code serves different purposes in the pharmacist's dispensing activity compared to the patient's intake activity.

In the act of dispensing and dealing with a precise prescription, the pharmacist must identify a precise medicine and dosage from a 'population' of medicines with various active ingredients, arranged in pharmacy drawers and shelves based on multiple criteria, such as pharmaceutical form and alphabetical order.

In the act of dispensing and based on the prescription, the pharmacist must identify a precise medicine and dosage, choosing from a 'population' of medicines with different active ingredients, whose arrangement and proximity in the pharmacy drawers and shelves is guided by various criteria, including pharmaceutical form and alphabetical order. The act of choosing consists of at least two distinct stages. First, the pharmacist distinguishes the medicine from other medicines based on the active ingredient and with the help of the graphic-visual elements that characterise the packaging (including colour). Once identified, the pharmacist chooses the proper dosage (also based on colour). Thus, there is at least a double stage in the pharmacist's choice: the first stage concerns the discrimination between the different medicines (where the visual impact of the brand name, colour contrasts, typefaces, etc. play an essential role); the second stage concerns the choice between the different dosages of the same medicine prescribed within the group of medicines having the same active ingredient. In this case, the pharmacist has to choose within a homogeneous group of medicines (where visual homogeneity is mainly entrusted to the brand image), and the choice of dosage, in addition to the numerical code, generally relies on a chromatic marking which emphasises the numerical data and allows the different dosages to be discriminated by comparison.

If we analyse this process from the perspective of the patient seeking medicine, we observe that the choice is made between medicines generally organised according to personalised criteria. For example, these are criteria aimed at distinguishing the treatment of patients living in the same house, grouping medicines according to the time of intake, dividing medicines for daily use from those for occasional use, etc. The alphabetical order, defining the pharmacist's field of choice, is not respected at home. Precisely for this reason, the colour code 'operates' with different logics both in the selection of medicines and (and this is not uncommon) in the choice of different dosages of the same medicine.

The risk is that the colour switches from being a visual reinforcement to a substitute for the numerical code, especially at the time of medicine intake, where there is an interplay of factors such as superficiality and distraction, automatic and repetitive gestures, non-analytical reading of medicine details, identification of the medicine by formal names, etc.

At a glance, the colour code is 'perceived' before the numerical code and may even progressively overshadow it. However, this type of substitution presupposes that the patient has memorised the correct colour-dose association.

The most appropriate solution to address this complexity seems to design—for the colour marking indicating the dosage—a fixed association between colour code and numeric code (e.g. dosage 2.5 mg is always associated with colour code X; dosage 5 mg is always associated with colour code Y, and so on) and this association must be standardised at supra-industry level. A standardised dose-colour association generates a limited number of combinations, which are easier to 'learn' and memorise by the user, be it the pharmacist or the patient.

To date, there is a lack of in-depth research to test the behaviour of different parties (i.e., industry, pharmacist, patient) in contexts of choice defined by other criteria. Likewise, there is a lack of careful thought as to whether or not the correct choice can be favoured, using contrasting colours, increasing colour scales as the dosage increases, etc.

22.7.4 Secondary Packaging: The Information Function of the Colour Code

As we have seen, the information elements constituting the 'registry' of a medicine, crucial for its unique identification, are numerous, and each must be prominently featured. Underestimating any one of these elements could lead to medicine mix-ups during dispensing or errors during intake. The multitude of active ingredients, varied dosages for each active ingredient, multiple pharmaceutical forms for the same active ingredient, and diverse doses per packet create a range of combinations in the pharmaceutical formulary, increasing the risk of errors.

To enhance the safety of the dispensing activity, which involves choosing between products with a high degree of similarity (even when not specific to LASA medicines), it is crucial to incorporate the following features during the design stage:

- principles of visual hierarchization: prioritize information elements based on their significance;
- creation of relationships: establish relationships between elements through proximity, colour, or other graphic means (e.g., the relationship between dosage and active ingredient);
- information redundancy: repeat essential information not only as required by law on several sides of the pack but also across the secondary pack, primary pack, and package leaflet. This redundancy ensures that critical information is emphasized and available through multiple sources.

The design of the text, both in verbal expression and visual translation, should focus on providing clear information for pharmacists to easily distinguish between different medicines during dispensing and for users to find the necessary information before purchase, after purchase and before use, during use, and at the end of the pack's life cycle.

The information on secondary packaging regarding the disposal of medicines is insufficient to indicate correct behavior. It necessitates differentiated disposal forms for secondary packaging, primary packaging, and any unused or expired medicine, which should be returned to the pharmacy in its primary packaging, and removed from the secondary packaging.

For the sake of completeness, it is essential to determine which information within the packaging should also be placed on the outside (i.e., on the secondary packaging) for the prescribing doctor, pharmacist, and patient during the purchase of the medicine. By way of example, characteristics of the pharmaceutical form (e.g., size and shape of the tablet), should be clearly represented on the outside of the packaging to avoid large tablets being prescribed and dispensed to patients with swallowing difficulties. Similarly, the intake route must be well indicated, especially for medicines such as drop preparations or sachet powders. These may contain ambiguities regarding their use, as they do not have a shape that unequivocally associates them with the intake route. Regarding the indication of the intake route, the legislation states 'if necessary' (Art. 54, Directive 2001/83/EC of the European Parliament and of the Council of 6 November 2001 on the Community code relating to medicinal products for human use). From our point of view, however, it should always be included.

Among the information inside the packaging, it is crucial to make available to the user, before purchase, details about categories of users for whom the use of the medicine is not recommended or prohibited, such as pregnant women, children, adolescents, and patients intolerant to specific substances. The legislation requires the packaging to include 'a list of excipients with known action or effect' (Art. 54, Directive 2001/83/EC of the European Parliament and of the Council of 6 November 2001 on the Community code relating to medicinal products for human use), but it does not specify the prominent position this information should have.

In the current packaging, these lists have an entirely secondary position and visibility and are useless in guiding the patient's purchasing decisions. This visibility is crucial for non-prescription medicines.

One important consideration concerns Braille lettering. Article 56(a) of Directive 2001/83/EC mandates that pharmaceutical product outer packaging must include the trade name of the medicine in Braille. Braille lettering results from overprinting. Although the regulations require that these inscriptions be placed in secondary packaging spaces devoid of written text, in many packages Braille lettering is superimposed on other information such as the dosage or pharmaceutical form due to lack of space or inappropriate design.

As outlined in Chap. 17, the textured surface resulting from Braille printing, combined with the use of shiny or semi-shiny cardboard common in pharmaceutical packaging, creates visual interference, impeding the readability of all information on the secondary packaging. Of particular concern is the overlapping of Braille lettering with vital details like active ingredient and dosage information.

We will forego an exhaustive examination of every individual element constituting 'labelling' to prioritize discussing the visual similarity between the names of two medicines: the limited number of medicines typically included in a patient's home therapy significantly reduces the likelihood of encountering medications with similar names. Even in cases of similarity, the name of the medicine is distinguished by additional factors like packaging size and colour, collectively aiding in easier differentiation.

The situation differs for the pharmacist, for whom the name is an indispensable element in correctly identifying the product to be dispensed based on the doctor's request. We recalled in Chap. 8, we revisited some errors encountered, especially in the prescription and dispensing phases, linked to the excessive similarity between two different names. This similarity involves the name itself, as well as its 'visual impression,' including factors like length, presence of uppercase consonants such as 'T' or 'L', or similar vowels such as lowercase 'o' and 'a'. The graphic definition of the name also plays a role in accentuating or attenuating the visual similarity of the two names.

In Appendix 3, we have included the complex approval procedure that a new name must follow to avoid similarity in the names of several medicines. In that context, we have observed various attempts to intervene with design hypotheses aimed at addressing the problem of similarity between names in terms of visual perception. It is important to note that, in the world of medicines, there are two very distinct types of names, as defined by Directive 2001/83/EC in Article 1, paragraphs 20 and 21:

- 20. Name of the medicinal product: The name, which may be either an invented name not liable to confusion with the common name, or a common or scientific name accompanied by a trade mark or the name of the marketing authorisation holder;
- 21. Common name: The international non-proprietary name recommended by the World Health Organization [NdR "International Common Name" (DCI) or "International Non-proprietary Name" (INN)], or, if one does not exist, the usual common name.

In designations consisting of a 'invented' name, this is supplemented by the dosage information immediately following the name, and the International Non-proprietary Name (i.e., active ingredient) which is usually placed below the medicine name. In cases where the name of the medicine coincides with the active ingredient (INN), this is supplemented by information on the name of the company or its logo or trademark. This is followed by dosage information. In its guidelines on the acceptability of names for human medicinal products, processed through the centralised procedure—Scientific guideline (European Medicines Agency 2014), the European Medicines Agency (EMA) sets out these aspects of the name definition in detail. This results in two cases:

- Invented name + dosage; the active ingredient is placed below the name;
- Name of the medicinal product coinciding with the active ingredient followed by the Name/Logo/Brand of the pharmaceutical company + dosage.

Two issues are mentioned here which will be revisited later:

- In the case of medicine with a invented name, the dosage is not connected to the Active Principle (to which it refers) but to the name of the medicine;
- In the case of a name coinciding with the Active Ingredient, this is followed by the Company Name, and generally, also thanks to the graphics used, these two distinct information elements, under their proximity and the use of identical typefaces, come to constitute a single information unit, becoming indistinguishable.

This aspect will be further explored in the paragraphs *Summary notes: Preface to recommendations* and *Secondary packaging: Recommendations* because, in addition to the similarity of names, these elements also contribute to complicating the reading of the medicine's identifying elements and their connections.

22.7.5 Secondary Packaging: The Information Function of the Colour Code

The readability of the medicine name may be compromised by:

- the use of different fonts within the name;
- the use of different colours within the name;
- the use of decorated or deformed fonts within the name;
- the excessive proximity of graphic elements or images that interfere with the clear reading of the name.

Although discouraged in the Guidelines and Recommendations, many medicines on the market still feature these negative elements, hindering easy readability.

Additional considerations include:

- when the name of the medicine coincides with the name of the active ingredient and is accompanied by the name or logo of the pharmaceutical company, especially when the name and/or logo correspond to an acronym, the two elements (medicine name/company name) become indistinguishable if they are both written in the same typeface and size. This has a twofold implication. On the one hand, the patient regards the active ingredient and the company name as identifying a specific medicine and, especially in the case of the elderly, does not readily accept replacing that medicine with another having the same active ingredient followed by another company's name. In other words, the name thus composed and unified, even more so by the uniform typographical treatment of the two terms, creates an improper patient loyalty to the brand. On the other hand, at the international level, where thousands of names of active ingredients, proprietary medicine names and pharmaceutical companies are available, it is not always easy to distinguish the naming part (i.e., the active ingredient) from the added part (i.e., company name/logo). In particular, the problem arises when the part added to the active ingredient is an acronym that can easily be mistaken for an extension of the active ingredient or its characterisation;
- the dosage is usually placed next to the name of the medicine, although it refers to the amount of active ingredient in the pack. Alternatively, to make it clear, it is written in an isolated area of the packet. There is no direct link between dosage and active ingredient in both cases. The association problem arises when there are several active ingredients and, therefore, several dosages;
- when the dosage is placed next to the name of the medicine, it is sometimes not sufficiently spaced, creating interference between the final letters of the name and the dosage numbers;
- company logos and brand names may overshadow the medicine name.

The outer packaging lacks or does not sufficiently display certain information useful to the patient before purchasing the medicine, such as:

- the shape and size of the medicine;
- categories of patients for whom the medicine is not recommended without medical advice;
- excipients known to create intolerances.

Additional notes concern:

- information in the Braille alphabet, which, if overwritten with other visual elements, may create visual interference or not allowing a proper reading of information;
- some images on the secondary packaging and certain company trademarks may lead to misunderstandings about the use of the medicine or the pharmaceutical form contained;
- the expression of the pharmaceutical form is not always adequate for patient understanding the implications relating to medicine grasping, manipulation, or intake;
- the notes placed on the outer packaging by patients to personalise the product and its use. A sign of the anonymity of the packaging that makes the patient uncomfortable. To date, systems facilitating these forms of personalisation are lacking (or scarcely present), even though the legislation recommendations (Art. 54(e), Directive 2001/83/EC). Furthermore, the Guideline on Checking the process of mock-ups and specimens of outer/immediate labelling and package leaflets of human medicinal products in the centralised procedure (European Medicines Agency 2006, p. 3) explicitly states that: "outer packaging must also include a space for the prescribed dose to be indicated (e.g. to affix the dispensing label or for hand-written pharmacist instructions)" [...];
- the package has no detachable parts to allow the patient to take all the information to be shown to the doctor for proper prescribing.

Concerning warnings:

- indications concerning Warnings lack a precise location in the packaging, with each company placing them based on its logic and space availability. This hinders the traceability of common information on the secondary packaging, emphasizing the need for regulated placement. The traceability of information is only possible if their location in the packaging is regulated;
- warnings employ various graphic elements such as colour, bold text, framing, etc., chosen by each company, leading to different graphic treatments for the same.

Warnings in different medicines. This inconsistency makes it challenging to give proper weight to different prescriptive indications;

- special warnings and those providing specific indications for a particular medicine are indistinguishable due to both their graphical treatment and the absence of a precise location in the packaging. Special Warnings are often confused with the standard warnings legally present in all medicines;
- warnings are not consistently spaced out to allow for autonomous reading, and they are not grouped into categories of meaning or placed at privileged moments for information use;
- unlike the guidelines, warnings are not always placed on the main sides of the package, sometimes appearing on minor faces, resulting in reduced font size and inadequate margins and spacing;

- warnings are written both horizontally and vertically, with the latter being difficult for correct reading;
- text/background contrast is not always guaranteed, both for the text colours and for the background colours affecting the reading of Warnings, which generally have a reduced font size;
- the contrast between text and background may be compromised by graphic effects such as textures, shading, etc.;
- in several medicines, consistent graphic elements between outer packaging, inner packaging, and the medicine itself are lacking. Establishing a visual identity through these elements, as suggested by legislation and guidelines, could aid in linking these three components;
- unlike other products where brand identity is expressed through elements like the brand, logo, associated colour, and page layout design, medicines require careful consideration. Inaccurate design could have negative effects on the correct choice of medicine during dispensing or sale.

22.7.6 Readability and Usability

At the outset of this chapter, we noted that while the legislation on medicines and their packaging addresses readability issues comprehensively, there's a lack of attention to usability. In this context, usability refers not only to the challenges of finding, reading, and understanding the information but also encompasses ergonomics, prehensibility, and the difficulties associated with actions and gestures required to access the package leaflet. This interpretation of usability is distinct from its understanding of pharmaceutical regulatory affairs. Instead, we are referring to the fact that the informations readability on the primary and secondary packaging and the package leaflet highly depends on design elements that may favour or hinder its access. For a more detailed discussion of these elements, please refer to Chap. 17.

Summarizing these elements with a few notes:

- the patient tends to consider the package leaflet as the only place to find information about medicine use. Consequently, the patient tends to ignore the information on the secondary packaging. In other words, an information traceability problem arises. On the secondary packaging, there is no one common place to find the various information: each company places it on different sides of the packaging, according to its communication design;
- establishing a temporal and logical connection between information, its location (i.e., secondary pack, primary pack, package leaflet), and the moment the patient needs the information for correct action is challenging;
- secondary packaging frequently lacks clear signs explicitly designed to guide the user to the correct opening side;
- secondary packaging is designed without a clear bias towards right-sided opening, neglecting the fact that a significant percentage of the population is right-handed;

- there is no designed relationship between the opening side and the side where the user should find the package leaflet, leading to uncertainty regarding the correspondence between the opening side and the presence of the package leaflet;
- similar to packages containing blister packs that open on one of the two short sides, packages opening from the top (e.g., syrups, eye drops, powder sachets) do not necessarily position the package leaflet at the top (i.e., the opening side), preventing the user from encountering it before taking the medicine;
- the folding of the package leaflet generates strong interferences with the secondary pack and the primary pack;
- interference between the package leaflet, secondary pack, and primary pack intensifies after opening the package leaflet when the user struggles to fold it correctly and to take out and reinsert the primary pack in the outer package.

22.7.7 Premises Towards a System of Recommendations to Improve the Secondary Packaging

[**Pack 1**] To enhance readability, it is recommended to use only one font and one colour in the medicine name. The use of decorated or distorted fonts should be avoided. These recommendations align with those in the Guideline on the Readability of the Labelling and Package Leaflet of Medicinal Products for Human Use (European Commission 2009), which states, *"Different colours in the name of the product are discouraged since they may negatively impact on the correct identification of the product name. The use of different colours to distinguish different strengths is strongly recommended. The similarity in packaging which contributes to medication error can be reduced by the judicious use of colour on the pack. The number of colours used on packs will need careful consideration as too many colours could confuse. Where colour is used on the outer pack it is recommended that it is carried onto primary packaging to aid identification of the medicine."* These detailed recommendations, however, are not consistently enforced at the 'marketing authorization' stage.

[**Pack 2**] It is recommended not to place any graphic elements near the name of the medicine that might alter its legibility.

[**Pack 3**] For medicines with a name consisting of the "International Nonproprietary Name" (INN), accompanied by the Name/Logo/Brand of the pharmaceutical company (See *Guideline on the Acceptability of Names for Human Medicinal Products Processed Through the Centralised Procedure—Scientific Guideline, EMA, 2014*), it is recommended that the Name/Logo/Brand of the pharmaceutical company be written while maintaining its visual identity. To avoid the logo being considered as part of the active ingredient (which can easily happen when the logo corresponds to an acronym), the fonts of the logo should not be the same as those of the active ingredient. Adequate spacing between the two elements is also advisable to help distinguish them (Fig. 22.27).

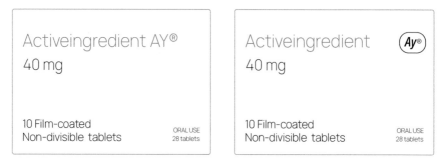

Fig. 22.27 In the two packs shown, the company logo (on the left) takes on the font and character body of the medicine name, blending in with it. On the right, the logo, although placed next to the medicine name, retains its distinctive graphic characteristics, thus differentiating itself from it

[Pack 4] According to current legislation, the dosage of the active ingredient follows the name of the medicinal product: "The name of the medicinal product followed by its strength and pharmaceutical form" (Art. 54(a), Directive 2001/83/EC—European Parliament and of the Council, 2001). However, this information element, referring to the active ingredient, should be placed next to it to form a 'unit of meaning' and make the information on the medicine to be dispensed more comprehensible (Fig. 22.28).

This shift of one of the most crucial pieces of information makes it possible to break down, in the (easily error-prone) act of dispensing, the moment of medicine choice into two distinct phases: the choice of Name and the choice of Dosage. Bringing the dosage indications closer to the active ingredient gives greater meaning to this information, making it more effective, mainly when the medicine contains more than one active ingredient. In this case, each active ingredient will have its own dosage next to it. In the case of medicines consisting of the name(s) of the active ingredient(s) + company name/logo, the dosage should be placed underneath, next to each active ingredient. It is also noted in the *Guideline on the Readability of the Labelling and Package Leaflet of Medicinal Products for Human Use*, taking up Art. 54(a) of Directive 2001/83, specifies: "Labelling must contain all elements required by Article 54 of Directive 2001/83/EC [...]. These items are 1) the name of the medicine; 2) strength and, where relevant, total content; and 3) route of administration. Where possible these should be brought together using a sufficiently large type size on the labelling. Having these items together in the same field of view should be considered to aid users" (Fig. 22.28).

[Pack 5] When the dosage is placed next to the name of the medicine, as is the current condition under Directive 2001/83/EC, Art. 54(a) (European Parliament 2001), it is recommended to maintain a correct distance between the two pieces of information so that the final letters of the name are not confused with the numbers that make up the dosage.

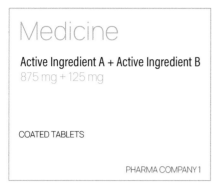
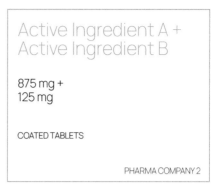

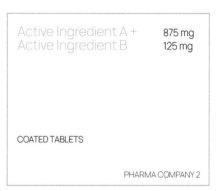

Fig. 22.28 In the two pictures on the left, the 'invented' name of the medicine is followed by the two active ingredients, next to which the respective dosage has been indicated, to create an 'information unit' (top is the version in use, bottom is the redesigned version). In the two images on the right, the name of the medicine consists of the two active ingredients. In this case, the dosage has been placed underneath, corresponding to the two active ingredients, to create, again, a completed 'information unit' (top the version in use, bottom the redesigned version)

[Pack 6] Careful design of colour when used as an identification code for different dosages is recommended. Currently, no studies have focused on this specific aspect and the effectiveness of colour coding in use by different users (pharmacists, patients, etc.) (Fig. 22.29).

[Pack 7] It is recommended that the name of the pharmaceutical company and/or its Logo or Brand should not overshadow the Name of the medicine.

[Pack 8] In addition to the labelling elements required by the regulations in force, on the front of the pack it is recommended that the following information should always be present to avoid mistakenly purchasing a medicine that cannot be taken by the patient:

- illustration of the medicine contained. Particularly in the case of oral solid forms, the medicine must be represented in its actual size, and, if possible, its size

Fig. 22.29 The three illustrations show different ways of signalling the increase in dosage of the active ingredient. Top, illustration of the colour codes of a medicine in use. In the middle, illustration of the same colour scale in crescendo. At the bottom, the colour code is supplemented with signs in progression. These are different ways of using colour to make the dosage of medicines recognisable through comparison

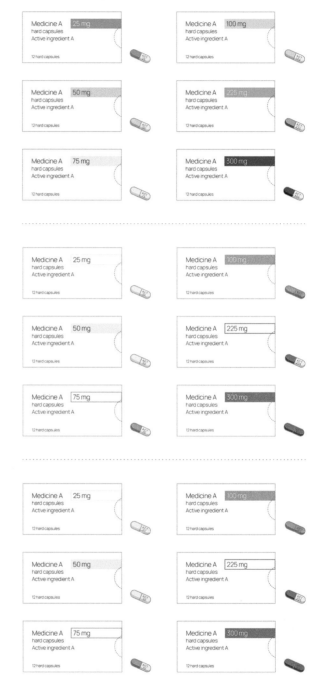

should be indicated. The representation should not be in perspective to avoid distorting the shape. This is necessary to avoid dysphagic patients purchasing medicines that they are then unable to take. The representation should also contain the colour characteristics and surface markings of the medicine, as this information can help the patient to identify tablets that may no longer be recognisable once removed from the package;
- indicating whether the medicine cannot be taken during pregnancy is always recommended. This applies especially to non-prescription medicines;
- it is recommended to indicate whether the medicine cannot be taken under or over a certain age. This applies especially to over-the-counter medicines;
- it is recommended that excipients contraindicated in specific patient groups (e.g., diabetics, coeliacs, lactose intolerant, etc.) be clearly indicated. It is not sufficient that this information is included in the medicine's list of excipients, even if it is highlighted in bold. This information element must be separately communicated and prominently highlighted. To catch the patient's attention, this information could be accompanied by visual information (e.g., pictograms). To facilitate the patient's understanding of the information provided, it is always helpful to supplement the scientific names of the components with terms the patient can understand. For example, if the excipients include sorbitol, explicitly cite the presence of sugar, in addition to the scientific name of the excipient (Fig. 22.30).

[**Pack 9**] It is recommended that information given using the Braille alphabet should not be imprinted on written elements (in particular, dosage and active ingredient) because they may alter or render the written information illegible. The guidelines already provide this indication, but it is currently largely disregarded.

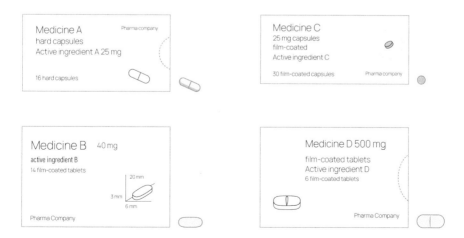

Fig. 22.30 Examples of realistic illustration of the medicine contained to avoid purchase by patients with swallowing difficulties

[**Pack 10**] It is recommended that the images on the secondary packaging, as well as company trademarks, should not give rise to ambiguous interpretations for the user that could lead to misunderstandings as to the pharmaceutical form contained or the manner of use of the medicine.

[**Pack 11**] It is recommended that the route of administration be indicated in a visible manner and language understandable to the user. When needed, this indication should complement more usual indications expressed in scientific language, useful for the doctor and the dispenser: for example, 'dissolvable in the mouth' should complement terms such as 'orosoluble', 'orodispersible', and 'sublingual.' In the case of oral solid forms, on the front of the packet, the terms 'crushable/non-crushable', 'divisible/non-divisible' should supplement terms such as 'film-coated', 'gastro-resistant', 'modified-release', which are useful for the doctor and the dispenser but not suitable for indicating to the patient that the medicine may or may not be manipulated. In the case of pharmaceutical forms that do not have an explicit connection with the route of administration (e.g., drops or powder preparations), it is recommended that the correct method of use be indicated on the outer packaging (Fig. 22.31).

[**Pack 12**] The strong need for personalization is a prevalent behaviour observed among patients in their relationship with their medicine. Notations made by patients on the medicine packaging have different nature but serve a unique purpose, supplementing the information on the packaging according to individual needs. The name of the medicine is one element 'enriched' by the patient with additional information. The name of the medicine does not always convey the reason for its prescription, leading to the first element of personalisation found in notations supplementing the name with user-assigned labels such as "for the heart," "for blood pressure," "diuretic," etc.

A second aspect of personalisation arises when multiple patients in the same household take medicines. Particularly in the elderly, the name of the patient or familial titles like 'mum', 'dad', 'granddad', etc., is often written on the pack, typically by family members.

Another piece of information added to the packet is the daily dosage (e.g., 1 tablet after meals at midday). Additionally, details such as the start date of therapy and/or the date on which the packet was opened are included. This information serves various purposes, including helping the patient track the total duration of

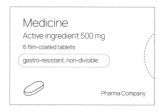

Fig. 22.31 Example of secondary packaging that indicates to the patient how the medicine may be taken

therapy, checking whether medicines have been taken daily, and determining the packet's opening date, which defines the expiry date.

In this context, a recommendation supported by current legislation (Art. 54(e), Directive 2001/83/EC, and European Medicines Agency (EMA) 2006, p. 3) suggests supporting the process of information integration. This can be a valuable tool to prevent medication errors. Consideration should also be given to inserting adhesive sheets inside the pack that can be easily filled in by the patient and then attached to the pack (e.g., in the space of the pharmacy's dispensing label, which fulfils its role in the pharmacy) (Fig. 22.32).

[**Pack 13**] The occurrence of patients not precisely recalling details about the medicine they need a prescription for or must purchase at the pharmacy is quite common. Some pharmaceutical companies have effectively addressed this challenge, as outlined in Directive 2011/62/EU (European Parliament 2011). They have adapted the opening/closing flaps of secondary packaging to comply with the directive, preventing tampering and counterfeiting of medicines. These companies have ingeniously incorporated a pre-cut flap that contains all the necessary data for the doctor to issue a correct prescription. The easy tear-off feature of the flap aligns with a behavior already practiced by patients, making the process more user-friendly. The pre-cut flap, providing the patient with essential identification data for the medicine, proves to be a valuable solution. It helps prevent errors during refill purchases and serves as a practical 'memo' at home, aiding the patient in therapy preparation. When affixed, for instance, to the treatment plan, it becomes a visual element directly associated with the medicine. Placed on the saucer where the therapy is prepared, it serves as a replacement when the medicine needs to be stored in the refrigerator until consumption, among other uses (Fig. 22.33).

[**Pack 14**] While the arrangement of the information elements constituting a medicine's biographical data on the main side of the packet and at least three other contiguous sides is strongly standardised, the organization of additional information and mandatory warnings for all medicines lacks equally precise definitions in legislation or guidelines. Pharmaceutical manufacturers may arrange these elements according to their criteria, with guidelines suggesting that the

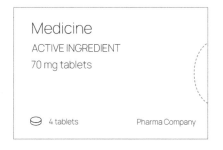 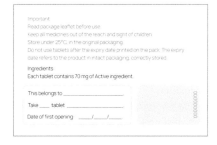

Fig. 22.32 Example of secondary packaging that allows the patient to personalise the therapy information

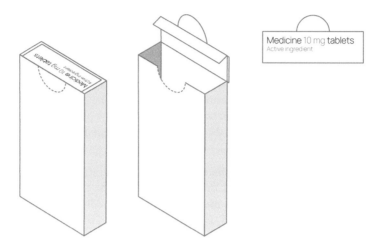

Fig. 22.33 Label with medicine information, easily separable from the secondary packaging thanks to the pre-cut. The example is taken from packaging already used by some pharmaceutical companies

wider sides of the pack are the most suitable placement (European Medicines Agency 2006). Recommendations also encourage the use of graphic elements to enhance text readability, such as font choice, minimum permitted size, line spacing, and the use of colour and bold for creating visual hierarchies. However, these recommendations are often ignored. Instead, when the package size allows, all necessary patient information and warnings should be placed on the two main sides—typically the front and back for horizontal secondary packaging (e.g., blister packs of tablets). The smaller sides, in turn, should be used to repeat labelling information and provide mandatory details like production batch, company name and address, A.I.C. number, expiry date, and price. It is generally recommended to treat warnings as independent texts, each having autonomy, instead of treating them as propositions within a single text. It is suggested to establish precise criteria for:

- the placement of the mandatory Warnings, to create the habit of identifying the information when sought by the patient;
- the use of the wider 'sides' of the package to allow proper spacing between the individual Warnings, making them readable in their individuality and giving each of them a stronger prescriptive force;
- the use of bold, italics, colours, etc. It has been observed that leaving these elements to the sole discretion of the companies does not produce such effective results;
- the use of vertically written text, which should be avoided, especially when sufficient space is available;
- the grouping of mandatory warnings according to categories of related issues (e.g. warnings concerning use, storage and disposal; special warnings concern-

ing characteristics or effects induced by the medicine), to create 'areas of meaning' that reinforce their ability to attract the interest of the patient;
- the distinction between the mandatory Warnings applied to all medicines and the Special Warnings specific to the individual medicine (e.g. storage temperature). The latter should have their location and established graphic treatment. The use of pictograms could be effective in drawing attention to the text and making it immediately comprehensible.

[**Pack 15**] The storage conditions must be clearly stated: the patients should read this information at purchase, not just at the time of use. Therefore, some time may pass before the patient reads it. This information is not given due prominence, considering it may vary between medicines. It is crucial for those whose active ingredient is temperature-sensitive (and therefore should be stored under temperature-controlled conditions) or light-sensitive (and therefore should be stored in the original, non-opened packaging).

To attract the patient's attention, pictograms are recommended to make the information visible and reinforce the textual message (Fig. 22.34).

[**Pack 16**] An indication that is often poorly emphasized, and therefore not very effective in conveying the correct behavior to the patient, concerns the disposal of the medicine. In most packages, patients encounter the phrase "do not dispose of the product in the environment" as guidance for the disposal phase. In rare cases, and usually in verbal form, instructions may be more comprehensive, such as: "dispose of the unused product using the collection systems provided in pharmacies. Do not dispose of glass in the environment after use". Although somewhat indistinct compared to other details on the back of the medicine, the latter information places more emphasis on the issue of waste and offers more precise instructions on how to handle it. More recent, albeit still sporadic, are positive examples of medicines that pay significant attention to disposal methods. In the example below, the table format effectively captures the patient's attention, providing a comprehensive message on how to dispose of each packaging component based on its material (Fig. 22.35).

[**Pack 17**] The expiry date of a sealed medicine is always indicated on the opening flap of the outer packaging. However, in some medicines, the active ingredient may

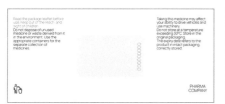
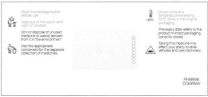

Fig. 22.34 The same type of information is communicated in a different way by intervening only on the interlineations between the different Warnings and by adding some pictograms to make the content more immediate

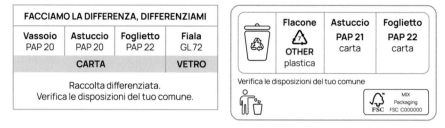

Fig. 22.35 Examples of medicine disposal information demonstrating a new sensitivity to environmental issues. The example is taken from medicines in use in Italy

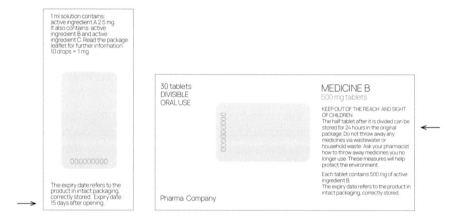

Fig. 22.36 On the left an example of important information on the duration of the medicine's efficacy after opening. Similarly, on the right, a secondary package of tablets showing the duration of the medicine's effectiveness after handling the tablet. This information is not made self-contained, and is therefore not distinguishable from the other warnings

lose effectiveness after a certain time interval since it was first opened. This interval varies for each medicine. This condition is well-known in ointments and eye drops but less recognized in other medicines like drops, syrups, or tablets, which may undergo an 'early decay' of the active ingredient's effectiveness after opening. Unfortunately, this information is generally not very visible, either due to its position or the lack of graphic reinforcement (such as the use of red, bold, etc.) that would draw attention to its importance. Below, we observe the information on a 20 ml packet of Bromazepam, a medicine that can have a very long shelf life for patients who take it occasionally or have mild anxiety symptoms. Conversely, the medicine is only valid for 16 days after it is first opened. However, the information does not receive the necessary visual prominence (Fig. 22.36).

In the realm of cosmetic products, the expiration date after first opening is typically conveyed through a pictogram featuring the acronym PAO (Period After Opening) (Fig. 22.37).

22 Compendium: Step Toward Design-Oriented Practices in the Pharma Industry...

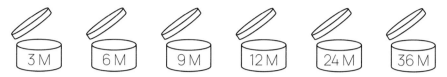

Fig. 22.37 A symbol has been introduced in cosmetic products to draw the user's attention to the expiry date after opening

Fig. 22.38 Introduction of forms of personalisation of the packaging to make the user aware of the shelf life of the product after it has been opened for the first time, achieved with minimal graphic interventions on the original packaging

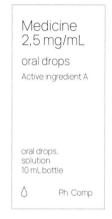
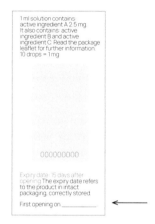

In the case of medicines, it would be advisable to consider the introduction of a similar pictogram designed to emphasize the importance of adhering to the validity interval after opening the medicine. Some companies have already incorporated the option to write the date of first opening and the subsequent expiry date on the packaging (e.g., "I will have to finish this medicine by..."). This allows users to personalize their packaging with the correct expiry date (Fig. 22.38).

[Pack 18] The guidelines provide direction on the necessary contrast between written text and background to enhance readability (Article 2, "Design and Layout of the Information," Guideline on the Readability of the Labelling and Package Leaflet of Medicinal Products for Human Use, European Commission 2009). Unfortunately, this recommendation is often overlooked. Merely having a correct colour contrast between the written parts and the background is not sufficient. It is essential to avoid images and background treatments, such as decorative effects, mottling, marbling, dithering, etc., that could impede the reading of individual vocabulary. Additionally, backgrounds with large, shaded areas should be avoided, and if present, measures should be taken to ensure that the text/background colour contrast remains effective in both the darkest and lightest parts (Fig. 22.39).

[Pack 19] The Guideline on the Readability of the Labelling and Package Leaflet of Medicinal Products for Human Use (European Commission 2009), particularly in Article 4—Labelling, Design, and Layout, expressly suggests making the graph-

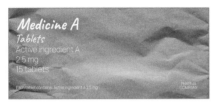
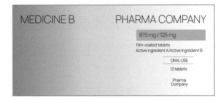

Fig. 22.39 Even though standards and guidelines are very clear in this respect, several medicines placed on the market do not observe elementary principles of readability such as the correct contrast between written text and background. These are fictitious examples simulating problems present in pharmaceutical products placed on the market

ics of the secondary pack coherent with those of the primary pack to ensure their recognition as two parts of the same product. Unfortunately, this recommendation is often disregarded. It is advisable to assess, during the approval phase, that the graphic elements defining the outer packaging (such as colour, font type, visual identity signs, etc.) are also consistently present on the primary pack and, whenever possible, on the medicine itself. For example, in oral solid forms, it can be beneficial to use the same colour as on the outer packaging to characterize the dosage.

[Pack 20] In contrast to most products on the market, the principles governing brand identity should be meticulously considered in the case of medicines. A robust brand identity can potentially result in confusion between different medicines from the same pharmaceutical company or even among pharmaceutical companies that employ similar graphic elements. It's worth noting the prevalent tendency to mimic the image of certain leading brands, heightening the risk of confusion in the choice of medicine (Fig. 22.40).

[Pack 21] It is advisable to position information on product usage as close as possible to the point of the product and the moment of action involved in taking the medicine. Some companies have already adopted good practices in this regard. For instance, directions on how to open a bottle are displayed on the flaps of the secondary pack. This ensures that the user encounters the information just before interacting with the cap, or when feasible, the instructions are placed directly on the bottle cap itself.

[Pack 22] It is recommended to clearly mark and highlight the side from which the pack should be opened. Additionally, placing the package leaflet on the right-hand side when opening the package is advised. This ensures that the user finds the package leaflet on that side, facilitating the correct sequence of actions—first reading the leaflet and then taking the medicine. Similarly, for top-opening packages, it is recommended to position the package leaflet on the top, guiding the patient to follow the correct sequence: open, read the package leaflet, and use the medicine (Fig. 22.41)

22 Compendium: Step Toward Design-Oriented Practices in the Pharma Industry... 503

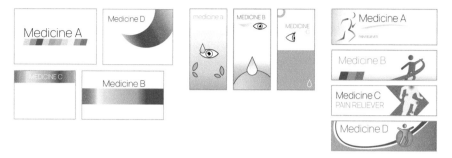

Fig. 22.40 Examples of medicines using similar and easily confused visual elements

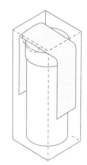

Fig. 22.41 Medicines with a clear indication of the opening side and correct positioning of the package leaflet

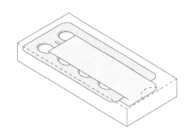

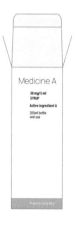

Fig. 22.42 Medicines with opening from the top (opening in the correct direction, bringing the flap from the front to the back) and with correct positioning of the package leaflet

[**Pack 23**] For packs that open from the top, it is recommended to design the cover flap opening from front to back. This design ensures that the user is not compelled to rotate the pack from front to back, thus avoiding the loss of sight of crucial information about the medicine being taken (Fig. 22.42).

[**Pack 24**] It is advisable to avoid types of openings that cannot be re-closed after the initial opening (some closure types, such as those sealed with hot-melt glue, may tear the cardboard flaps, preventing the pack from resealing). This could have adverse effects on both storage (an open package may fail to protect the enclosed medicine from light sources) and the easy inspection of contents, particularly by children.

[**Pack 25**] It is recommended that LASA (Look-Alike Sound-Alike) and FALA (For-All-Limited-Age groups) Medicines should not be packaged in shapes that hinder the visual recognition of identifying elements (e.g., cylindrical containers).

[**Pack 26**] Secondary packaging of OTC medicines must include specific additional information.

22.8 Package Leaflet

The package leaflet, a relatively recent and intricate communication artefact, has evolved significantly over its 45-year history. It has experienced substantial modifications in both content and format. The development of the package leaflet faced considerable obstacles and resistance. Prevailing beliefs suggested that Patient Information Leaflets (PIL) could potentially induce in patients unwarranted anxiety, encourage inappropriate self-medication, suggest side effects to patients, invite patients to detect side effects by suggestion, make patients more demanding, induce a refusal in patients to beneficial medicine treatment, increase the exchange of prescription medicines between patients by 'de-mystifying' medicines and reducing the placebo effect (van der Waarde 2008, p. 38).

Among the diverse information elements accompanying patient medication, the package leaflet stands out as the most regulated. Regulatory pressures have driven substantial revisions, primarily focusing on enhancing content accessibility. Legislative attention has been directed towards several key aspects:

- precision: Legislation demands the elimination of ambiguous indications in the information for the users (e.g., "for the shortest possible time," "small quantity").
- comprehensibility: Requirements include supplementing medical terms and technical-scientific language with user-friendly explanations.
- readability: Criteria regarding text, character body, and interlineations have been established, emphasizing the construction of short sentences.
- traceability: Standard structures have been proposed to facilitate easy navigation for patients in search of information. Typography has been strategically employed to create a visual hierarchy of content through distinct headings, paragraphs, and sub-paragraphs. Verbal text has been made more immediate using pictograms, as mandated by regulations.

The Guideline on the packaging information of medicinal products for human use authorized by the Union (European Medicines Agency—EMA 2021) includes an annex containing country-specific pictograms permitted for use. These pictograms

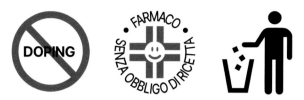

Fig. 22.43 For Italy, from the left: a doping pictogram; a smile pictogram for non-prescription medicinal products; a pictogram on waste disposal

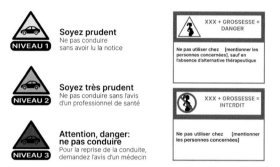

Fig. 22.44 For France, from the left: pictograms on the dangers of medicine-dependent driving

contribute to the visual enhancement of information traceability and adhere to regulatory guidelines (Figs. 22.43 and 22.44).

Despite refinements, the package leaflet continues to pose challenges since it is still a complex and dense document. Although the language has been 'updated' in favour of the user, its comprehensibility requires a high level of education and basic knowledge of pharmacology and medicine that most patients do not possess.

Caratti et al. (2021), defined the language of the package leaflet as "a matter of an articulated and hypertrophic linguistic system" and attributed the persistence of a de-personalised character, not aimed at the patient but addressed, at least in form, to the doctor and medicine specialists, to the persistence of a problematic accessibility of its contents.

In Chap. 19, Dionigi pointed out that, even in terms of usability, the package leaflet remained cumbersome, difficult to fold and store due to its format. In addition, the structure of the text, as well as the size of the font, continued to make it unclear and difficult to read in all its parts. In this way, the medicine produced for everyone, is not inclusive for some users, such as the elderly, the visually impaired, the poorly educated, and those who, as 'foreigners', find themselves having to seek treatment outside their own country. The density of information and difficulty in finding, understanding, and remembering it put the patient at risk of taking the medicine without having acquired all the prior knowledge for its correct use.

In Chap. 10, Caratti pointed out the absence of a reflection on the communication of non-prescription medicines (OTC). For these, the same typology, sequence of contents and location are maintained, even though we are dealing with a different product from the medicine that a doctor prescribes. In this case, the user purchases the medicine without the doctor's support. The package leaflets of OTC medicines comply with the Ministerial Decree of 1997. It states that the package leaflet must have an introductory section specifying that it is a self-medication medicine aimed at treating mild or transient ailments and that medical intervention is appropriate if the problem is not resolved. There may also be a section entitled 'Health Education Notes' for patient information. In the case of leaflets for OP medicine (with a doctor's prescription), it is possible to find specialised information at the end of the sections aimed at doctors and healthcare professionals (Di Pace 2019, pp. 33–34). While the readability of the text and comprehensibility of the contents have improved after the introduction of very punctilious regulations, much remains to be done regarding the usability of the package leaflet, meaning, in this context, the ease with which users relate to it. It is well known that an attitude of rejection has developed towards the package leaflet.

Karen van der Waarde highlights inherent limitations, noting that package leaflets are not universally suitable, especially in hospital settings for managing multiple medicines, and in digital contexts. They are not accessible to all patients, particularly those who are functionally illiterate. The volume of information within them is often overwhelming, leading patients to seek online information. Unfortunately, the use of package leaflets has shown little improvement in patient knowledge and has minimal impact on medicine-taking behavior (van der Waarde 2008, p. 40).

Thus, part of the problems with package leaflets is related to the textual content (e.g., fears nurtured by reading the side effects; rejection nurtured by the length of the text, etc.); part of the problems stem from the reading and comprehension difficulties, which are not always easy, and despite the efforts mentioned above have not yet been entirely resolved.

Furthermore, problems are also encountered with the physical artefact: the leaflet itself. For example, this presents manageability problems: the leaflet is often oversized. It uses very different reading formats to provide the necessary information from those we are familiar with.

These formats include leaflets folded and closed with a label or glue dot (offering a large print area but challenging to fold), small-folded leaflets integrated into the medicine label, leaflets integrated into the pouch as large sheets folded several times (increasing production costs and complicating reinsertion into the pack), and bound sheets in booklet format (suitable for multilingual content and storage inside the pack). The variability in format and size impacts information reading and physical handling of the leaflet.

The act of reading the package leaflet involves frequent movement of the paper support to follow the written lines of text with the eyes. Opening and, particularly, closing the sheet are complex operations, often leading users to discard the package leaflet or store it separately, rather than returning it to its packaging after the initial opening. This challenge is especially pronounced with blister packs but applies to other packaging formats as well.

Moreover, the characteristics of the paper itself contribute to difficulties in reading. The paper is extremely light to fit within the medicine packaging, occupying minimal space. However, this lightness creates problems of visual interference, as the transparency of the leaflet allows a glimpse of the text on the back, significantly reducing readability. The sheet does not present itself as a flat page due to the necessity of folding it for packaging, imprinting folds on the sheet, sometimes coinciding with the lines of the text. These folds introduce a multidimensionality that complicates the reading process.

Chapter 17 underscores a prevalent issue: a lack of a logical relationship between information on the secondary pack, primary pack, and the package leaflet. The packaging of medicine in its secondary pack often fails to guide users through the correct sequence of actions, hindering access to the package leaflet immediately after opening the pack and before accessing the medicine in the primary pack. In various packs, users may not notice the package leaflet upon opening because it is positioned on the opposite side of the opening side. This occurs in packs with horizontal openings (common with blister packs) and those with top openings (typical for bottles, vials, and sachets, see Chap. 17). The optimal arrangement, ensuring a clear indication of the opening side on the secondary pack, placing the package leaflet on the opening side, and then presenting the primary pack, at the very least, encourages users to follow the correct sequence of actions when taking the medicine.

Sachet preparations exemplify a notable challenge regarding the placement of the package leaflet. Placing the package leaflet at the base of the packaging is discouraging, requiring users to remove all the sachets from the secondary packaging to access it. To enhance and promote the reading of the package leaflet, it is crucial for companies to strategically design its placement, guiding and facilitating the sequence of actions that users would typically undertake. This thoughtful design can significantly improve the user experience and ensure that essential information is easily accessible without unnecessary inconvenience.

Certain types of sheets and their folding can significantly contribute to a better user experience. For instance, sheets that allow for a compact and space-saving format when closed, especially when sealed with a glue dot or label, enable placement on top of blister packs or the side of secondary packs for easy access without removing the primary pack.

In evaluating the package leaflet's usability, the evolving lifestyles of medication users, who often take medicines away from home for work, study, or travel reasons, must be considered. Convenience often leads patients not to carry all the elements of the package (e.g., primary pack, secondary pack, package leaflet and medicine), risking the omission of crucial information during medication intake.

While technologies like QR codes can address some issues, the transition to electronic formats should be approached cautiously, especially for the elderly who currently has the highest use of medicines and the lowest access to digital technologies. Consideration should be given to potential challenges or concerns with the transition, such as data privacy, accessibility, and user acceptance. The European Medicines Agency (EMA), the European Network of Regulatory Agencies (HMA), as well as the European Community, have published a list of principles aimed at harmonizing the process of introducing electronic Product Information-ePI of medicines (European Commission, EMA, HMA 2020) to make electronic medicine information systems interoperable with other electronic health care systems such as electronic prescriptions and electronic health records.

The introduction of the electronic package leaflet may facilitate access to up-to-date information on the medicine and promote its safer use. Some experiences in this respect are already underway, with one of the early examples being the eLeaflet® from myHealthbox (Editorial, 30 March 2013). Today, many packages carry codes that can be read by a smartphone, allowing the information in the package insert to be downloaded. In Chap. 19, Dionigi pointed out the availability of the electronic document offers numerous advantages: the text can be enlarged; it can facilitate the search for specific information; it can allow the medicine information to be updated over time; it can provide access to the text in other languages; it can show videos and animations, etc.

However, each of these potentials brings with it problems that should not be underestimated. Below, we indicate just a few of them, to give a glimpse of the complexity of a translation operation:

- Multilingual translation is complex because it involves not just transcribing content into another language but also presupposing knowledge of attitudes and cultures related to medicine and treatment. These may vary in different geographical contexts and may require that the content of some information be supplemented or modified.
- The facilitated search for information, according to the interests and needs of the user, presupposes the autonomy of reading and the possibility of choosing in-depth paths that the digital package leaflet allows and favours. This autonomy, however, may lead to using the information contained in the package leaflet in a fragmented way when the effectiveness of its role lies in the text.
- the digital format lends itself to supplementing the written text with information conveyed through diagrams, pictograms, symbols, illustrations, realistic photos, and even videos. However, there is a lack of in-depth studies on the comprehensibility and effectiveness of images in providing information, descriptions, and indications of a prescriptive nature in a segment of the population that possesses, by training, a predominantly verbal and textual culture.

22.8.1 Premises Towards a System of Recommendations to Improve Package Leaflet

[**Package Leaflet 1**] Observation of users' processes of use highlights the frequency with which they throw away the package leaflet. This occurs for several reasons, but primarily because harmful interference is created between the primary packaging, the secondary packaging, and the package leaflet during use. There are several types of package leaflets on the market; among them, the 'C' folded type is the most common but also the most problematic. It is recommended that pharmaceutical companies favour using the 'folded' type of leaflet with a glue point closure, preferably with a resealable adhesive label.

[Package Leaflet 2] The leaflet can be in the classic 'open C' folded format that wraps around the blister pack. It can also be folded with a glue dot in the 'compact' format. In this case, it is recommended that the package leaflet, and possibly the information sheet with special warnings (if provided), be placed on top of the blister and not underneath. For some pharmaceutical products, where reading the package leaflet is particularly important, the 'booklet' format of the package leaflet allows easier reading. Some pharmaceutical companies offer the package leaflet in 'book form' in conjunction with the primary packaging so that one simultaneously takes out the primary packaging and the leaflet.

[Package Leaflet 3] It is recommended that the user always re-inserts the leaflet into the packaging so that all the information required for proper use is always available. Alternatively, following good practice adopted by some users, it is recommended to read the package leaflet at the start of treatment and to keep all the package leaflets of the medicines that make up the daily therapy neatly in a dedicated folder. This folder should be kept near the medicines so that all information is available.

[Package Leaflet 4] Since the leaflet is not read in its entirety by the patient, it is recommended to anticipate intake patterns at the beginning of the leaflet also integrating it with those indications that may direct the patient towards the correct behaviour to adopt during therapy. For example, whether the intake on a full or empty stomach or whether the patient should avoid particular foods or drinks (e.g., milk, grapefruit, alcohol, etc.). In this context, it is also helpful to provide the patient with information about effects that may affect daily activities: drowsiness, photosensitivity, etc. Alternatively, while the intake mode should remain in its current position to induce the patient to read all the information before intake, this information should also be easily traceable and made evident through pictograms or graphic expedients that highlight this information.

[Package Leaflet 5] Position the package leaflet on the opening side of the pack, clearly marked on the secondary pack for easy access.

[Package Leaflet 6] For some medicines, it has become good practice to include a card in the packaging in addition to the package leaflet. This card contains the primary 'basic' information about the medicine, the reasons for its use, how to take it and the main precautions that the patient should take (e.g. not to consume alcohol, not to expose oneself to light in the case of photosensitive medicines, not to consume food and/or drinks that may enhance or reduce the effectiveness of the active ingredient, etc.). The usefulness of the information card is not only linked to the fact that it puts in the 'foreground' information that is immediately useful for correct user behaviour. In card format, the card also responds to needs increasingly felt by patients, such as the need to carry medicines safely away from home, where the user generally does not take the entire packet with them. If also designed for this purpose, in addition to being informative, the card could also act as a protective element of the blister portion, possibly separated from the overall pack, to cope with outdoor use.

[Package Leaflet 7] Follow Package Leaflet Readability Guidelines, ensuring that text lines and fold lines do not overlap to enhance readability. It is recommended to design the spacing of the leaflet text and the spaces between paragraphs so that written parts never coincide with the folds of the leaflet, as this coincidence interferes with the reading of the information contained.

[Package Leaflet 8] Patients are reluctant to read the package leaflet, partly because they are discouraged by the side effect information. It is recommended to balance the long list of side effects that accompanies the indications on the use of the medicine, with positive hints on correct lifestyles that may favour the successful outcome of the treatment and that may have a preventive function (e.g. in the case of blood pressure medication, positive rules such as limiting the use of salt in food, practising sport, etc.).

[Package Leaflet 9] It is recommended to mark the parts of the package leaflet whenever possible, identifying those mainly addressed to the patient and those addressed to doctors and pharmacists. This promotes writing in differentiated language and helps patients identify the parts that are most interesting to them.

[Package Leaflet 10] In the package leaflet, in addition to the directions for use prohibiting tablet breakage or fragmentation, it is recommended that alternative pharmaceutical forms (e.g. syrup, granules, drops, etc.) commercially available for that active ingredient be indicated as a substitute for the solid form. The purpose of this indication is to prevent the patient with swallowing problems or with a need to customise the dosage of the medicine from deciding to fragment the medicine despite the prohibition and to be supported with information on accessible alternatives of choice. This good practice is already in use in some pharmaceutical companies.

[Package Leaflet 11] Especially for oral solid forms, the leaflet should include more specific and effective instructions on storing the medicine outside the package.

[Package Leaflet 12] The leaflet should provide the patient with all the information on the medicine's characteristics, its pharmaceutical function, and the effects that altering the pharmaceutical form may produce, preceded by details of what the patient can and cannot do when handling the medicine. For example, *"Tablets should not be cut, crushed, or chewed, as this may lead to an increased risk of adverse effects, including convulsions. Biperiden hydrochloride is an extended-release formulation. Splitting the tablet alters the mode of release (pharmacokinetics) of the active substance"* or *"Capsules should not be opened. The active ingredient Minocycline is highly irritating to the oesophagus. Capsules should be swallowed with an adequate amount of water, in an upright* *or sitting position, and at least 1 hour before going to bed*". It is also advisable to explicitly inform the patient whether the fragments can be kept for later use (and within how long after the medicine has been split) or whether they should be disposed of.

[Package Leaflet 13] Ensure the leaflet contains instructions and procedures for reporting side effects and defects in the purchased product.

[Package Leaflet 14] Redesign package leaflets for non-prescription medicines with specific additional information.

[Package Leaflet 15] Printed package leaflets should provide the basic information in a concise form combining verbal and visual language, allowing for digital extension.

[Package Leaflet 16] Package leaflets should offer digital expansion options, including different languages and alternative visual or auditory codes, alternative to the textual form.

[Package Leaflet 17] In the transition to digital formats, allow the comparison of package leaflets for medicines with the same active ingredient.

22.9 Medicines and the "Minute Techniques" of Everyday Life. Educating in Caring Behaviour

The legislation tasked with overseeing the procedures and technical specifications of medicine, along with its packaging, employs terms such as 'immediate packaging' and 'outer packaging' to denote the packaging in direct contact with the medicine and the outermost packaging, respectively. These terms are confined to the regulatory sphere and are not used outside this context.

In the realm of pharmaceutical companies and the project field, these terms transform, becoming known as primary packaging and secondary packaging, respectively. However, these designations are unfamiliar in the user's world, where descriptive language about everyday items such as ampoules, bottles, and vials is used to define primary packaging, while terms like box, tin, and case are employed for secondary packaging. Notably, terms like blister or strip are not commonly used. Furthermore, users often do not name the packaging itself, referring directly to the medicine and distinguishing it by its type, such as tablets, suppositories, syrup, and so on.

If we reflect on the use of the adjectives 'primary' and 'secondary' coined by the packaging industry—not only pharmaceutical packaging—it becomes evident that a sense of primacy is attributed to the object being protected by the packaging, as opposed to the subject using it. When viewed from the user's perspective, it appears logical to reverse the meaning of these terms. Thus, one might consider referring to the outer packaging (encountered first by the user) as the primary pack and the inner packaging (seen later or possibly not at all if the product is not purchased or used) as the secondary pack.

For the user, temporal logic is shaped by the sequence of accessing the product, prompting them to observe, read, and handle the packages from the outermost to the innermost. What may initially seem like linguistic sophisms ultimately signify the underlying perspective that propels the design of packaging objects. Sophisticated preservation and protection techniques, anti-tampering solutions, package traceability, environmental sustainability in packaging, and the growing influence of digital technologies, even in the realm of medicine packaging, are all highly pertinent for ensuring the contemporary integrity of pharmaceutical product packaging. However, it is within the minutiae of the details, encompassing both the packaging itself and the information apparatus, that one discerns a still modest inclination to move closer to the patient-user and address their discomfort, needs, and cultural context.

Unlike other packaging that enters our homes relatively anonymously in everyday products, medicines evoke a sense of intangibility and otherness. Users approach these objects through a process of *familiarisation*, as discussed in Chap. 15. Approximation strategies involve employing a familiar lexicon shared among family members, using indicative appellations such as 'the little blue box' and 'the box with the stripes' instead of the medicine's name. Alternatively, medicines are referred to by translating their technical-scientific names into common terms such as 'the one for the heart,' 'the white one,' 'the bitter one,' etc., replacing the medicine's name with its characteristics and purpose of use. At times, users adopt pet names or diminutives (such as 'squirt,' 'breather,' 'tin,' 'tablet,' etc.), which we recognize as an affectionate way of expressing emotional closeness to the object in question.

But the approach to the user's sphere of use then takes place through a process of appropriation of the medicine: a true personalisation that is expressed by writing the user's name, the daily dose of use, notes on use, starting therapy, etc. on the packaging.

The process of personalization, manifested in the writing of notations directly on the medicine package, extends beyond the package itself. Particularly in the context of complex therapies, this personalization extends to diaries, calendars, and therapy plans, which are often crafted by the patient (and occasionally by family members, but rarely by a doctor). These documents serve to recall the various activities associated with the medicine treatment, including examinations, visits, prescriptions, and pharmacy refills.

Furthermore, we have observed instances where the patient rewrites the entire therapy, restructuring the data for specific purposes. This results in different versions, each serving a distinct function. For instance, there is a 'daily calendar' script organized by grouping medicines according to daily intake times. Another script takes the form of a list, encompassing all the essential data of the medicine, including the pharmaceutical company's brand name, and is used for repurchases. Additionally, there is a script tailored for visits with specialists, associating medicines with the pathology and including information on intolerances or indications for occasional use.

A further aspect of the familiarisation process involves drawing upon practical aspects from everyday domesticity, including gestures, rituals, manners, and the use of tools, and applying them to the sphere of medicine and therapy. Items such as knives, chopping boards, small saucers, containers, bags for storing food in the freezer, adhesive film, and even domestic tools such as steak beaters, tongs, and screwdrivers indicate that the worlds of food and small routine maintenance tasks are significant sources of practical experience. Reflecting on the transfer of experience across dissimilar contexts, we have emphasized how reckless is it to introduce improper actions in the management of therapy. Additionally, we have warned against neglecting certain attitudes within the domestic sphere. Everyday life is characterized by simplicity, informality, automatism, a 'personal way' of accomplishing tasks, and behaviours that is crucial not to transfer indiscriminately to the realm of medicine, which represents, or should represent, a domain of precision.

Instead, preparing the therapy several days before use; storing all the unblistered and already fragmented tablets together according to the therapeutic plan; using one's own and improper aids such as chopping boards and knives to fragment the tablets, which are then used for other foods, are just some of the many examples of how even medicine—an object of science—once introduced into the frugal activities inherent to everyday life, becomes itself frugal and trivialized. It enters the realm of the obvious, becoming an object within reach, akin to others in the home that can be used with ease. These examples also underscore the need for additional information and, more importantly, education in care.

We have mentioned—although this reflection, which here remains at the level of a note, would deserve a broader analysis—how the mechanics, automatisms, unconscious, instinctive, and even careless gestures that characterize routine everyday actions can be reconverted by the patient into 'rituals' or practices through which even the recurring and seemingly meaningless gesture becomes particular, acquiring meaning and memory. Contributing to this process of 'particularisation' of what is generic and indistinct are the 'place' where the medicine is positioned and the accompanying 'objects' that can take on quasi-sacred values. For example, the choice of 'framing' the space of the cure, using trays, doilies, and dedicated boxes, as well as the selection of memorable objects (the odd cup that survived the 'wedding service', the favour box, the small boxes with sacred images imprinted on them) to contain the day's tablets, contributes to a shift—mostly unnoticed—from the level of practices to the symbolic level (see Chaps. 13 and 15 in this text; Pizzocaro and Penati 2021).

These are small examples that nonetheless make one realize how, from the world of home care, one can also learn a great deal through the codification and transfer of management techniques, memory techniques, and effective organisational forms. Indeed, in the process of familiarising oneself with medicines, we also find ways of personalising therapy, strategies for defining an autonomous storage space, expedients for distinguishing one's medicines from those of others, and in-use medicines from 'reserve' ones. These experiences are rarely collected and shared because, like most everyday techniques, they arouse little interest. Those of the everyday, as de Certeau (2001) puts it, are "minute techniques".

In addition to techniques for managing therapy and organization, which provide valuable insights into the challenges associated with medication adherence—particularly in patients undergoing polypharmacy—and the emergence of innovative do-it-yourself solutions, attention should also be directed towards other care techniques. Techniques, rarely educated in a formal way, remain largely unknown to those involved in home care.

In addition to organisational techniques, in Chap. 14, we introduced the concept of 'techniques of the body.' According to Mauss (2017 [1936]), the ability to use the body effectively in performing specific tasks is cultivated through the observation and imitation of 'chainings' and 'sequences of actions' carried out proficiently by others. Starting from an early age, the body undergoes a process of domestication and training to achieve particular performances. Even within nursing, there exist 'body techniques'. While caregivers share knowledge about body techniques derived from training and professional experience, the realm of users lacks structured and recognized knowledge. Self-learning appears to be the primary mode through which individuals engage with the medical sphere.

There is a noticeable underestimation of the potential contribution of 'techniques of the body' in easing the administration of medicines. Professionals in the health sector are well-versed in the correct procedures to alleviate this discomfort, offering numerous descriptions of the sequences of actions and gestures necessary for administering various types of medicine.

For each of these actions, appropriate procedures, expedients, gestures, and body postures have been defined, whether it involves breaking a vial, giving an injection, taking a capsule, instilling eye drops, and so forth. The Italian Ministry of Health has established specific 'Recommendations' for certain pharmaceutical forms that include descriptions of actions and gestures falling within the category of 'techniques of the body in treatment'. However, these recommendations are directed at healthcare personnel who are already familiar with the fundamental principles of care practices. Conversely, patients receive no education, suggestions, or recommendations that should ideally be part of a foundational understanding of the body, illness, and care (Borgna 2005).

Finally, user observation reveals the use of memory techniques. Here, too, we encounter personal strategies aimed at addressing contingent problems that distress the patient. Although not highly advanced in technical development, the analysis of these strategies reveals valuable insights for reflecting on the project. For examples, one realizes from the solutions implemented by the observed patients, how much recourse is made to 'spatialised memory': examples of this include the movement on a plane—from left to right, for instance—of the medicines already taken, thus separating them from those yet to be taken. Another technique involves placing the medicine in points of the house where one is sure to pass at the scheduled time for consumption. Further methods leverage the concept of the 'parasite object', entailing 'attaching' medicines to objects (e.g., food packages) habitually used precisely at the time corresponding to the medication schedule. Some methods associate the medicine with activities (e.g., washing dishes after lunch) carried out at the scheduled therapy time, and so forth. The observation of organizational techniques, body techniques, and memory techniques can bring out and provide important contributions. These contributions still need to be deepened with more extensive and structured analyses. In the art of self-organization, the user prepares solutions, even approximate ones. However, recognizing these solutions and their underlying principles can be the starting point to fuel the design process leading to innovation.

References

AA VV (2023) Prontuario farmaceutico 2023 [Pharmaceutical formulary 2023]. Edizioni Minerva Medica, Milano

Abrate P, Castellino L, Brunitto C, Leone F, Cavalli R, Cattel R (eds) (2016) Valutazione della divisibilità e frantumabilità di forme farmaceutiche orali solide [Evaluation of divisibility and breakability of solid oral pharmaceutical forms]. I manuali SIFO, Società Italiana di Farmacia Ospedaliera e dei Servizi Farmaceutici delle Aziende Sanitarie. ISBN 978-8-86528-363-9. Retrieved from: https://www.sifoweb.it/images/pdf/pubblicazioni/altre-edizioni/Farmacista_Dipartimento/SIFO_Valutazione_della_divisibilit%C3%A1.pdf

Aldughayfiq B, Sampalli S (2021) A framework to lower the risk of medication prescribing and dispensing errors: a usability study of an NFC-based mobile application. Int J Med Inform 153:1–10

Al-Khani S, Moharram A, Aljadhey H (2014) Factors contributing to the identification and prevention of incorrect medicine prescribing errors in outpatient setting. Saudi Pharm J 22:429–432

Berman A (2004) Reducing medication errors through naming, labeling, and packaging. J Med Syst 28(1):1–29

Borgna P (2005) Sociologia del corpo [Sociology of the body]. Laterza, Milano

Campmans Z, van Rhijn A, Dull RM, Santen-Reestman J, Taxis K, Borgsteede SD (2018) Preventing dispensing errors by alerting for medicine confusions in the pharmacy information system. A survey of users. PloS One 13(5) Retrieved August, 17, 2022 from https://doi.org/10.1371/journal.pone.0197469

Caratti E, Penati A, Bucchetti V (2021) Translation design for medicine leaflets. Research and innovation. In: Design culture(s). Cumulus conference proceedings, vol 2, Roma

Chen Y-F, Neil KE, Avery AJ, Dewey ME, Johnson C (2005) Prescribing errors and other problems reported by community pharmacists. Ther Clin Risk Manag 1(4):333–342

Collina L (2005) Design e metaprogetto: Teorie, strumenti, pratiche [Design and meta-design: theories, tools, practices]. Polidesign, Milano

Comelli M (2021) Cur@. Personalizzare la terapia riconfigurando processi e oggetti per il paziente politerapico [C@re. Personalising therapy by reconfiguring processes and objects for the polytherapy patient]. Master' Thesis, Rapporteur prof. Penati A; co-rapporteur prof. Lavizzari F. School of Design, Politecnico di Milano, Milan

de Certeau M (2001) L'invenzione del quotidiano. EdizioniLavoro, Roma. [L'invention du quotidien. Arts de faire (1990) Èditions Gallimard, Paris].

Deserti A (ed) (2003) Metaprogetto: riflessioni teoriche ed esperienze didattiche [Metaproject: theoretical reflections and didactic experiences]. Polidesign, Milano

Di Pace L (2019) La lingua del bugiardino. Il foglietto illustrativo tra linguaggio specialistico e linguaggio comune [The language of the leaflet. The package leaflet between specialist and everyday language]. Franco Cesati Editore, Firenze

Dyck A, Deschamps M, Taylor J (2005) Pharmacists' discussions of medication side effects: a descriptive study. Patient Educ Couns 56:21–27

Editorial (30 march 2013) Farmaci. Il "bugiardino" diventa elettronico [Medicines. The package leaflet becomes electronic], Quotidianosanitàit. Retrieved from: https://www.quotidianosanita.it/scienza-e-farmaci/articolo.php?articolo_id=14190#:~:text=30%20marzo%20%2D%20 Si%20chiama%20eLeaflet,modo%20semplice%2C%20veloce%20e%20puntuale

European Commission (The) (Revision 1, 12 January 2009) Guideline on the readability of the labelling and package leaflet of medicinal products for human use. Retrieved from https://health.ec.europa.eu/system/files/2016-11/2009_01_12_readability_guideline_final_en_0.pdf

European Commission, EMA, HMA (2020) Key principles for the use of electronic product information for EU medicines. Retrieved from https://www.ema.europa.eu/en/documents/press-release/key-principles-use-electronic-product-information-eu-medicines_en.pdf

European Medicines Agency (EMA) (2006, 4th edn 2022) Checking process of mock-ups and specimens of outer/immediate labelling and package leaflets of human medicinal products in the centralised procedure. Retrieved from https://www.ema.europa.eu/en/documents/regulatory-procedural-guideline/checking-process-mock-ups-specimens-outer/immediate-labelling-package-leaflets-human-medicinal-products-centralised-procedure_en.pdf

European Medicines Agency (EMA) (2011) QRD recommendation on Pack design and labelling for centrally authorised non-prescription human medicinal products (Draft). QRD Recommendations pack design & labelling non-prescription CP (europa.eu)

European Medicines Agency (EMA) (2014) Guideline on the acceptability of names for human medicinal products processed through the centralised procedure—Scientific guideline 22 May 2014 EMA/CHMP/287710/2014—Rev. 6 Committee for Medicinal Products for Human Use (CHMP). Retrieved from https://www.ema.europa.eu/en/documents/regulatory-procedural-guideline/guideline-acceptability-names-human-medicinal-products-processed-through-centralised-procedure_en.pdf

European Medicines Agency (EMA) (2021) Guideline on the packaging information of medicinal products for human use authorised by the Union. Retrieved from https://health.ec.europa.eu/system/files/2021-04/2018_packaging_guidelines_en_0.pdf

European Parliament and of the Council (The) (2001) Directive 2001/83/EC of 6 November 2001 on the Community code relating to medicinal products for human use. Off J Eur Communit 28(11):2001. Retrieved from https://eur-lex.europa.eu/legal-content/EN/TXT/PDF/?uri=CELEX:32001L0083

European Parliament and of the Council (The) (2004) Directive 2004/27/EC of 31 March 2004 amending Directive 2001/83/EC on the Community code relating to medicinal products for human use. Off J Eur Union 30(4):2004. Retrieved from https://eur-lex.europa.eu/LexUriServ/LexUriServ.do?uri=OJ:L:2004:136:0034:0057:en:PDF

European Parliament and of the Council (The) (2011) Directive 2011/62/EU of 8 June 2011 amending Directive 2001/83/EC on the Community code relating to medicinal products for human use, as regards the prevention of the entry into the legal supply chain of falsified medicinal products Text with EEA relevance. Off J Eur Union 1(7):2011. Retrieved from https://eur-lex.europa.eu/legal-content/EN/TXT/PDF/?uri=CELEX:32011L0062

Good Practice Guidance on the Procurement and Supply of Pharmaceutical Specials (Giugno 2011) http://www.rpharms.com/support-pdfs/good-practice-guidance-proc-supply-pharm-specials-%287%29.pdf. Last accessed Dec 2019

Gruppo regionale sul rischio clinico da farmaci (agosto 2015) Corretta gestione delle forme farmaceutiche orali [Proper management of oral pharmaceutical forms]. Documento tecnico regionale per la sicurezza nella terapia farmacologica n.4, Regione Emilia-Romagna

Hoxsie DM, Keller AE, Armstrong EP (2006) Analysis of community pharmacy workflow processes in preventing dispensing errors. J Pharm Pract 19(2):124–130. https://doi.org/10.1177/0897190005285602

James LK, Barlow D, McArtney R, Hiom S, Roberts D, Whittlesea C (2009) Incidence, type and causes of dispensing errors: a review of the literature. Int J Pharm Pract 17:9–30. https://doi.org/10.1211/ijpp/17.1.0004

Kahan B, Goodstadt M (2001) The interactive domain model of best practices in health promotion: developing and implementing a best practices approach to health promotion. Health Promot Pract 2(1):43–54. http://www.idmbestpractices.ca

Kennedey AG, Littenberg P, Callas PW, Carney JK (2011) Evaluation of a modified prescription form to address prescribing errors. Am J Health-Syst Pharm 68:151–157

Lai F (2023) Le Compresse rivestite [The coated tablets], Modulo di Tecnologia Farmaceutica. Retrieved from https://www.unica.it/static/resources/cms/documents/Lezione14LeCompresserivestiteeControlliCompresse.pdf on 11 May 2023

Lizano-Díez I, Figueiredo-Escribá C, Piñero-López MA, Lastra CF, Mariño EL, Modamio P (2020) Prevention strategies to identify LASA errors: building and sustaining a culture of patient safety. BMB Health Serv Res 20(63):1–5

Mauss M (2017) Le tecniche del corpo. Edizioni ETS, Pisa. [Les Techniques du Corps (1936) Journal de psychologie XXXII(3–4)]

Ministero della salute—Direzione generale della programmazione sanitaria—Ufficio III (September 2018) Raccomandazione n. 18—Raccomandazione per la prevenzione degli errori in terapia conseguenti all'uso di abbreviazioni, acronimi, sigle e simboli [Recommendation for the prevention of errors in therapy resulting from the use of abbreviations, acronyms, acronyms and symbols]. Retrieved from https://www.salute.gov.it/imgs/C_17_pubblicazioni_2802_allegato.pdf

Ministero della salute—Direzione generale della programmazione sanitaria—Ufficio III (October 2019) Raccomandazione n. 19—Raccomandazione per la manipolazione delle forme farmaceutiche orali solide [Recommendation 19—Recommendation for the handling of solid oral pharmaceutical forms]. Retrieved from https://www.salute.gov.it/imgs/C_17_pubblicazioni_2892_allegato.pdf

Ministero della salute—Direzione generale della programmazione sanitaria—Ufficio III ex DGPROGS. (December 2014). Raccomandazione n. 17—Raccomandazione per la riconciliazione della terapia farmacologica [Recommendation No. 17—Recommendation for medicine therapy reconciliation]. Retrieved from https://www.salute.gov.it/imgs/C_17_pubblicazioni_2354_allegato.pdf

Norman DA (1997) La caffettiera del masochista. Psicopatologia degli oggetti quotidiani. Giunti, Firenze. [The psychology of everyday things (1988) Basic Books, New York]

Nusair MB, Guirguis LM (2017) How pharmacists check the appropriateness of medicine therapy? Observations in community pharmacy. Res Social Adm Pharm 13:349–357

Pizzocaro S, Penati A (2021) The in-home use of medications: in pursuit of design-driven knowledge. Home Cultures 17(3):153–171. https://doi.org/10.1080/17406315.2021.1916225

Royal Pharmaceutical Society (2011) Pharmaceutical issues when crushing, opening or splitting oral dosage forms. Retrieved from http://www.rpharms.com/supportpdfs/pharmaceuticalissuesdosagefor ms-%282%29.pdf. ultimo accesso dicembre 2019

van der Waarde K (2008) Designing information about medicine for people. InfoDesign Revista Brasileira de Design da Informação 5(3):37–47. ISSN 1808-5377

Weir NM, Newham R, Bennie M (2020) A literature review of human factors and ergonomics within the pharmacy dispensing process. Res Social Adm Pharm 16(5):637–645. https://doi.org/10.1016/j.sapharm.2019.08.029

Open Access This chapter is licensed under the terms of the Creative Commons Attribution 4.0 International License (http://creativecommons.org/licenses/by/4.0/), which permits use, sharing, adaptation, distribution and reproduction in any medium or format, as long as you give appropriate credit to the original author(s) and the source, provide a link to the Creative Commons license and indicate if changes were made.

The images or other third party material in this chapter are included in the chapter's Creative Commons license, unless indicated otherwise in a credit line to the material. If material is not included in the chapter's Creative Commons license and your intended use is not permitted by statutory regulation or exceeds the permitted use, you will need to obtain permission directly from the copyright holder.

Addendum 1 Regulatory References

Antonella Valeria Penati

In this appendix, we present the main regulatory texts currently in use. We would like to emphasise that the regulatory reference, for the reader who has no specific knowledge of the constraints to which the design of products in this type of industry is subject, is intended here to emphasise the importance of certain principles whose scope transcends the time span of the individual regulations which, of course, are subject to continuous updating.

As mentioned in Chap. 2, as far as the packaging of pharmaceuticals is concerned, the reference legislation at European level is, first and foremost, the Directive 2001/83/EC *on the Community code relating to medicinal products for human use* (European Parliament and of the Council 2001a).

This first regulatory level has been implemented by the individual states through the issuing of legislative decrees. As far as Italy is concerned, for example, (the country of reference for the authors of this volume), the law transposing the European Directive is Legislative Decree No 219 of 2006, Implementation of Directive 2001/83/EC (and subsequent amending directives) on a community code relating to medicinal products for human use.

This was followed by laws to regulate safety aspects and to prevent the introduction of falsified medicinal products into the legal supply chain. These laws provide for the introduction of a unique identifier and tamper-evident systems on the packaging of medicinal products to enable their identification and authentication.

The European legislation was later amended by Directive 2004/27/EC—*Directive 2004/27/EC of 31 March 2004 amending Directive 2001/83/EC on the Community code relating to medicinal products for human use* (European Parliament and of the Council 2004) and supplemented by the Delegated Regulation 2016/161, *Commission delegated regulation (EU) 2016/161 of 2 October 2015 supplementing*

A. V. Penati
Department of Design, Politecnico di Milano, Milan, Italy
e-mail: antonella.penati@polimi.it

Directive 2001/83/EC of the European Parliament and of the Council by laying down detailed rules for the safety features appearing on the packaging of medicinal products for human use (European Parliament and of the Council [The] 2016) entered into effect as of 9 February 2019 for all Member States except Belgium, Greece and Italy, for which application is postponed to 9 February 2025 (see Chap. 2 of this volume).

The Basic Regulation has also been supplemented by norms concerning the reduction of packaging due to its environmental implications (*Legislative Decree No. 116 of 3 September 2020—Implementation of Directive (EU) 2018/851 amending Directive 2008/98/EC on waste and implementation of Directive (EU) 2018/852 amending Directive 1994/62/EC on packaging and packaging waste*—(2020) [Legislative Decree No. 116 of 3 September 2020—Implementation of Directive (EU) 2018/851 amending Directive 2008/98/EC on waste and implementation of Directive (EU) 2018/852 amending Directive 1994/62/EC on packaging and packaging waste].

In Italy, these standards were supplemented by Guidelines of 27/7/2022, which came into effect on 1 January 2023 (Ministry of Ecological Transition 2022). It is useful to emphasise that the legislation, at both Community and national level, is aimed exclusively at companies that produce and market medicines, regulating the characteristics of the medicine, its packaging and the package leaflet.

In addition to the Community and national regulations, over time Guidelines issued at Community level and Recommendations issued at local level have been added, aimed at specifying and providing technical-operational indications to supplement the regulatory provisions to facilitate their correct interpretation.

1.1 Guidelines

Guidelines are a widely used tool to reinforce, on a technical level, the regulatory dictate. Guidelines indicate rules and principles aimed at guiding the behaviour of the drug developer based on indications drawn up from systematic review processes of data collected in the literature or opinions of eminent experts. Compared to tools such as Protocols, which, being a manual of rules to be followed, have a greater degree of cogency and rigidity, Guidelines are less restrictive: they direct a process of action towards behaviour deemed optimal. If the drug developer intends to deviate from the Guidelines, he must justify in detail the reasons for differing choices. The relevant aspect of the Guidelines is that they contain rules and criteria derived from established practices that have proven to be effective in their field of action. As such, they presuppose—or should presuppose—constant monitoring of the situation, to retroactively influence the Guidelines themselves, modifying or integrating them where they prove to be deficient or ineffective in directing ways, actions, decisions and behaviour. They tend to be accredited by a scientific community of reference and, as such, they enjoy credibility with the community that produced them and, for this reason, they are respected even though they do not have strict regulatory value. Guidelines are drawn up both at EU level and at the level of individual states. Like the regulations, it is useful to point out that the Guidelines are addressed exclusively to the drug manufacturing companies and are aimed at making the law operative through concrete indications on the product characteristics and the approval process.

In the case of drugs, the main Guidelines that must be considered in the submission procedure of a new drug, for its introduction on the European market, are the following:

- Brand name: *Guideline on the acceptability of names for human medicinal products* (European Medicines Agency [EMA] 2014a);
- Packaging: *Guideline on the packaging information of medicinal products for human use authorised by the Union* (European Medicines Agency [EMA] 2021);
- Readability of information: *Guideline on the readability of the labelling and package leaflet of medicinal products for human use* (European Commission [The] 2009a).

In addition to the Regulatory Guidelines, formats are prepared indicating the documents to be filed to apply for approval of the brand name, packaging, and package leaflet:

- Mock-up evaluation of packaging materials: *Checking process of mock-ups and specimens of outer/immediate labelling and package leaflets of human medicinal products in the centralised procedure* (European Medicines Agency [EMA] 2006, 4th edn. 2022);
- Name request form: https://www.ema.europa.eu/en/name-review-group-form;

In this regard, the instructions that EMA provides to companies on specific and recurring questions are also supportive: see, in this regard, Section 3, *Preparing the dossier* (2016, last update July 2023).

1.2 Recommendations

In addition to the Guidelines, each individual government, through its Ministries of Health, has published specific Recommendations. In common parlance, the recommendation is the exhortation, the advice, to do or not to do something.

It can take on the character of an invitation, a suggestion, but it can also take on the authoritative character of a warning. In the legislative sphere, recommendations are of a technical nature and generally contain rules intended to make laws and regulations clearer and more comprehensible. They tend not to have a binding character but constitute an invitation to adhere to a certain behaviour or to take certain measures.

The Italian Ministry of Health, for example, has made significant use of Recommendations with the intention of raising the awareness of health professionals to pay attention and take the necessary actions to prevent those clinical and care conditions that are potential causes of adverse events because they are exposed to a high risk of error.

To this end, it has drawn up, with the support of experts and stakeholders, the Recommendations listed below, i.e. specific indications aimed at providing tools to prevent adverse events. These can occur in the use of medicines at the different stages of prescription, dispensing and use. In the case of use, the Recommendations are addressed exclusively to healthcare professionals, with the aim of raising awareness in the professional sphere that operates, at different levels, in the activities of care. The Recommendations do not touch the world of pharmaceutical companies, let alone the sphere of use of the end user. As we will argue in the concluding chapter, the dissemination of some of the contents in them, if expressed in a less technical language and closer to the culture of the user, could help to avoid many errors in the management of therapy at home.

The Recommendations concerning medicines, for Italy, are as follows:

- Recommendation no. 7—*Recommendation for the prevention of death, coma or serious harm resulting from errors in therapy Medicines* (Ministry of Health March 2008);
- Recommendation No. 12—*Recommendation for the prevention of errors in drug therapy look-alike/sound-alike* (Ministry of Health August 2010);
- Recommendation no. 14—*Recommendation for the prevention of errors in therapy with antineoplastic drugs* (Ministry of Health October 2012);
- Recommendation No. 17—*Recommendation for drug therapy reconciliation* (Ministry of Health December 2014);
- Recommendation No. 18—*Recommendation for the prevention of errors in therapy resulting from the use of abbreviations, acronyms, acronyms and symbols* (Ministry of Health September 2018);
- Recommendation No. 19—*Recommendation for the handling of oral solid pharmaceutical forms* (Ministry of Health October 2019).

Addendum 2 Medication Errors Data

Carlo Emilio Standoli

This addendum deals with medication errors, specifically focusing on errors in the domestic context, where a person/patient has to manage even complex pharmacological therapies. Medication errors have been defined as '*any preventable event that may cause or lead to inappropriate use of the drug or harm to the patient while the drug is under the control of the healthcare professional, patient or consumer*' (National Coordinating Council for Medication Error Reporting and Prevention 2015). Such events can be related to professional practice, healthcare products, procedures, and systems, including prescribing, reporting the order, product labelling, packaging and nomenclature, compounding, dispensing, distribution, administration, education, monitoring, and use (National Coordinating Council for Medication Error Reporting and Prevention 2015).

There is a substantial difference between errors committed in a hospital environment and an extra-hospital context. In the former case, the error may be committed by healthcare personnel without the patient being aware; therefore, the patient is passive in drug selection, management, and administration.

In the case of the extra-hospital setting, the person/patient has an active role: if correctly informed and aware of their treatment, they should be able to distinguish errors committed by others (e.g. pharmacist, caregiver, etc.) or by themselves in the management and administration of the drug. In this case, medical literacy—or proper communication between doctor, pharmacist, and patient—may be associated with greater confidence in handling medication, and, thus, better therapeutic adherence (Dionisi et al. 2022).

Between the hospital context and the extra-hospital context, we can identify the moments of *Transition of Care*, in which, following a patient's admission to the hospital, the discharge, or transfer between departments of the same facility or to

---

C. E. Standoli
Department of Design, Politecnico di Milano, Milan, Italy
e-mail: carloemilio.standoli@polimi.it

another healthcare facility, unintentional errors may emerge in the process of drug therapy management; these may be committed both by the patient and by healthcare personnel (Carollo 2016). This moment is crucial for correctly managing the information transfer, both in terms of completeness and clarity—especially when informing the patient. The World Health Organisation (WHO) recommends interventions to prevent errors in treatment resulting from inadequate knowledge of current therapies. It considers Medication Reconciliation one of the best strategies to ensure quality of care (WHO 2014).

In 2017, the WHO launched a global initiative to reduce severe and preventable harms associated with medicines by 50% in all countries over 5 years (WHO 2017). The Global Patient Safety Challenge on Medication Safety aims to improve how drugs are prescribed, dispensed, and consumed to increase patient awareness of the risks associated with the misuse of medicines. The Global Challenge actions will focus on four areas: patients and the public; healthcare professionals; medicines as products; and medication systems and practices. The aim is to analyse and improve each stage of the medicines use process, including prescribing, dispensing, administration, monitoring, and use (WHO 2017).

In the Italian context, with Recommendation No. 17, the Ministry of Health defines 'Pharmacological Therapy Reconciliation' (*Riconciliazione farmacologica/ Reconciliation*) as "*a formal process that allows, clearly and completely, to detect and know the pharmacological therapy followed together with other information related to the patient and allows the prescribing physician to carefully evaluate whether to continue, vary or interrupt it in whole or in part*" (Ministero della Salute 2014). This recommendation mainly concerns error in the hospital setting. Still, much of the information and guidelines can be applied in the extra-hospital environment, from the relationship with the general practitioner, to the pharmacist to the home setting.

The Recommendation outlines three fundamental stages: the recognition, namely the collection of data in a structured form on the medicinal treatments taken by the patient; the reconciliation, namely the comparison made by the physician between the current therapies with the new provisions, to verify possible inconsistencies, such as overlaps, omissions, interactions, contraindications, confounding due to *Look-Alike/Sound-Alike* (LASA) drugs; the communication, namely the continuous dialogue between health professionals and patients, to explain the motivations, processes and actions of the therapy and the verification of the actual understanding (Ministero della Salute 2014). Therapeutic reconciliation thus appears to be a tool to reduce medication-related errors.

Therefore, this section aims to highlight the leading causes of errors, starting from existing literature, to understand how to intervene from a design point of view, beginning with the drug form and ending with the primary and secondary packaging and the package leaflet. This collection does not pretend to be exhaustive. Still, it takes its cue from the literature—which is rich in the case of errors committed within hospital facilities but extremely rare in the case of errors committed in the domestic context, because they are difficult to monitor, trace and recognise—and tries to bring together data from different social and cultural contexts, in which drugs are also managed differently, such as in the prescription, sale and storage process in the domestic context (Dionisi et al. 2022). In fact, a fundamental difference between the hospital and extra-hospital context is the data collected in a structured form regarding medicine management and use. In the former case, due to regulations and defined management and accountability processes, error data are known and historicised. In the case of the domestic context, the collection of data on medication handling and use errors is not so structured, for example, because the patient may not be aware of the error made because it caused no serious harm or because the error, when detected, was not reported to the pharmacist, doctor or pharmaceutical authority.

Errors in the practice of drug management can be divided into prescription errors (e.g. due to unclear prescription writing, wrong drug selection, unclear verbal communication and orders, etc.), distribution and administration errors (e.g. due to not understanding the prescription, wrong drug selection, etc.), or management errors (e.g. order, transcription, communication, product categorisation, packaging and nomenclature, composition, distribution).

An Italian research from 2005, on a sample of 1369 calls made to the *Centro Anti Veleni* (CAV) at *Niguarda* Hospital, revealed several recurrent error patterns in the out-of-hospital setting (Moro et al. 2005).

The error occurs in the following ways:

- in the dosage (44.3%)
- by exchange of drugs (37.7%);
- in the route of administration (4.4%);
- by expiry of the drug (3.6%);
- in the method of preparation (1%);
- by incorrect reading by the pharmacist (0.3%).

Again, in the same study (Moro et al. 2005), over 60% of these errors relate to repeatable prescription drugs, while errors with non-prescription (SOP) and over-the-counter (OTC) drugs account for 15.8% and 12.6%, respectively. Of these, the drugs most frequently involved in the genesis of errors were:

- respiratory drugs (19%);
- anti-inflammatory, analgesic and antipyretic drugs (18.2%);
- central nervous system drugs (13.6%);
- antimicrobials (13.22%);
- gastrointestinal drugs (8.47%);
- dermatological drugs (5.3%);
- vitamins (3.6%);
- drugs of the genito-urinary system (2.8%);
- antihypertensives (2.3%);
- drugs of the cardiovascular system (2%).

Other epidemiological research from North America (USA and Canada) estimates that many adverse events and errors in therapy management occur within the home setting (Forster et al. 2003). For example, out of a sample of three million patients receiving home healthcare, 13% reported errors in therapy management (Madigan 2007). Even in Canada, out of every 100 cases of home care, about 13% report having experienced adverse events (Sears et al. 2013). And among the most common adverse events are those related to medication management.

An epidemiological analysis conducted in Ireland in 2011 indicates a sample of 2348 people who committed and then reported errors to the *National Poisons Information Centre*. Of these, 1220 children and adolescents under the age of 18. Furthermore, of these reported cases, 2279 were related to errors in the home setting, and the majority related to incorrect drug administration (Cassidy et al. 2011).

In their literature review, Parand et al. (2016) highlight many causes and potential contributing factors to committing medication errors (Table 1).

A closer look is needed at LASA medicines, meaning all those errors can occur when medicines have similar names or formal characteristics (e.g., from the shape and colour of the medicine to the appearance of the packaging). For example, LASA errors often occur due to similarities in the letters that make up the names of different medicines or products, at the beginning, middle or end of the name (WHO 2023). Or LASA errors can occur due to confusion of name combinations, such as generic-generic names, brand-brand names, or brand-generic names (WHO 2023).

LASA errors are estimated to be responsible for 6.2–14.7% of all medication errors. LASA errors often lead to administering the wrong medicine at the wrong or incorrect dose of the intended medicine, leading to toxic effects or other adverse effects (Aronson 2009; Alteren et al. 2018).

To clearly understand, dimension, and quantify, the various national drug agencies have defined procedures and ways to report adverse event or medication error. For example, the Italian Medicines Agency (AIFA), through its website, gives the possibility to report errors committed by both healthcare professionals and ordinary citizens, whether patients or caregivers (AIFA 2023). Or like the Medicines and Healthcare products Regulatory Agency, which through its *YellowCard* website allows reporting suspected side effects to medicines, vaccines, e-cigarettes, medical device incidents, defective or falsified (fake) products (MHRA 2019). Unfortunately, in many cases, the request for detailed information (e.g. from patient data, current treatment, medication taken and adverse reactions, up to report on the treating physician, etc.) makes it challenging to fill out, thus leading to a paucity of recorded data on the misuse of medicines in the domestic context.

Table 1 Example and data of some common causes and potential contributing factors in the management of pharmacological treatment

Contributory factor	Contributory sub-factor	Evidence
Individual care recipient factor	Age of child	Being a care-recipient child below the age of 5 years was found to be a significant predictor of an increased risk for a MAE.
		Infants were found to be significantly more likely to receive an incorrect dose of medication than older children.
		Underdosing was most commonly noted in both younger and lighter children. The mean age and weight of the children were significantly less in the underdosed group and overdosed group compared with the appropriate dose group.
		Surpassing the recommended maximum number of doses was more likely with increasing age of the child care-recipient.
		From the age of 12 months, administration of the recommended dose declined with the increasing age of the child (regardless of an increase in dosage given): 1–2 years (81%), 2–3 years (65%), 4–6 years (55%), 6–8 years (43%). Of those between the age of 4 ± 11 months 62% gave a recommended dose
		Children aged between 1 ± 4 most frequently had unintentional overdoses and 10 times the rate in other (older and younger) age groups (3.2 versus 0.3 ADEs per 1000 persons).
		71% (10 of 14) children under 10 years old (all receiving multiple overdoses by parents) had a severe toxic condition of the liver, compared with 31% (18 of 59) in the older group.
Individual carer factor	Age of carer	More medication errors were reported by older carers (>65 years), despite fewer older caregivers in the study sample
	Educational level of carer	Carers with less education reported more MAEs.
		Carers with a low educational level (below 12th grade $\pm$ school aged around 17 ± 18) had complied less with medication prescriptions.
	Carer's time and other responsibilities	Carers who continued to work or who had other family/caregiving responsibilities reported more missed doses, regardless of their administration schedules.
		Following a treatment regimen in between everyday activities or special occasions was raised as a potential contributor to missing administration.
	Language of carer	In English speaking countries:
		Non-English speaking parents gave the recommended dose of paracetamol less frequently than English-speaking parents.
		Accuracy of dosage differed across language groups, with Spanish speakers less accurate in dosing than English speakers, however this was found to be not significant.
		Bottle labels in English contributed to MAEs for non-English speakers, despite a consultation in the mother tongue of the carer.
	Health of carer	Carers with poorer health reported more MAEs than those with better health.
	Carer marital status	Single mothers had lower compliance with prescription administration compared with married mothers (p = .004).

(continued)

Table 1 (continued)

Contributory factor	Contributory sub-factor	Evidence
Medication factors	Polypharmacy	Children with multiple prescriptions were at a significant increased risk of having a preventable ADE.
		Medication errors increased with the number of administered medications.
		Taking more than one medication increased the risk of a MAE (odds ratio: 1.60, 95% confidence interval).
		20% of parents were reluctant to give more than one medication at a time.
	Type of medication	The most common drugs involved in preventable ADEs in paediatric outpatients were amoxicillin/amoxicillin-clavulanate, inhaled steroids, topical anti-fungals, antihistamines, and inhaled bronchodilators.
		More cough and cold medication-related emergency visits involved medication errors (e.g. administering an overdose) than visits from all other medications combined.
		MAEs were most prevalent, in nebulised therapy, followed by oral antibiotics.
		More errors were found with non-chemotherapy medications rather than chemotherapy medication.
	Route of administration	Paracetamol given via the rectal route of administration had a significantly greater rate of supratherapeutic doses than oral administration (9/28 [32%] versus 39/149 [26%]), respectively (95% CI = 0.14 to 0.48).
	Medication supply	25% of 20 parents who did not administer diazepam did not have any diazepam (25%).
		Parents raised the issue of being given incorrect products.
		Carers created complex strategies to maintain their supply when faced with a host of different sources (e.g. pharmacies, samples, and mail order), various reimbursement sources and variable doses.
		A double dose of senna was identified due to two filled prescription bottles.
		Not replacing spilled medication or broken medication bottles that resulted from difficulty in administering the medication.
Environmental factors	Storage	Families that reported MAEs said they had not stored the products in their original container.
		Inappropriate places of storage included under the sink, in the refrigerator or bathroom. Few stated they stored them in a locked cupboard.
	Equipment	Use of inappropriate measuring equipment was often identified as potential contributory factors, particularly the use of teaspoons.
		A 100% dosage accuracy was found in the group that received their prescription along with a syringe that had a line marked at the correct dose, compared to 37% correct dosage accuracy from a group that only received a prescription and verbal instruction. 83% accuracy in dose was found when a group with provided with the syringe, prescriptions, and demonstration alone.
		Percentage of incorrect use for the following measuring aids were: Dosing spoons 44% (used by 20% of carers), teaspoons 100% (used by 17%), syringes 60% (used by 17%), and droppers 100% (used by 10%).
		The mean dose given with an infant dropper was lower (6.4 mg/kg per dose, $p < 0.0002$) than the mean doses given with other measuring devices.
		Parents reported difficulties in using IV lines and nebulizers/inhalers, and the supply of incorrect equipment.
		Parents sometimes deviated their administration technique from the doctor's instructions because they did not have the proper equipment.
		3.6% (12) carers stated that they did not know how to open child safe containers.

Addendum 2 Medication Errors Data

Contributory factor	Contributory sub-factor	Evidence
Prescription communication factors	Communication with healthcare professionals & carers' understanding of instructions or medication/illness	In a case study example, lisinopril and amlodipine were prescribed at discharge; however, the daughter did not understand that the mother was to take the drugs.
		Of 20 parents who did not administer diazepam when they should, 60% reported it was due to the complicated administration information, 35% said they were unaware, and 2% potentially had misinformation on dosage.
		Inadequate and erroneous understanding by parents about their children's medications/illness was identified, however no significant relationship was found between this understanding and MAEs.
		Advice to parents on administration was not associated with MAEs.
		The source of information on medication amount was not significantly different between the correct group and the incorrect group.
		Parental MAEs resulted from misunderstanding instructions, disregarding medication labels or following them rather than other given instructions
		Carers who said that medication dose is based on weight were significantly less likely to give an incorrect dose of medication (RR 0.71, $p = 0.03$).
		The mean administered dose of paracetamol was 62% of that recommended when the calculation was made based on the care-recipient's age, and 64% when it was calculated by body weight.
		Miscalculation of dose was found to be a factor in wrong dose errors.
		Three causes of MAEs were due to a new carer being unfamiliar with medications.
		More errors occurred where medication labels did not specify dosage but directed carers to consult a healthcare professional.
		25.3% (84) of carers did not know how to administer medicine to their child, 7.2% (24) forgot what their pharmacist or doctor told them to take note of at administration and 5.4% (18) reported that they found it difficult to understand medicine information pamphlets.
	Dosage change	Becoming accustomed to a medication and consequently not reading new instruction labels was identified.
		Administration errors were most often caused by confusion regarding a change in dose of a medication.
		Unnoticed expired medicines used by parents were usually PRN (taken as needed).
Psycosocial factors	Panic / Cognitive failure	20% of 20 parents who did not administer diazepam when they should have, reported that they panicked at the time it was needed, while 15% said it did not occur to them.
	Fear of spillage	Mothers reported not filling the entire spoon due to fear of spilling the medication, particularly when dosage was half or three quarters of a spoonful rather than one whole spoonful.
	Carer-to-carer communication	In 89 (18.1%) cases a lack of communication between two carers resulted in both giving a dose to the child. In 80 of these cases, the carers were both parents. Poor communication between parents was reported 97 times, 10 times between parents and grandparents, and 4 times between other carers.

Source: Parand et al. (2016)
MAE(s) medication administration error(s), *ADE(s)* adverse drug event(s)

Addendum 3 The Name of Medicines: LASA Medicines

Antonella Valeria Penati, Annabella Amatulli, and Lamberto Dionigi

"According to Article 1(20) of Directive 2001/83/EC, it should be noted that the name of the medicinal product *"may be either an invented name not liable to confusion with the common name, or a common name or scientific name accompanied by a trade mark or the name of the marketing authorisation holder"*. It is also understood by legislation that a common name is, according to Article 1(21) of Directive 2001/83/EC, as amended, "The international non-proprietary name (INN) recommended by the World Health Organization, or, if one does not exist, the usual common name." […]

The checking of the (invented) name is part of the EMA's role in evaluating the safety of medicinal products within the authorisation procedure, as the proposed (invented) name(s) could create a public- health concern or potential safety risk. Such an evaluation should be performed based on best available evidence and research.

Proposals for invented names as well as for names submitted with the 'INN + company/brand name' formula will be subject to EMA review.

[…]

4.1.3. The (invented) name of a medicinal product should not be misleading with respect to the composition of the product.

4.1.4. Consideration should be given to the phonetics and the potential difficulties a proposed (invented) name may create in terms of pronunciation in the different EU official languages. […]" (EMA 2014b, Revision 7, di December 2021)

A. V. Penati
Department of Design, Politecnico di Milano, Milan, Italy
e-mail: antonella.penati@polimi.it

A. Amatulli
AlfaSigma S.p.A., Milan, Italy

L. Dionigi
Zambon S.p.A., Italy

The cited passage from the Guideline on the acceptability of names for human medicinal products makes direct reference to the articles of Directive 2001/83/EC that regulate the naming of medicinal products. In particular, Art.1 (part. 20 and 21) and Art. 54 specify:

- *Art.1, 20. Name of the medicinal product:*
  The name given to a medicinal product, which may be either an invented name or a common or scientific name, together with a trade mark or the name of the manufacturer; the invented name shall not be liable to confusion with the common name.
- *Art.1, 21. Common name:*
  The international non-proprietary name recommended by the World Health Organization, or, if one does not exist, the usual common name.
- *Art. 54*
  The following particulars shall appear on the outer packaging of medicinal products or, where there is no outer packaging, on the immediate packaging: (a) the name of the medicinal product followed by the common name where the product contains only one active substance and if its name is an invented name; where a medicinal product is available in several pharmaceutical forms and/or several strengths, the pharmaceutical form and/or the strength (baby, child or adult as appropriate) must be included in the name of the medicinal product [...].

The need to arrive at the design of an international system for the validation of new drug names and a common global authorisation policy is present in several studies (Weir et al. 2020; Lizano-Díez et al. 2020a). Unlike other forms of error, those generated by the similarity between different drug names are not solely dependent on the prescribing physicians, dispensing pharmacists, or nurses or care givers administering the drugs. In this type of error, responsibilities involve the manufacturers, the regulators, and the naming bodies. According to Bryan et al. (2020), the literature does not pay much attention to the role played by senior actors in the approval procedures, nor to the fallout in terms of error dependent on the cumbersome nature of approval procedures. While some authors have drawn attention to the establishment of standards that limit confusion in the naming and labelling of pharmaceutical products (Berman 2004), others have noted the lack of internationally valid guidelines and regulatory requirements (Galanter et al. 2014).

In the study by Bryan et al. (2020) it is argued that vague and inconsistently applied guidelines are unable to intercept *Look Likee/Sound Like* (LASA) drugs in the pre-marketing phase. All medicines must be authorised before they can be marketed and made available to patients. Adrien Berman (2004) gives an account of the complicated procedure that must be followed in the US for the approval of the name of new drugs:

- the chemical name is coined by the International Union of Pure and Applied Chemistry and identifies the molecular structure and configuration of the active ingredient. It is rarely used in the clinical field;

- the generic name, is used in the health sector, and is assigned by the United States Adopted Name Council (USC) is intended to give an indication of the chemical and/or therapeutic characteristics of the drug;
- the official title of a drug is determined by the USP Nomenclature Committee;
- the proprietary name, trademark, or trade name, is determined by the pharmaceutical company to promote brand loyalty and facilitate recognition;
- the U.S. Patent and Trade Office examines the similarity between new and existing marks in terms of printed appearance, with the goal of preventing new brand names from infringing existing marks;
- the FDA (Office of Post-Marketing Drug Risk Assessment) examines proprietary names, including the way they appear when handwritten, and regulates the labelling of drugs that use generic or proprietary names;
- at the international level, the World Health Organisation (WHO) coordinates the naming and nomenclature of individual countries.

Bryan et al. (2020) report on the methods used to define the nomenclature of the active ingredients of drugs, with the aim of making their names unambiguous throughout the world. The most common ways include:

- development of a name around a root derived from classical languages;
- construction of a name by combining several roots derived from the classical languages;
- use of acronyms or abbreviations especially in the prefix or suffix part.

The aim is to reduce the risk of confusion and ensure that the names are easy to remember, understand, and correlate with the chemical composition, pharmacological action and/or therapeutic use of the active ingredient. The authors, however, noted a certain ineffectiveness of pharmacological names in responding to the stated principles, as well as verifying that approximately one fifth of the names are distinguishable from others by only a single letter, creating a high potential for confusion.

Lizano-Díez et al. (2020a) point out that the approval procedures for innovative drug names (so-called specialities) do not follow a common policy at the international level, nor are there any coordinated procedures in the authorisation steps between the different countries of the world, for which different levels of complexity in terms of linguistics and phonetics have to be addressed. Added to this, the authors point out, is the idiomatic character of names, signs, symbols typical of the cultural variability of different countries.

Only for marketing in the countries of the European Union, the European Medicines Agency (EMA) has a working group made up of representatives from each national agency that ensures that the names of these innovative drugs do not give rise to conflicts in any country.

In the European Union, there are two main routes for authorising medicines: a centralised route and a national route. Under the centralised authorisation procedure, pharmaceutical companies submit a single marketing-authorisation application to EMA; this procedure is applicable and mandatory only to certain medicines that fall under categories as for example: medicines containing a new active substance; human immunodeficiency virus; cancer; diabetes etc. (EMA 2015)

However, in the case of authorisation procedures other than centralised ones, the drug agencies of each country independently check the names that are proposed and reject them when they are like other products marketed in their own country. This mechanism increases the variability of names between Member States.

Numerous studies, conducted mainly in the United States but also in the United Kingdom, Australia, Brazil, Hong Kong, India, Iran, Israel, South Africa, return, precisely because of the non-alignment of international approval procedures, several examples of names of active ingredients or registered brand names, approved almost simultaneously in different countries, despite their obvious similarity: Cefuroxima Cefotaxima; Doxorubicin Daunorubicin; Adderall®, Inderal®; PD-Mox®, PD-Rox®; Clomine®, Clozine®; etc. (Lizano-Díez et al. 2020a)

Evident symptoms of a deficient procedure in determining the names of drugs can be found:

- in the presence of drugs with confusing names (LASA) because they are poorly differentiated;
- in the presence of active ingredients that give rise to dozens of different pharmaceutical names company by company;
- in the presence of active ingredients that, for marketing reasons, give rise to different names even within the same company following the logic of 'specialisation';
- in the presence of medicines with different active ingredients but identical brand parts;
- in the presence of medicines that have similar names to medical devices and food supplements.

This proliferation is at the origin of many prescription and dispensing errors, and among these should not be forgotten the erroneous prescription, by the doctor, of an active ingredient, already present in the patient's therapy, but with a trade name not recognised by the prescribing doctor. The result of this non-recognition is to introduce into therapy a drug that is in fact already present. Which entails, for that patient, taking the same active ingredient twice.

These few reminders support a different naming validation procedure that would bring order to what already exists and initiate unambiguous approval paths at supranational level. A pathway certainly with many complexities to be resolved because, for example, the use of the same name in several countries runs into trademark problems, as well as problems with the 'meaning' of the word defining the brand in different countries.

1.1 Drug Confusability: Name, Label Elements, Graphic Image of the Packaging

The possibility of confusing different drugs with each other is high, especially in the dispensing phase in pharmacies and hospital wards, with regard to emergency units. In Chap. 8, we saw that, about confusability between drugs, particular attention was paid to the category of drugs called LASA (look alike/sound alike). Attention to these drugs arose, in the first instance, from the visual or acoustic similarities that can be found in the names (e.g. names of drugs with the same prefix or suffix; names of drugs with a common root; the sound of the name of a drug that can be confused with that of another drug), but immediately afterwards, interest was extended to all the elements that make up the drug's labelling, starting with the dosage, and ending with the overall graphics of the packaging. It was seen how packs with a very similar visual impression (as is typical in packs of drugs of the same brand name) put users (pharmacist and patient) at a particularly high risk of error. Precisely because of their dangerousness, due to the ease of confusion and exchange between drugs, a vast collection of examples, case studies, and even experiments aimed at mitigating the negative effects induced by similarity are available on LASA errors. Several areas of study have been, and are, involved in the search for solutions, starting mainly with the need to reduce the error produced by similarity of names. These include, for example, experiments on spelling, re-design of packaging and communication, regulatory affairs, and clinical management, each looking for ways to influence the perception, attention, operational and organisational behaviour of those involved in the process and limit errors. The resulting solutions are mainly:

- in the area of organisation with regard to the criteria for arranging drugs in pharmacies and hospital wards;
- in the technological area, which includes the computerisation of the prescription process; the connection between prescription and medical records; the introduction of warning signals; the automation of dispensing activities (Spinks et al. 2017); the use of reading devices such as barcodes, radio frequency identification tags, packaging serialisation, etc.;
- in the area of graphics with, for example, experiments on the visual differentiation that can be achieved by intervening on typographic fonts, etc.

While the literature provides many examples of this multidisciplinary focus, it at the same time offers few cases of implementation of recommendations from pilot projects that are useful for verifying the positive impact of each of these interventions (Ciociano and Bagnasco 2014).

Ciociano and Bagnasco (2014) collected numerous experiments aimed at identifying which conditions and factors are involved in the processes that generate orthographic and phonetic similarity between similar nouns and how much these may affect the ability to distinguish between similar elements. The authors report on numerous experiments aimed at establishing the degree of similarity between drug names, using computer algorithms to measure the orthographic similarity produced by bigrams and trigrams (i.e. groups of two or three letters with a single sound) or to measure the similarity between images or texts. These studies have been used to identify possible confusable pairs of drugs in pharmaceutical formularies due to excessive similarity in spelling.

Still other tests have been applied to identify drugs with high phonetic similarity. Similarity which, in languages where the written word differs from the spoken word, is not always evident based on the written word alone. Again, the review by Ciociano and Bagnasco (2014) exemplifies the various graphic and typographic experiments that give visual form to the name of drugs, such as: content, composition/layout, typography, colour and graphics, evaluating, in particular, how readability changes by introducing typographic variations (switching from lower to upper case characters; contrast in font weight from standard to bold; contrast between black characters and white characters on a black background, etc.).

One of the most studied and used graphic intervention strategies is the one that makes use of Tall Man Lettering (Campmans et al. 2018). After being approved by the Food and Drug Administration (FDA), the Institute for Safe Medical Practices (ISMP), and the Joint Commission, this practice has become common, although evidence of a beneficial effect of this technique is limited (Lambert et al. 2016).

Tall Man Lettering is a writing system that seeks to visually maximise the difference between similar names by playing on the combination of small and capital letters. The technique is used in the labelling of packaged drugs at pharmacies; in stickers accompanied by safety symbols or pictograms on the drug's packaging; in labels on shelves and drawers where the drug is stored; in warnings in the computer system of doctors and pharmacists to support both the prescription and dispensing phases, etc. (Lizano-Díez et al. 2020a; Van de Vreede et al. 2008) (Fig. 1).

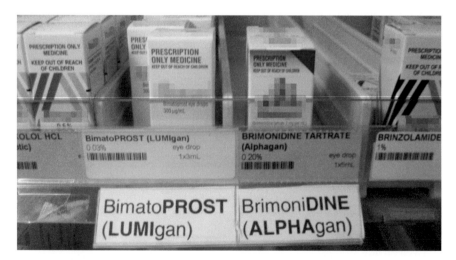

Fig. 1. Packaging components. Example of Tallman letter labelling in the pharmacy department's inpatient dispensary. (Van de Vreede et al. 2008, p. 264)

In some experiments, Tall Man inscriptions were introduced directly on the drug packaging (Lizano-Díez et al. 2020a) with the aim of assessing their ability to prevent and reduce the risk of errors when choosing similarly named drugs. The Tall Man technique resulted in readability verification studies using different graphic combinations:

- all drug names in capital letters;
- capitalise only the letters or the portion of the name that differs (e.g. DOBUTamine and DOPamine) (Ciociano and Bagnasco 2014).

In addition to Tall Man Lettering, the impact of further graphic alternatives was evaluated: use of white on a black background; use of black on a white background; use of colour; use of round/grass; use of round and italic; use of fonts with different weights etc. These tests tried to focus on different levels of the problem:

- how graphic changes can be more or less effective in assessing whether the names being tested are the same or different;
- how graphic changes are able to reduce the time needed to verify similarities and differences between names;
- how graphic changes may affect memory processes in subsequent recognition.

The result of these experiments shows that highlighting parts of a word through graphic treatment on fonts has varying degrees of effectiveness (Al-Khani et al. 2014). But this effectiveness occurs almost exclusively if the test participants are aware of the purpose of the experiment. Zhong et al. (2016) also concluded that these different experiments are vitiated by methodological shortcomings and that one of the problematic elements is whether the user is aware that he is confronted with a graphic experiment. Interventions on graphics only seem to function as warnings, regardless of the visual expedient used, if they are first communicated as such, i.e. as signalling devices (Lambert et al. 2016; Zhong et al. 2016). A limitation of effectiveness has also been found in situations with a high risk of confusion (such as Emergency Departments). Confusion that cannot be mitigated by typographical interventions alone (Lizano-Díez et al. 2020a).

In addition to the graphic treatment, several studies have been interested in the use of technology to overcome the problems of exchange between similar drugs. A study conducted in a group of Dutch pharmacies found a reduction in LASA errors in drug dispensing due to alert signalling in computerised prescription/dispensing systems (Campmans et al. 2018). This same study, however, also warned against 'alert fatigue', a state caused by an excessive number of alert signals leading to ignoring messages, urging that the benefits of error prevention be weighed against the risk of fatigue caused by alert signal overload. The recommendation from this study is to use these signals only for drugs/doses that incur frequent or severe confusions. Malhotra et al. (2016) report that the cancellation rate of alerts exceeds 90%, significantly limiting their potential impact on healthcare professionals.

Even in this study, most respondents did not feel that Tall Man characters enhanced the warning notice, but that it was the warning itself that triggered more attention.

We close this section on the errors that can be generated by visual or sonorous similarity between names, and the experiments that have attempted to address the problem by intervening in the lettering of names, with a reflection.

The ineffectiveness of graphic interventions, on LASA drug names, must be considered within the framework of the great variety that currently characterises, precisely from a graphic point of view, the names of medicinal products. In fact, there is no standard regulating the use, in the naming of medicines, of colour, capital letters, bold type, etc. The extreme graphic variety is one of the elements that does not allow any distinctive typographical features intended for a specific purpose to emerge: for example, to indicate classes of medicines, or to serve as a warning sign.

The introduction of certain rules and restrictions in the use of fonts, and their graphic treatments (italics, bold, capital letters, colour, etc.) to define the name of drugs (especially those that present a low risk of error in the prescription and dispensing phases), could be a first indication to bring out those drug names whose graphic characterisations are specifically introduced to indicate particular categories to be cautioned against (e.g. LASA, FALA, etc.).

As we said at the beginning of this paragraph, and as we analysed in Chap. 8, the interest in errors arising from LASA drugs has allowed us to extend our attention to the problems of distinguishability of all those 'elements' that should unambiguously identify the individual drug: in addition to the name, therefore, also the active ingredient(s), the dosage(s), the unit of measurement, the packaging graphics and the shape of the packaging itself.

Many medication mix-ups, in fact, result from the plurality of information elements that, instead of being read in their individuality (name of the drug; active ingredient; pharmaceutical form; dosage; number of doses per pack, etc.), are weakened by the 'appearance' or overall graphic/orthographic impression of the packaging.

Examples of the difficulty in unambiguously distinguishing the information elements of the packaging due to inappropriate graphic treatment include dosages of the same drug that can be confused because they are similar and not made sufficiently distinguishable graphically. In the case of dosage, it is not only the graphic 'treatment' that affects the possibility of error. Many problems can arise due to the inconsistent way the same data is presented to the user. Here are some possible causes:

- use of different units of measurement to express the dosage;
- different dosage of the active ingredient when switching between different pharmaceutical formulas;
- need to convert the dosage measurement units when passing from solid to liquid formula (mg, ml);
- different dilution ratios with which concentrations of the active ingredient are expressed. (Berman 2004)

The packaging and its graphic elements (the shape and size of the packaging in addition to the graphic-visual elements that make up its graphic layout) can

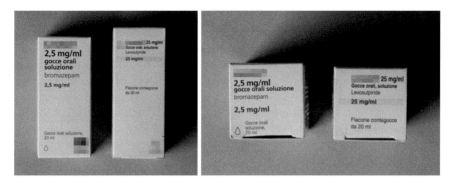

Fig. 2 Example of drugs that start with the same letter of the alphabet and have almost identical graphics, despite being from two different pharmaceutical companies. On the left the two drugs seen from the front where the only thing that differentiates them 'at a glance' is the height of the packaging; on the right the two drugs seen from above. The latter view is particularly important for the pharmacist because it is the one most frequently seen when looking for the drugs in the drawers during dispensing

contribute to accentuate the similarities between packages: this is what, for example, happens in secondary packaging of different drugs, but produced by the same pharmaceutical company, in which the visual elements (e.g., font, colour, arrangement of the information elements on the page, distinctive graphic signs, etc.), used as brand identification elements, increase the level of similarity between packages (Fig. 2).

1.2 The Name of the Medicine

We have mentioned, in this part of the chapter on packaging and labelling, how delicate the naming of a new drug is and how complex the approval procedure is. We have also seen, on several occasions, how many difficulties arise regarding the name during use.

These difficulties are related to the marketing of similar drug names, even if they are not based on the same active ingredient. We have seen that this similarity may be due to:

- names that share identical parts (prefixes, suffixes and desinences, etc.);
- names that are distinguished by only one or a few letters, although they do not arise from shared roots;
- names that are characterised by the presence of similar vowels and consonants even if arranged in a different order
- names that have similar sounds and may lead to confusion even if spelled differently.

But problems in use also arise from:

- fancy names or names that coincide with the active ingredient that do not refer to a meaning that the user can connect to a pathology and memorise. Lizano-Díez et al. (2020a), have highlighted the artificiality of these names to which only a community of experts is able to attribute meaning, while for the majority of users (the patient in particular) they are meaningless. This difficulty in connecting the name of the drug to the pathology, for example, precludes the patient from exercising conscious control over the drugs he buys and does not even help to better manage the taking of the drug at home;
- active ingredients corresponding to a plurality of names given by different companies or even by the same company;
- 'proprietary' names that are used in different medicines with minor variations (e.g. because they are known to consumers) even though they contain only partially the same active ingredients.

The written form (font, font body, colour) also contributes to the problem, especially with names of the same length creating a perceptual impact of similarity that overrides the effort of careful reading.

Many of these aspects should be handled more attentively before the drug is placed on the market. Even at the European level alone, the existence of local and EU procedures, for example, is already an obvious limitation in moving towards the reduction of existing names and the prior verification of newly marketed names. A first order of action should, however, necessarily involve the manufacturing industries, the regulatory bodies and the standardisation bodies, committing the former to avoid a forced diversification of names where it is not useful—and indeed counterproductive—for the patient; the latter to greater rigour (especially in local procedures); and the third to provide for supplementing the standards where there are shortcomings in this respect.

Standards, Guidelines and Recommendations constitute a well-designed system of rules. And yet, the presence on the market of packaging that clearly contradicts the regulatory framework suggests that some loopholes can be found in the approval procedure. Or, they suggest that Recommendations and Guidelines have insufficient regulatory power.

After marketing, it is the personnel who operate in different roles along the process of prescribing, dispensing, storing, and administering medicines, who have an important role that requires both great scrupulousness in respecting the procedures that regulate the different activities, and in reporting any errors and the reasons why these errors occurred (Van de Vreede et al. 2008).

The intervention level on Regulatory Authorities and Regulatory Organisms is the most appropriate for a reformulation of criteria and procedures that can work on names, addressing 'content' issues.

But to reduce errors generated by indistinguishable drug names, it is also important to address issues of 'form'. Berman (2004) emphasised the importance of typographic interventions to maximise the readability of the name and the degree of distinguishability of different names and reduce the errors that similarity produces

Addendum 3 The Name of Medicines: LASA Medicines

as much as possible. We have introduced some of these suggestions in the recommendations that follow.

However, we would like to make a general remark here: there are no specific criteria on the use of typographic characters when writing the name of a medicine other than its legibility. Criteria that rule, at most, the choice of font, its size, and certain prohibitions on the manipulation of the font format always aimed at ensuring maximum readability.

The great formal variety that can be achieved, while still complying with Standards and Guidelines, as we have already mentioned, makes the possible introduction of graphic characterisations to distinguish classes of drugs ineffective. We have seen, for example, that in the case of LASA drugs the use of Tall Man Lettering is not totally effective. The user only recognises and evaluates the effectiveness of the typographical artifice introduced to distinguish two LASA drugs if he is warned that he is dealing with a typographical experiment. The use of capital letters to characterise certain parts of a term can only be a distinctive mode if this typographical device is able to create a perceptible difference. But the names of medicines are written indifferently in capital letters, in small letters, in small letters with an initial capital letter, but we also find names with some characters in capital letters and others in small letters. In such variety it is difficult for this typographic element to become distinctive (Fig. 3).

The same applies to other forms of typographical experimentation (e.g., use of boldface, use of white on black, use in black on white, use of colour, etc.) which, as we have seen, have had alternating results. To make the differences, introduced on a typographical level, effective and readable, it is necessary to act on a level ground of uniformity. And to achieve uniformity, common rules must be enacted. Purely by way of example: if all drugs, which do not present problems of recognisability, distinguishability, etc., are written in lower case and black font, it may become effective to use capital letters, in LASA drugs, to differentiate the names to which attention needs to be drawn. Still about examples, red typefaces can be used to

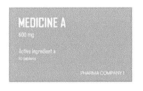
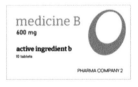
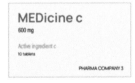
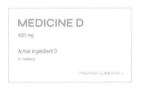
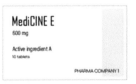
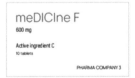

Fig. 3 The use of the Tall Man Lettering technique is not particularly effective in distinguishing drugs with similar names or parts of names with the same root or desinence

indicate FALA drugs (High Alertness Level Drugs). But even in this case, the distinctiveness achieved through colour 'works' only by difference. These are, of course, and we repeat, two examples that need in-depth studies of typographic design and experimentation with users. But the effectiveness of these interventions is achieved by generating perceptible differences from a homogeneous base and using a distinctive criterion to identify specific classes of drugs. Let us recall, in closing, Berman again (2004) for his hypothesis not to entrust the task of creating distinction to the visual register alone, but to examine the hypothesis of introducing other sensory registers—e.g. the use of touch—in the design of packages containing drugs belonging to categories considered critical.

Addendum 4 Methods of User Involvement

Antonella Valeria Penati, Annabella Amatulli, and Lamberto Dionigi

Involvement of patients in the readability testing of the package leaflet is required by current legislation. It is the *Guideline on the readability of the labelling and package leaflet of medicinal products for human use* (European Commission 2009a) that not only provides guidance on how to ensure that the information contained in the labelling and package leaflet is accessible and comprehensible, but also includes guidance on consultations with groups of 'target patients' to test the readability of the package leaflet.

In the standard, we note two elements deserving further in-depth analysis. The first, we find in the fact that patient involvement is aimed at testing the 'readability' of the package leaflet only. The procedure, in fact, does not provide for the readability of the information on the primary and secondary pack to be assessed as well. The readability of the primary and secondary packs is subject to assessment by the commission appointed by the EMA for marketing procedures, in the case of an EU centralised procedure (see EMA 2022b).

Undoubtedly, the EMA has taken the potential positive effects of user involvement in readability tests very seriously (see in this respect Kim Sherwood https://www.ema.europa.eu/en/documents/presentation/presentation-user-test_en.pdf where the various steps of the procedure and the expected aims are explained).

But the exclusion from these tests of such an important object of observation as the secondary pack is one of the shortcomings that produces, as an effect, its poor informative capacity, as the many examples of medicines on the market today prove. For example, many warnings and indications, contained in the secondary pack, do

---

A. V. Penati
Department of Design, Politecnico di Milano, Milan, Italy
e-mail: antonella.penati@polimi.it

A. Amatulli
AlfaSigma S.p.A., Milan, Italy

L. Dionigi
Zambon S.p.A., Italy

not have a precise and fixed location. This makes it difficult for the user to find the information they consider important. Not only that. The regulations prescribe that, as a priority, the warnings must be on the wider sides of the packaging. Whereas, contrary to the regulations, warnings are frequently found on the smaller sides of the package. This does not allow for the necessary space to separate the different contents, just as it does not allow for an adequate font for reading. In fact, the information does not have the right autonomy, nor visibility.

The standards require that there be the right contrast between text and background, but the many examples of medicines collected show that sometimes the text is illegible precisely because of the lack of visual contrast. The standards stipulate that there must be spacing (line spacing) between different contents. In this respect, too, we noted the design deficiency of several marketed medicines.

It is also necessary to make the user perceive the prescriptive nature of the information contained, and basic education on medicines and their use by the user should contribute to this. At present, however, the warnings do not have a proper graphic treatment that enhances their prescriptive function.

A second regulatory deficiency is related to the fact that the procedure provided for is limited to testing readability and not the sequence of actions that the user must perform to start reading the package leaflet. It is noted here that taking a medicine is a far more complex activity than merely reading the accompanying information. And one must consider that the reading activity is indeed facilitated by the readability of the text, but this constitutes one of the elements that must be considered.

The series of actions/operations that the user must perform in the right sequence to start the therapy correctly depend in the first instance on the patient's interest, convictions, and reluctance to read the package leaflet. Readiness to read can be stimulated through specific 'invitations' to read designed to draw the user's attention. The predisposition to reading, in fact, is also the result of designing the packaging and package leaflet in such a way as to facilitate usability, meaning by this term the inclusion of all those expedients able to make the various actions that the patient must perform simple and intuitive, including the action of reading the information before using the medicine. A rather neglected aspect.

Finally, there is a lack of opportunities for the user to be proactive and for the company to collect problems and suggestions brought by the user and his user experience. Many of these problems are the subject of attention, for example, by the U.S. Food and Drug Administration, as returned by L. Sterrett (2023) in his *Us-Related Risk Analysis (URRA) and Human Factors (HF) Protocol Reviews: What to submit for an efficient Review*.

These new and important attentions may constitute the fundamental step to enrich the evaluation procedure of the readability of the P.L. by the users, widening the experience of the involvement of the end user up to the reading of the information reported on the primary pack and on the secondary pack. In a perspective of greater realism of the evaluation experience, it proves useful to recruit not only the patient but also doctors, pharmacists, care givers. A final element requiring attention is the context in which the test is carried out: it is important to simulate domestic situations, unprotected by ambient noise, with not necessarily adequate light and, above all, with the individual medicine in interaction with all the medicines that make up the patient's therapy. Many errors, or difficulties in understanding, in fact arise from the complexity generated by the set of medicines that make up the therapy and the sequences of organisational activities, memory, manipulation given by the mixture of intake constraints, usage behaviour etc. that are different for each medicine.

Addendum 5 Undesirable Effects or Product Defects Reporting Procedures

Antonella Valeria Penati and Annabella Amatulli

Reducing errors, at all stages of the medicine lifecycle, starting with prescription and pharmaceutical dispensing, is possible if error reporting is encouraged.

Lizano-Díez et al. (2020b) analysed "the most common types of reported medication" and found, in the prescriptive act alone, "*errors of wrong dose, wrong drug, wrong duplicate prescription of the same active substance; wrong duration, wrong patient, unauthorised/non-approved drug prescribed, wrong or unspecified dosage form*" (2020b, tab. 1).

Errors, which, as we have seen, punctuate the entire cycle from prescription to taking the medicine, can only be detected if they are reported or self-reported. LASA pairs, for example, may only become apparent after the error has been reported. But the literature notes the strong reluctance to report errors. It also notes that the most frequently reported errors are those occurring at the prescribing stage, because they are reported by pharmacists. This is an indication that third-party monitoring favours the emergence of errors. On the other hand, errors occurring in the dispensing phase (Franklin and O'Grady 2007) and in the use phase are underestimated.

The rate of reporting problems, which may occur during medicine dispensing, suffers from a punitive error culture. Encouraging error reporting and sharing information about problems that are encountered (before they become errors) can help people learn from the errors themselves (Chen et al. 2005). Starting with James Reason's (1991) theory of human error, two distinct research approaches have been developed: one is focused on the person making the error and focuses on the role of the practitioner. This approach implies negligence, carelessness, incompetence, lack/lack of knowledge or inadequate professional training. The second approach,

---

A. V. Penati
Department of Design, Politecnico di Milano, Milan, Italy
e-mail: antonella.penati@polimi.it

A. Amatulli
AlfaSigma S.p.A., Milan, Italy

© The Editor(s) (if applicable) and The Author(s) 2025
A. V. Penati (ed.), *In-Home Medication*, Research for Development,
https://doi.org/10.1007/978-3-031-53294-8

on the other hand, is concerned with the context within which the error is committed, leading to an assessment of the non-human factors, circumstances and latent causes in the organisation that generated it: work overload; chaotic situations with poor or incorrect organisation and division of tasks; day of the week or time of day when the error occurred; workload, etc. It has been shown that an approach that does not blame, but searches for explanations in external causal factors, encourages workers to report the error also through self-reporting (Lizano-Díez et al. 2020b).

The patient also has a tendency not to report the error except when adverse events have occurred.

Many errors, then, depend on a lack of communication between doctor and pharmacist and also on a lack of collaboration, the result of a lack of mutual trust. The presence of trust or mistrust is what, when faced with the same problem, can produce very different decisions: for example Chen et al. (2005) verified how, when faced with an incomplete prescription, the trust relationship between doctor and pharmacist can lead to the following different outcomes the pharmacist refers the patient to the doctor to complete the prescription and the medicine is not dispensed; the pharmacist telephones the doctor and completes the prescription with his support before dispensing the medicine; the pharmacist dispenses the medicine anyway and completes the prescription himself; the pharmacist dispenses the medicine and completes the prescription with the doctor's support after dispensing; the pharmacist dispenses the medicine and subsequently sends the prescription to the dispensing clinic. Almost all these steps contain procedural errors, but what is interesting to note here is how communication and the predisposition to cooperate constitute the behaviour that most encourages efficient and safe modes of action.

The sharing of experience, between pharmacy professionals and prescribing physicians, is considered the necessary basis for setting up procedures and protocols of action based on good practice. Large pharmacies in the United States are required to report dispensing incidents (Szeinbach et al. 2007).

Avoiding punitive behaviour; activating forms of incentive to report; encouraging 'confidential' forms of reporting; providing an environment focused on learning from errors (Hoxsie et al. 2006): error reporting procedures as well as error review bodies should favour an approach that aims at learning from individuals and the system as a whole.

Specifically regarding reports that may arise from the user's experience of use, two cases can be identified with different channels and modalities: reports on undesirable effects; reports on product quality.

In the first case, the patient may report an undesirable effect through the doctor or pharmacist or directly to the authorities. In the latter case, the patient will find a link and instructions for reporting the side effect/adverse event in the package leaflet of the medicine under section 4 'Possible side effects'. In the EU countries this procedure is harmonised and each country has in the P.L. the link to the respective regulatory authority. In Italy, the patient will find the following in the package leaflet under *'Reporting undesirable effects'*: *"If you experience any undesirable effect, please contact your doctor or pharmacist. This advice also applies to any side effects not listed in this package leaflet. You can also report side effects directly through the national reporting system https://www.aifa.gov.it/content/segnalazioni-reazioni-avverse. By reporting side effects, you can help to provide more information on the safety of this medicine".*

Through specific databases, the company can analyse the reports and assess whether the package leaflet needs to be updated (e.g. by adding a new side effect).

Regarding reports on the quality or non-conformity of the product, these can be made to the doctor or pharmacist, who will contact the company to report any defects.

Each company has its own internal procedures for handling these reports. Pharmacovigilance bodies monitor these reports to exclude problems that may have an impact on the safety of the product (e.g. a quality problem or non-conformity of a device that may lead to an overdose of medicine).

The company, which is obliged to keep counter-samples of all batches produced, performs appropriate analyses depending on the defect reported on both the sample received and the counter-samples kept.

Both types of reporting (reporting of side effects; reporting of non-compliance) are not particularly familiar to patients and, there is no procedure codifying the closure of the reporting process by leading the company or the competent authorities to provide the patient with the outcome of the report made.

There is at least one further shortcoming in the reporting procedures: there is currently no procedure for detecting the discomfort that the patient or care giver feels when using the product because they do not understand how to use the product or do not understand the information on its use. This meandering discomfort is often the cause of intake errors or poor adherence to therapy.

References

References for Addendum 1

European Commission (Revision 1, 12 2009a) Guideline on the readability of the labelling and package leaflet of medicinal products for human use. Retrieved from https://health.ec.europa.eu/system/files/2016-11/2009_01_12_readability_guideline_final_en_0.pdf

European Commission, EMA, HMA (2020) Key principles for the use of electronic product information for EU medicines. Retrieved from https://www.ema.europa.eu/en/documents/press-release/key-principles-use-electronic-product-information-eu-medicines_en.pdf

European Medicines Agency (EMA) (2006, 4th edn. 2022) Checking process of mock-ups and specimens of outer/immediate labelling and package leaflets of human medicinal products in the centralised procedure. Retrieved from https://www.ema.europa.eu/en/documents/regulatory-procedural-guideline/checking-process-mock-ups-specimens-outer/immediate-labelling-package-leaflets-human-medicinal-products-centralised-procedure_en.pdf

European Medicines Agency (EMA) (2011) QRD recommendation on Pack design and labelling for centrally authorised non-prescription human medicinal products (Draft). QRD recommendations pack design & labelling non-prescription CP (europa.eu)

European Medicines Agency (EMA) (2014a) Guideline on the acceptability of names for human medicinal products processed through the centralised procedure—Scientific guideline 22 May 2014 EMA/CHMP/287710/2014—Rev. 6 Committee for Medicinal Products for Human Use (CHMP). Retrieved from https://www.ema.europa.eu/en/documents/regulatory-procedural-guideline/guideline-acceptability-names-human-medicinal-products-processed-through-centralised-procedure_en.pdf

European Medicines Agency (EMA) (2016, last update July 2023) Section 3: Preparing the dossier retrieved from https://www.ema.europa.eu/en/human-regulatory/marketing-authorisation/pre-authorisation-guidance#3.1-product-name,-product-information-and-prescription-status-section

European Medicines Agency (EMA) (2021) Guideline on the packaging information of medicinal products for human use authorised by the Union. Retrieved from https://health.ec.europa.eu/system/files/2021-04/2018_packaging_guidelines_en_0.pdf

European Parliament and of the Council (The) (2001a) Directive 2001/83/EC of 6 November 2001 on the Community code relating to medicinal products for human use. Off J Eur Communit 28(11):2001. Retrieved from https://eur-lex.europa.eu/legal-content/EN/TXT/PDF/?uri=CELEX:32001L0083

European Parliament and of the Council (The) (2003) Directive 2003/15/EC of 27 February 2003 amending Council Directive 76/768/EEC on the approximation of the laws of the Member States relating to cosmetic products. Off J Eur Union 11(3):2003. Retrieved from https://eur-lex.europa.eu/legal-content/EN/TXT/PDF/?uri=CELEX:32003L0015

European Parliament and of the Council (The) (2004) Directive 2004/27/EC of 31 March 2004 amending Directive 2001/83/EC on the Community code relating to medicinal products for human use. Off J Eur Union 30(4):2004. Retrieved from https://eur-lex.europa.eu/LexUriServ/LexUriServ.do?uri=OJ:L:2004:136:0034:0057:en:PDF

European Parliament and of the Council (The) (2011) Directive 2011/62/EU of 8 June 2011 amending Directive 2001/83/EC on the Community code relating to medicinal products for human use, as regards the prevention of the entry into the legal supply chain of falsified medicinal products Text with EEA relevance. Off J Eur Union 1(7):2011. Retrieved from https://eur-lex.europa.eu/legal-content/EN/TXT/PDF/?uri=CELEX:32011L0062

European Parliament and of the Council (The) (2016) Commission delegated regulation (EU) 2016/161 of 2 October 2015 supplementing Directive 2001/83/EC of the European Parliament and of the Council by laying down detailed rules for the safety features appearing on the packaging of medicinal products for human use. Off J Eur Union 9(2):2016. Retrieved from https://eur-lex.europa.eu/legal-content/EN/TXT/PDF/?uri=CELEX:32016R0161

Ministero della salute—Dipartimento della qualità—Direzione generale della programmazione sanitaria, dei livelli di assistenza e dei principi etici di sistema—Ufficio III (march 2008) Raccomandazione n. 7—Raccomandazione per la prevenzione della morte, coma o grave danno derivati da errori in terapia farmacologica [Recommendation 7—Recommendation for the prevention of death, coma or serious harm resulting from medication errors]. Retrieved from https://www.salute.gov.it/imgs/c_17_pubblicazioni_675_allegato.pdf

Ministero della salute—Dipartimento della qualità—Direzione generale della programmazione sanitaria, dei livelli di assistenza e dei principi etici di sistema—Ufficio III (August 2010) Raccomandazione n. 12—Raccomandazione per la prevenzione degli errori in terapia con farmaci "lookalike/sound-alike" [Recommendation 12—Recommendation for the prevention of errors in look-alike/sound-alike drug therapy]. Retrieved fromhttps://www.salute.gov.it/imgs/C_17_pubblicazioni_1307_allegato.pdf

Ministero della salute—Dipartimento della programmazione e dell'ordinamento del servizio sanitario nazionale—Direzione generale della programmazione sanitaria—Ufficio III ex DGPROGS (October 2012) Raccomandazione n. 14—Raccomandazione per la prevenzione degli errori in terapia con farmaci antineoplastici [Recommendation 14—Recommendation for the prevention of errors in antineoplastic drug therapy]. Retrieved fromhttps://www.salute.gov.it/imgs/C_17_pubblicazioni_1861_allegato.pdf

Ministero della salute—Direzione generale della programmazione sanitaria—Ufficio III ex DGPROGS (December 2014) Raccomandazione n. 17—Raccomandazione per la riconciliazione della terapia farmacologica [Recommendation No. 17—Recommendation for drug therapy reconciliation]. Retrieved from https://www.salute.gov.it/imgs/C_17_pubblicazioni_2354_allegato.pdf

Ministero della salute—Direzione generale della programmazione sanitaria—Ufficio III (September 2018) Raccomandazione n. 18—Raccomandazione per la prevenzione degli errori in terapia conseguenti all'uso di abbreviazioni, acronimi, sigle e simboli [Recommendation for the prevention of errors in therapy resulting from the use of abbreviations, acronyms, acronyms and symbols]. Retrieved from https://www.salute.gov.it/imgs/C_17_pubblicazioni_2802_allegato.pdf

Ministero della salute—Direzione generale della programmazione sanitaria—Ufficio III (October 2019) Raccomandazione n. 19—Raccomandazione per la manipolazione delle forme farmaceutiche orali solide [Recommendation 19—Recommendation for the handling of solid oral pharmaceutical forms]. Retrieved from https://www.salute.gov.it/imgs/C_17_pubblicazioni_2892_allegato.pdf

Ministero della transizione ecologica (2022 Provvedimento entrato in vigore il 1° gennaio 2023) Linee Guida sull'etichettatura degli imballaggi ai sensi dell'art. 219 comma 5 del D.Lgs. 152/2006 e ss.mm, del 27/7/2022 [Packaging Labelling Guidelines]. Retrieved from https://www.mase.gov.it/sites/default/files/archivio/normativa/rifiuti/Linee_guida_etichettatura_ambientale_27.09.2022.pdf

Presidente della Repubblica (2006) Decreto Legislativo 24 aprile 2006, n. 219—Attuazione della direttiva 2001/83/CE (e successive direttive di modifica) relativa ad un codice comunitario concernente i medicinali per uso umano [Community code relating to medicinal products for human use], entrata in vigore il 6-7-2006, Gazzetta Ufficiale n.142 del 21-06-2006—Suppl. Ordinario n. 153. Retrieved from https://www.gazzettaufficiale.it/eli/id/2006/06/21/006G0237/sg

Presidente della Repubblica (2014) Decreto legislativo 19 febbraio 2014, n. 17—Attuazione della direttiva 2011/62/UE, che modifica la direttiva 2001/83/CE, recante un codice comunitario relativo ai medicinali per uso umano, al fine di impedire l'ingresso di medicinali falsificati nella catena di fornitura legale [Community code relating to medicinal products for human use, in order to prevent falsified medicines from entering the legal supply chain]. Gazzetta Ufficiale n. 55 del 07.03.2014. Retrieved from https://www.normattiva.it/uri-res/N2Ls?urn:nir:stato:decreto.legislativo:2014;017

Presidente, della Repubblica (2020) Decreto legislativo 3 settembre 2020, n. 116 –Attuazione della direttiva (UE) 2018/851 che modifica la direttiva 2008/98/CE relativa ai rifiuti e attuazione della direttiva (UE) 2018/852 che modifica la direttiva 1994/62/CE sugli imballaggi e i rifiuti di imballaggio [Packaging and Packaging Waste Directive]. Gazzetta Ufficiale Serie Generale n. 226 del 11-09-2020. Retrieved from https://www.gazzettaufficiale.it/eli/id/2020/09/11/20G00135/sg

References for Addendum 2

AIFA—Agenzia Italiana del Farmaco (2023) Form per la segnalazione di una reazione avversa a farmaci e/o vaccini. Retrieved at: https://servizionline.aifa.gov.it/schedasegnalazioni

Alteren J, Hermstad M, White J, Jordan S (2018) Conflicting priorities: observation of medicine administration. J Clin Nurs 27(19-20):3613–3621

Aronson JK (2009) Medication errors: EMERGing solutions. Br J Clin Pharmacol 67(6):589

Carollo A (2016) Commento alla Raccomandazione n. 17 Riconciliazione Terapeutica. Bollettino SIFO 62(5):283–287

Cassidy N, Duggan E, Williams DJ, Tracey JA (2011) The epidemiology and type of medication errors reported to the National Poisons Information Centre of Ireland. Clin Toxicol 49(6):485–491

Dionisi S, Di Simone E, Liquori G, De Leo A, Di Muzio M, Giannetta N (2022) Medication errors' causes analysis in home care setting: a systematic review. Public Health Nurs 39:876–897

Forster AJ, Murff HJ, Peterson JF, Gandhi TK, Bates DW (2003) The incidence and severity of adverse events affecting patients after discharge from the hospital. Ann Intern Med 138(3):161–167

Madigan EA (2007) A description of adverse events in home healthcare. Home Healthc Now 25(3):191–197

MHRA—Medicines and Healthcare products Regulatory Agency (2019) Yellow Card Scheme: making medicines safer. Guidance on adverse drug reactions. Retrieved at: https://yellowcard.mhra.gov.uk

Ministero della Salute (2014) Raccomandazione n.17—Raccomandazione per la riconciliazione della terapia farmacologica. Retrieved at: https://www.salute.gov.it/imgs/C_17_pubblicazioni_2354_allegato.pdf

Moro A, Modena T, Colombo G (2005) L'errore terapeutico: quando umano e quando diabolico. Bollettino d'informazione sui farmaci, pp 162

National Coordinating Council for Medication Error Reporting and Prevention (2015) What is a medication error? National Coordinating Council for Medication Error Reporting and Prevention. Retrieved at: http://www.nccmerp.org/about-medication-errors

Parand A, Garfield S, Vincent C, Franklin BD (2016) Carers' medication administration errors in the domiciliary setting: a systematic review. PloS One 11(12):e0167204

Sears N, Baker GR, Barnsley J, Shortt S (2013) The incidence of adverse events among home care patients. International J Qual Health Care 25(1):16–28

World Health Organization (2014) The High 5s Project—standard operating protocol for medication reconciliation. World Health Organization, Geneva

World Health Organization (2017) WHO launches global effort to halve medication-related errors in 5 years Available in: https://www.who.int/news-room/detail/29-03-2017-who-launches-global-effort-to-halvemedication-related-errors-in-5-years.

World Health Organization (2023) Medication safety for look-alike, sound-alike medicines

References for Addendum 3

Al-Khani S, Moharram A, Aljadhey H (2014) Factors contributing to the identification and prevention of incorrect drug prescribing errors in outpatient setting. Saudi Pharm J 22:429–432

Berman A (2004) Reducing medication errors through naming, labeling, and packaging. J Med Syst 28(1):1–29

Bryan R, Aronson GK, Williams A, Jordan S (2020) The problem of look-alike, sound-alike name errors: drivers and solutions. Br Pharmacol Soc 87:386–394

Campmans Z, van Rhijn A Dull RM, Santen-Reestman J, Taxis K, Borgsteede SD (2018) Preventing dispensing errors by alerting for drug confusions in the pharmacy information system. A survey of users. Plos One 13(5). Retrieved August, 17, 2022 from https://doi.org/10.1371/journal.pone.0197469

Cheung K, Bouvy ML, De Smet P (2009) Medication errors: the importance of safe dispensing. Br J Clin Pharmacol 67(6):676–680

Ciociano N, Bagnasco L (2014) Look alike/sound alike drugs: a literature review on causes and solutions. Int J Clin Pharm 36:233–242. https://doi.org/10.1007/s11096-013-9885-6

European Medicines Agency (EMA) (2014b) Guideline on the acceptability of names for human medicinal products processed through the centralised procedure—Scientific guideline 22 May 2014 EMA/CHMP/287710/2014—Rev. 6 Committee for Medicinal Products for Human Use (CHMP). Retrieved from https://www.ema.europa.eu/en/documents/regulatory-procedural-guideline/guideline-acceptability-names-human-medicinal-products-processed-through-centralised-procedure_en.pdf

European Medicines Agency (EMA) (2015) The centralized procedure at EMA. Retrieved at: https://www.ema.europa.eu/en/documents/presentation/presentation-centralised-procedure-european-medicines-agency_en.pdf

EMA (2022a) Human Medicines Division Checking process of mock-ups and specimens of outer/immediate labelling and package leaflets of human medicinal products in the centralised procedure. Retrieved at: https://www.ema.europa.eu/en/documents/regulatory-procedural-guideline/checking-process-mock-ups-specimens-outer/immediate-labelling-package-leaflets-human-medicinal-products-centralised-procedure_en.pdf

European Parliament and of the Council (The) (2001b) Directive 2001/83/EC of 6 November 2001 on the Community code relating to medicinal products for human use. Off J Eur Communit 28(11):2001. Retrieved from https://eur-lex.europa.eu/legal-content/EN/TXT/PDF/?uri=CELEX:32001L0083

Galanter WL, Bryson ML, Falck S et al (2014) Indication alerts intercept drug name confusion errors during computerized entry of medication orders. PLoS One 9(7):e101977

Lambert BL, Schroeder SR, Galanter WL (2016) Does Tall Man lettering prevent drug name confusion errors? Incomplete and conflicting evidence suggest need for definitive study. BMJ Qual Saf 25(4):213–217

Lizano-Díez I, Figueiredo-Escribá C, Piñero-López MA, Lastra CF, Mariño EL, Modamio P (2020a) Prevention strategies to identify LASA errors: building and sustaining a culture of patient safety. BMB Health Serv Res 20(63):1–5

Malhotra S, Cheriff AD, Gossey JT, Cole CL, Kaushal R, Ancker JS (2016) Effects of an e-Prescribing interface redesign on rates of generic drug prescribing: exploiting default options. J Am Med Inform Assoc 23(5):891–898. Retrieved September, 18, 2022 from https://doi.org/10.1093/jamia/ocv192

Spinks J, Jackson J, Kirkpatrick CM, Wheeler A (2017) Disruptive innovation in community pharmacy—impact of automation on the pharmacist workforce. Res Social Adm Pharm 13(2):394–397

van de Vreede M, McRae A, Wiseman M, Dooley MJ (2008) Successful introduction of Tallman letters to reduce medication selection errors in a hospital network. J Pharm Pract Res 38(4):263–266

Weir NM, Newham R, Bennie M (2020) A literature review of human factors and ergonomics within the pharmacy dispensing process. Res Social Adm Pharm 16(5):637–645. https://doi.org/10.1016/j.sapharm.2019.08.029

Zhong W, Feinstein JA, Patel NS et al (2016) Tall man lettering and potential prescription errors: a time series analysis of 42 children's hospitals in the USA over 9 years. BMJ Qual Saf 25:233–240

References for Addendum 4

European Commission (Revision 1, 12 2009b) Guideline on the readability of the labelling and package leaflet of medicinal products for human use. Retrieved from https://health.ec.europa.eu/system/files/2016-11/2009_01_12_readability_guideline_final_en_0.pdf

EMA (2022b) Human Medicines Division Checking process of mock-ups and specimens of outer/immediate labelling and package leaflets of human medicinal products in the centralised procedure. Retrieved at: https://www.ema.europa.eu/en/documents/regulatory-procedural-guideline/checking-process-mock-ups-specimens-outer/immediate-labelling-package-leaflets-human-medicinal-products-centralised-procedure_en.pdf

Sherwood K. User test. https://www.ema.europa.eu/en/documents/presentation/presentation-user-test_en.pdf

Sterrett L (2023) Use-Related Risk Analysis (URRA) and Human Factors (HF) protocol reviews: what to submit for an efficient review. Vd. Use-Related Risk Analysis (URRA) and Human Factors (HF) protocol reviews: what to submit for an efficient (fda.gov)

References for Addendum 5

AIFA (n.d.) Come segnalare una reazione avversa. https://www.aifa.gov.it/content/segnalazioni-reazioni-avverse

Chen Y-F, Neil KE, Avery AJ, Dewey ME, Johnson C (2005) Prescribing errors and other problems reported by community pharmacists. Ther Clin Risk Manag 1(4):333–342

Franklin BD, O'Grady K (2007) Dispensing errors in community pharmacy: frequency, clinical significance and potential impact of authentication at the point of dispensing. Int J Pharm Pract 15:273–281. https://doi.org/10.1211/ijpp.15.4.0004

Hoxsie DM, Keller AE, Armstrong EP (2006) Analysis of community pharmacy workflow processes in preventing dispensing errors. J Pharm Pract 19(2):124–130. https://doi.org/10.1177/0897190005285602

Lizano-Díez I, Figueiredo-Escribá C, Piñero-López MA, Lastra CF, Mariño EL, Modamio P (2020b) Prevention strategies to identify LASA errors: building and sustaining a culture of patient safety. BMB Health Serv Res 20(63):1–5

Reason J (1991) Human errors. Cambridge University Press, Cambridge

Szeinbach S, Seoane-Vazquez E, Parekh A, Herderick M (2007) Dispensing errors in community pharmacy: perceived influence of sociotechnical factors. Int J Qual Health Care 19(4):203–209